Atlas of Thyroid Surgery

Alexander Shifrin
Editor

Atlas of Thyroid Surgery

Springer

Editor
Alexander Shifrin
Atlantic Health Oncology Service and Department of Surgery
CentraState Health System
Atlantic Health Partner
Freehold, NJ, USA

ISBN 978-3-030-93672-3   ISBN 978-3-030-93673-0 (eBook)
https://doi.org/10.1007/978-3-030-93673-0

This Springer imprint is published by the registered company Springer Nature Switzerland AG
The registered company address is: Gewerbestrasse 11, 6330 Cham, Switzerland

In memory of my father, Leonid Shifrin, the inventor of thromboelastographs, and my uncle, pediatric surgeon, Vadim Shifrin.

To my mother, Margarita Shifrina, for her love and endless support.

To my beloved children, Michael, Daniel, Benjamin, Julia, Christian, and Liam, who continue to provide perspective on what is truly important in life.

To the love of my life, Svetlana L. Krasnova, for her love, patience, and encouragement.

Preface

> No volume which deals with the treatment of the thyroid gland would be complete without a statement regarding our obligation to Theodor Kocher…. because of his skill as a surgeon and his sound reasoning as a scientific physician as to the nature, diagnosis, and treatment of every form of goiter, to Theodore Kocher, as to no other man, is due the credit for writing the chapter on goiter in the history of medicine. George Crile

The aim of the atlas is to illustrate different techniques of successful thyroid surgery. Each author, an expert in the field of thyroid surgery, presented their own specific way on how to perform a successful thyroid surgery. The atlas illustrates thyroid lobectomy, total thyroidectomy, thyroidectomy for substernal goiter, thyroidectomy with central neck lymph nodes dissection and lateral neck dissection, video-assisted thyroidectomy, endoscopic total thyroidectomy via bilateral axillo-breast approach (BABA), and transoral endoscopic total thyroidectomy via vestibular approach (TOETVA). A separate chapter is dedicated to describing a safe thyroidectomy in developing countries. Each chapter presents a case description that defines the main aspect of surgery. Each picture, which is taken intraoperatively, is accompanied by corresponding drawings for an easier understanding of the anatomical structures and steps of the procedure. In addition, most of the authors provided a video of the same case as it is depicted in the chapter, which is annotated and can be accessed online via SpringerLink (link.springer.com). The atlas includes common pitfalls of the procedure in an effort to avoid complications and improve patient outcomes. I hope this atlas will provide an indispensable source of knowledge to all surgeons, those who just started their career, and those who are in more advanced stages of their practice and are learning new techniques of thyroidectomy.

> To carry out successfully the technique [of thyroidectomy]…it is clear that the operation cannot be performed by the surgeon alone, but by a team, of which the surgeon is the captain. George Crile

Freehold, NJ, USA — Alexander Shifrin

Acknowledgments

The creation of this atlas, covering the entire scope of thyroid surgery, was dependent on team effort, which was possible only with the support and enthusiasm of the many individuals who contributed to this book, Sanziana A. Roman, Julie Ann Sosa, Travis McKenzie, Janice Pasieka, Sarah E. Carty, Benzon M. Dy, Melanie L. Lyden, Miguel Francisco Herrera Hernández, Richard A. Hodin, Mark Sywak, Andreas Machens, Henning Dralle, Marco Raffaelli, Carmela De Crea, Rocco Bellantone, Joon-Hyop Lee, Sihoon Lee, Young Jun Chai, Gustavo Fernández-Ranvier, Schelto Kruijff, Marco S. Demarchi, Frédéric Triponez, and Hyunsuk Suh, my colleagues who trusted me and dedicated their time and effort to make it happen, without whom this atlas would have never come to life! To my surgical team, Tara Corrigan, George Kunak, and Pedro Garcia.

I am very thankful to my teachers, who dedicated their lives and efforts to the science of surgery. Those who made me into a surgeon and inspired me to produce this atlas: William Inabnet, MD, John Chabot, MD, Ali Bairov, MD, Steven Raper, MD, and Jerome Vernick, MD.

Special thanks to the artists who worked on this atlas at Springer. To Executive Editor Richard Hruska, who believed in me, and Senior Editor Lee Klein of Springer for his hard work and dedication.

Finally, I would like to thank the entire staff at Springer, who were very supportive from the first idea of this atlas and maintained their enthusiasm until the end.

Contents

1 **Right Thyroid Lobectomy** 1
Alexander Shifrin

2 **Open Right Thyroid Lobectomy** 23
Jina Kim, Sanziana A. Roman, and Julie Ann Sosa

3 **Thyroid Lobectomy** 31
Trenton Foster and Travis McKenzie

4 **Left Thyroid Lobectomy** 43
Caitlin T. Yeo, Adrian Harvey, and Janice L. Pasieka

5 **Total Thyroidectomy** 53
Ujas S. Shah, Kristina J. Nicholson, and Sally E. Carty

6 **Total Thyroidectomy for Substernal Goiter** 69
Benzon M. Dy and Melanie L. Lyden

7 **Left Thyroid Lobectomy as Completion of Total Thyroidectomy with Central Neck Lymph Node Dissection on the Left** 75
Alexander Shifrin

8 **Total Thyroidectomy** 97
Rafael Humberto Pérez-Soto, Alicia Maybí Trolle-Silva, and Miguel F. Herrera

9 **Left Thyroid Lobectomy and Isthmusectomy** 109
Rajshri M. Gartland and Richard A. Hodin

10 **Total Thyroidectomy and Ipsilateral Central Lymph Node Dissection for the Management of Papillary Thyroid Carcinoma** 117
Adam Ofri and Mark Sywak

11 **Hemithyroidectomy with *en bloc* Ipsilateral Central Node Dissection for Low-Risk Papillary and Medullary Thyroid Cancer** 129
Frank Weber, Andreas Machens, and Henning Dralle

12 **Video-Assisted Thyroidectomy** 143
Marco Raffaelli, Carmela De Crea, Francesco Pennestrì, Celestino Pio Lombardi, and Rocco Bellantone

13 **Robotic Total Thyroidectomy via Bilateral Axillo-Breast Approach (BABA)** 163
Hyunsuk Suh

14 **Transoral Endoscopic Total Thyroidectomy via Vestibular Approach (TOETVA)** 173
Joon-Hyop Lee, Sihoon Lee, and Young Jun Chai

15 Transoral Endoscopic Thyroidectomy via Vestibular Approach (TOETVA) 181
Gustavo Fernández-Ranvier, Ghayth Al Awwa, and Daniela Guevara

16 Safe Thyroidectomy in Low- and Middle-Income Countries 191
Schelto Kruijff, Marianne Roberta Frederiek Bosscher, and Pim Johan Bongers

17 Total Thyroidectomy with Comprehensive Central and Lateral Neck Dissection for Differentiated Thyroid Carcinoma 199
Marco Raffaelli, Carmela De Crea, Luca Sessa, and Rocco Bellantone

18 Thyroidectomy for Substernal Goiter 219
Marco S. Demarchi and Frédéric Triponez

Index 233

Contributors

Ghayth Al Awwa, MD Department of Surgery/Division of Metabolic, Endocrine, and Minimally Invasive Surgery, Icahn School of Medicine at Mount Sinai, New York, NY, USA

Rocco Bellantone, MD Center of Endocrine and Obesity Surgery, Fondazione Policlinico Universitario Agostino Gemelli IRCCS, Università Cattolica del Sacro Cuore, Rome, Italy

Pim Johan Bongers, MD, PhD Department of Surgical Oncology, University Medical Center Groningen, Groningen, The Netherlands

Marianne Roberta Frederiek Bosscher, MD, PhD Department of Surgical Oncology, University Medical Center Groningen, Groningen, The Netherlands

Sally E. Carty, MD, FACS Division of Endocrine Surgery, Department of Surgery, University of Pittsburgh School of Medicine, Pittsburgh, PA, USA

Young Jun Chai, MD, PhD Department of Surgery, Seoul Metropolitan Government-Seoul National University, Boramae Medical Center, Seoul, Republic of Korea

Carmela De Crea, MD Division of Endocrine and Metabolic Surgery, Fondazione Policlinico Universitario Agostino Gemelli IRCCS, Università Cattolica del Sacro Cuore, Rome, Italy

Marco S. Demarchi, MD Department of Thoracic and Endocrine Surgery, Geneva University Hospitals and University of Geneva, Geneva, Switzerland

Henning Dralle, MD Department of General, Visceral and Transplantation Surgery, Section of Endocrine Surgery, University of Duisburg-Essen, Essen, Germany

Benzon M. Dy, MD Division of Endocrine and Metabolic Surgery, Mayo Clinic, Rochester, MN, USA

Gustavo Fernández-Ranvier, MD, PhD Garlock Division of Surgery, Mount Sinai Hospital, New York, NY, USA

Trenton Foster, MD Department of Surgery, Mayo Clinic, Rochester, MN, USA

Rajshri M. Gartland, MD, MPH Department of Surgery, Massachusetts General Hospital, Boston, MA, USA

Daniela Guevara, MD The Garlock Division of General Surgery, Icahn School of Medicine at Mount Sinai Hospital, New York, NY, USA

Adrian Harvey, MD Section of General Surgery and Surgical Oncology, Department of Surgery, Faculty of Medicine, Foothills Medical Center, University of Calgary, Calgary, AB, Canada

Miguel F. Herrera, MD, PhD Department of Surgery, Division of Endocrine and Advanced Laparoscopic Surgery, Instituto Nacional de Ciencias Médicas y Nutrición, Salvador Zubirán, Tlalpan, Mexico City, Mexico

Richard A. Hodin, MD Department of Surgery, Massachusetts General Hospital, Boston, MA, USA

Jina Kim, MD Department of Surgery, Inova Health System, Fairfax, VA, USA

Schelto Kruijff, MD, PhD Department of Surgical Oncology, University Medical Center Groningen, Groningen, The Netherlands

Joon-Hyop Lee, MD Department of Surgery, Gachon University College of Medicine, Gil Medical Center, Incheon, Republic of Korea

Sihoon Lee, MD, PhD Gachon Medical Research Institute, Gachon University College of Medicine, Gil Medical Center, Incheon, Republic of Korea

Celestino Pio Lombardi, MD Division of Endocrine Surgery, Fondazione Policlinico Universitario Agostino Gemelli IRCCS, Università Cattolica del Sacro Cuore, Rome, Italy

Melanie L. Lyden, MD Division of Endocrine and Metabolic Surgery, Mayo Clinic, Rochester, MN, USA

Andreas Machens, MD Department of Visceral, Vascular and Endocrine Surgery, Martin Luther University Halle-Wittenberg, Halle (Saale), Germany

Travis McKenzie, MD Department of Surgery, Mayo Clinic, Rochester, MN, USA

Kristina J. Nicholson, MD, MSc Department of Surgery, University of Pittsburgh School of Medicine, Pittsburgh, PA, USA

Adam Ofri, BMed, MS, FRACS School of Medicine, University of New South Wales, St Leonards, NSW, Australia

Department of Surgery, Royal North Shore Hospital, St Leonards, NSW, Australia

Janice L. Pasieka, MD, FRCSC, FACS Division of Surgical Oncology and General Surgery, Department of Surgery, University of Calgary, Calgary, AB, Canada

Francesco Pennestrì, MD Division of Endocrine and Metabolic Surgery, Fondazione Policlinico Universitario Agostino Gemelli IRCCS, Rome, Italy

Rafael Humberto Pérez-Soto, MD Department of Surgery, Division of Endocrine and Advanced Laparoscopic Surgery, Instituto Nacional de Ciencias Médicas y Nutrición, Salvador Zubirán, Tlalpan, Mexico City, Mexico

Marco Raffaelli, MD Division of Endocrine and Metabolic Surgery, Fondazione Policlinico Universitario Agostino Gemelli IRCCS, Università Cattolica del Sacro Cuore, Rome, Italy

Sanziana A. Roman, MD, FACS Department of Surgery, Division of Surgical Oncology, University of California, San Francisco, San Francisco, CA, USA

Luca Sessa, MD Division of Endocrine and Metabolic Surgery, Fondazione Policlinico Universitario Agostino Gemelli IRCCS, Rome, Italy

Ujas S. Shah, MD Division of Endocrine Surgery, Department of Surgery, University of Pittsburgh School of Medicine, Pittsburgh, PA, USA

Alexander Shifrin, MD, FACS, FACE, ECNU, FEBS, FISS Atlantic Health Oncology Service and Department of Surgery, CentraState Health System, Atlantic Health Partner, Freehold, NJ, USA

Julie Ann Sosa, MD, MA, FACS, MAMSE, FSSO Department of Surgery, University of California San Francisco (UCSF), San Francisco, CA, USA

Hyunsuk Suh, MD Suh Scarless Thyroid Surgery Center, Norman/Clayman Endocrine Institute, Hospital for Endocrine Surgery, Tampa, FL, USA

Mark Sywak, MBBS, MMed Sci(Clin Epi) University of Sydney Endocrine Surgery Unit, Royal North Shore Hospital, St Leonards, NSW, Australia

Department of Endocrine and Oncology Surgery, Royal North Shore Hospital, St Leonards, NSW, Australia

Frédéric Triponez, MD Department of Thoracic and Endocrine Surgery, Geneva University Hospitals and University of Geneva, Geneva, Switzerland

Alicia Maybí Trolle-Silva, MD Department of Anatomical Pathology, National Institute of Medical Sciences and Nutrition Salvador Zubirán, Mexico City, Mexico

Frank Weber, MD Department of General, Visceral and Transplantation Surgery, Section of Endocrine Surgery, University of Duisburg-Essen, Essen, Germany

Caitlin T. Yeo, MD Section of General Surgery and Oncology, Department of Surgery, Cumming School of Medicine, University of Calgary, Calgary, AB, Canada

Right Thyroid Lobectomy

1

Alexander Shifrin

Introduction

Right thyroid lobectomy (also known as a hemithyroidectomy) is the removal of the right thyroid lobe, including the isthmus and a pyramidal lobe, leaving the left thyroid lobe intact. The removal of the isthmus and pyramidal lobe is indicated to avoid the possibility of recurrent laryngeal nerve (RLN) injury on the operative side in case completion of a total thyroidectomy would be warranted in the future. If isthmus and a pyramidal lobe would be left behind, there would be a possibility of a partial regrowth (regeneration) of an isthmus and a pyramidal lobe toward the previously operated side and over the RLN, which may result in injury of the nerve during the completion of total thyroidectomy. Meticulous surgical technique and attention to detail are pertinent in performing a successful thyroidectomy. The main goal of thyroid surgery is not only to remove the diseased thyroid gland or lobe but also to prevent complications, such as RLN injury and the incidental removal of parathyroid glands. The complications of thyroidectomy by themselves could be more devastating than the disease that it was intended to cure. Therefore, the procedure of thyroidectomy or thyroid lobectomy involves, first, the identification, full exposure, and safe dissection of the RLN, then the identification and preservation of all parathyroid glands, followed by performing an indicated removal of the thyroid lobe [1, 2]. Almost all our thyroidectomies are performed as outpatient procedures with a 5-hour observation stay for lobectomy and 6 hours for a total thyroidectomy [3–6]. Patients with severe medical comorbidities, those who travel from out of state or from a distance, as well as those who require modified radical neck dissection or sternotomy need to stay overnight for observation (patients with sternotomy may stay longer until the chest tube is removed). All patients are evaluated with an assessment of the vocal cord function through flexible laryngoscopy prior to and right after the procedure. Intraoperative RLN monitoring (IONM) has gained widespread acceptance as an adjunct to the gold standard of identification and visualization of the nerve [7–10]. We perform IONM for all thyroidectomy and parathyroidectomy procedures in our practice. In addition, monitoring of the external branch of the superior laryngeal nerve (EBSLN) is performed for all patients who require extra attention to their voice, such as singers, teachers, public speakers, and so on. Thyroidectomy is considered a clean surgical procedure, and no preoperative antibiotics are required. For extra precaution, we do give preoperative antibiotics only to patients with implantable metal devices, immunosuppressed patients, and patients who require sternotomy or a prolonged (over 4 hours) procedure, such as total thyroidectomy with modified radical neck dissection.

Supplementary Information The online version contains supplementary material available at [https://doi.org/10.1007/978-3-030-93673-0_1].

A. Shifrin (✉)
Atlantic Health Oncology Service and Department of Surgery, CentraState Health System, Atlantic Health Partner, Freehold, NJ, USA

Anatomical Considerations

Recurrent (Inferior) Laryngeal Nerve (RLN)

It is important to know anatomical variations in the position and location of the RLN. The right RLN comes off the main trunk of the right vagus nerve on the level of the right subclavian artery, hooks around the artery, and ascends up into the neck to enter into the cricothyroid muscle. The right RLN is usually positioned more obliquely and laterally to the tracheoesophageal groove compared to the left RLN (Fig. 1.1) [10, 11]. A surgeon should always keep in mind the possibility of a nonrecurrent laryngeal nerve (NRLN) on the right side, which occurs in about 1% of patients (Fig. 1.2). In this case, the NRLN will come directly from the vagus nerve laterally at the level of the cricothyroid muscle and go directly transverse to enter the cricothyroid muscle from the lateral location rather than inferiorly. If NRLN is not recognized, it can be easily injured. In the

A. Shifrin (ed.), *Atlas of Thyroid Surgery*, https://doi.org/10.1007/978-3-030-93673-0_1

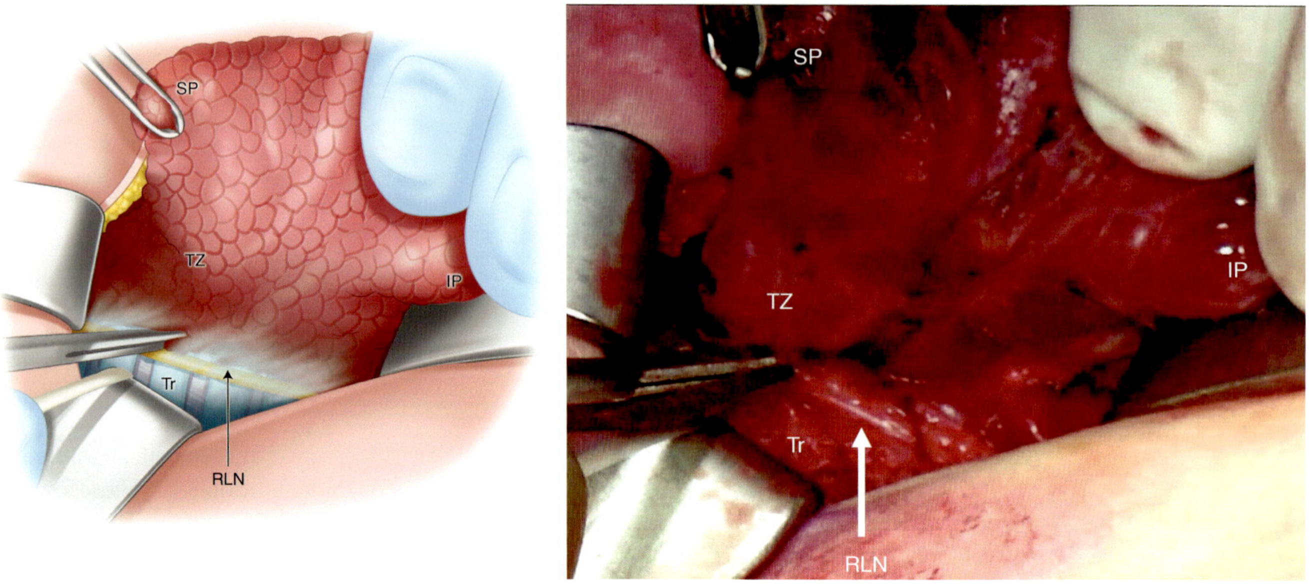

Fig. 1.1 Normal anatomy of the recurrent laryngeal nerve (RLN) on the right side. The right RLN is usually positioned more obliquely and laterally to the tracheoesophageal groove compared to the left RLN. Left side of the screen – cephalad; right side of the screen – caudal. Arrow is pointing at the recurrent laryngeal nerve (RLN). Tr – trachea, SP – superior pole of the right thyroid lobe, IP – inferior pole of the right thyroid lobe, TZ – tubercle of Zuckerkandl

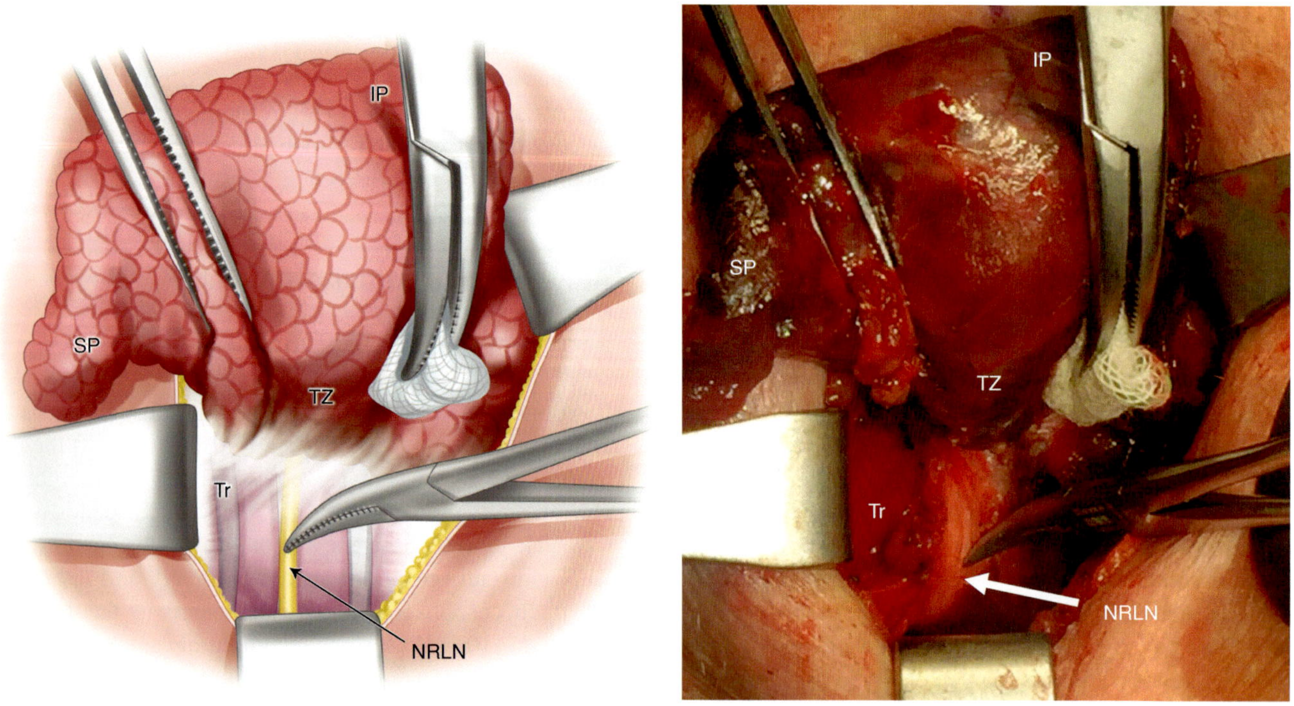

Fig. 1.2 Nonrecurrent laryngeal nerve (NRLN) on the right side. RLN is seen as nonrecurrent (NRLN) (arrow) coming off the vagus nerve from the carotid sheath laterally toward the cricothyroid muscle, rather than from the inferior direction, as in Fig. 1.1. Left side of the screen – cephalad; right side of the screen – caudal. Arrow and mosquito are pointing at the nonrecurrent laryngeal nerve (NRLN). Tr – trachea, SP – superior pole of the right thyroid lobe, LP – inferior pole of the right thyroid lobe, TZ – tubercle of Zuckerkandl

majority of cases, the presence of NRLN is associated with an aberrant right subclavian artery [1, 12].

The RLN can have up to six branches [11]. Bifurcation of the RLN was reported on the right side in between 26% and 33% of cases, and on the left side in 19–23% of cases with bilateral bifurcation reported in about 8.9% of patients. The RLN bifurcates into two branches in about 70% of cases on the right side and 67% of cases on the left and more than two branches in about 30% of cases on the right side and 33% of cases on the left side. It is important to dissect the entire length of the neck part of the RLN during the thyroidectomy since it can bifurcate at more than 2 cm inferior to the larynx in 33% of patients on the right side and 58% of cases on the left side. The most important anatomical considerations are given to the functional aspect of the RLN. The vocal cords' adduction and abduction are controlled exclusively by motor fibers located in the anterior (the more medial) branch of the RLN, and none are present in the posterior (or lateral) branch(es) of the RLN. That is the reason why the exposure of the entire RLN during a surgical dissection is required in order to detect all branches of the nerve. Intraoperative monitoring of the RLN can help with nerve identification, mapping, and evaluation of function. IONM is especially helpful with the branching nerve. Losing the RLN IONM signal on one side during the dissection can influence the surgeon's decision to proceed to the other side with a total thyroidectomy [12, 13].

Inferior Thyroid Artery

The anatomical relationship and variation between the position of the inferior thyroid artery (ITA) and the RLN are important for safe dissection of the RLN. Most commonly, the RLN runs posterior to the ITA in about 76% of patients on both sides, anterior to the ITA in 19% of patients on the right side and 24% of patients on the left side, and in between the branches of the RLN in about 3.3% of patients on the right side and less than that on the left side [1, 14]. If the RLN runs in between the branches of the ITA, retracting the thyroid lobe up and medially may cause pressure from one of the ITA branches, causing "strangulation injury" of the RLN, and may result in transient neural paralysis. To prevent this, the identification and transection of this branch of the ITA earlier during the dissection of the RLN may be necessary to eliminate this complication.

Tubercle of Zuckerkandl

Tubercle of Zuckerkandl, a posterior extension of the lateral lobes of the thyroid gland, is more obvious on the right side (83% of cases) than on the left side (69% of cases) and was reported to be larger than 1 cm in 31% of cases on the right side and 23% of cases on the left side [15–17].

Parathyroid Glands

The typical location of a superior parathyroid gland is usually 1 cm cranial to the crossing of the RLN and ITA and within 1 cm of the cricothyroid cartilage (in 80% of cases). The inferior parathyroid gland usually locates 1 cm lateral, inferior, or posterior to the inferior pole of the right thyroid lobe in about 50% of cases. Potentially, it could be intrathyroidal or subcapsular [1, 10].

Instruments Set (Fig. 1.3)

1. Gemini right angle forceps (8″)
2. Gemini right angle forceps (5-1/8″)

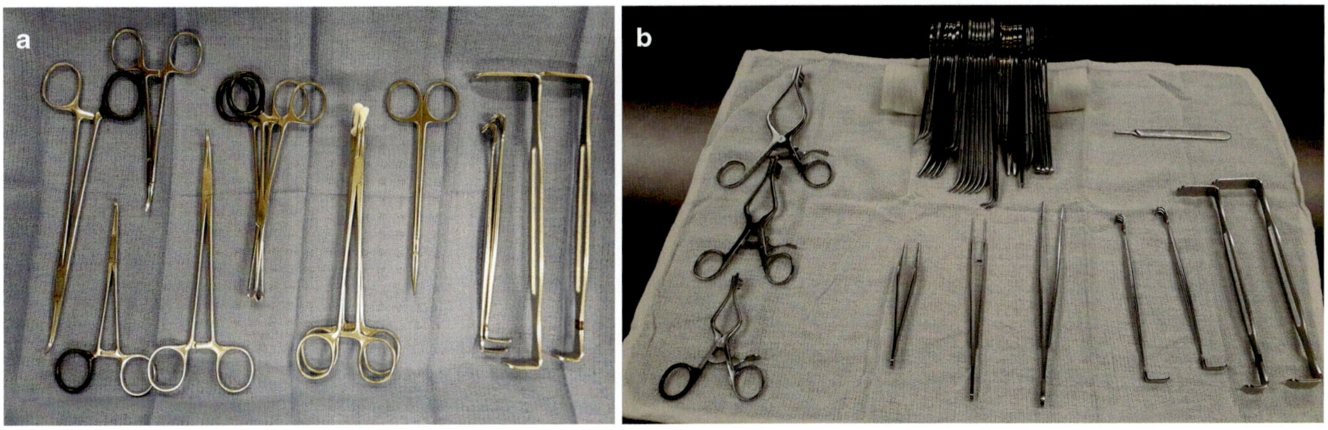

Fig. 1.3 (**a**) Essential instruments set (left to right): 1. Gemini right angle forceps (8″). 2. Gemini right angle forceps (5-1/8″). 3. Micro Halstead mosquito (5″). 4. Adson delicate tonsil forceps (7-1/4″). 5. Allis clamps (6″). 6. Adson delicate tonsil forceps with peanut (7-1/4″). 7. Nerve dissecting scissors (6″). 8. Miller Senn retractor blunt double-ended (6-1/4″). 9. Army/navy retractors. (**b**) Extended instruments set: 1. Weitlaner self-retaining retractors; sharp and dull, different sizes (left). 2. Adson delicate tonsil forceps (7-1/4″). 3. Adson toothed tissue forceps (middle left). 4. Gerald forceps (middle). 5. Debakey forceps (middle right). 6. Energy-based vessel-sealing devices, such as Harmonic Focus or LigaSure device. 7. No. 15 scalpel

3. Micro Halstead mosquito forceps (5″)
4. Adson delicate tonsil forceps (7-1/4″)
5. Allis clamps (6″)
6. Adson delicate tonsil forceps with peanut (7-1/4″)
7. Nerve dissecting scissors (6″)
8. Miller Senn retractor blunt double-ended (6-1/4″)
9. Army/navy retractors
10. Weitlaner self-retaining retractors; sharp and dull, different sizes (left)
11. Adson delicate tonsil forceps (7-1/4″)
12. Adson toothed tissue forceps (middle left)
13. Gerald forceps (middle)
14. Debakey forceps (middle right)
15. Energy-based vessel-sealing device, such as Harmonic Focus or LigaSure device
16. Surgical loupes (help in identifying the RLN and parathyroid glands and are essential for the operation).

Patient's Case

A 29-year-old female was presented with incidental findings of a 3-cm right thyroid nodule, with no significant symptoms, no history of radiation exposure, and no significant family history. Ultrasound-guided fine-needle aspiration biopsy showed findings suspicious for follicular neoplasm (Bethesda category 4). She was consented for a right thyroid lobectomy. The possibility of complications was discussed, such as a 1% chance of injury to the RLN, the development of infection, or hematoma. The possibility of a total thyroidectomy, including central neck lymph nodes dissection, was also discussed in the event a cancer would be detected during the surgery by intraoperative frozen section evaluation with findings of aggressive features, such as extrathyroidal extension with invasion and/or findings of metastatic lymph nodes.

Patient's Preparation, Intubation, and Positioning

The patient is taken to the operating room and placed in a supine position. Sequential compression devices are placed on the lower extremities bilaterally for deep venous thrombosis prophylaxis. General anesthesia is administered, and the patient is intubated using a 7.0 endotracheal tube (ET tube) with the electrodes for IONM. Both arms are tucked at the patient's sides, ensuring the padding of pressure points is given close attention to mitigate brachial and ulnar nerve injury. A shoulder roll is placed under the shoulders for neck hyperextension to promote the visibility of the surgical site; however, it should not be hanging. The head is placed in a foam head cradle. Of note is if the patient has a history of cervical spine injury or vocalizes preoperatively the symptoms of neck pain with hyperextension, the positioning could be performed prior to intubation while the patient is awake, therefore highlighting the limitations of neck extension. The alternative approach that we use is to perform intraoperative upper extremity motor nerve monitoring using the same technique and by the same technician who performs IONM for the thyroidectomy. Then flexible laryngoscopy is performed to position the ET tube IONM electrode over the vocal cords, the ET balloon is inflated, and the ET tube is secured in place. The patient is prepped with chlorhexidine surgical skin prep and draped with blue sterile paper drape towels and strips of an IOBAN antimicrobial adhesive drape to box off the paper drapes for a tight seal of the field. This is done to prevent accidental gas leaks from the anesthesia ventilation (to avoid fire hazards from using a Bovie cautery in the presence of oxygen) and for sterility of the field. Preoperative antibiotics are not usually given unless the patient is immunosuppressed or has metal implantable devices (joint replacements, heart valves, defibrillator, and so on), or other risk factors for infection (for example, the history of splenectomy), and in the presence of a large substernal goiter.

Procedure Step by Step

1. Skin, muscle incision, and access to the thyroid gland (lobe)
2. Lateral mobilization of the thyroid lobe with transection of the middle thyroid vein
3. Mobilization and transection of the superior pole vessels with identification and preservation of the external branch of the superior laryngeal nerve (EBSLN)
4. Identification and preservation of the inferior parathyroid gland
5. Identification, dissection, and preservation of the right recurrent laryngeal nerve
6. Identification, dissection, and preservation of the right superior parathyroid gland
7. Transection of Berry's ligament
8. Dissection of the thyroid lobe off the trachea with isthmus and pyramidal lobe
9. Muscle and skin closure

Skin Mark, Muscle Incision, and Access to the Thyroid Gland (Lobe)

Skin mark and skin incision are placed in the natural skin fold, preferably at the level of the thyroid isthmus (Fig. 1.4). The platysma muscle is separated at midline

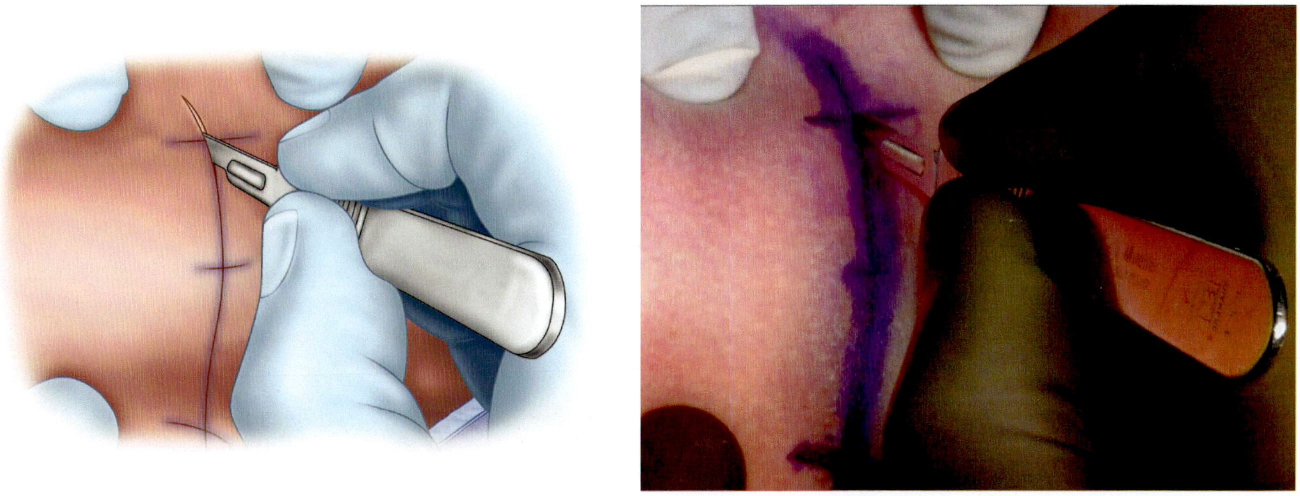

Fig. 1.4 Skin mark and skin incision are placed in the natural skin fold, preferably at the level of the thyroid isthmus

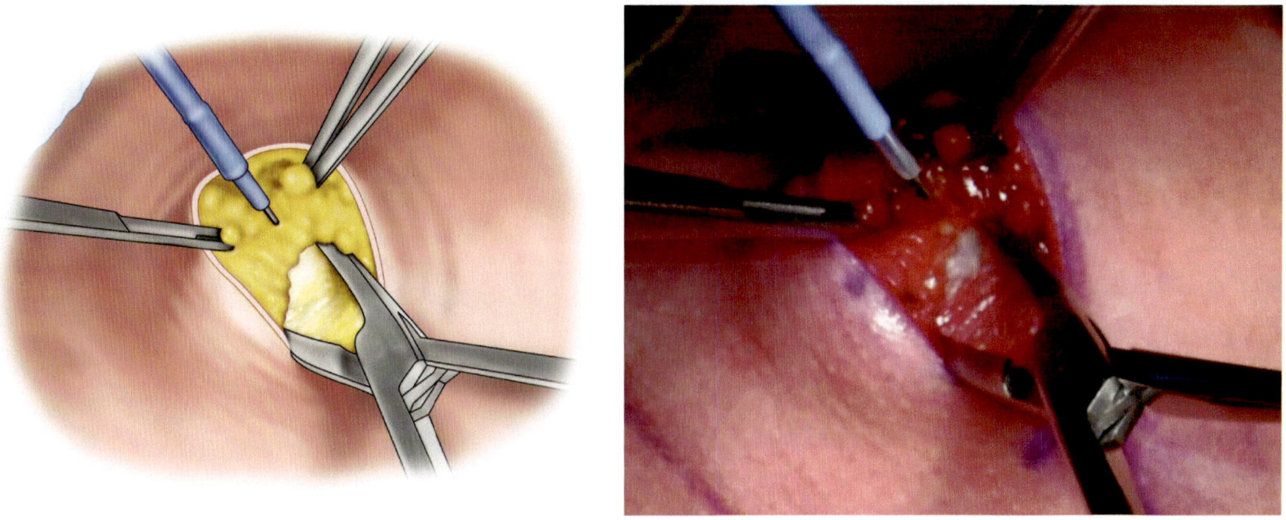

Fig. 1.5 The platysma is separated at midline using a Bovie cautery

using a Bovie cautery (Fig. 1.5). Holding the platysma with Adson tonsil forceps and Debakey forceps, subplatysmal flaps are created inferiorly (Fig. 1.6) and superiorly (Fig. 1.7) by using a Bovie cautery. The superior flap should be smaller than the inferior flap in order to avoid denervation of the skin flap, which could be presented as postoperative skin numbness at the level of the lower chin. Weitlaner self-retaining retractors are used to spread the skin and the platysma muscle edges to expose strap muscles at the midline (Fig. 1.8). By using Adson forceps, space is created under the strap muscles. Then by using the Bovie cautery, strap muscles are split at the midline along the *linea alba* (Fig. 1.9) (Video 1.1).

Lateral Mobilization of the Thyroid Lobe with Division of the Middle Thyroid Vein

The next step is the mobilization of the thyroid lobe off the strap muscles laterally. Two army/navy retractors are placed to retract the skin, the platysma, and strap muscles laterally and inferiorly. When performing lateral retraction, be very careful not to cause significant pressure over the carotid artery in elderly patients or those with a history of carotid artery disease (calcifications and occlusion) to avoid accidental carotid plug dislodgement, which can lead to the liberation of the plug into the circulation, which can, in turn, result in a stroke. By using

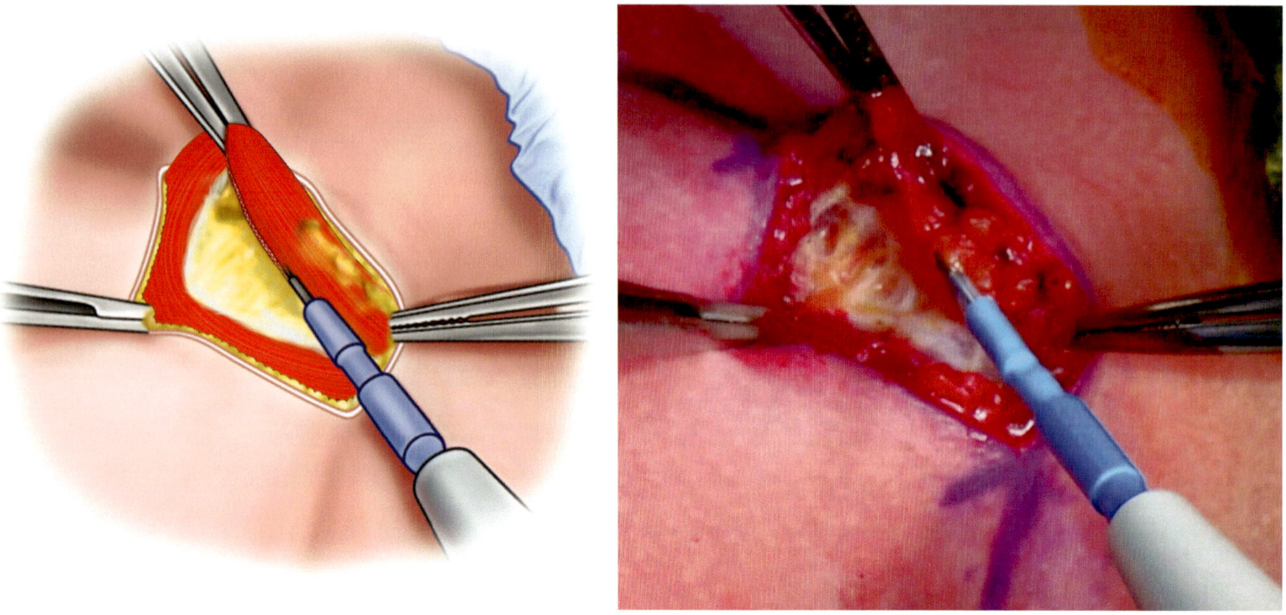

Fig. 1.6 Subplatysmal flap is created inferiorly by using a Bovie cautery and holding the platysma with Adson tonsil forceps and Debakey forceps

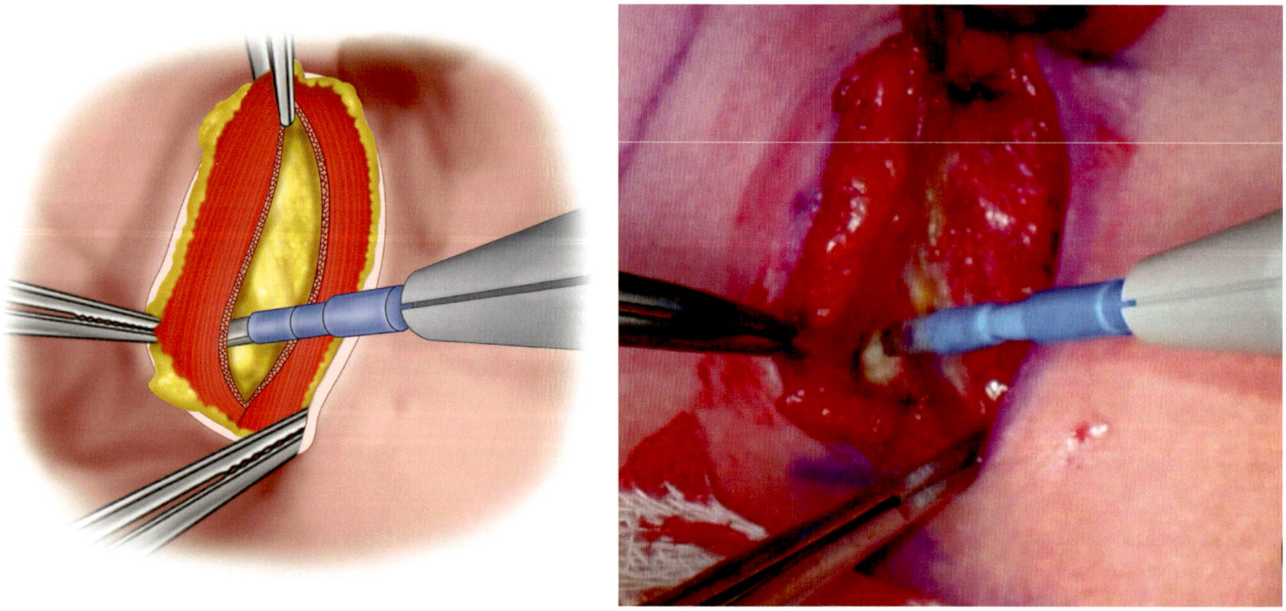

Fig. 1.7 Subplatysmal skin flap is created superiorly by using a Bovie cautery and holding the platysma with Adson tonsil forceps and Debakey forceps

Adson forceps with peanut, the thyroid lobe is retracted medially. Army/navy retractors are used to pull the strap muscles and skin laterally to create contra tension, while Debakey forceps are used to pull some of the muscle fibers off the thyroid lobe laterally to under the army/navy retractors (Fig. 1.10). The middle thyroid vein is mobilized circumferentially with Adson forceps. It is important to dissect the vein off the underlying carotid artery and jugular vein to prevent any injuries to them. When the vein is mobilized, the small Gemini right angle forceps are inserted under the middle thyroid vein to elevate it off the carotid sheet. Then the middle thyroid vein is transected in between the jaws of the small Gemini right angle forceps by using the Harmonic Focus device (Fig. 1.11). It is important to always keep the vein elevated up and away from the carotid sheet with the use of the small Gemini right angle forceps during this maneuver.

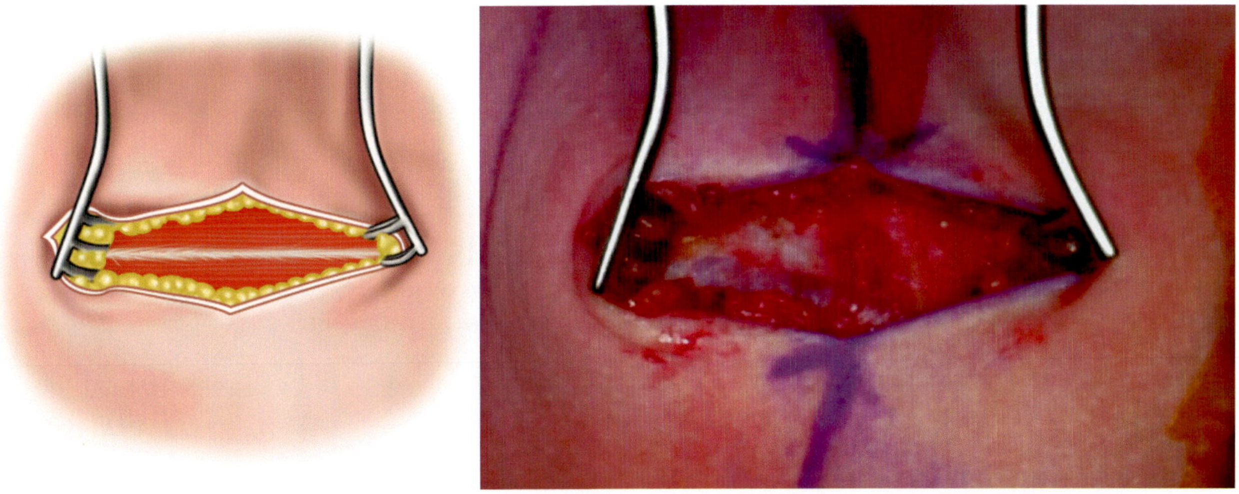

Fig. 1.8 Weitlaner self-retaining retractors are used to spread the skin and the platysma muscle edges to expose strap muscles at midline

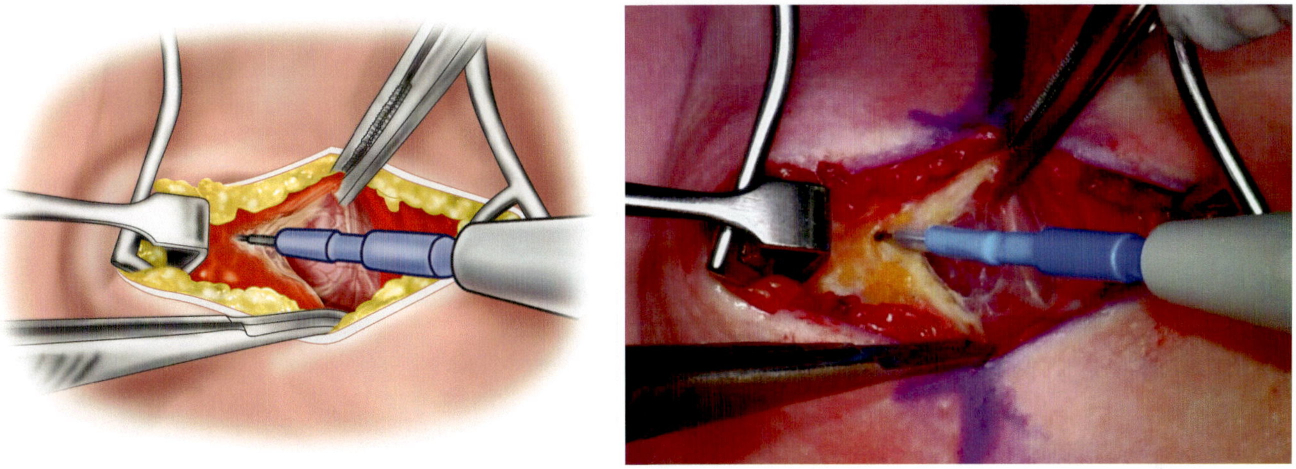

Fig. 1.9 Strap muscles are split at midline along the *linea alba*

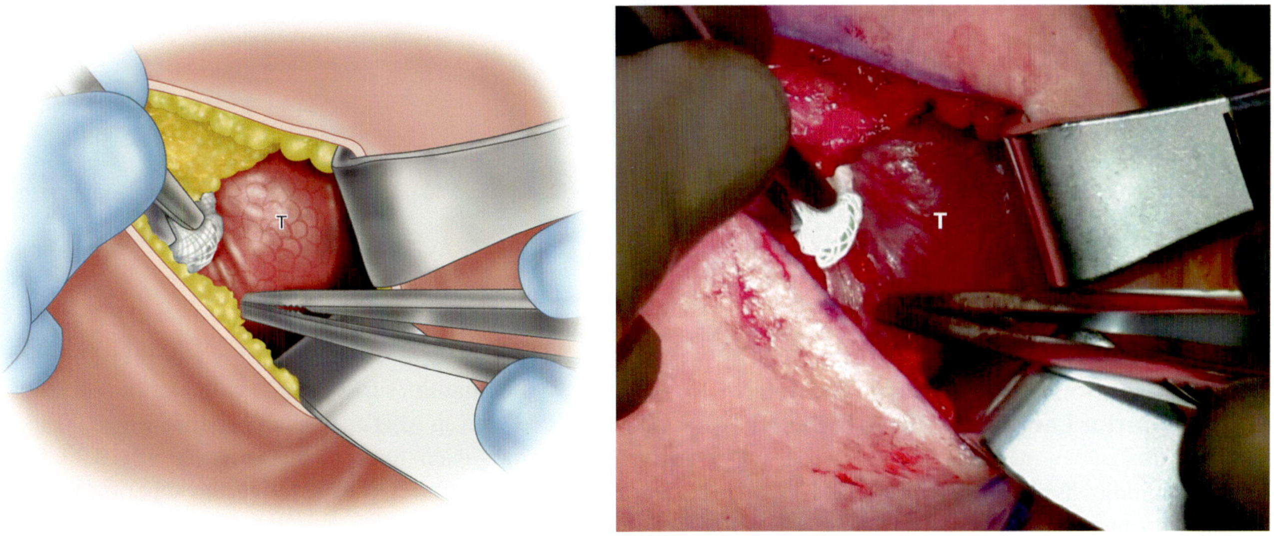

Fig. 1.10 Mobilization of the thyroid lobe off the strap muscles laterally. Two army/navy retractors are placed to retract the skin, the platysma, and strap muscles laterally and inferiorly. By using Adson forceps with peanut, the thyroid lobe is retracted medially. Army/navy retractors are used to pull the strap muscles and skin laterally to create contra tension, while Debakey forceps are used to pull some of the muscle fibers off the thyroid lobe laterally to under the army/navy retractors. T – right thyroid lobe

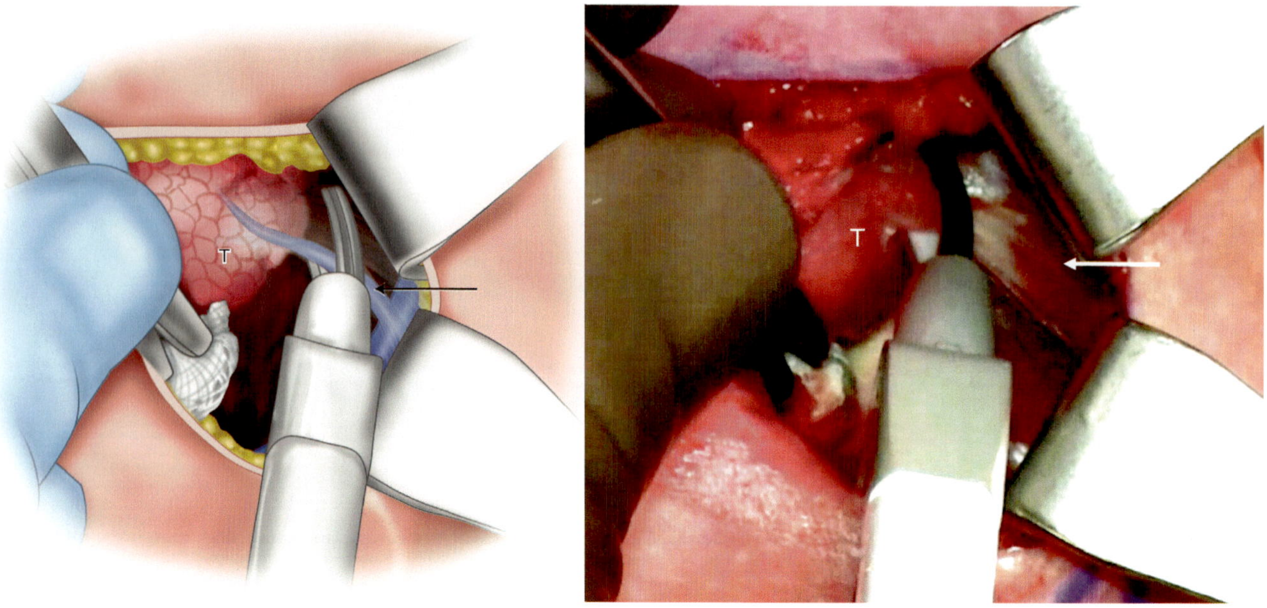

Fig. 1.11 The middle thyroid vein is transected by using the Harmonic Focus device. Arrow at the middle thyroid vein (in this case, the vein has several branches that are transected simultaneously). T – right thyroid lobe

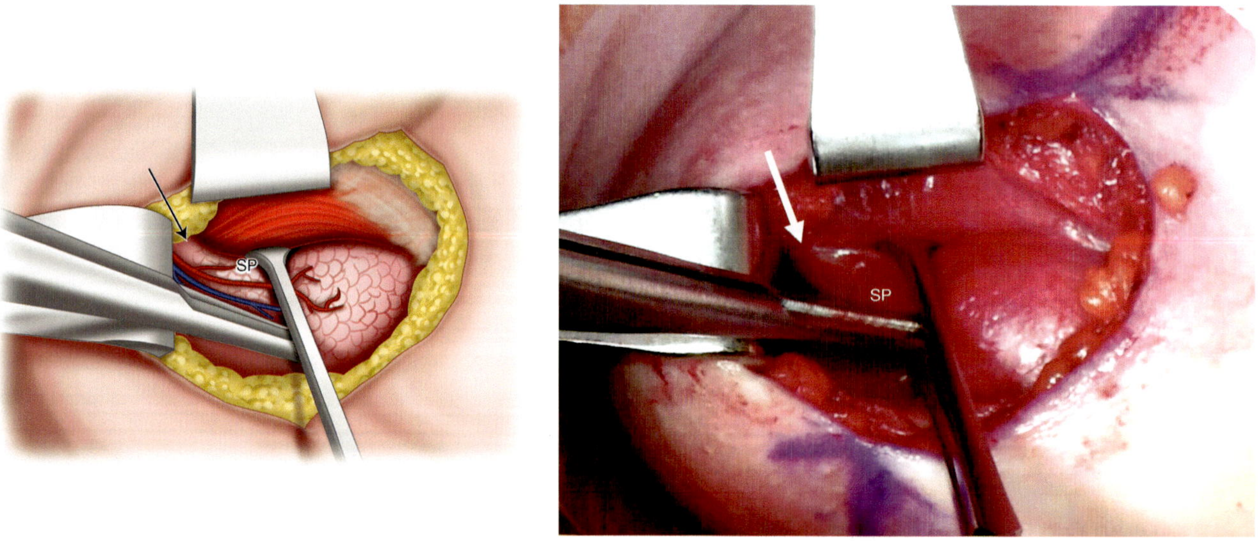

Fig. 1.12 By holding the superior pole with Debakey forceps, it is grabbed with an Allis clamp and pulled inferiorly. Arrow pointing at the superior pole vessels. SP – superior pole

Mobilization and Transection of the Superior Pole Vessels with Identification and Preservation of the External Branch of the Superior Laryngeal Nerve (EBSLN)

After the middle thyroid vein is transected, two army/navy retractors are moved superiorly. The first army/navy retractor is placed lateral to the superior pole with the deep end in, and the second is medial to the superior pole with the short end in. By holding the superior pole with Debakey forceps, it is grabbed with an Allis clamp and pulled inferiorly (Fig. 1.12). By using Adson forceps, the avascular space of Reeve is entered and dissected to separate the superior pole vessels from the cricothyroid muscles (Fig. 1.13). Keeping this

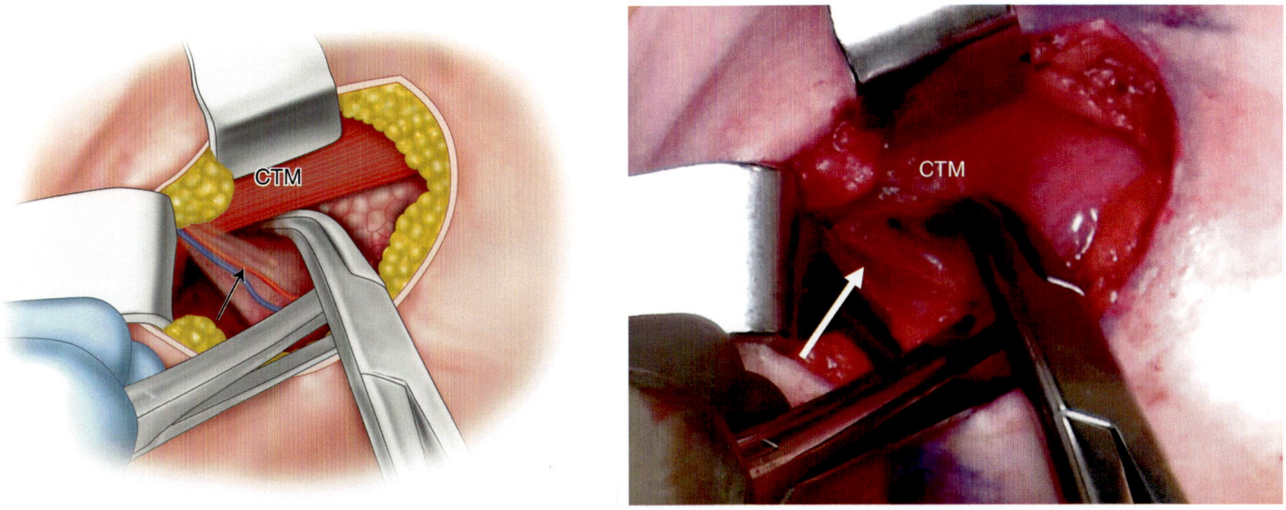

Fig. 1.13 Avascular space of Reeve is entered and dissected to separate the superior pole vessels from the cricothyroid muscles. Arrow pointing at the superior pole vessels. CTM – cricothyroid muscle

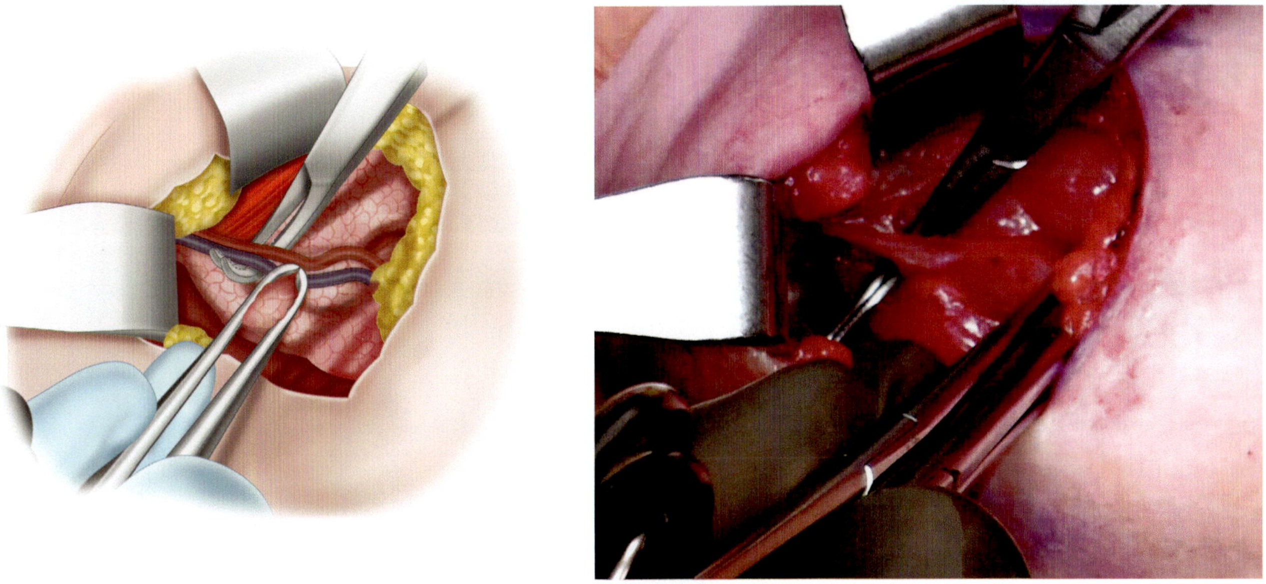

Fig. 1.14 Gemini right angle forceps are used to dissect and elevate superior pole vessels

space dry is crucial for the safe dissection and prevention of injury to the external branch of the superior laryngeal nerve (EBSLN). The EBSLN usually lies medially on or in between the fibers of the cricothyroid muscle. By using small Gemini right angle forceps, several superior pole vessels are dissected and elevated up (Fig. 1.14). It is important to stay as close to the thyroid lobe as possible to avoid injury to the EBSLN. These steps are repeated until all superior pole vessels are transected (Figs. 1.12, 1.13, 1.14, 1.15, 1.16, and 1.17). Nerve stimulation can also be used to determine the location and integrity of the EBSLN (Fig. 1.16). Then superior pole vessels are transacted using the Harmonic Focus device in between the jaws of a small Gemini right angle forceps (Figs. 1.15 and 1.17). To avoid incidental injury to the RLN, dissection should not be conducted too deep in the proximity to the RLN entrance site into the cricothyroid muscle. Significant traction on the superior pole may result in traction on the RLN, neural stretch, and temporary paralysis.

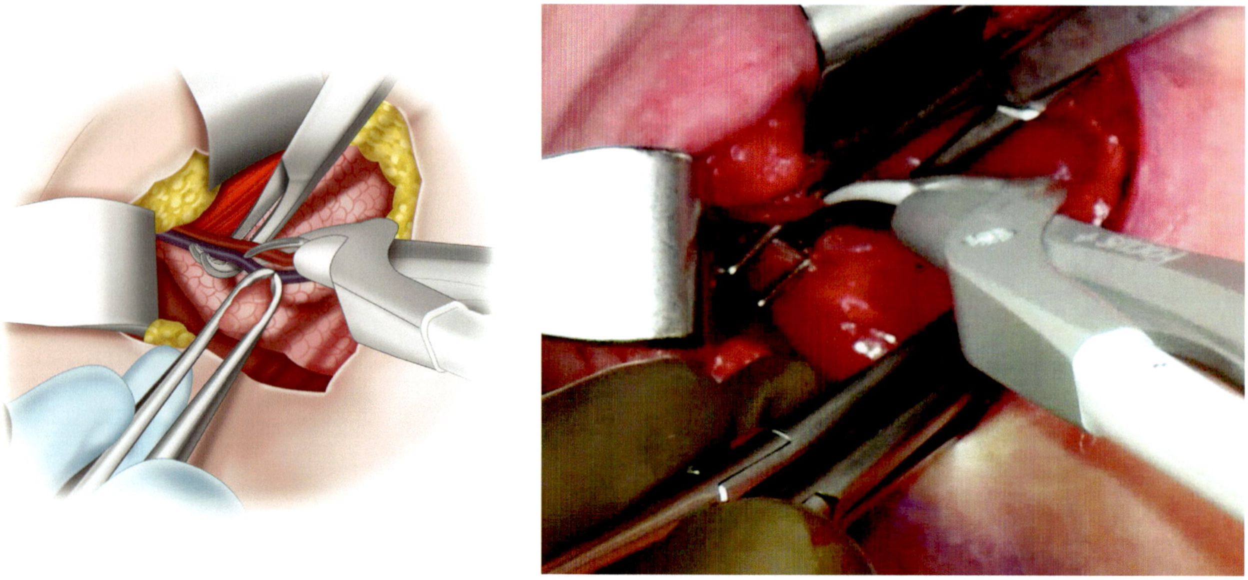

Fig. 1.15 Superior pole vessels are transected using the Harmonic Focus device

a

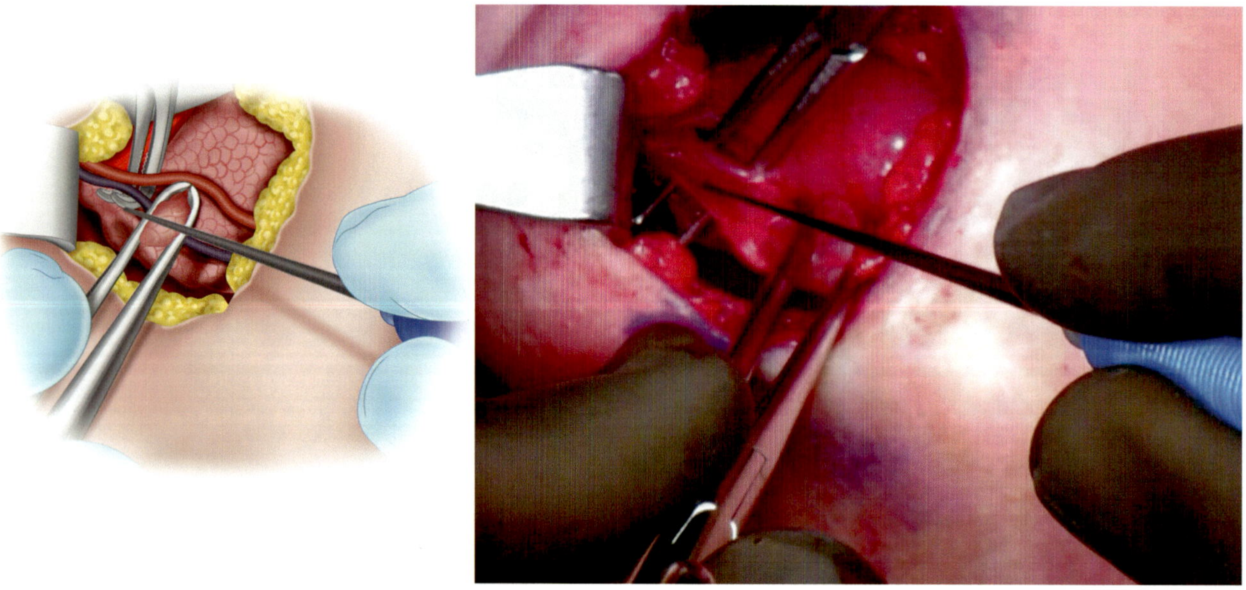

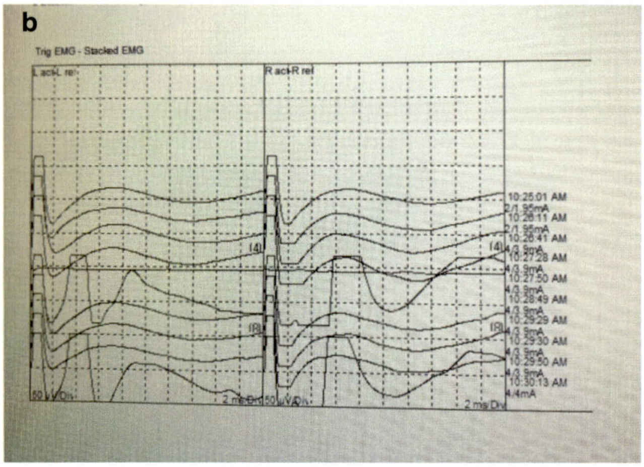

Fig. 1.16 (**a**) External branch of the superior laryngeal nerve (EBSLN) monitoring is used to determine the location and integrity of the EBSLN. (**b**) Electromyography (EMG) monitoring of the EBSLN showing normal waveform responses from the endotracheal tube (ET) electrode during EBSLN stimulation

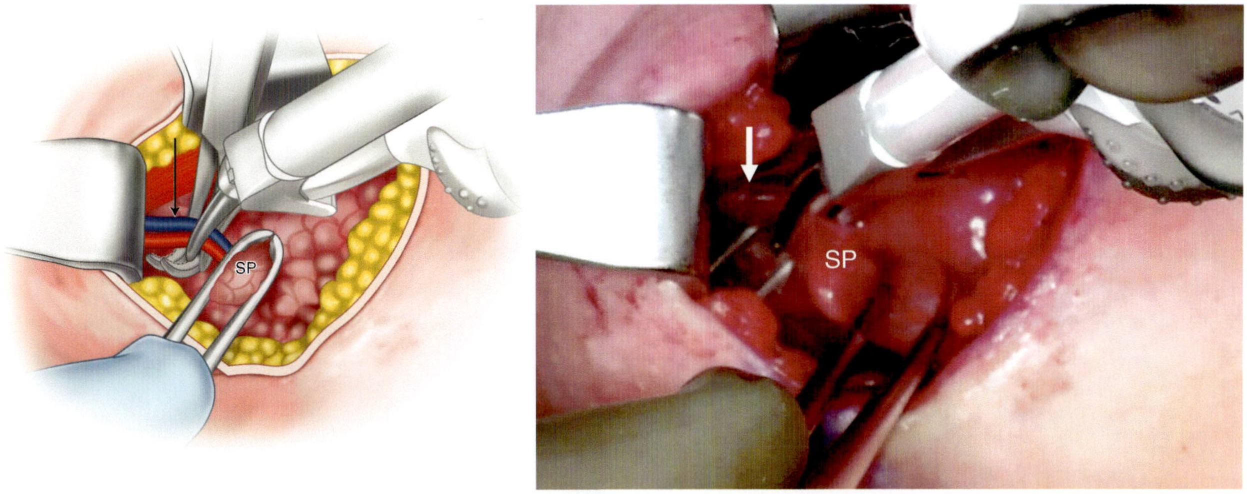

Fig. 1.17 Transection of superior pole vessels using the Harmonic Focus device. Arrow at superior pole vessels. SP – superior pole of the right thyroid lobe

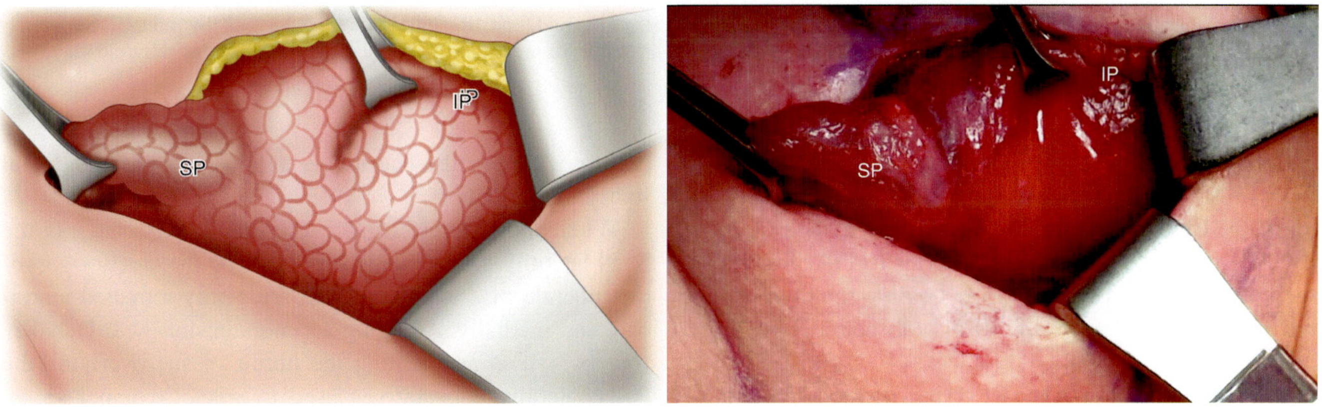

Fig. 1.18 Keeping the superior Allis clamp on the superior pole (SP) of the thyroid lobe, the second Allis clamp is placed on the inferior pole (IP) of the right thyroid lobe to retract the thyroid lobe medially

Identification and Preservation of the Inferior Parathyroid Gland

After the superior pole vessels are completely transacted, army/navy retractors are replaced laterally and inferiorly. Keeping the superior Allis clamp on the superior pole of the right thyroid lobe, the second Allis clamp is placed on the inferior pole of the right thyroid lobe. Be careful to not accidentally grab the inferior parathyroid gland during placement of the Allis clamp on the inferior pole. Next, the thyroid lobe is retracted medially and anteriorly with the Allis clamps (Fig. 1.18), along with a finger over the gauze (Fig. 1.19), or by using peanuts on Adson tonsil forceps. After the inferior parathyroid gland is identified (arrow), it is dissected off the thyroid by mosquito. The Harmonic Focus device is used to transect the attachments between the right inferior parathyroid gland and the inferior pole of the right thyroid lobe (Fig. 1.19). To prevent devascularization and injury to the parathyroid gland, the traction should be very gentle.

Identification, Dissection, and Preservation of the Right Recurrent Laryngeal Nerve

The thyroid lobe is retracted medially. In the presented case, we immediately visualized the right RLN along the right side of the trachea (appearing as a white cord). The nerve stimulator is used to confirm the integrity of the RLN (Fig. 1.20). If the nerve is not visualized right away (in most case scenarios), Debakey forceps are used to pull the fibrous tissue overlying the inferior thyroid artery (ITA) laterally. The RLN is identified by dissecting these tissues with mosquito along the course of the ITA and then under the ITA and inferiorly

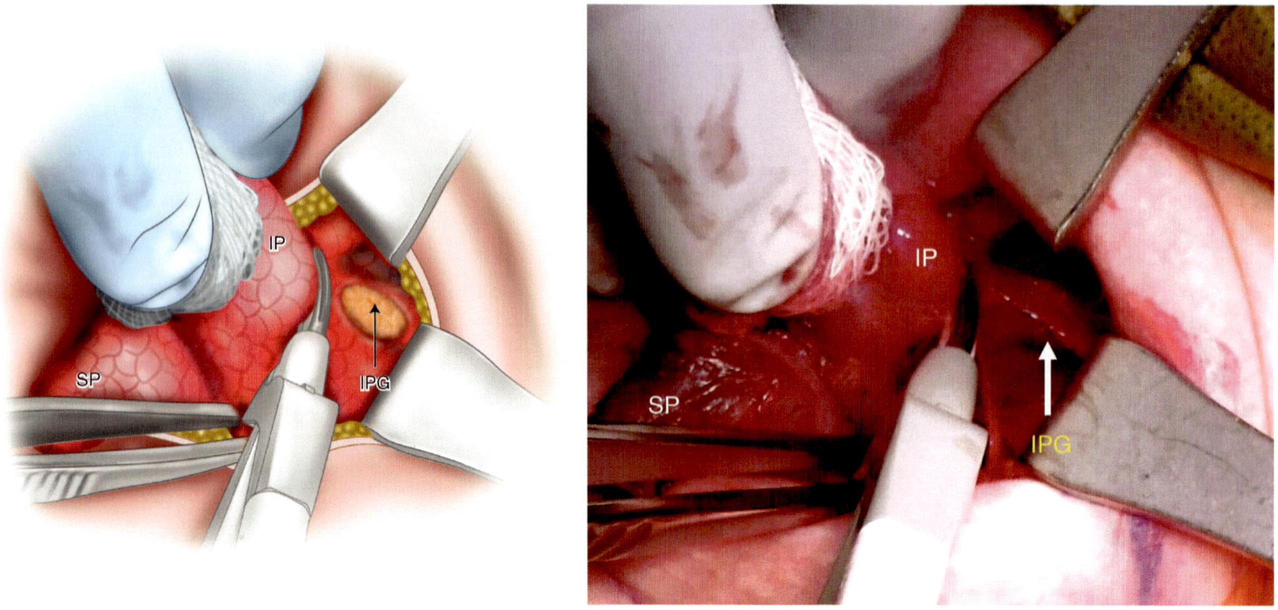

Fig. 1.19 After the inferior parathyroid gland (IPG) is identified (arrow), the Harmonic Focus device is used to transect the attachments between the right inferior parathyroid gland and inferior pole (IP) of the right thyroid lobe. IP – inferior pole of the right thyroid lobe, SP – superior pole of the right thyroid lobe, IPG – inferior parathyroid gland

to Berry's ligament. Meticulous dissection and magnification with surgical loupes make it easier to identify the position of the RLN and its branches, in relation to the ITA, since in 19% of cases the RLN runs anterior to ITA. Significant traction on the Allis clamps while holding the thyroid lobe may result in traction on the RLN with neural stretch and temporary paralysis.

Upon identification of the RLN, it is dissected with mosquito up toward the insertion site into the cricothyroid muscle and then down along its course (Fig. 1.21). This is done in order to identify the branching of the RLN. The most medial and anterior branch would be the motor branch. The integrity of the RLN is confirmed by the nerve stimulator (Fig. 1.22). When the exact positioning of the RLN is confirmed, the inferior thyroid pole attachment to the trachea can be dissected with mosquito and safely transected by using the Harmonic Focus device (Fig. 1.23). In the case presented, the tubercle of Zuckerkandl is overlying the RLN within the right side. By using the Debakey forceps, fibrous tissues overlying the RLN and the tubercle of Zuckerkandl are retracted laterally. A tunneled space is created over the RLN by mosquito forceps. Without replacing the Debakey forceps while holding this fibrous tissue, gentle traction is applied up and laterally while inserting the lower jaw of the Harmonic Focus device into the tunneled space. Keeping the RLN in full view, the superficial layer of these fibrous tissues is transected, unroofing the tunneled space (Fig. 1.24). ITA or its branches will be divided at the same time by the Harmonic Focus device. It is critical to know the exact position of the Harmonic jaw tips to avoid incidental injury to the RLN.

When the tubercle of Zuckerkandl is dissected off the RLN laterally, Allis clamps are placed on the anterior part of the tubercle of Zuckerkandl and are gently retracted anteriorly and medially. Applying a gentle tension with Debakey forceps, which are holding the fibrous tissue overlying the RLN laterally, mosquito is used to create a tunnel space. Mosquito is placed with its tips up and its curved back lying right on the RLN. Gently sliding up on the RLN and spreading mosquito jaws, the tunneled space is created (Fig. 1.25). Without replacing the Debakey forceps by holding the fibrous tissue, gentle traction is applied up and laterally while inserting the lower jaw of the Harmonic Focus device into the tunneled space. Keeping the RLN in full view all the time, the superficial layer of these fibrous tissues is transected, opening the tunneled space (Fig. 1.26). These steps can be repeated until you can clearly visualize the insertion site of the RLN into the cricothyroid muscle. Under no circumstances should the RLN be manipulated or grabbed with instruments. During every step of the procedure, the surgeon should always be aware of the exact location of the RLN.

Identification, Dissection, and Preservation of the Right Superior Parathyroid Gland

The right superior parathyroid gland is identified anteriorly and laterally under the superior pole of the thyroid lobe,

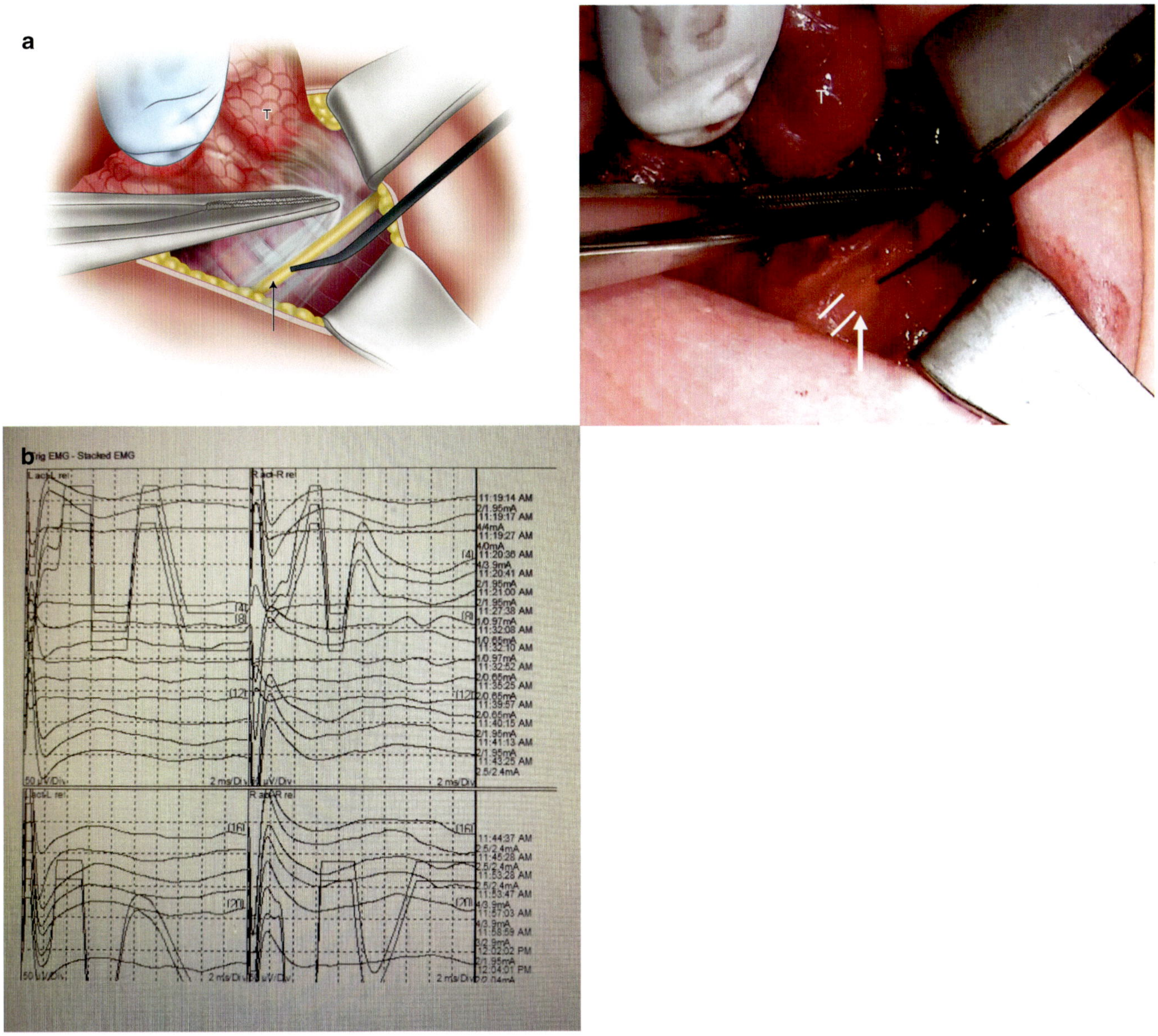

Fig. 1.20 (**a**) The right RLN is visualized along the right side of the trachea. A nerve stimulator is used to confirm the integrity of the RLN. The nerve stimulator and the arrow are pointing at the right RLN; it is also outlined by two white lines. (**b**) EMG monitoring of the right RLN showing a normal waveform response from the endotracheal tube (ET) electrode during RLN stimulation. See the difference in waveform appearance between EBSLN (see Fig. 1.16b) and RLN stimulation. T – thyroid

attached to the tubercle of Zuckerkandl. By using the Debakey forceps, fibrous tissues attaching the right superior parathyroid gland to the tubercle of Zuckerkandl are retracted laterally. A tunneled space is created under these attachments by using mosquito, similar to the prior steps. Without replacing the Debakey forceps by holding this fibrous tissue with gentle traction up and laterally, the lower jaw of the Harmonic Focus device is inserted into the tunneled space and the superficial layer of these fibrous tissues is transected detaching the parathyroid gland from the tubercle of Zuckerkandl (Fig. 1.27). Always keep the RLN in full view. Do not apply significant traction on the parathyroid gland to prevent its detachment and devascularization.

Transection of Berry's Ligament

By using the Debakey forceps, fibrous tissues attaching Berry's ligament to the trachea are retracted laterally. A tunneled space is created under these attachments by using mosquito (Fig. 1.28). Without replacing the Debakey forceps by holding these fibrous tissues, gentle traction is applied up

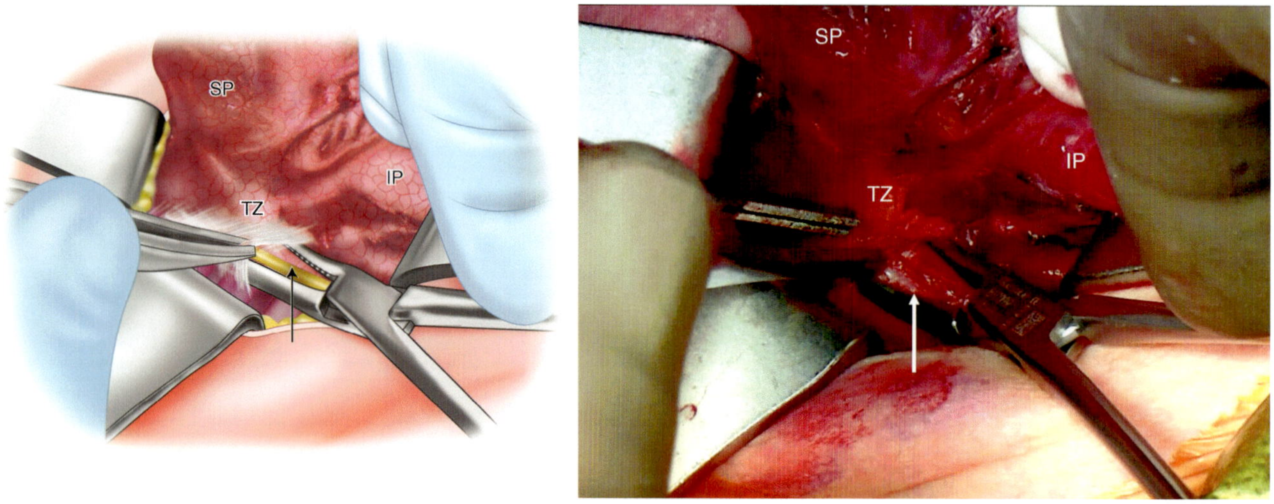

Fig. 1.21 Upon identification of the RLN, it is dissected down with mosquito and then up to its insertion site into the cricothyroid muscle. Arrow pointing at the right RLN. SP – superior pole of the right thyroid lobe, IP – inferior pole of the right thyroid lobe, TZ – tubercle of Zuckerkandl

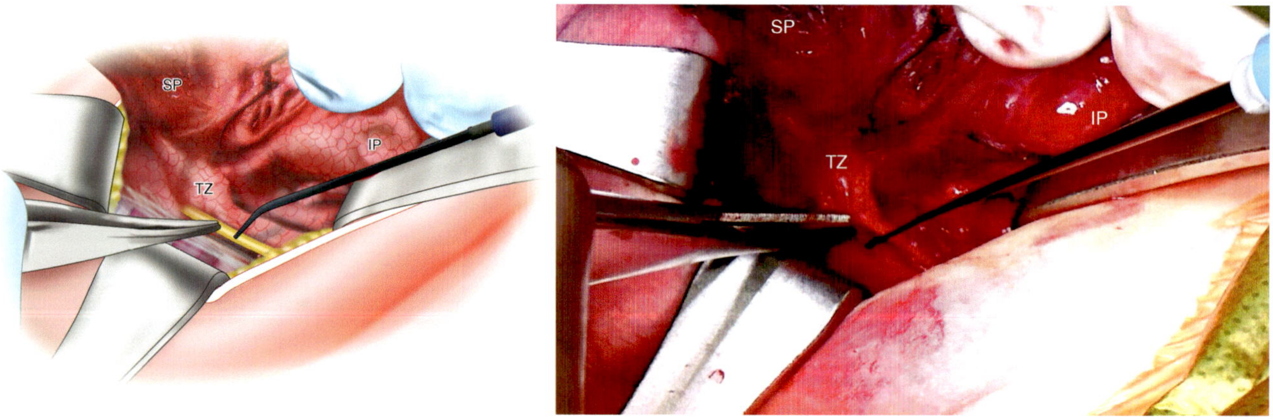

Fig. 1.22 The integrity of the RLN is confirmed with nerve stimulation. SP – superior pole of the right thyroid lobe, IP – inferior pole of the right thyroid lobe, TZ – tubercle of Zuckerkandl

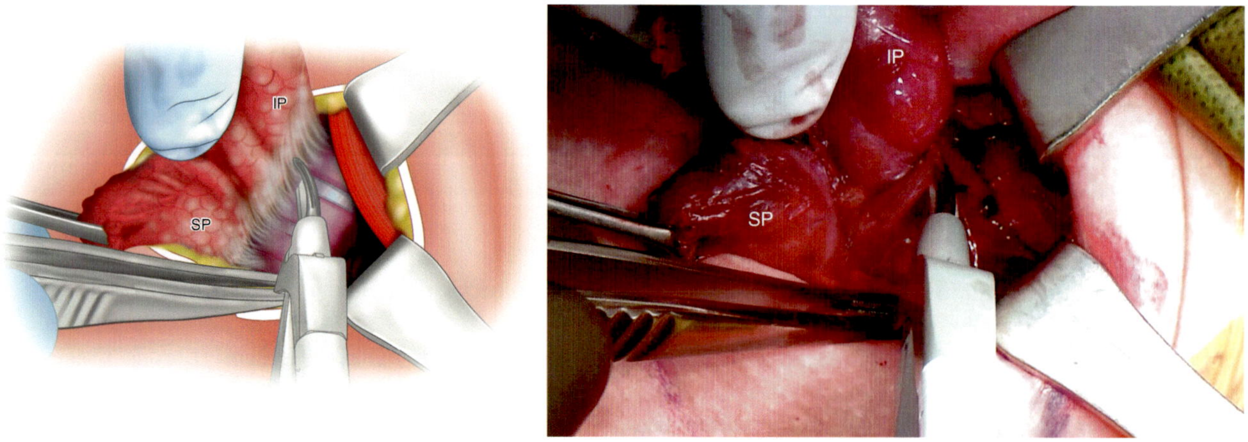

Fig. 1.23 The attachments between the inferior pole of the right thyroid lobe and the trachea are transected using the Harmonic Focus device. SP – superior pole of the right thyroid lobe; IP – inferior pole of the right thyroid lobe

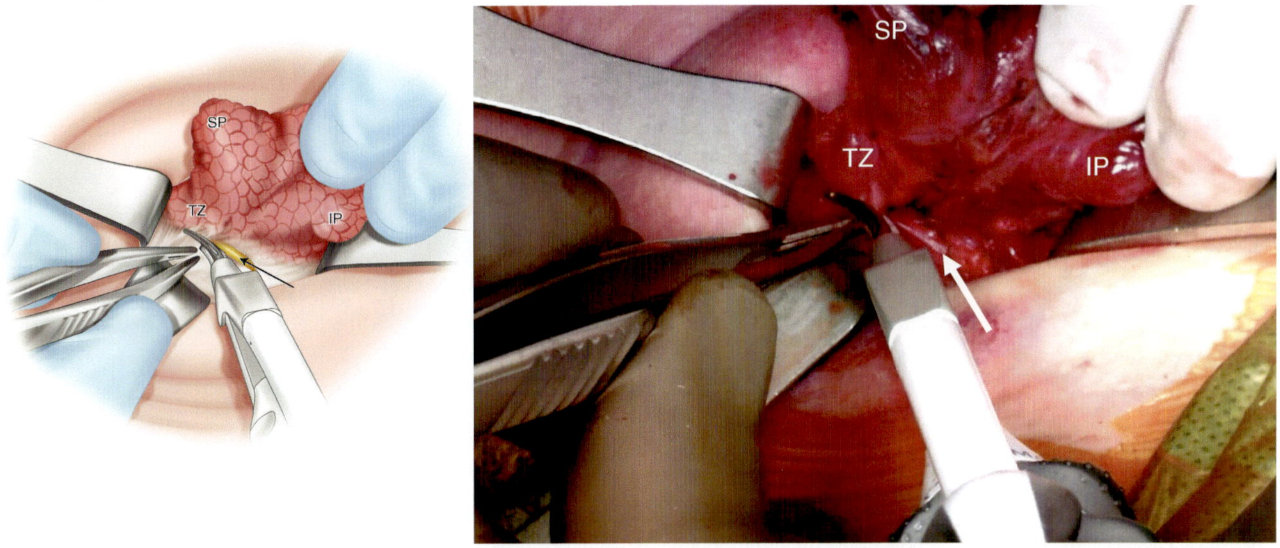

Fig. 1.24 Dissection of the tubercle of Zuckerkandl using the Harmonic Focus device. Arrow pointing at the right RLN. TZ – tubercle of Zuckerkandl, SP – superior pole of the right thyroid lobe, IP – inferior pole of the right thyroid lobe

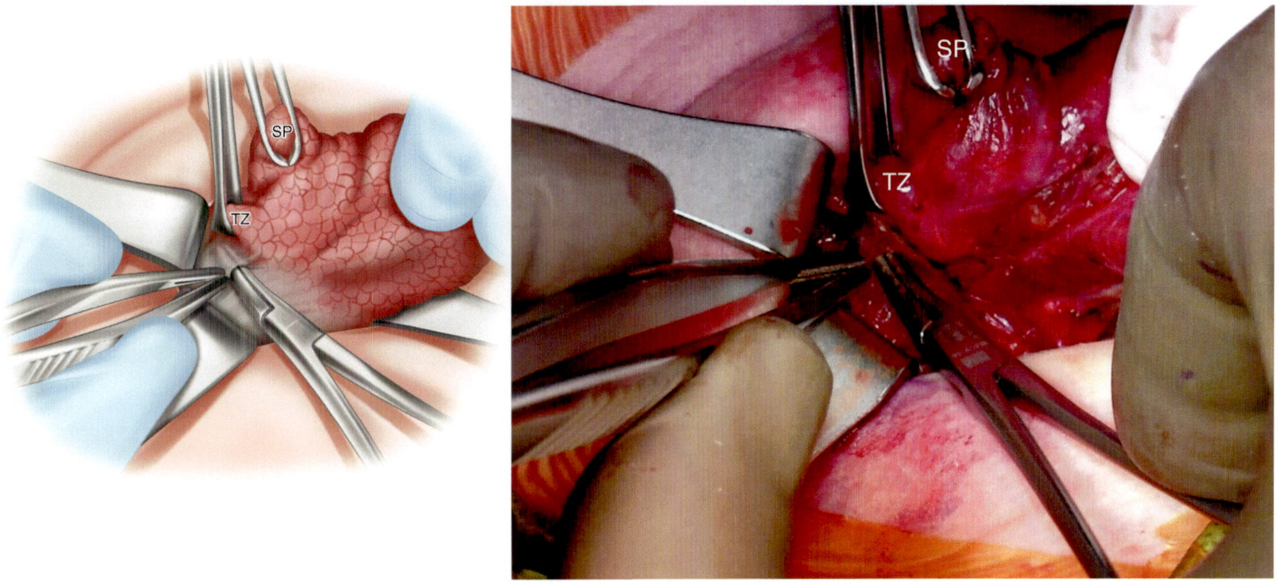

Fig. 1.25 Mosquito forceps are used to create a tunnel space above the RLN. TZ – tubercle of Zuckerkandl; SP – superior pole of the right thyroid lobe

and laterally while inserting the lower jaw of the Harmonic Focus device into the tunneled space. Always keep the RLN in full view. The superficial layer of these fibrous tissues is transected, opening the tunneled space (Fig. 1.29). These steps can be repeated until Berry's ligament is completely detached from the trachea. Berry's ligament can wrap the trachea to the posterolateral surface in between the cartilaginous and membranous part of the trachea or at the lower edge of the cricoid cartilage and the first tracheal rings. This is the most vulnerable part of the trachea as it is where it can be injured.

Dissecting the Thyroid Lobe Off the Trachea with Isthmus and Pyramidal Lobe

By using mosquito, a space in between the thyroid lobe and trachea is created. The lower jaw of the Harmonic Focus device is inserted into that space, and the thyroid lobe attachments to the trachea are divided superiorly (Fig. 1.30) and then inferiorly (Fig. 1.31). While dissecting the isthmus superiorly, the pyramidal lobe, if present, should also be dissected off. In this case, the patient did not have a pyramidal lobe. Then using the Harmonic Focus device, the thyroid isthmus is transected

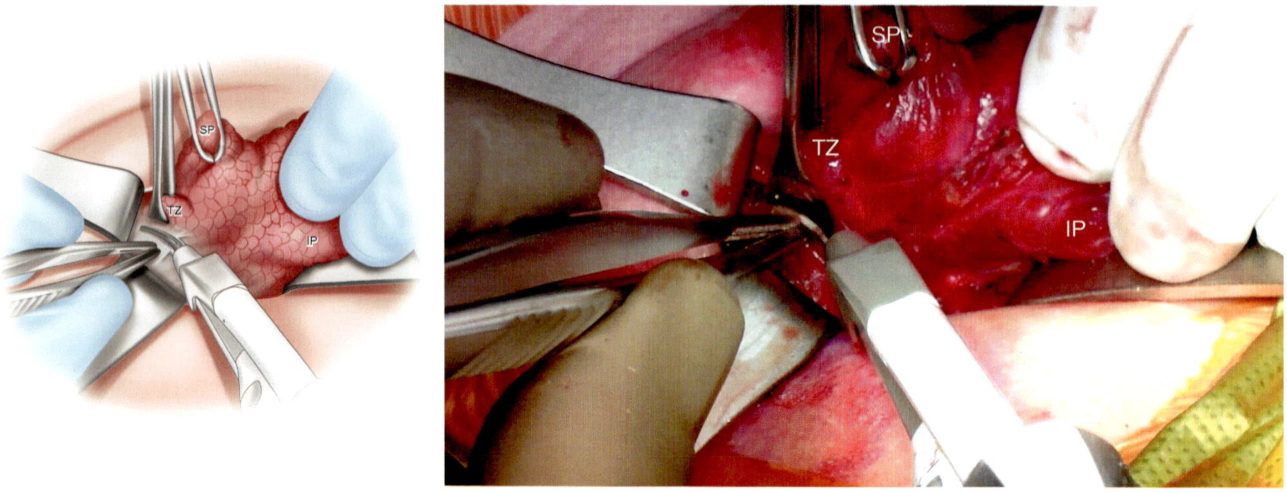

Fig. 1.26 Superficial layer of fibrous tissue overlying the RLN is transected using the Harmonic Focus device opening the tunnel space. TZ – tubercle of Zuckerkandl, SP – superior pole of the right thyroid lobe, IP – inferior pole of the right thyroid lobe

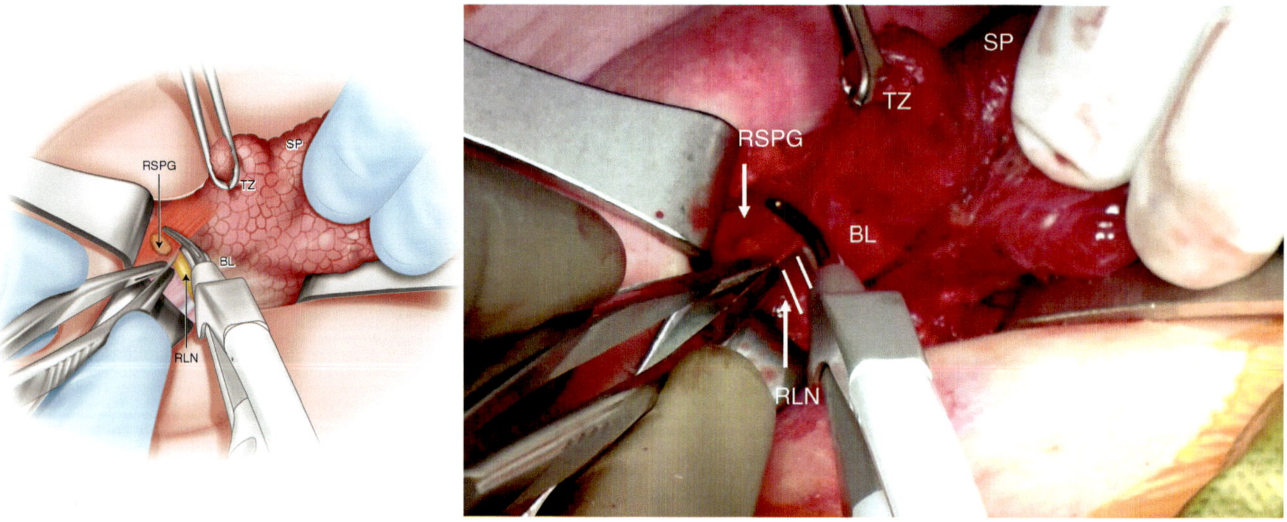

Fig. 1.27 The Harmonic Focus device is used to transect attachments between the tubercle of Zuckerkandl and the right superior parathyroid gland. Arrow pointing down – right superior parathyroid gland (RSPG), arrow pointing up and outlined with two white lines – RLN, SP – superior pole of the right thyroid lobe, TZ – tubercle of Zuckerkandl, BL – Berry's ligament, RSPG – right superior parathyroid gland, RLN – recurrent laryngeal nerve

in between the left thyroid lobe and isthmus, keeping the whole right lobe with the isthmus as a specimen (Fig. 1.32).

Muscle and Skin Closure

After the thyroid lobe is removed, a stitch is placed at the superior pole to orient the specimen during pathological evaluation. The wound is irrigated with sterile saline solution or sterile water. Valsalva maneuver is performed to create a positive intrathoracic pressure, which helps to visualize any bleeding vessels and confirm the absence of any air leak indicating tracheal injury. Small pieces of Fibrillar (absorbable hemostatic agent) are placed in the cavity. We do not use drains. Then the wound is closed by layers with interrupted 3.0 Vicryl to the strap muscles, leaving the lower part of the strap muscles open (Fig. 1.33). Placing interrupted sutures, rather than running, and leaving the lower part of the muscle open help manage potential hematoma or seroma without opening the entire incision. This could be done in the office without going to the operating room. Then the platysma muscle is closed with interrupted 4.0 Vicryl (Fig. 1.34), followed by the skin with a single running 5.0 Monocryl (Fig. 1.35a, b). Dermabond is placed on the wound, and the ends of the Monocryl stitch are cut to the level of the skin without leaving any nodes (Fig. 1.36).

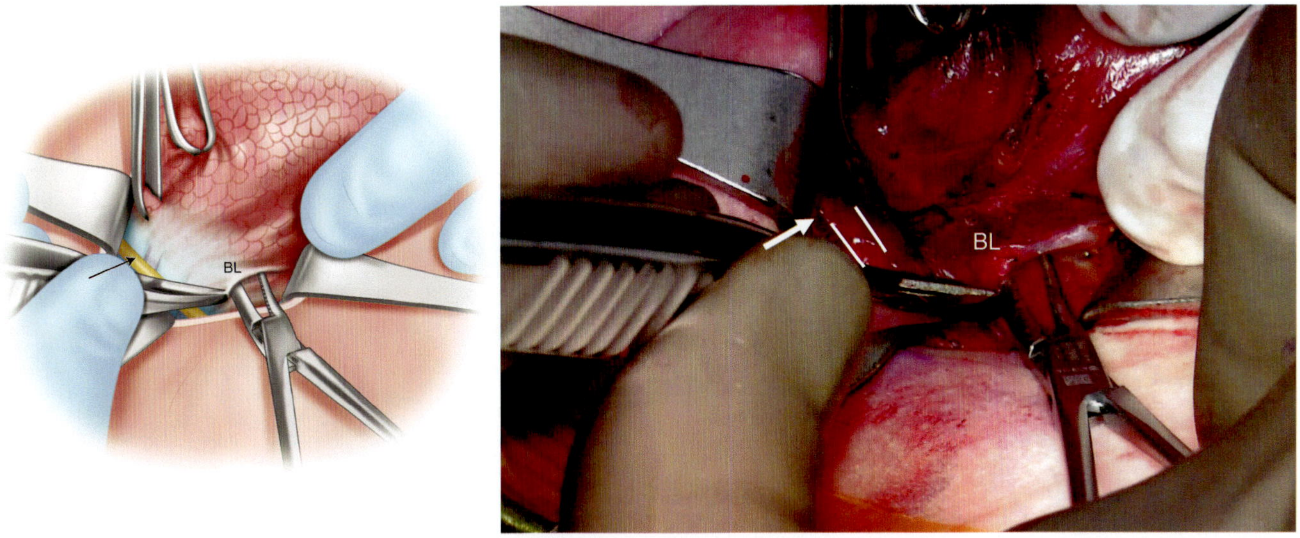

Fig. 1.28 Space is created between Berry's ligament and the trachea by using a mosquito. Arrow is pointing at the RLN, which is also outlined by white lines; BL – Berry's ligament

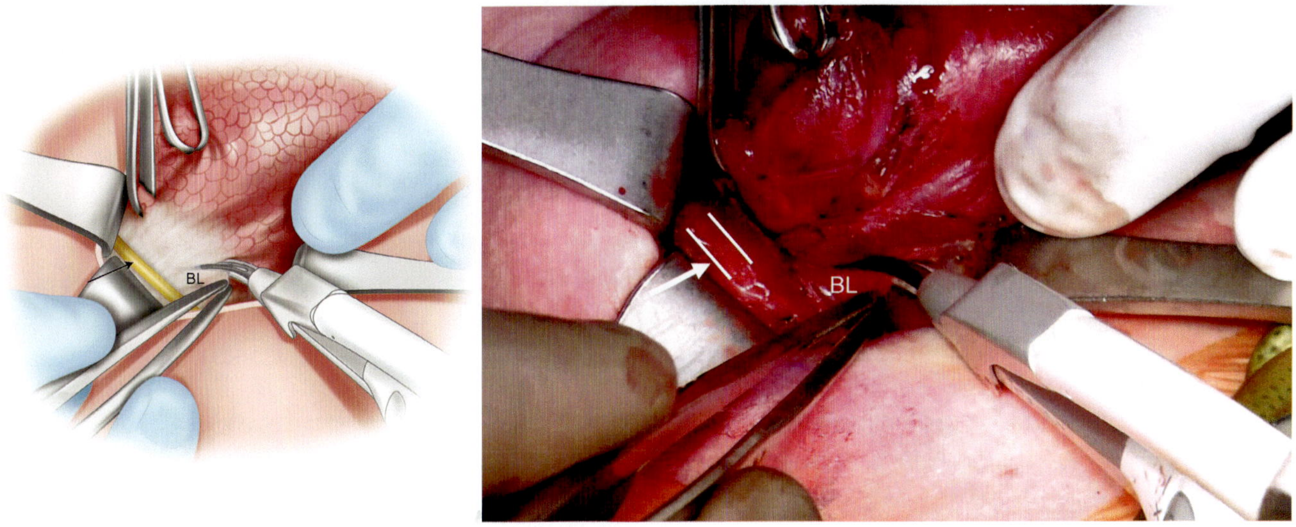

Fig. 1.29 Harmonic Focus device is used to transect attachments of Berry's ligament to the trachea. Arrow is pointing to the RLN, which is also outlined with two white lines; BL – Berry's ligament

After the patient is extubated, a flexible laryngoscopy is performed to confirm the normal function of the vocal cords. An ice pack is placed on the neck over the towel in the recovery room. The patient is observed for approximately 5–6 hours in an outpatient recovery unit and monitored to make sure there are no hematoma developments. Approximately 2 weeks later, the patient follows up in the office for a postoperative wound check and to review pathology results.

Surgical Pearls

1. Always evaluate thyroid imaging studies prior to surgery. In case of a significant enlargement of the thyroid gland/lobe on ultrasound imaging, CT scan without contrast should be ordered to evaluate the patient for substernal mediastinal or intrathoracic extension of the thyroid gland/lobe. If present, appropriate preoperative surgical arrangements should be made to include the possibility of sternotomy (thoracic surgical instrument tray with a saw and/or thoracic surgeon consult)
2. Preoperative evaluation of the vocal cord function is pertinent, especially in a preoperative diagnosis of thyroid cancer or suspicion for thyroid cancer as well as suspicion for involvement of the RLN (voice hoarseness). Preoperative evaluation of vocal cords is also important in patients with a prior history of neck surgery (thyroid, parathyroid, or C-spine surgery).

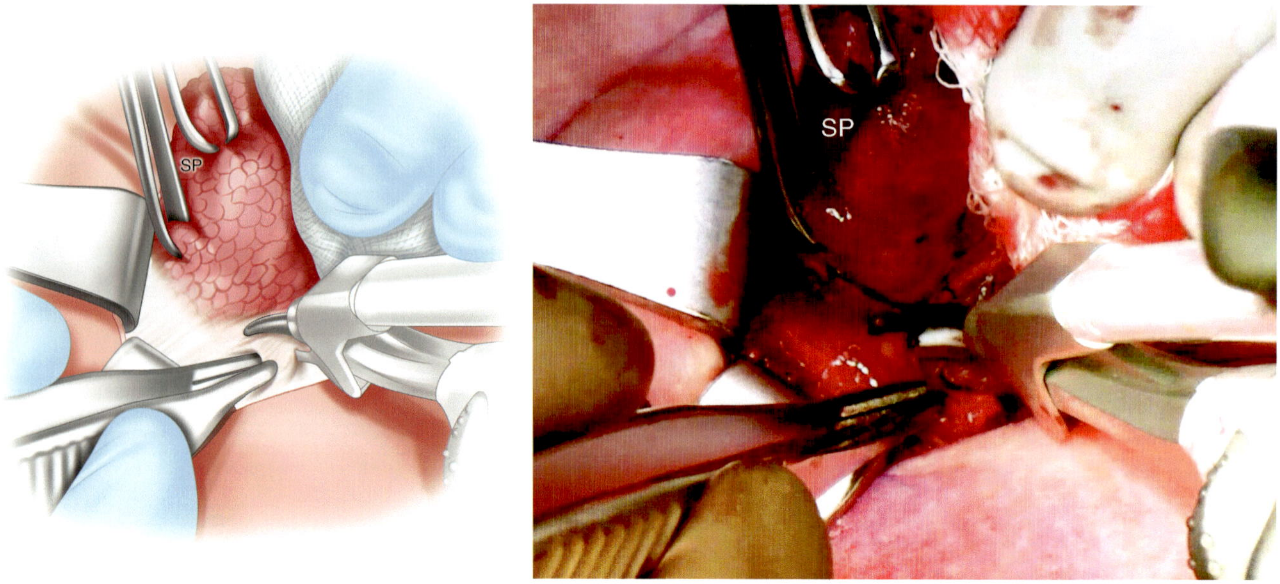

Fig. 1.30 By using mosquito, a space is created in between the thyroid lobe and trachea superiorly; then using the Harmonic Focus device, superior attachments between the thyroid and trachea are transected. SP – superior pole of the right thyroid lobe

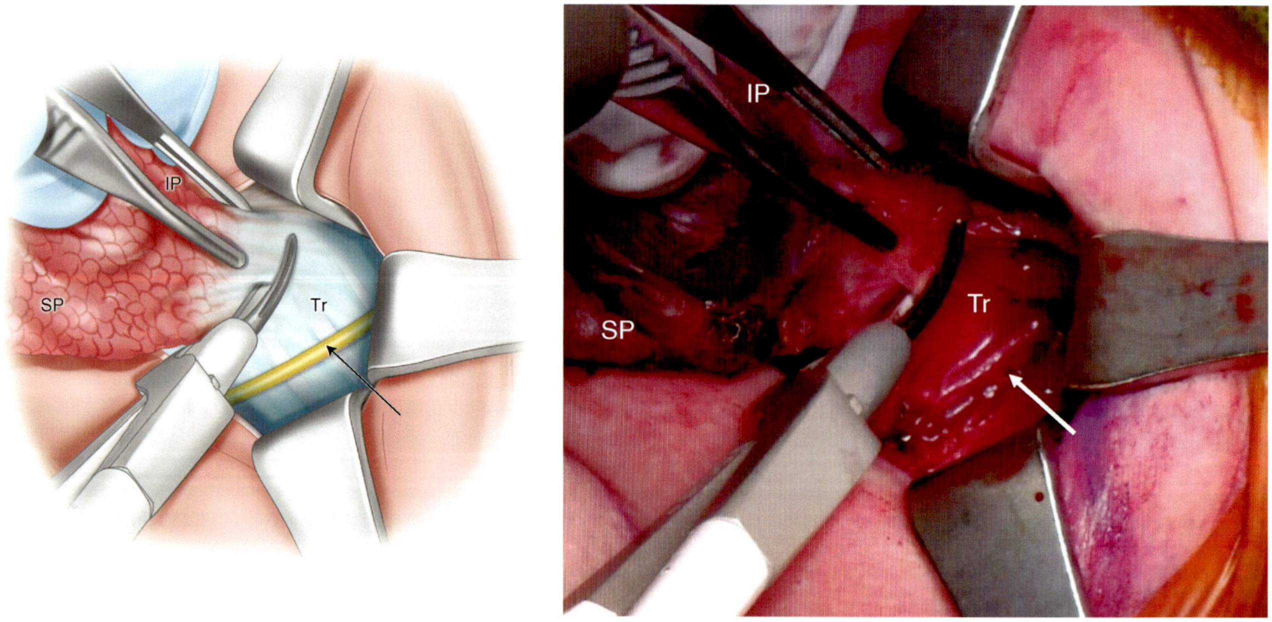

Fig. 1.31 By using mosquito, a space is created in between the thyroid lobe and trachea inferiorly; then using the Harmonic Focus device, inferior attachments between the thyroid and trachea are transected. Arrow is pointing at the RLN. SP – superior pole of the right thyroid lobe, IP – inferior pole of the right thyroid lobe, Tr – trachea

3. Preoperative antibiotics are not usually needed. But they should be considered in the following circumstances: patients with implantable metal devices; immunosuppressed patients; concerns for systemic infection, large intrathoracic goiter, or intra-mediastinal thyroid gland; and patients who require sternotomy or a prolonged (over 4 hours) procedure, such as total thyroidectomy with modified radical neck dissection.
4. Make sure to keep the surgical field bloodless. Any blood-staining impairs the ability to identify the RLN and parathyroid glands. By using gentle pressure with dry gauze, all small areas of blood oozing can be controlled. In case

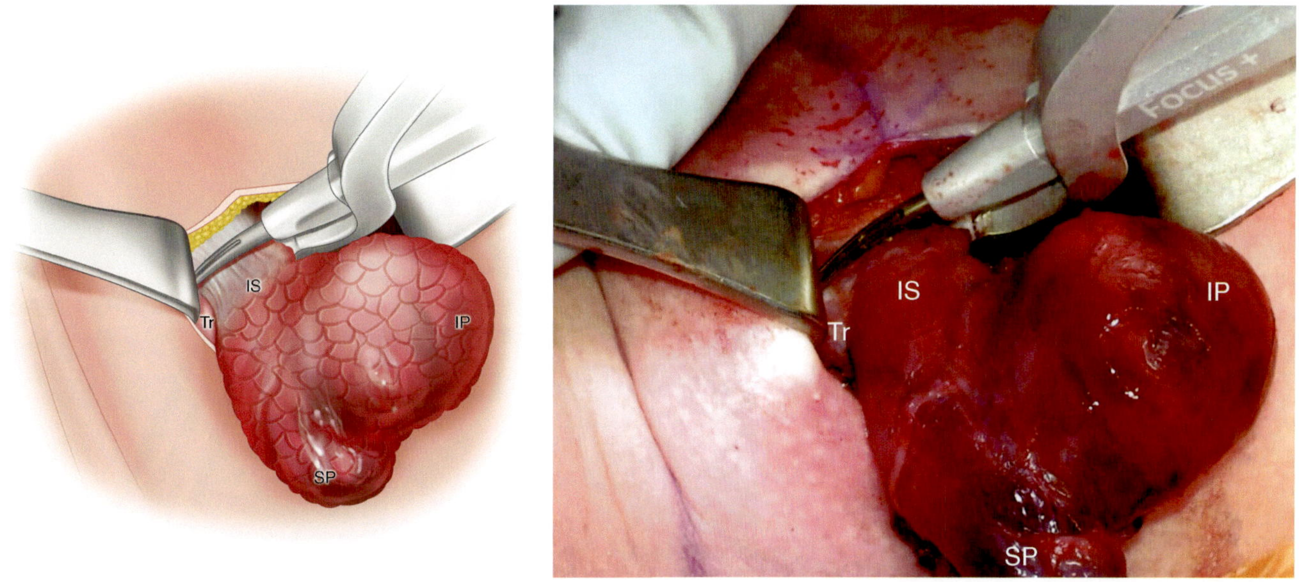

Fig. 1.32 By using the Harmonic Focus device, thyroid isthmus is transected in between the left thyroid lobe and isthmus, keeping the whole right thyroid lobe with the isthmus as a specimen. IS – isthmus, SP – superior pole of the right thyroid lobe, IP – inferior pole of the right thyroid lobe with nodule, Tr – trachea

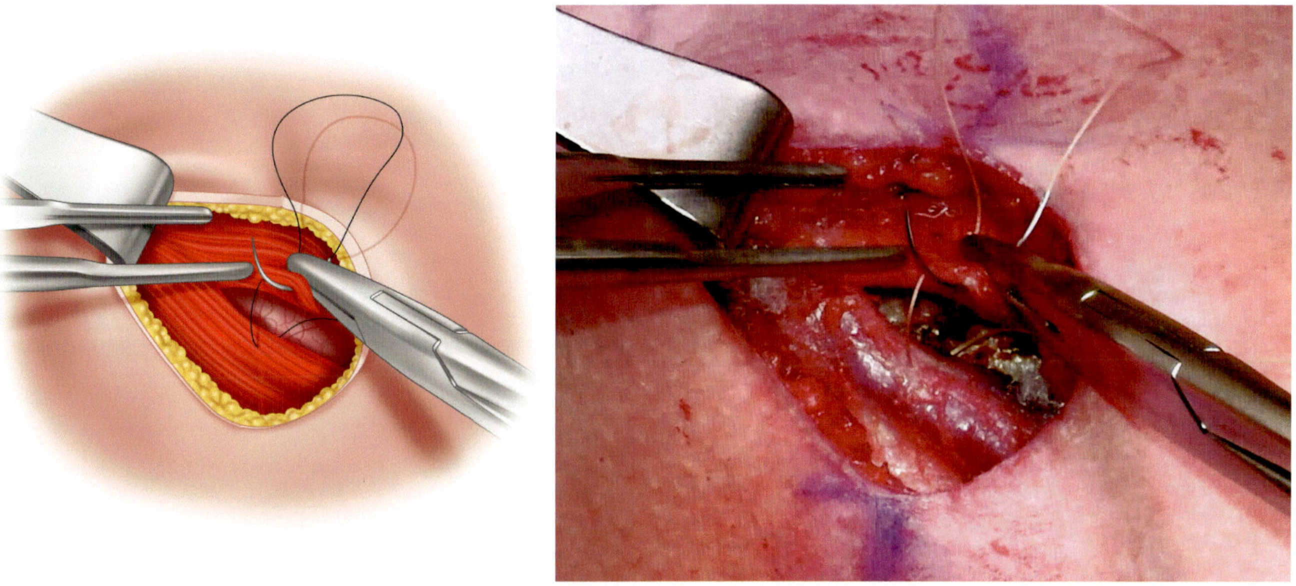

Fig. 1.33 After the wound is irrigated and Valsalva maneuver is performed, Fibrillar is placed into the wound and then the strap muscles are approximated with interrupted 3.0 Vicryl, leaving the lower part of the wound open

of more significant bleeding, the following maneuvers can be performed. Hold the pressure with a dry gauze over the bleeding area. Slowly start unrolling the gauze off the bleeding area. When the bleeding vessel is clearly visualized, grab it with Debakey forceps, release the gauze, and clip the vessel with a 5-mm clip. Alternatively, vessel-sealing devices, such as the Harmonic Focus device or LigaSure device, can be used to coagulate the vessel. The bleeding vessel also can be grabbed with mosquito and ligated with a tie. Avoid using Bovie cautery in the proximity to the RLN or parathyroid gland to prevent burning injury.

5. The RLN should always be identified and dissected along its entire course up to its insertion site into the cricothyroid muscle. It should be evaluated for possible branch-

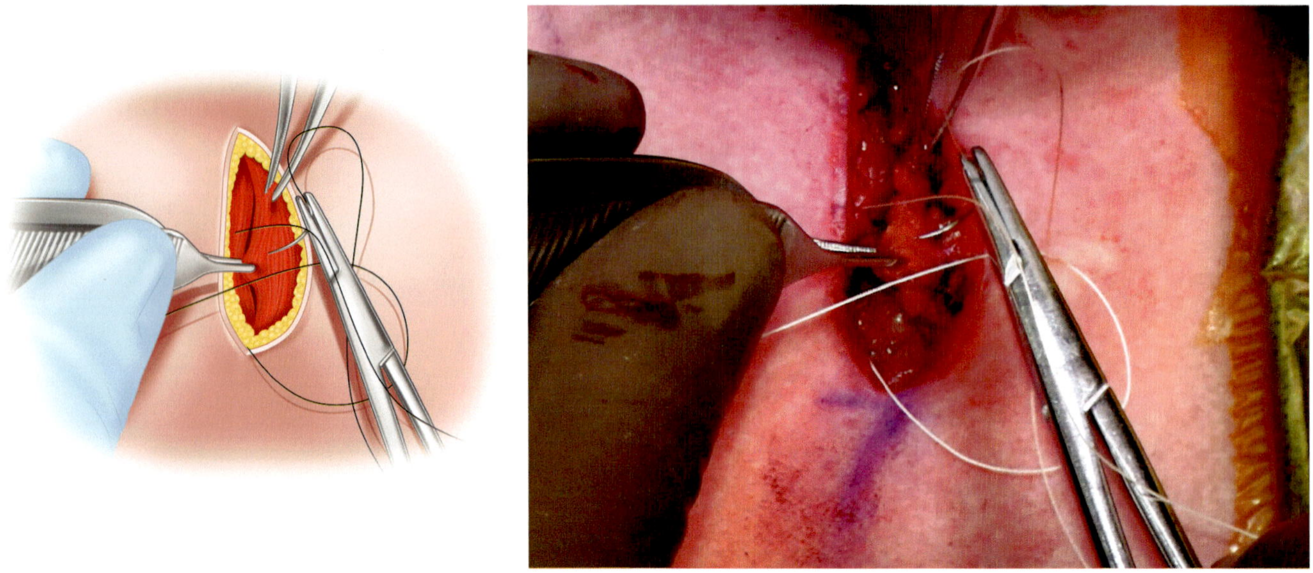

Fig. 1.34 The platysma is closed with interrupted 4.0 Vicryl

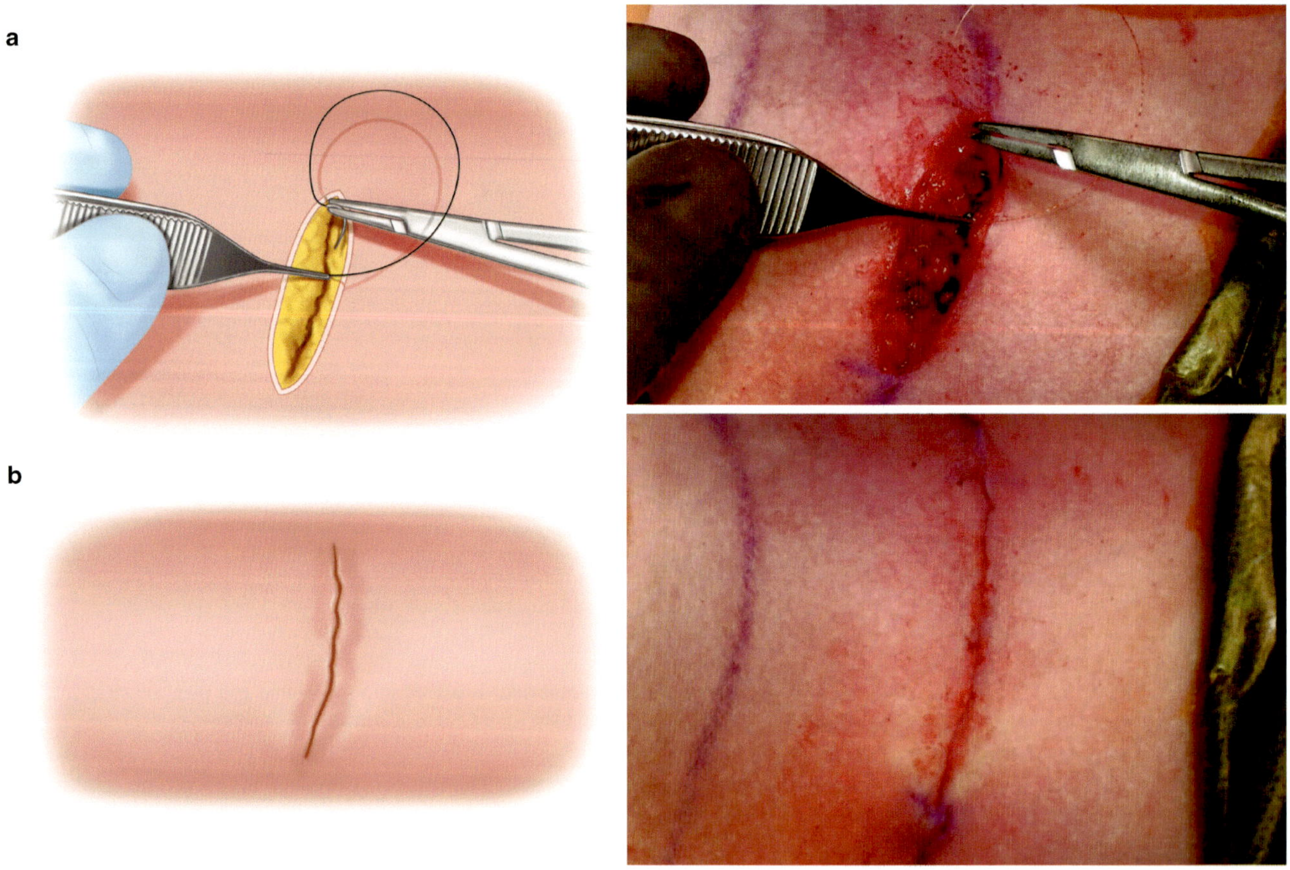

Fig. 1.35 (**a**, **b**) Skin is closed with a single running 5.0 Monocryl (**a**), leaving the ends of the stitch on both sides of the incision without nodes (**b**)

ing. The most anterior and medial branch is a motor branch.

6. Avoid significant traction on the thyroid lobe during the dissection. Significant traction on the thyroid may also result in traction on the RLN with neural stretch and temporary paralysis.
7. Do not apply significant tension on the parathyroid gland to prevent its detachment and devascularization.

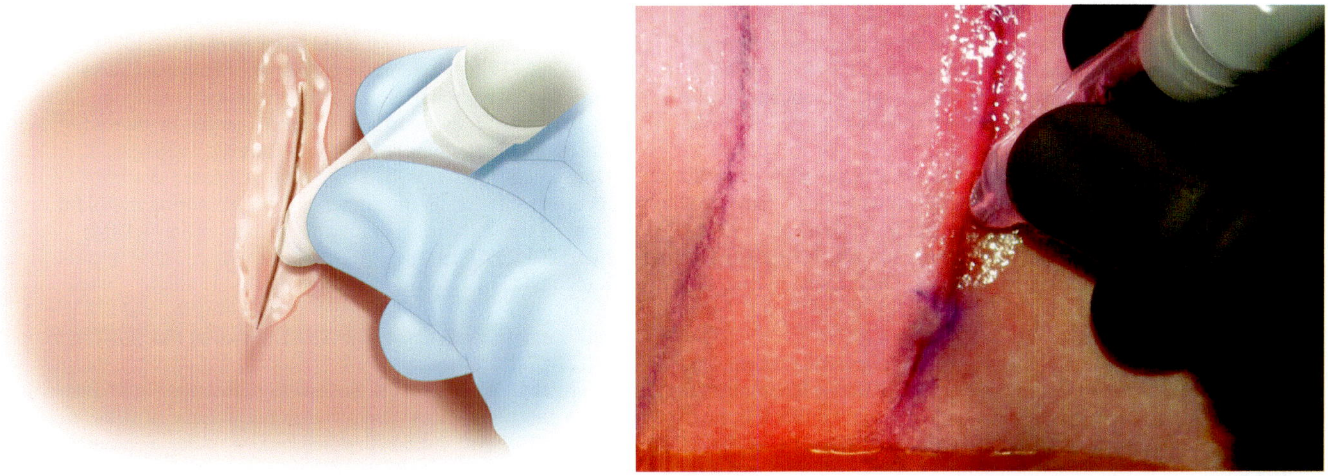

Fig. 1.36 Dermabond is placed on the wound, and the ends of the Monocryl stitch are cut at the level of the skin without leaving any nodes

8. Perform the Valsalva maneuver prior to closing the wound. It helps to identify any bleeding vessels and air leaks in the event of tracheal injury.

Management of Complications

Hematoma

The development of acute postoperative hematoma during the immediate postoperative period requires an urgent exploration in the operating room. If severe stridor develops, an incision should be opened at the bedside and the hematoma should be drained, followed by immediate reexploration in the operating room to control the bleeding.

Delayed postoperative hematoma or seroma (several days after the surgery) can be managed in an outpatient setting. This could be done by ultrasound-guided drainage by using a sterile technique with 20G or 18G needle on a 20-cc syringe. The other option would be opening the corner of the incision, draining the hematoma, and then packing the opening with iodoform gauze loosely into the wound.

Postoperative Hypocalcemia

It is almost impossible to develop acute hypocalcemia after a thyroid lobectomy, considering that the opposite side has normal parathyroid glands, unless the patient had a prior surgery on the opposite side. Nevertheless, younger patients may develop transient hypocalcemia, which could be easily controlled by the administration of oral calcium carbonate with vitamin D (Oscal) 1000 mg every 6–8 hours for 1–2 weeks.

RLN Injury

Injury to the RLN could be a devastating complication of a thyroid lobectomy. Damaging consequences of the RLN injury are especially noticeable in older patients, who, in addition to severe voice hoarseness, may also develop dysphagia with aspiration, especially liquids.

Transient Injury to the RLN RLN injury can be due to the traction of the thyroid, which results in neural stretch and temporary paralysis. This usually resolves within days to weeks after surgery.

Complete Transection of the RLN This specific technique is addressed in another publication [18]. Briefly, if the RLN injury is recognized intraoperatively, there are several options for immediate repair that can be accomplished. If both ends of the RLN are visible and can be approximated, it should be repaired by a direct approximation of the RLN ends. If there is a segment of the RLN loss, flipping the end of the *ansa cervicalis* to the proximal end of the RLN, or vagus-RLN anastomosis, may be done or free nerve grafting can be used.

References

1. Randolph GW. Surgery of the thyroid and parathyroid glands. 2nd ed. Philadelphia, PA, USA: Elsevier; 2012.
2. Terris DJ, Duke W, editors. Thyroid and parathyroid diseases: medical and surgical management. 2nd ed. New York, NY, USA: Thieme; 2016.

3. Inabnet WB, Shifrin AL, Ahmed L, Sinha P. Safety of same day discharge in patients undergoing sutureless thyroidectomy: a comparison of local and general anesthesia. Thyroid. 2008;18(1):57–61.
4. Terris DJ, Snyder S, Carneiro-Pla D, et al. American thyroid association statement on outpatient thyroidectomy. Thyroid. 2013;23:1193–202.
5. Snyder SK, Hamid KS, Roberson CR, et al. Outpatient thyroidectomy is safe and reasonable: experience with more than 1,000 planned outpatient procedures. J Am Coll Surg. 2010;210:575–82, 582–4.
6. Terris DJ, Moister B, Seybt MW, et al. Outpatient thyroid surgery is safe and desirable. Otolaryngol Head Neck Surg. 2007;136:556–9.
7. Randolph GW, Dralle H, International Intraoperative Monitoring Study Group, Abdullah H, Barczynski M, Bellantone R, Brauckhoff M, Carnaille B, Cherenko S, Chiang FY, Dionigi G, Finck C, Hartl D, Kamani D, Lorenz K, Miccolli P, Mihai R, Miyauchi A, Orloff L, Perrier N, Poveda MD, Romanchishen A, Serpell J, Sitges-Serra A, Sloan T, Van Slycke S, Snyder S, Takami H, Volpi E, Woodson G. Electrophysiologic recurrent laryngeal nerve monitoring during thyroid and parathyroid surgery: international standards guideline statement. Laryngoscope. 2011;121 Suppl 1:S1–16.
8. Barczyński M, Randolph GW, Cernea CR, Dralle H, Dionigi G, Alesina PF, Mihai R, Finck C, Lombardi D, Hartl DM, Miyauchi A, Serpell J, Snyder S, Volpi E, Woodson G, Kraimps JL, Hisham AN, International Neural Monitoring Study Group. External branch of the superior laryngeal nerve monitoring during thyroid and parathyroid surgery: International Neural Monitoring Study Group standards guideline statement. Laryngoscope. 2013;123 Suppl 4:S1–14.
9. Phelan E, Potenza A, Slough C, Zurakowski D, Kamani D, Randolph G. Recurrent laryngeal nerve monitoring during thyroid surgery: normative vagal and recurrent laryngeal nerve electrophysiological data. Otolaryngol Head Neck Surg. 2012;147(4):640–6.
10. Randolph GW. The recurrent and superior laryngeal nerves. 1st ed. Springer. Switzerland: Springer International Publishing; 2016.
11. Rustad WH. The recurrent laryngeal nerves in thyroid surgery. Hardcover. Springfield, MO, USA: Thomas; 1956.
12. Donatini G, Carnaille B, Dionigi G. Increased detection of non-recurrent inferior laryngeal nerve (NRLN) during thyroid surgery using systematic intraoperative nerve monitoring (IONM). World J Surg. 2013;37(1):91–3.
13. Randolph GW, Kamani D. Intraoperative electrophysiologic monitoring of the recurrent laryngeal nerve during thyroid and parathyroid surgery: experience with 1,381 nerves at risk. Laryngoscope. 2017;127(1):280–6.
14. Wojtczak B, Kaliszewski K, Sutkowski K, Bolanowski M, Barczyński M. A functional assessment of anatomical variants of the recurrent laryngeal nerve during thyroidectomies using neuromonitoring. Endocrine. 2018;59(1):82–9.
15. Wojtczak B, Sutkowski K, Kaliszewski K, Forkasiewicz Z, Knychalski B, Aporowicz M, Bolanowski M, Barczyński M. Voice quality preservation in thyroid surgery with neuromonitoring. Endocrine. 2018;61(2):232–9.
16. Serpell JW, Yeung MJ, Grodski S. The motor fibers of the recurrent laryngeal nerve are located in the anterior extralaryngeal branch. Ann Surg. 2009;249(4):648–52.
17. Randolph GW, Kobler JB, Wilkins J. Recurrent laryngeal nerve identification and assessment during thyroid surgery: laryngeal palpation. World J Surg. 2004;28(8):755–60.
18. Ito Y, Miyauchi A. Recurrent laryngeal nerve paralysis – management of recurrent laryngeal nerve injuries. In: Shifrin A, editor. Endocrine emergencies. 1st ed. Philadelphia, PA, USA: Elsevier; 2021. ISBN 0323760988 (ISBN13: 9780323760980).

Open Right Thyroid Lobectomy

2

Jina Kim, Sanziana A. Roman, and Julie Ann Sosa

Introduction

Surgery of the thyroid gland spans back to medieval times, with the first known operation dating back to 952 AD, when Abu al-Qasim (a renowned surgeon of the Middle Ages) performed the first goiter resection. In the mid-nineteenth century, thyroid surgery was considered so perilous that it was banned by the French Academy of Medicine. Over the next century, many prominent surgeons advanced techniques in thyroidectomy. For example, William Stewart Halsted was a strong advocate of distal vessel ligation to preserve blood supply to the parathyroid glands, and Frank Lahey described the identification and preservation of the recurrent laryngeal nerve [1]. More recently, technological advances such as bipolar energy devices and intraoperative nerve monitoring have become important adjuncts to thyroid surgery. In modern times, thyroid surgery is considered one of the most efficient and safest operations when performed by high-volume surgeons.

Thyroid lobectomy is considered to be an appropriate surgical management option for cases of toxic adenoma, indeterminate thyroid nodules, papillary thyroid microcarcinomas, and low-risk differentiated thyroid cancers. Compared to total thyroidectomy, thyroid lobectomy eliminates the risk of postoperative hypocalcemia as the contralateral parathyroid glands are spared from exposure to surgical risk. Thyroid lobectomy also avoids the risk of bilateral recurrent laryngeal nerve injury and is associated with lower overall morbidity. Thyroid lobectomy can be performed as an outpatient procedure for the majority of patients.

Procedure

A 35-year-old euthyroid woman presents to the surgery clinic with a right thyroid nodule, which she first noticed on self-examination. Ultrasound confirms a 2.2-cm right intrathyroidal nodule without associated cervical lymphadenopathy. Fine needle aspiration demonstrates Bethesda III cytology. Subsequent molecular testing indicates a 50% risk of malignancy. Preoperatively, a thorough discussion of the risks and benefits of thyroid lobectomy is shared with the patient. Risks of thyroid lobectomy include hoarseness, change in voice, pain, bleeding, infection, scar, need for reoperation, need for thyroid hormone replacement, and risks related to anesthesia. The patient elects to undergo diagnostic right thyroid lobectomy and signs a surgical consent.

In the preoperative holding area, the patient's neck is marked to indicate the appropriate laterality. She is transferred to the operating room, where general anesthesia is induced and a neural integrity monitor (NIM) electromyogram endotracheal tube is placed. In the majority of cases, we recommend a 7.0-mm endotracheal tube for women and 8.0-mm for men. A slightly larger NIM tube than a regular endotracheal tube is generally preferred to improve the approximation of the vocal cords to the electromyographic pads. An orogastric tube should be placed in the esophagus to allow the easy palpation of the esophagus during the process, thereby more easily delineating the tracheoesophageal groove and thus the likely path of the recurrent laryngeal nerve. This will make the surgery faster and easier. Antibiotics are not indicated for thyroid surgery, but preoperative steroids should be administered. A single preoperative dose of dexamethasone 8 mg has been shown to reduce nausea and pain postoperatively [2]. A time-out to confirm patient name, procedure, and laterality is performed.

Supplementary Information The online version contains supplementary material available at [https://doi.org/10.1007/978-3-030-93673-0_2].

J. Kim (✉)
Department of Surgery, Inova Health System, Fairfax, VA, USA

S. A. Roman
Department of Surgery, Division of Surgical Oncology, University of California, San Francisco, San Francisco, CA, USA

J. A. Sosa
Department of Surgery, University of California San Francisco (UCSF), San Francisco, CA, USA

A. Shifrin (ed.), *Atlas of Thyroid Surgery*, https://doi.org/10.1007/978-3-030-93673-0_2

For optimal positioning, the patient is placed supine on the operating table with both arms tucked and a shoulder roll placed transversely beneath the shoulder to extend the neck. Hyperextension should be avoided. A 1-l pressure infusion bag can be used as an adjustable, inflatable shoulder roll. A gel donut headrest is placed under the occiput to stabilize the head during surgery. The patient is placed in semi-Fowler's position to help extend the neck further and bring the head above the heart level, thus reducing the venous pressure in the head and neck. For intraoperative nerve monitoring, leads are placed in the subcutaneous tissues of the arm or chest.

Once the patient's neck is prepped with sterile cleaning solutions, it is draped in such a fashion that visual symmetry of the neck is maintained. A transverse curvilinear incision is made ideally in a natural skin crease, preferably just below the cricoid cartilage, which approximates the level of the ligament of Berry. At the ligament of Berry, the thyroid is densely attached to the trachea, and the recurrent laryngeal nerve enters the larynx. To accurately center the incision, the midline can be marked with a silk suture extending from the chin to the sternal notch. The length of the incision will depend on the size of the thyroid gland to be removed. Typically, a 4–6-cm incision suffices for most thyroid surgeries (Fig. 2.1). Starting with a smaller incision, but extending it if needed, is a good approach to minimize its length, but the surgeon should be mindful about safety and adequate visualization.

Once the incision is marked, it is incised sharply with a #15 blade and deepened through the subcutaneous tissues with electrocautery. Subplatysmal flaps are then raised, superiorly and inferiorly (Fig. 2.2). Double-armed skin hooks are used to elevate the subplatysmal flaps. The anterior jugular veins that overlie the sternohyoid muscles should be preserved if possible to avoid bleeding. The fascia of the sternohyoid muscles should remain with the muscle to preserve natural tissue planes during flap creation. The median raphe is incised with cautery to separate the sternohyoid muscles and expose the thyroid gland beneath (Fig. 2.3).

We then turn our focus to the right lobe. The sternohyoid and sternothyroid muscles are dissected away from the anterior aspect of the right thyroid lobe with electrocautery, and they are retracted laterally. The fascia of the sternohyoid

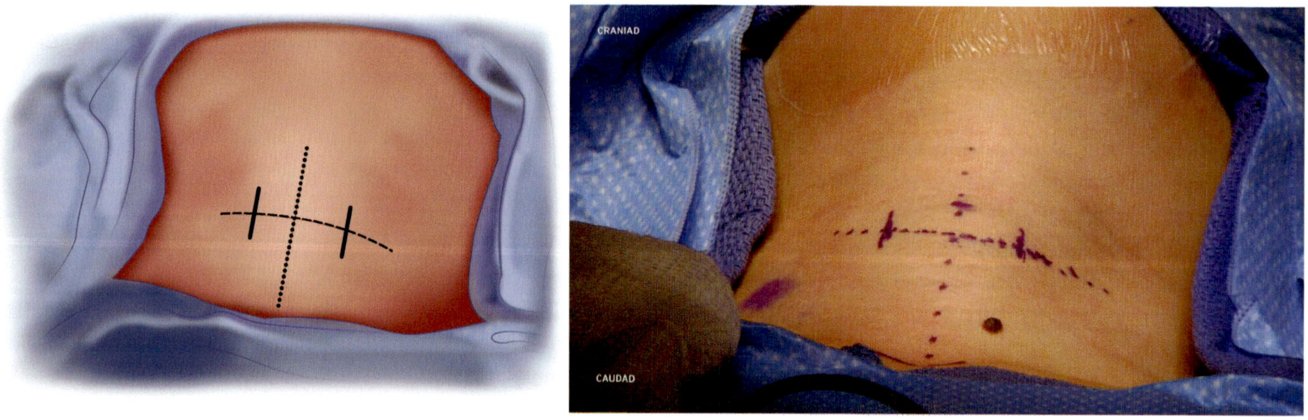

Fig. 2.1 Incision is marked on the neck, approximately two fingerbreadths above the sternal notch, ideally in a natural skin crease

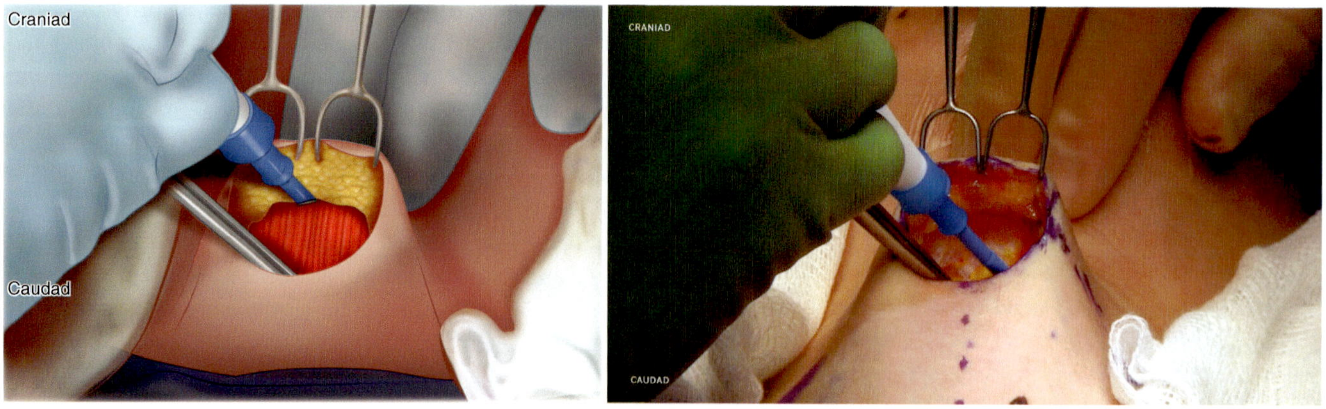

Fig. 2.2 Once the incision is deepened through skin and subcutaneous tissues, subplatysmal flaps are raised

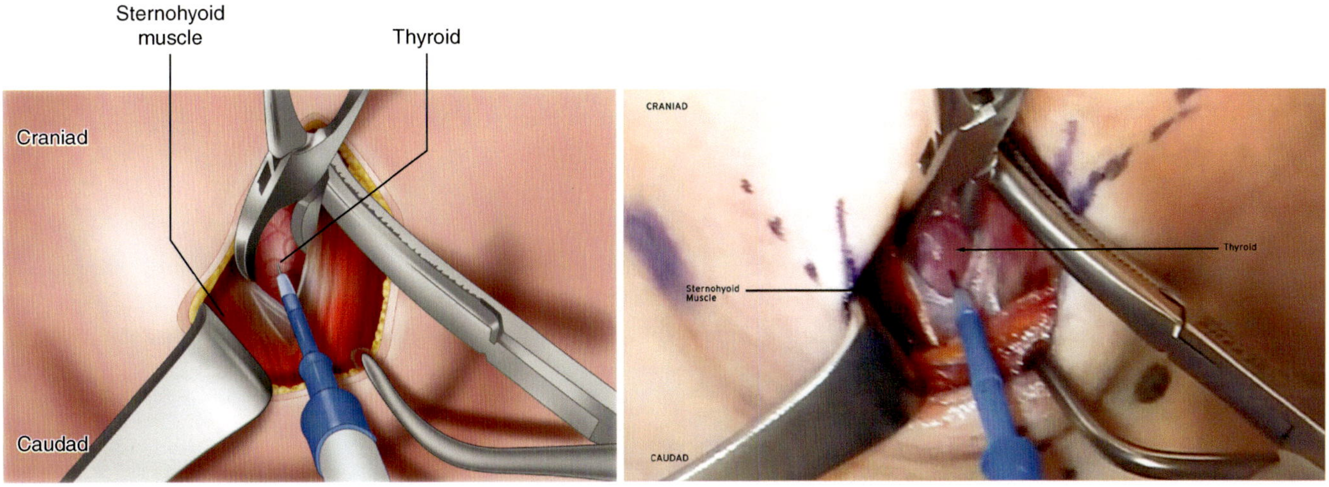

Fig. 2.3 The median raphe is incised to separate the sternohyoid muscles and expose the thyroid underneath

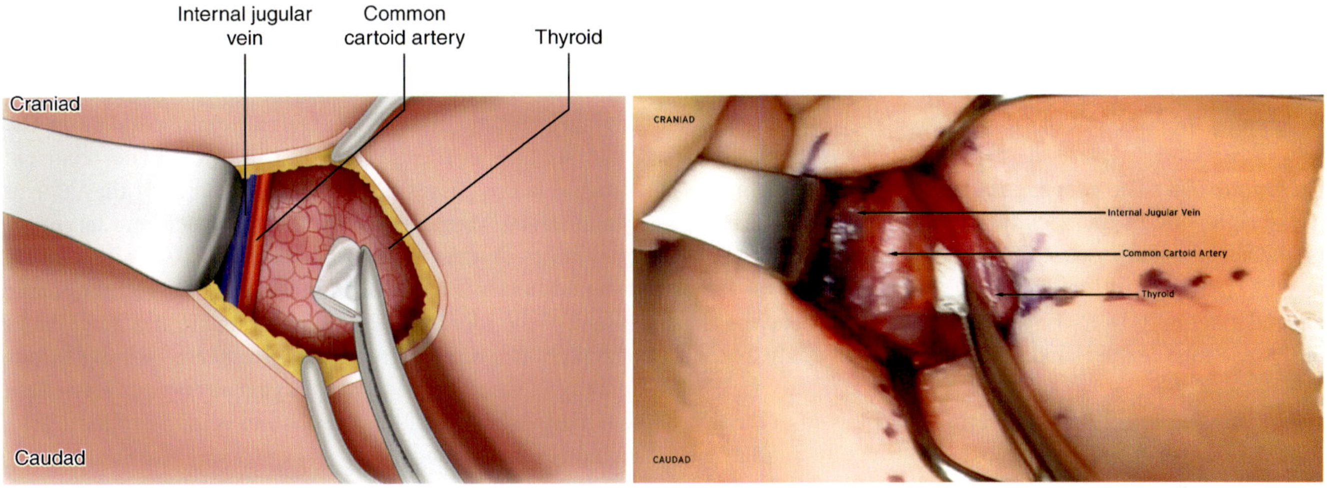

Fig. 2.4 Areolar tissue between the thyroid and common carotid artery is bluntly cleared, exposing the common carotid artery

muscles should remain with the muscle to preserve natural tissue planes during flap creation. The sternothyroid muscle can be divided at the level of the cricoid cartilage for additional exposure of the upper pole. The areolar tissue between the thyroid gland and the common carotid artery can then be cleared using blunt dissection and cautery (Fig. 2.4). The internal jugular vein is visualized adjacent to the common carotid artery; the vagus nerve lies between the internal jugular vein and the common carotid artery. The vagus nerve can be identified with the nerve monitor.

Technique Tip Care should be taken with the nerve monitor probe to avoid puncture or trauma to the carotid sheath; the authors routinely bend the tip of the probe to make it blunt. Touching the vagus in the carotid sheath low in the neck and obtaining a good NIM signal can indicate normal recurrent laryngeal nerve anatomy. If the signal cannot be obtained low in the carotid sheath, but rather is found high at the level of the upper pole, there is potential for a nonrecurrent laryngeal nerve. When seen, nonrecurrent laryngeal nerves are more commonly identified on the right. This maneuver can help plan the dissection of the nerve and alert the surgeon to potential variable anatomy.

The middle thyroid vein, which is the primary venous drainage of the thyroid gland, is seen in 70% of patients. The middle thyroid vein runs anterior to the carotid artery; it can be easily identified and ligated with 2-0 silk without concern [3]. The thyroid lobe then is mobilized anteromedially by

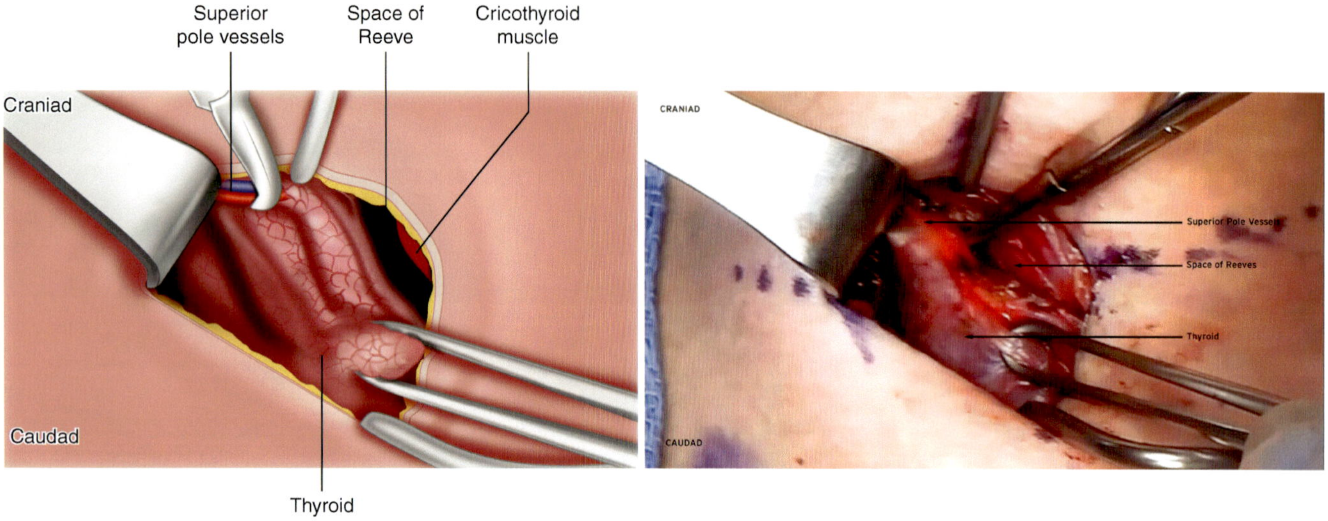

Fig. 2.5 The superior pole vessels are individually dissected and ligated with 2-0 silk ties

applying traction. A peanut sponge can be useful for applying traction and improving visualization in a small incision by keeping the hand out of the way.

Technique Tip The esophagus should be gently mobilized to the right side of the neck to allow better exposure of the tracheoesophageal groove. This can be done by gently pushing the right thyroid lobe medially and the thyroid cartilage pushed externally from the left side of the neck. Having the orogastric tube in the esophagus makes it easily palpable.

We turn our attention to the right superior pole of the thyroid. The superior pole is exposed with gentle caudal and lateral traction. Working medially to laterally, the avascular space of Reeves between the superior pole of the thyroid gland and cricothyroid muscle is opened, taking care to avoid injury to the external branch of the superior laryngeal nerve, which innervates the cricothyroid muscle and usually passes medial to the superior pole vessels. The external branch of the superior laryngeal nerve can be identified with the intraoperative nerve monitor. The superior pole vessels are individually ligated with 2-0 silk sutures and divided with a vessel-sealing device (Fig. 2.5). The right upper parathyroid gland also should be identified; parathyroid tissue is often orange-brown in color. The right upper parathyroid gland is preserved by incising the thyroid capsule and leaving behind extracapsular tissue surrounding the parathyroid gland.

Technique Tip In thyroid surgery, water is typically used for irrigation as it helps lyse red blood cells and clears the field quickly, allowing for the use of natural tissue color to identify structures.

With the superior pole freed, we turn our attention to the identification of the recurrent laryngeal nerve. The nerve can be visualized by dissecting anteriorly and parallel to the nerve, starting in the thyrothymic ligament. The recurrent laryngeal nerve passes between the branches of the inferior thyroid artery. More frequently, the right recurrent laryngeal nerve has an oblique trajectory compared to the left recurrent laryngeal nerve (Fig. 2.6). Intraoperative nerve monitoring can aid in the identification of variations in the nerve anatomy, such as a nonrecurrent laryngeal nerve (see *Technique Tip* above). Once the recurrent laryngeal nerve is identified, the tertiary branches of the arteries and veins surrounding the thyroid can be divided.

Technique Tip Use the lowest cautery settings necessary. When dissecting near the nerve or parathyroid glands, use bipolar cautery or no cautery.

By remaining close to the surface of the thyroid, the blood supply to the parathyroid glands can be better preserved. The right upper and lower parathyroid glands should be visualized and preserved by dissecting them away from the thyroid gland (Fig. 2.7). The thyroid lobe is dissected away from the recurrent laryngeal nerve. At the two upper tracheal rings, the recurrent laryngeal nerve embeds in the posterior portion of the ligament of Berry, which attaches the thyroid to the trachea. This area is where the recurrent nerve is most vulnerable to injury [4]. Undue medial traction on the thyroid gland can also injure the recurrent laryngeal nerve by stretching it, so care should be taken to avoid hard and prolonged rotation. At the ligament of Berry, the thyroid tissue is ligated with 2-0 silk sutures and cauterized

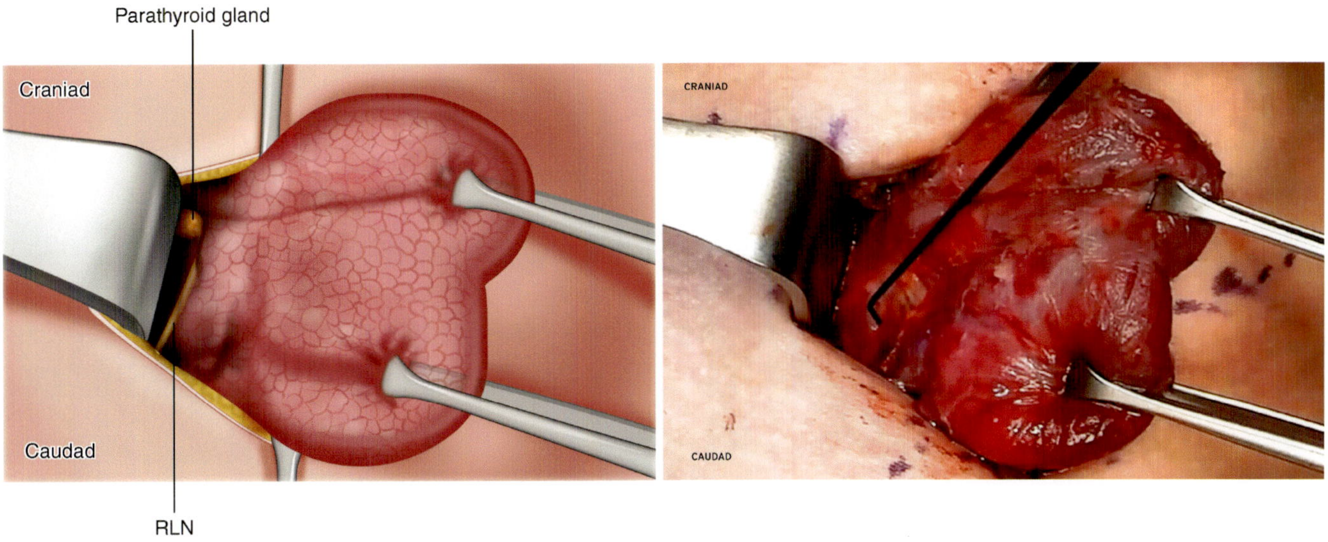

Fig. 2.6 With the thyroid retracted medially, intraoperative nerve monitoring is used to identify the recurrent laryngeal nerve, which generally has a more oblique trajectory on the right

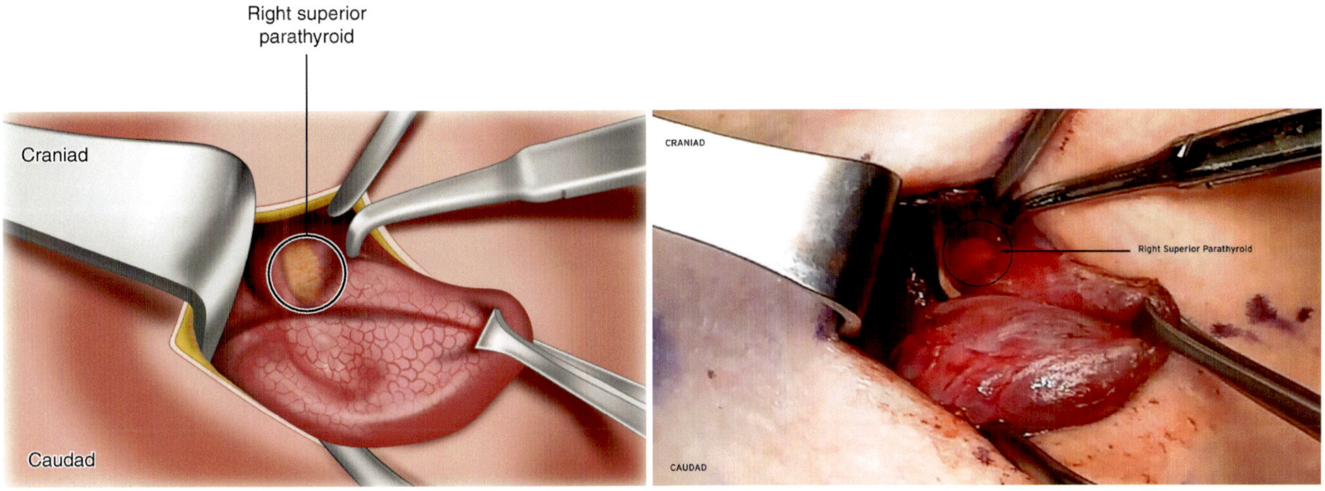

Fig. 2.7 The superior and inferior parathyroid glands should be visualized and preserved. The superior parathyroid gland will be posterior to the recurrent laryngeal nerve, while the lower parathyroid gland will be anterior to it

using bipolar energy to avoid injury to the recurrent laryngeal nerve (Fig. 2.8).

Technique Tip If a parathyroid gland is removed during thyroid surgery, it can be autotransplanted. First, the candidate parathyroid gland should be confirmed by frozen section to be indeed parathyroid tissue. Then it is minced with a #15 blade into 1-mm pieces and autotransplanted into a pocket of the adjacent sternocleidomastoid muscle. This pocket is closed with nonabsorbable suture.

Once the thyroid lobe has been separated from the recurrent laryngeal nerve, it is retracted medially and the trachea is exposed (Fig. 2.9). The isthmus is separated from the trachea using cautery. The pyramidal lobe should be resected at this point. The authors advise having the pyramidal lobe resected always at the first operation (lobectomy) as resecting it at a later time is very difficult, given the scarring, and may lead to remnant thyroid tissue in the neck.

A Kelly clamp is placed across the medial aspect of the contralateral thyroid lobe, which allows us to remove the isthmus with the thyroid lobe at the first operation. The thyroid is divided with a vessel-sealing device. The cut thyroid edge is then oversewn with interlocking horizontal mattress 2-0 silk sutures to compress the parenchyma and control the venous drainage of the thyroid (Fig. 2.10) [5].

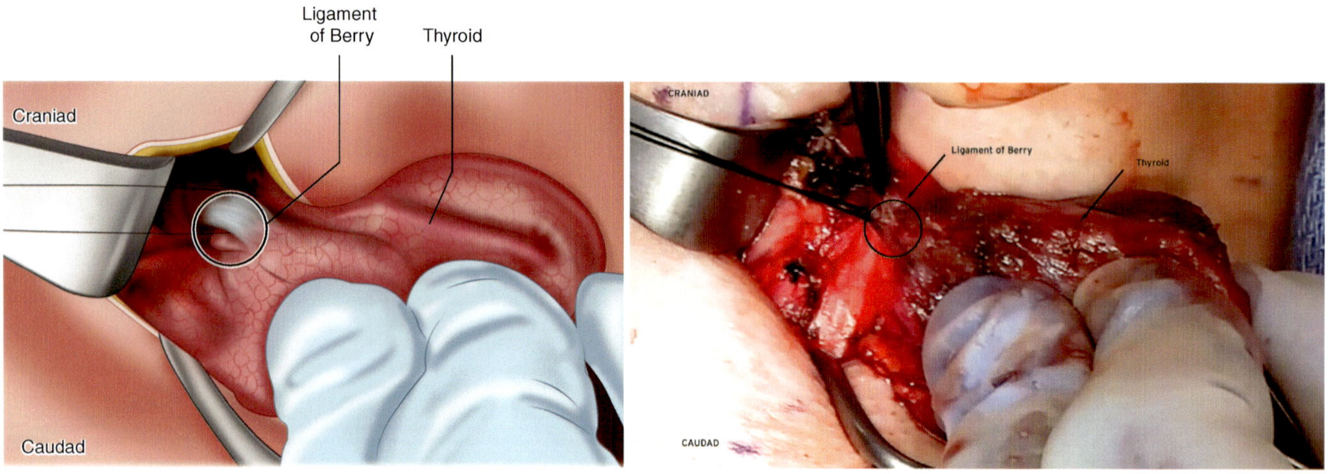

Fig. 2.8 At the ligament of Berry, the thyroid tissue is ligated with silk suture and cauterized with bipolar energy. Care should be taken to avoid injury to the recurrent laryngeal nerve with this maneuver

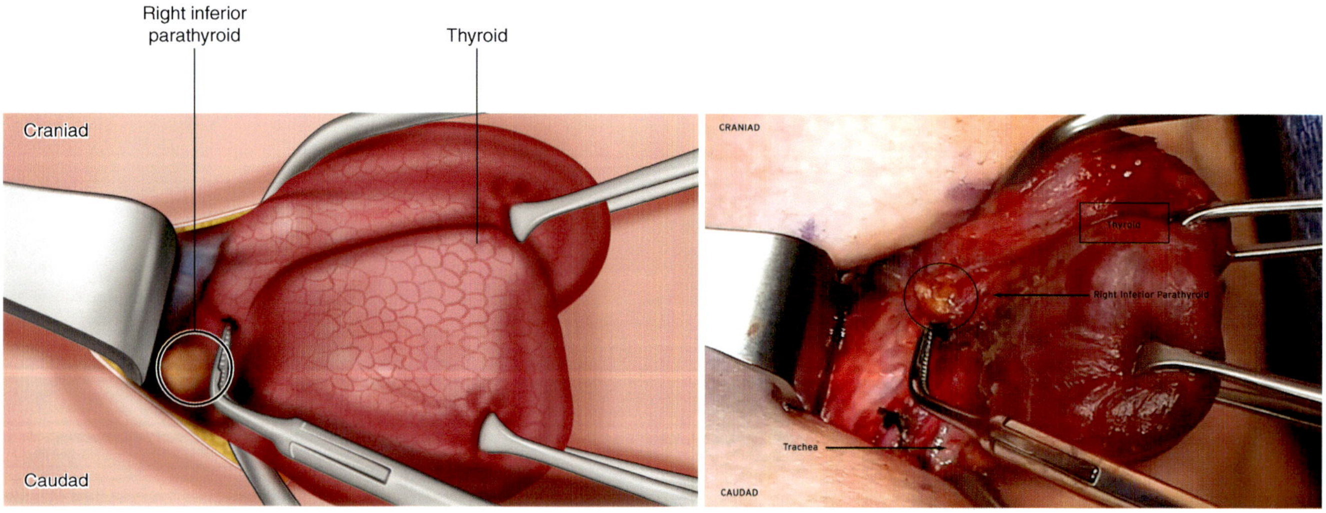

Fig. 2.9 Once the parathyroid glands and recurrent laryngeal nerve are dissected away from the thyroid, the lobe can be retracted medially to expose the trachea

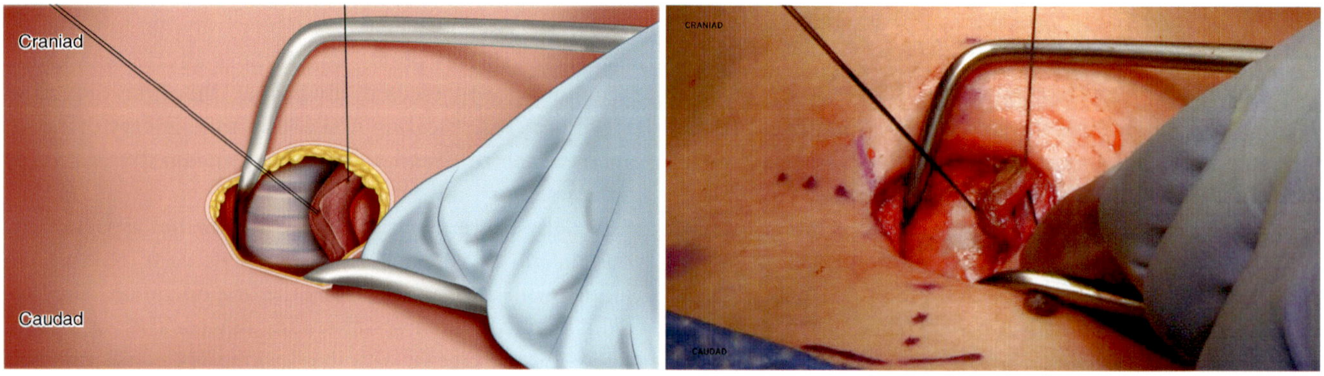

Fig. 2.10 Once the thyroid lobe is freed from the trachea and divided, the cut thyroid edge is oversewn with silk sutures for hemostasis

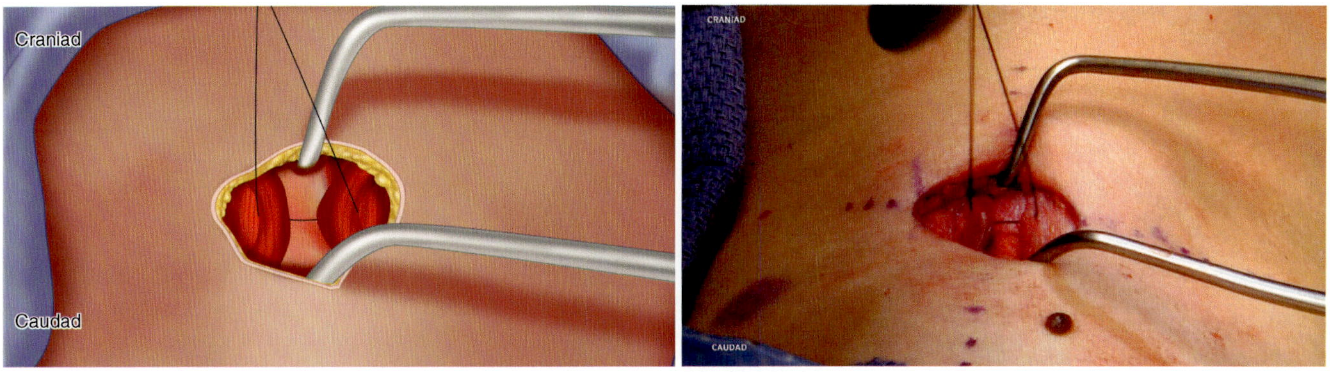

Fig. 2.11 After hemostasis of the thyroidectomy bed is assured, the sternohyoid muscles are reapproximated with silk sutures. If a complete thyroidectomy is required in the future, these nonabsorbable sutures will aid reidentification of the midline

The resection bed is irrigated with water and then examined for bleeding. Any bleeding points are controlled with cautery. The RLN should be tested again to assure that the NIM signal has been maintained. Hemostatic agents can be placed in the resection bed. The sternohyoid muscles are reapproximated in the midline. We recommend using nonabsorbable sutures, such as 3-0 silk, which will aid in the identification of the midline in the future if a complete thyroidectomy is required (Fig. 2.11). If the anterior jugular veins are very close to the midline, the authors recommend closing muscle from underneath the veins to allow the veins to roll away laterally from the midline incision. This will avoid injury and unnecessary bleeding if reoperation is needed in the future. If the sternothyroid muscle was divided, reapproximation is not necessary. The inferior aspect of the sternohyoid muscles is left open; if bleeding occurs postoperatively, blood can decompress through this open space. Using absorbable sutures, the platysma is reapproximated with a running, locking stitch, and the skin is closed with a subcuticular stitch. A final dressing, either with skin glue or adhesive bandage, is applied.

Technique Tip A running, locking stitch in the platysma avoids having the incision purse-string and misalign, with better cosmetic results.

After right thyroid lobectomy, the patient is awakened from anesthesia. After recovery in the postanesthesia care unit and an adequate observation period, the patient can be discharged home. Nowadays, thyroid surgery is often same-day surgery at many institutions, but the risk of bleeding can extend to 72 hours after thyroid surgery [6]. Thus, at discharge, patients should be provided with thorough postoperative instructions and appropriate contact information to reach the surgeon in cases of emergency.

Final surgical pathology demonstrates a benign thyroid nodule. This information is shared with the patient at her postoperative visit, approximately 2 weeks after surgery. Thyroid function tests should be measured at 6–8 weeks postoperatively to determine the need for a supplemental thyroid hormone (Video 2.1).

Disclosures JAS is a member of the Data Monitoring Committee of the Medullary Thyroid Cancer Consortium Registry supported by GlaxoSmithKline, Novo Nordisk, AstraZeneca, and Eli Lilly. She receives institutional research funding from Exelixis and Eli Lilly.

References

1. Hannan SA. The magnificent seven: a history of modern thyroid surgery. Int J Surg. 2006;4:187–91.
2. Worni M, Schudel HH, Seifert E, Inglin R, Hagemann M, Vorburger SA, et al. Randomized controlled trial on single dose steroid before thyroidectomy for benign disease to improve postoperative nausea, pain, and vocal function. Ann Surg. 2008;248:1060–6.
3. McHenry CR. Thyroidectomy for nodules or small cancers. In: Duh Q-Y, Clark OH, Kebebew E, editors. Atlas of endocrine surgical techniques. Saunders: Philadelphia, PA. 2010. p. 3–24.
4. Henry J-F. Surgical anatomy and embryology of the thyroid and parathyroid glands. In: Clark OH, Duh Q-Y, Kebebew E, Gosnell JE, Shen WT, editors. Textbook of endocrine surgery, 3rd ed. Jaypee Brothers Medical Publishers: New Delhi, India. 2016. p. 11–21.
5. Roman S. Right thyroid lobectomy. USA: GIBLIB; 2020.
6. Farooq MS, Nouraei R, Kaddour H, Saharay M. Patterns, timing and consequences of post-thyroidectomy haemorrhage. Ann R Coll Surg Engl. 2017;99:60–2.

Thyroid Lobectomy

3

Trenton Foster and Travis McKenzie

Thyroid lobectomy may be utilized for benign thyroid nodules, indeterminate thyroid nodules, or low-risk malignant thyroid nodules less than 4 cm in size, as recommended by the 2015 American Thyroid Association guidelines [1]. Thyroid preservation is desirable in appropriate settings to reduce the surgical risks of recurrent laryngeal nerve injury and postoperative hypoparathyroidism and can allow many patients to avoid the need for life-long thyroid replacement hormones.

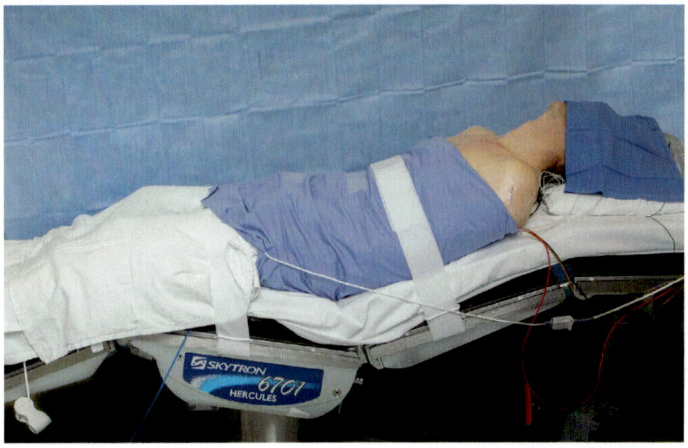

Fig. 3.1 Patient positioning with neck extended and head supported

Procedure

A 52-year-old gentleman presents for surgical management of a 2-cm indeterminate thyroid nodule (Hurthle cell neoplasm) located within the left thyroid lobe. He is euthyroid and without concerning nodules in the contralateral lobe. Diagnostic left thyroid lobectomy is pursued.

The patient is placed under general anesthesia using an endotracheal tube. The authors prefer the routine use of an endotracheal tube capable of intraoperative nerve monitoring to aid in the dissection of the recurrent laryngeal nerve in all thyroid operations. The patient is then positioned supine with an inflatable cushion under the scapulae. The cushion is inflated to maximize cervical extension while maintaining appropriate support of the occiput. Bean bags are placed laterally to the left and right of the head to ensure stability and avoid rotation. The bed is placed in a beach chair position with a slight reverse Trendelenburg (Fig. 3.1). The surgical field is widely prepared with clear ChloraPrep from the lower lip to the mid sternum laterally to the shoulders and allowed to dry. The field is then sterilely draped from chin to clavicles (Fig. 3.2). If a lateral neck dissection is planned, a wider field is draped. In the case of a substernal goiter, the anterior chest is also prepped into the field. Once draped, the necessary instruments are opened (Fig. 3.3) and a confirmatory pause is performed. Preincisional antibiotics are generally not utilized unless the patient is immunosuppressed.

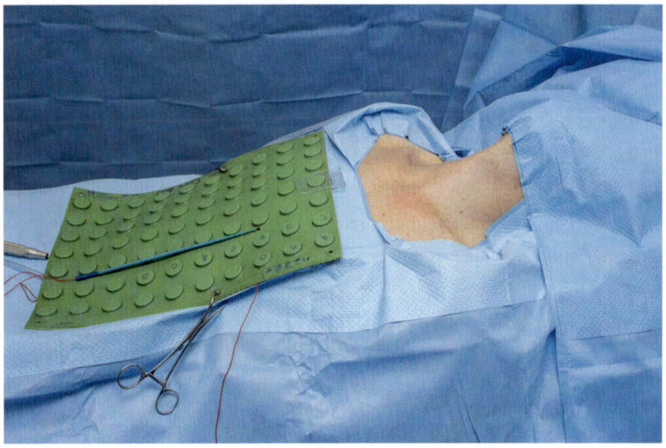

Fig. 3.2 Patient draping with adequate exposure from clavicles to chin

The incision is positioned over the thyroid isthmus, which is reliably located 1–2 cm caudal to the cricoid cartilage. This will be approximately two fingerbreadths above the

T. Foster (✉) · T. McKenzie
Department of Surgery, Mayo Clinic, Rochester, MN, USA
e-mail: Foster.Trenton@mayo.edu

A. Shifrin (ed.), *Atlas of Thyroid Surgery*, https://doi.org/10.1007/978-3-030-93673-0_3

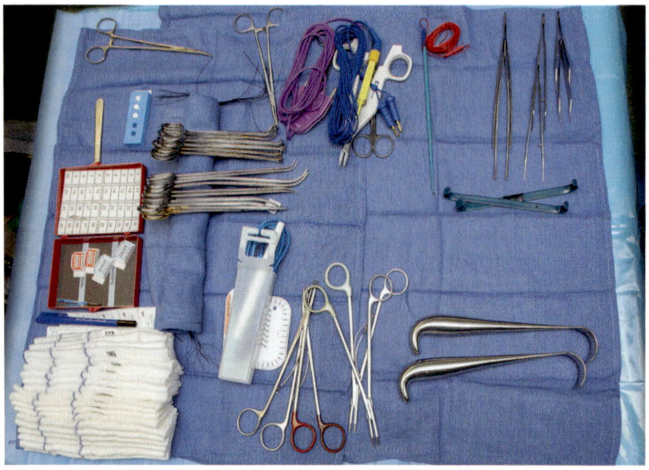

Fig. 3.3 Surgical instruments for retraction and fine dissection; ties, clips, and hemostatic energy devices are prepared

sternal notch in most patients, although this distance may vary in those with exceptionally short or long necks. If there is a skin crease present within this vicinity, the skin crease is utilized as the incisional site to enhance the cosmetic outcome. The incision length is guided by the underlying pathology, generally kept at 6 cm or less. The incision is marked and measured to ensure symmetry (Fig. 3.4). The incision is made with a 15-blade scalpel through the epidermis and dermis. The electrocautery of the dermis is avoided to prevent hypertrophic scarring. The platysma is divided with the use of electrocautery. The upper cut border of the platysma is grasped with Allis clamps and lifted. Counter traction is placed on the upper neck. The superior flap is developed with electrocautery in the subplatysmal plane. The subcutaneous fat and platysma muscle is elevated, while the fascia of the strap muscles and associated anterior jugular veins remain down. If injury to an anterior jugular vein occurs, the vein is ligated with a 3-0 Vicryl suture. The superior flap is developed to the level of the thyroid cartilage notch and laterally beyond the anterior border of the sternocleidomastoid muscles (Fig. 3.5). An inferior subplatysmal flap is similarly developed extending to the level of the clavicles and sternal notch (Fig. 3.6). Insulated band retractors are utilized to retract the flaps, and the midline is opened at the median raphe between the right and left sternohyoid muscles. This plane is typically avascular, although a small venous branch between anterior jugular veins can be encountered, especially near the sternal notch. The median raphe can be opened with electrocautery or LigaSure™ (Fig. 3.7). The sternothyroid muscles are bluntly swept off the midline to expose the isthmus. Prelaryngeal and pretracheal tissues are dissected to expose the larynx and trachea above and below the isthmus,

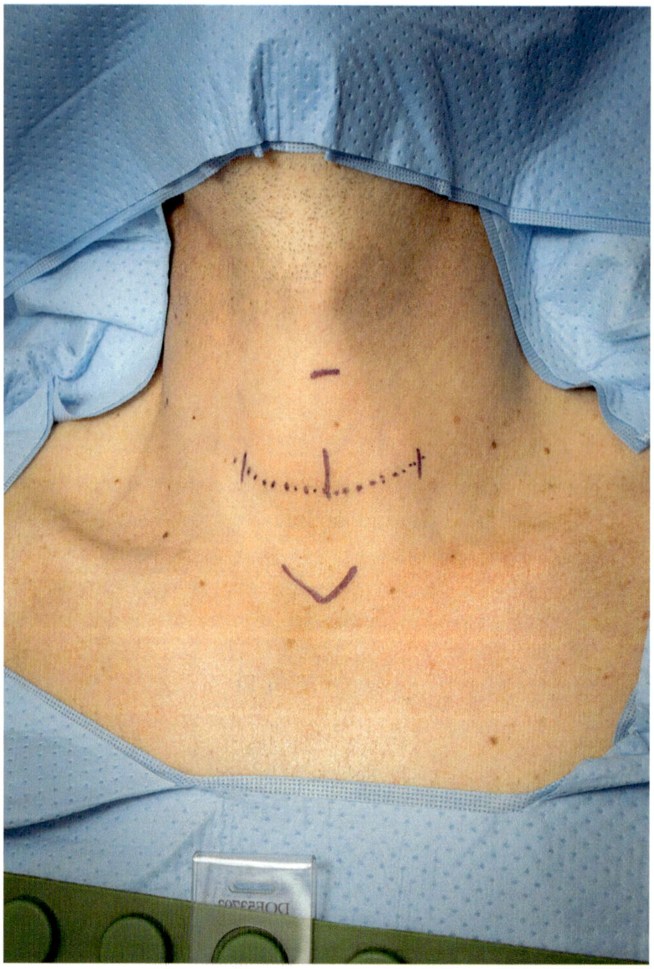

Fig. 3.4 Anatomic landmarks, including the sternal notch and cricoid cartilage, are identified. A symmetric midline skin incision is planned following the contours of the skin

respectively (Fig. 3.8). If a pyramidal lobe is encountered, it is dissected to remain with the thyroid. In the setting of suspected or confirmed malignancy, the Delphian lymph node is evaluated and resected if suspicious. Superior and inferior thyroid veins may be encountered anterior to the larynx and trachea and are divided with clips and LigaSure™. With the larynx and trachea exposed, a tunnel is created bluntly beneath the thyroid isthmus (Fig. 3.9). The thyroid isthmus is divided with LigaSure™ along its junction with the contralateral (right) lobe of the thyroid gland (Fig. 3.10). The isthmus is grasped with an Allis clamp and pulled to the right. The sternohyoid and sternothyroid muscles are dissected off the left thyroid lobe with a combination of electrocautery and blunt dissection. As the thyroid is pulled to the right, the middle thyroid vein, if present, will come into view (Fig. 3.11). The middle thyroid vein is clipped and then

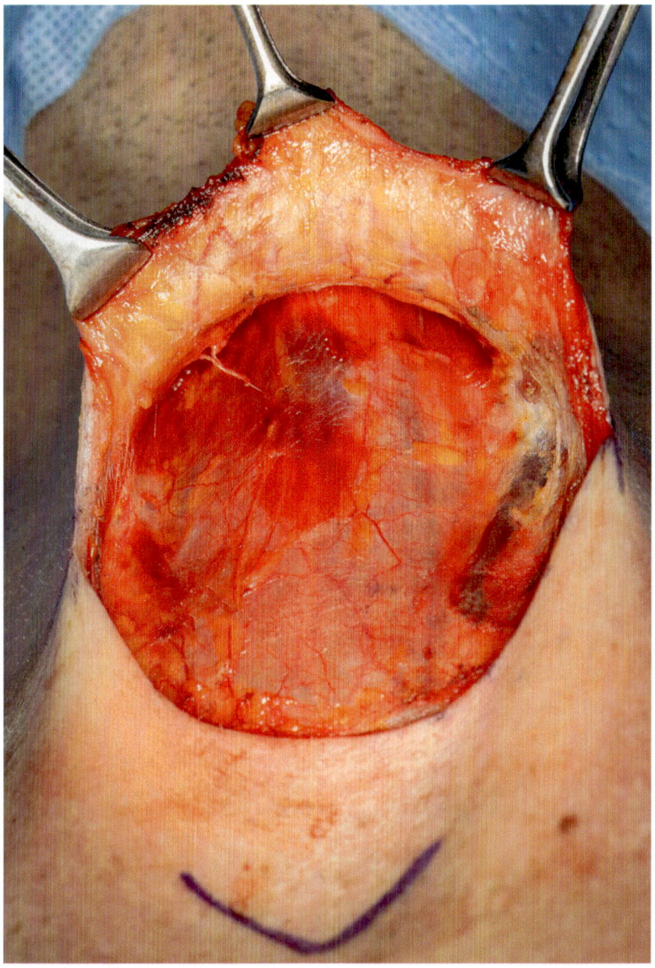

Fig. 3.5 Superior subplatysmal flap is developed to the level of the thyroid cartilage

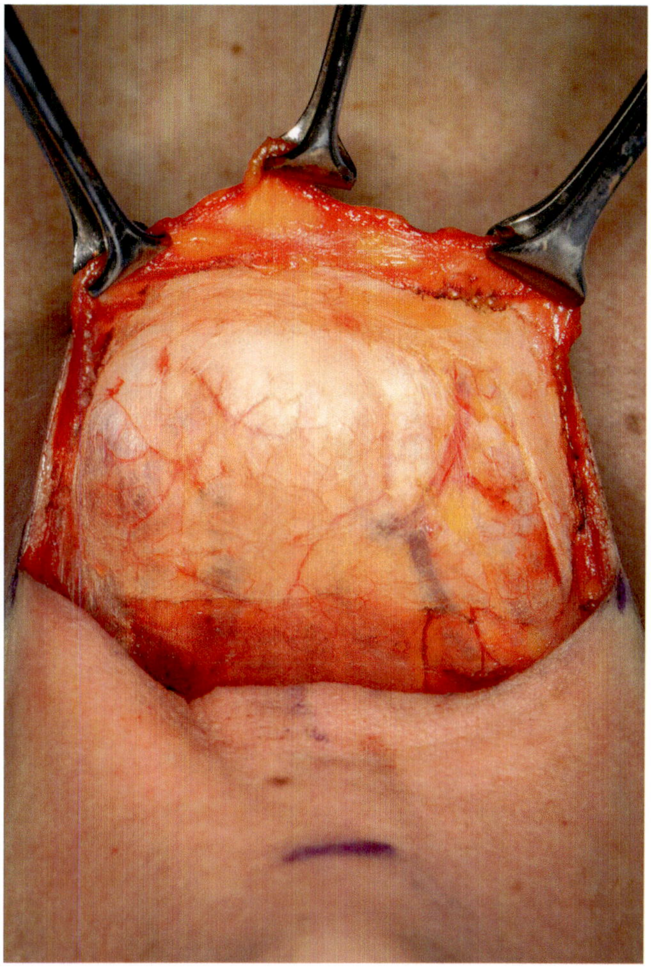

Fig. 3.6 Inferior subplatysmal flap is developed to the level of the sternal notch and clavicles

divided on the specimen side with LigaSure™ in a plane anterior to the carotid artery. Dissection over the anterior surface of the common carotid artery continues until the anterior adventitia of the carotid artery is fully exposed. Exposure of the common carotid artery allows all tissues between the carotid artery and thyroid lobe to fall away, thereby deepening the field of dissection to the level of the vertebral body. Care is taken to keep the dissection directly ventral to the carotid artery as the only structure that crosses ventral to the carotid artery in this region of the neck is the middle thyroid vein, which can be sacrificed. The recurrent laryngeal nerve will not cross ventral to the carotid artery, even in nonrecurrent situations. The vagus nerve is stimulated lateral and deep to the common carotid artery to confirm that the neurologic circuit is intact and the nerve monitoring device is functioning appropriately.

An Allis clamp is placed on the upper thyroid lobe, and the upper pole is retracted laterally (Fig. 3.12). This pulls the superior thyroid vessels away from the cricothyroid muscle, allowing the surgeon to fully open the avascular space of Joll with a straight Jacobson Schnidt (Fig. 3.13). Once the thyroid vessels are pulled away from the cricothyroid muscle, the surgeon examines the upper pole for the presence of a low external branch of the superior laryngeal nerve, which can be as low as the superior pole thyroid parenchyma. If identified, the nerve is dissected away from the superior pole of the thyroid. Once the surgeon is confident the external branch of the superior laryngeal nerve is protected, the upper pole vessels are ligated and divided using LigaSure™ along the superior most extent of the thyroid capsule (Fig. 3.14).

The thyroid can now be fully rotated medially and to the right with gentle traction (Fig. 3.15). With this field of view,

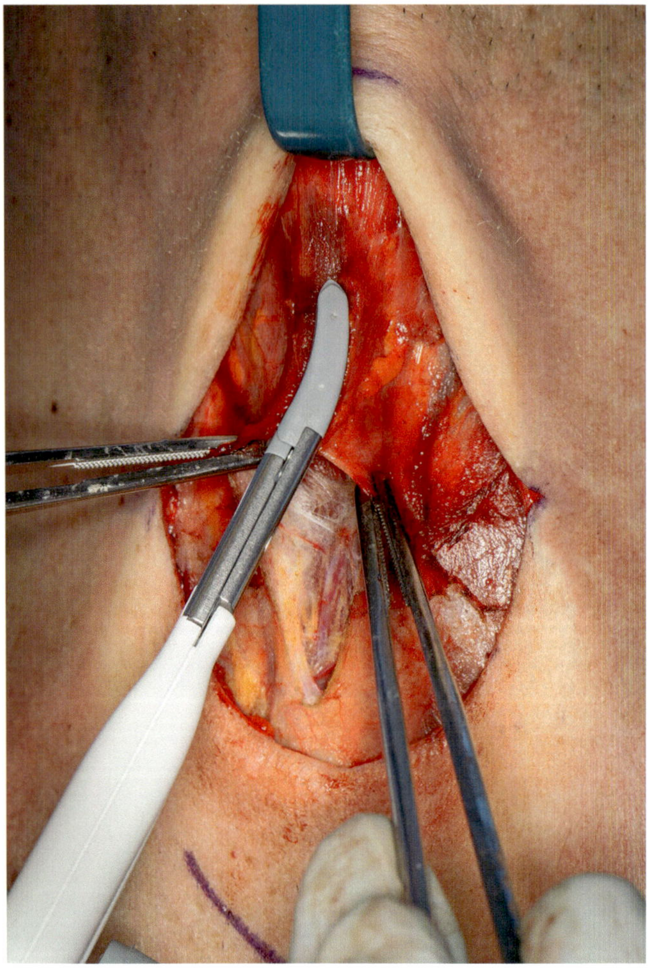

Fig. 3.7 The median raphe between strap muscles is opened using cautery or LigaSure™

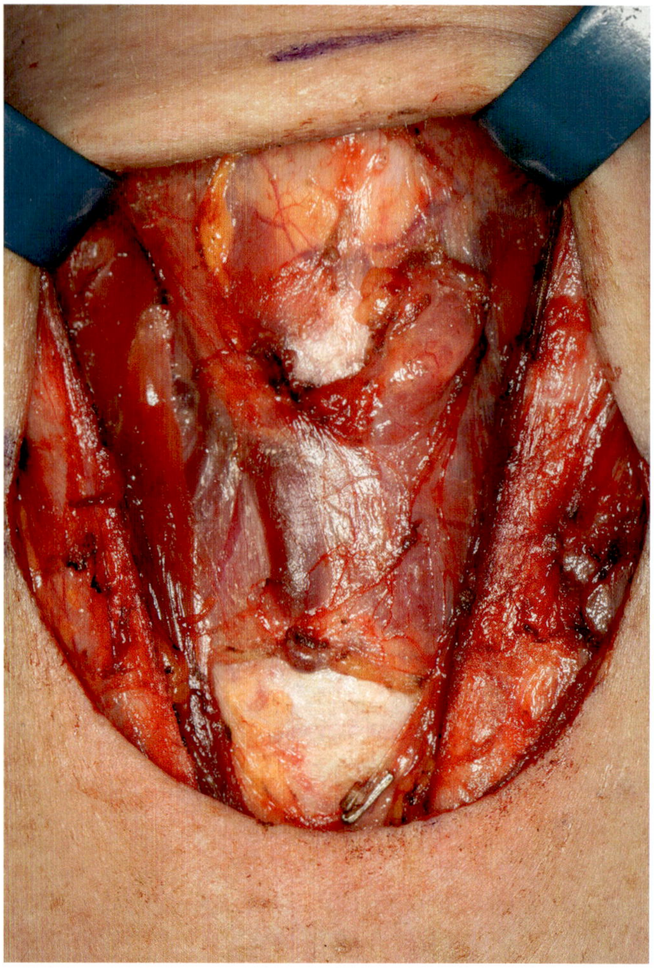

Fig. 3.8 The prelaryngeal space is developed along the superior aspect of the thyroid isthmus, and a pretracheal space is developed along the inferior aspect of the thyroid isthmus

the surgeon can identify the carotid artery, jugular vein, and inferior thyroid artery and should begin to identify the location of the left recurrent laryngeal nerve and superior and inferior parathyroid glands. The recurrent laryngeal nerve on the left is identified in the tracheoesophageal groove immediately caudal to where the inferior thyroid artery traverses the thyroid bed to insert on the thyroid capsule. The nerve is gently but fully exposed in this region. Intraoperative nerve monitoring can be utilized to assist with this portion of the procedure as needed. Once the recurrent laryngeal nerve is identified, the anterior surface of the nerve is carefully dissected from caudal to cranial while dividing tissue anterior to the nerve. This maneuver continues to fully expose the recurrent laryngeal nerve along its course. It should be noted that the blood supply to the recurrent laryngeal nerve is through the vasa nervorum running along the nerve and that there is no vessel that runs external to internal. Therefore, the nerve can be dissected anteriorly, and all tissues ventral to the nerve can be divided with the jewelers bipolar forceps. The inferior thyroid artery can have a variable relationship to the recurrent nerve, but the nerve most commonly runs deep to the artery. The artery is dissected away from the nerve and preserved. If the artery is divided proximally, the surgeon risks the devascularization of the parathyroid glands. At this point, the surgeon identifies the inferior and superior parathyroid glands and plans the final portion of dissection. With the recurrent laryngeal nerve and parathyroid glands directly in view, the inferior pedicle is ligated and divided along the thyroid capsule with

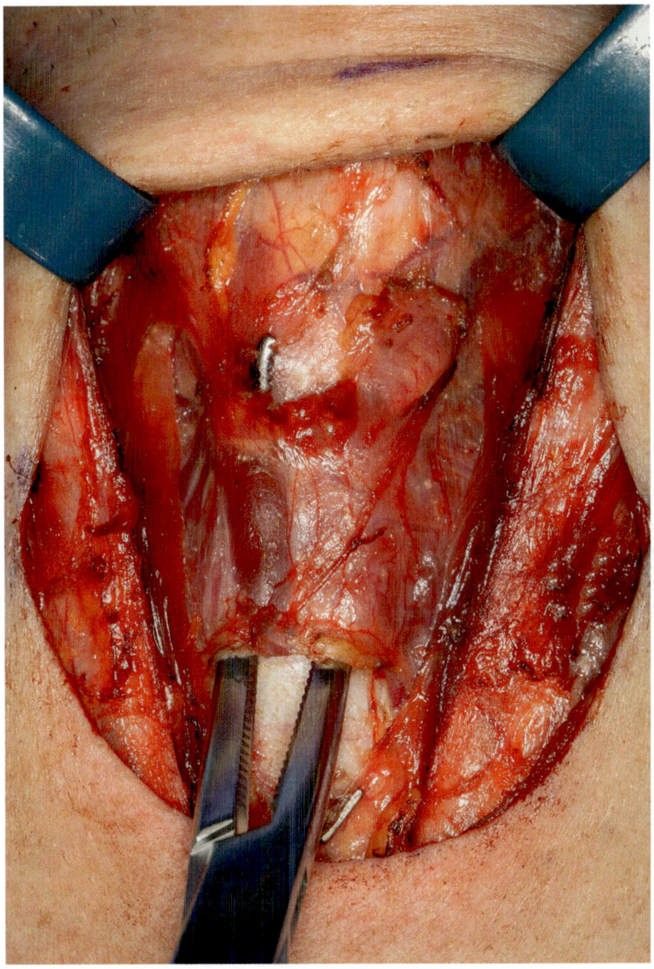

Fig. 3.9 The thyroid isthmus is mobilized off the anterior surface of the trachea with blunt dissection

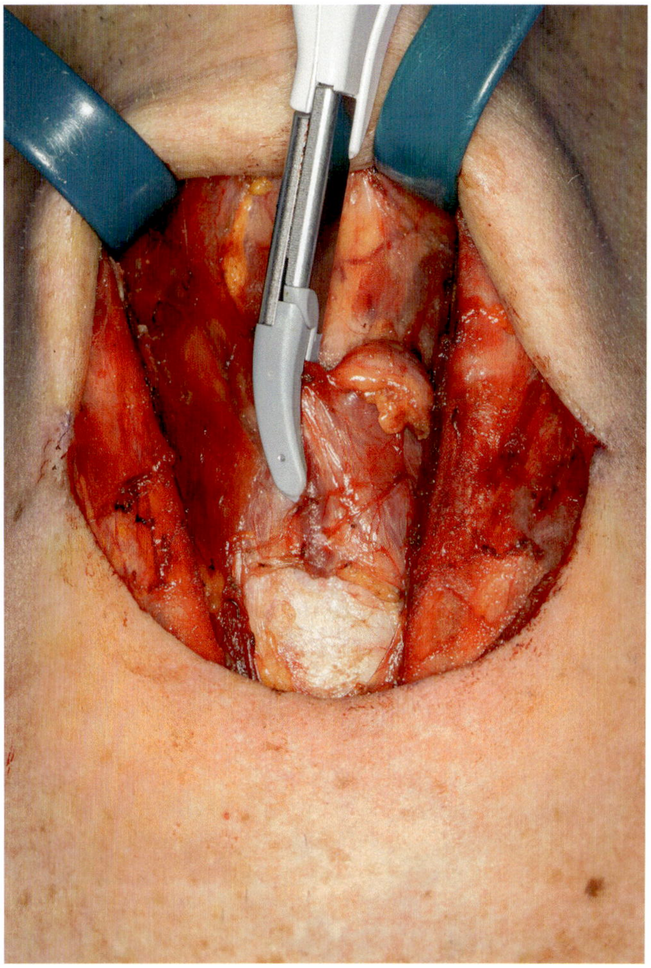

Fig. 3.10 The thyroid isthmus is divided at its junction with the contralateral lobe of the thyroid gland using LigaSure™

LigaSure™ (Fig. 3.16). Capsular dissection then ensues with the use of clips and bipolar in order to drop the inferior and superior parathyroid glands off the thyroid capsule while preserving their native vascular supply (Fig. 3.17). The thyroid is then carefully mobilized off the trachea at the ligament of Berry with the use of clips and bipolar parallel to the recurrent laryngeal nerve while keeping the nerve directly in view (Fig. 3.18). If necessary, near total thyroidectomy can be performed by placing clips on the thyroid parenchyma and dividing the thyroid tissue with the use of bipolar or LigaSure™. The specimen is oriented for pathological review. The operative field is then inspected (Fig. 3.19), and complete hemostasis is confirmed with a Valsalva maneuver while the operative bed is submerged in sterile water. Topical hemostatic may be placed in the operative bed as desired. The strap muscles are closed in the midline with 3-0 Vicryl in an interrupted fashion. Care is taken to leave an approximately 1-cm opening at the inferior aspect of the closure to serve as a "blowhole," allowing blood to decompress into the superficial compartment in the event of cervical hematoma (Fig. 3.20). The platysma is closed with interrupted 3-0 Vicryl. The dermis is infiltrated with 10 mL of 0.25% bupivacaine. The skin is closed with running 4-0 Monocryl in a subcuticular fashion. A Steri-Strip™ is placed horizontally over the incision (Fig. 3.21). The patient is then extubated and discharged home after a period of observation.

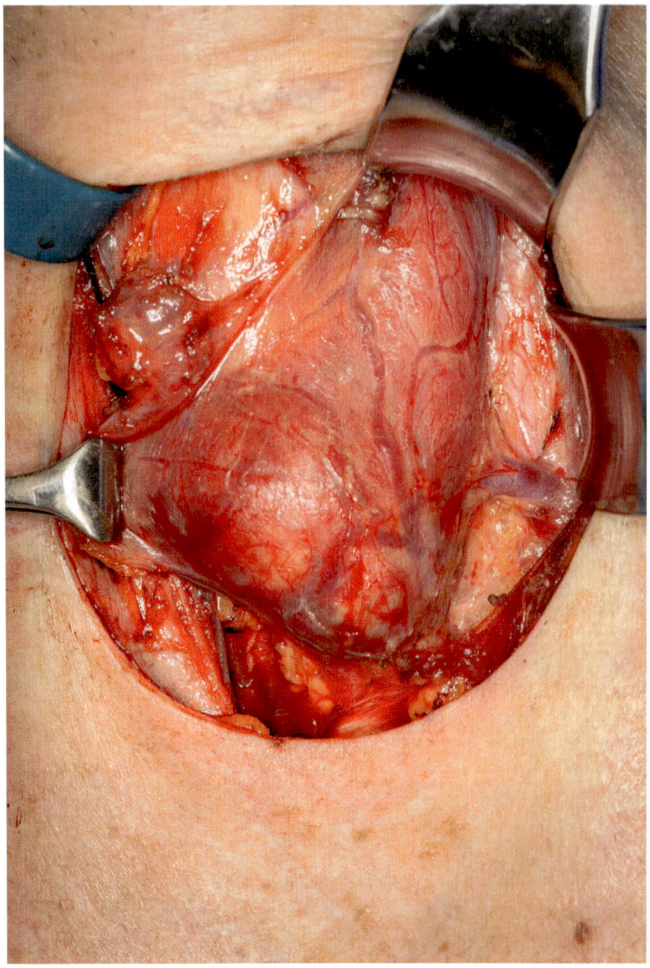

Fig. 3.11 The thyroid gland is pulled medially with an Allis clamp to expose the middle thyroid vein

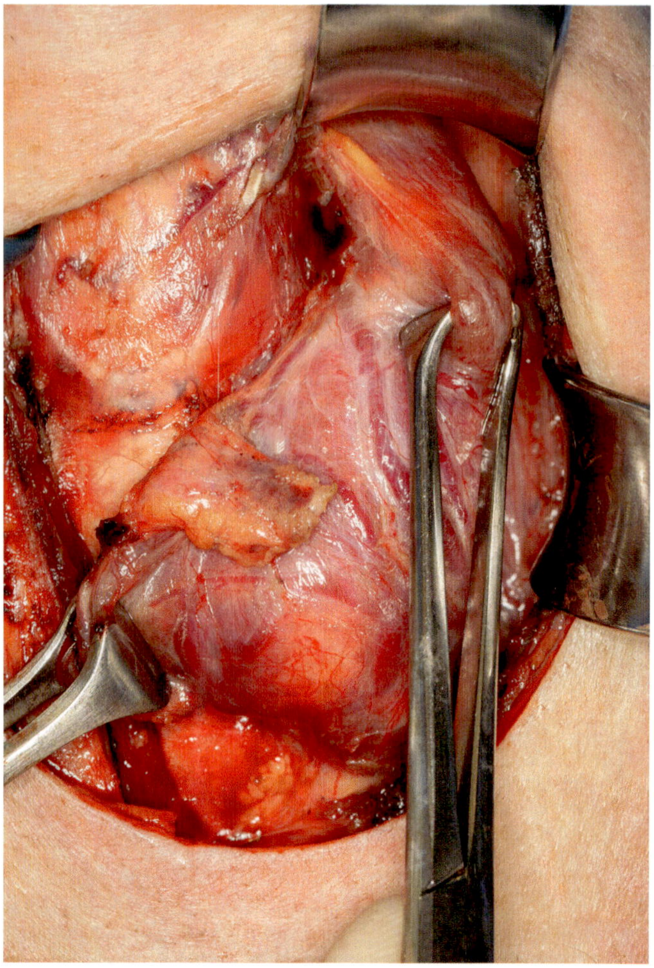

Fig. 3.12 The upper pole of the thyroid is grasped and pulled laterally

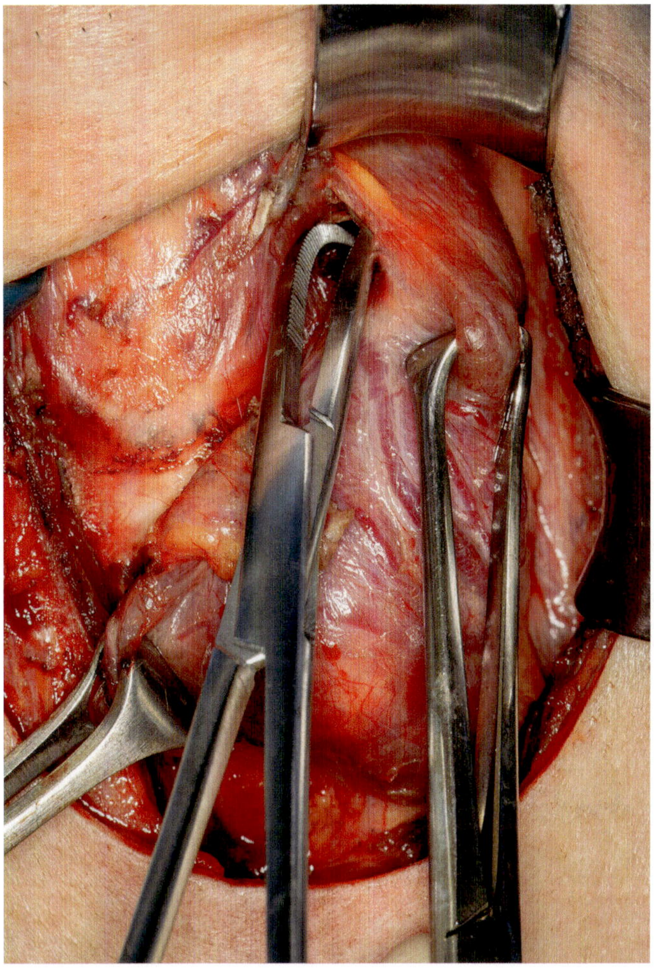

Fig. 3.13 The avascular space of Joll is opened, taking care to protect the external branch of the superior laryngeal nerve

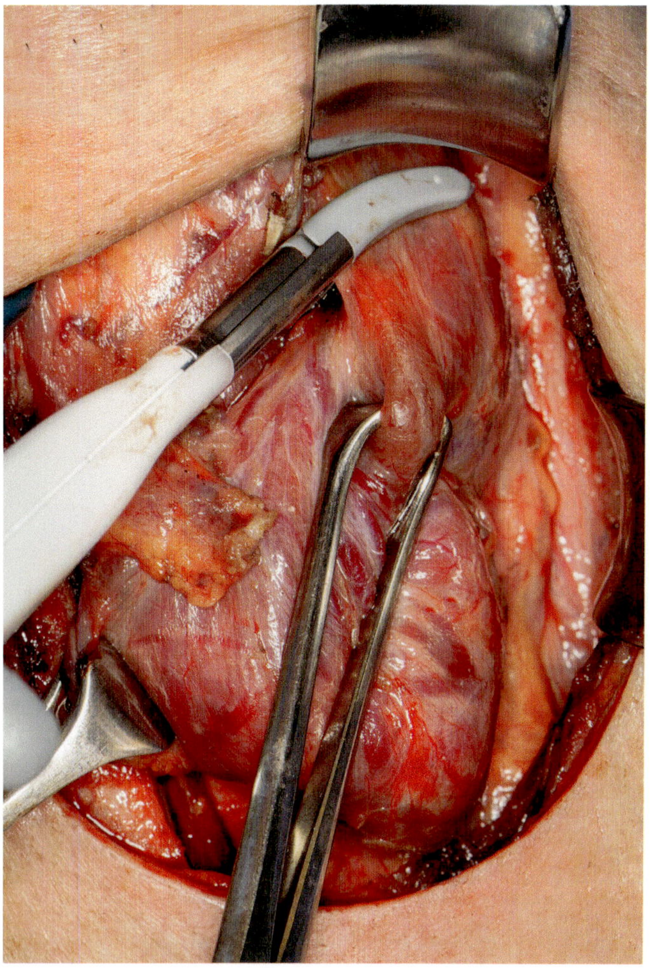

Fig. 3.14 The upper pole vessels are ligated with LigaSure™ along the superior most extent of the thyroid capsule

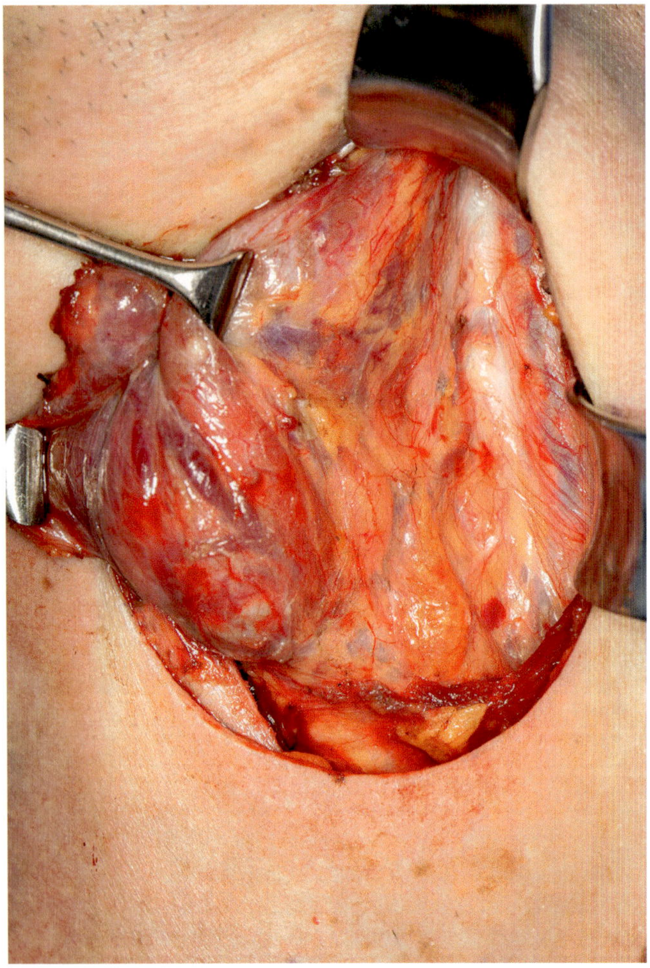

Fig. 3.15 The thyroid gland is pulled medially to reveal the carotid artery, jugular vein, and expected regions of the inferior thyroid artery, superior and inferior parathyroid glands, and recurrent laryngeal nerve

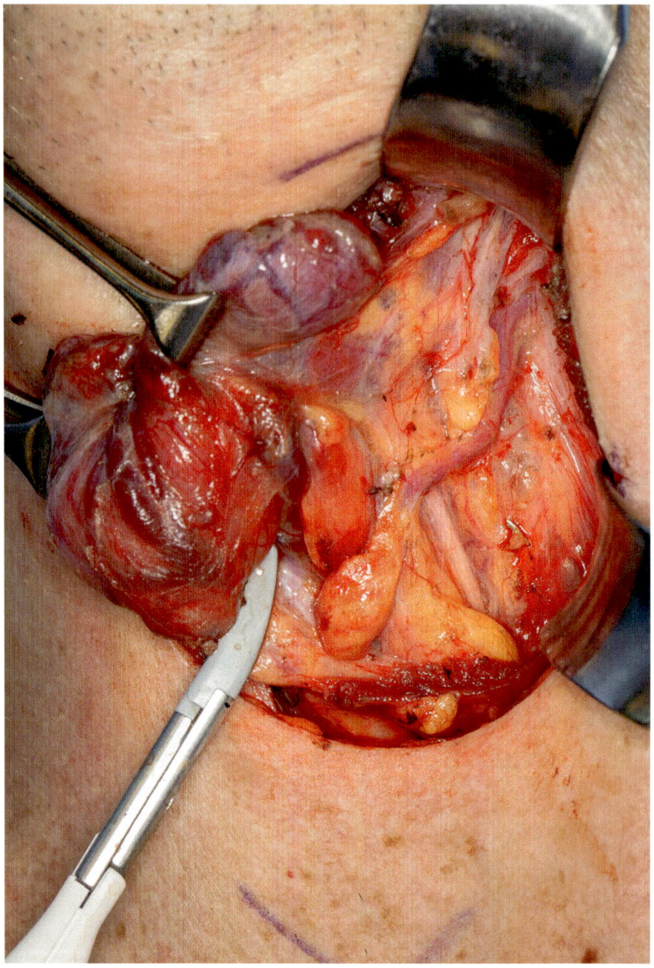

Fig. 3.16 The inferior vascular pedicle is divided using LigaSure™ while keeping the recurrent laryngeal nerve in view and the parathyroid glands protected

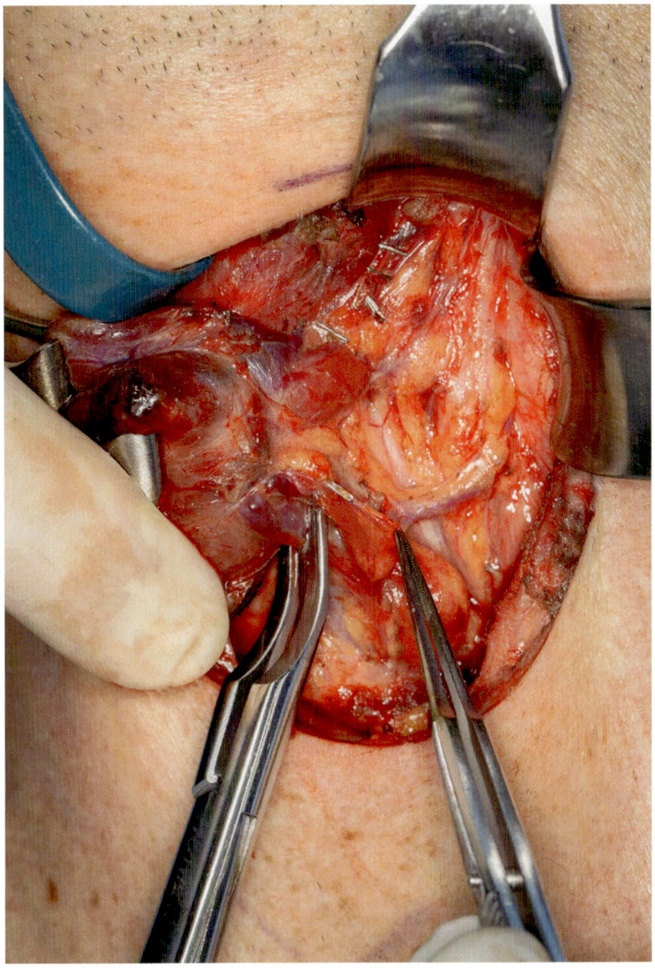

Fig. 3.17 The superior and inferior parathyroid glands are dissected away from the thyroid gland while taking care to preserve their vascular supply

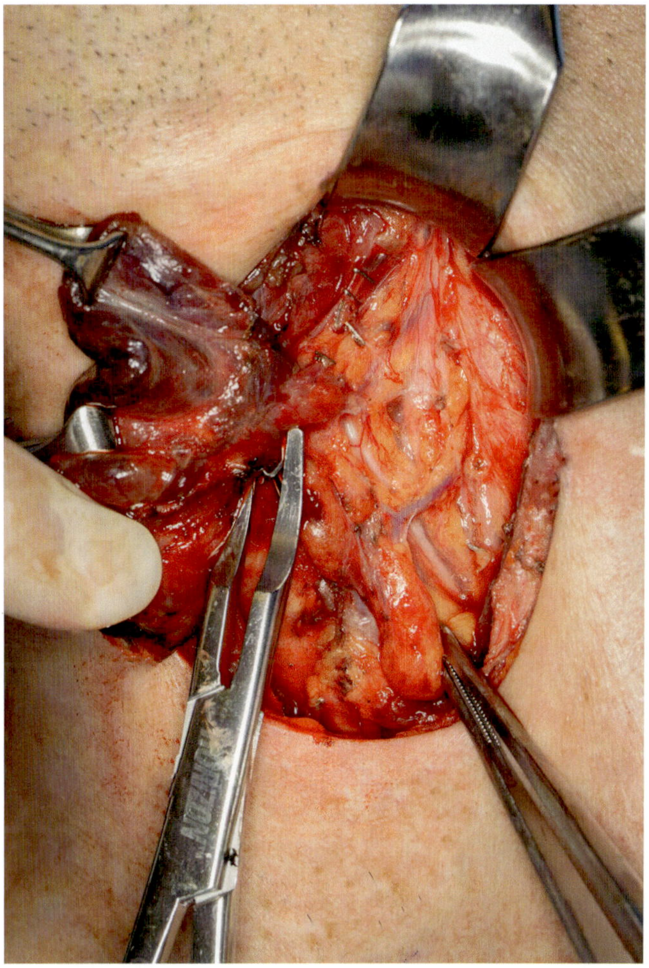

Fig. 3.18 The thyroid is dissected off the trachea while working parallel to the recurrent laryngeal nerve using clips and bipolar cautery

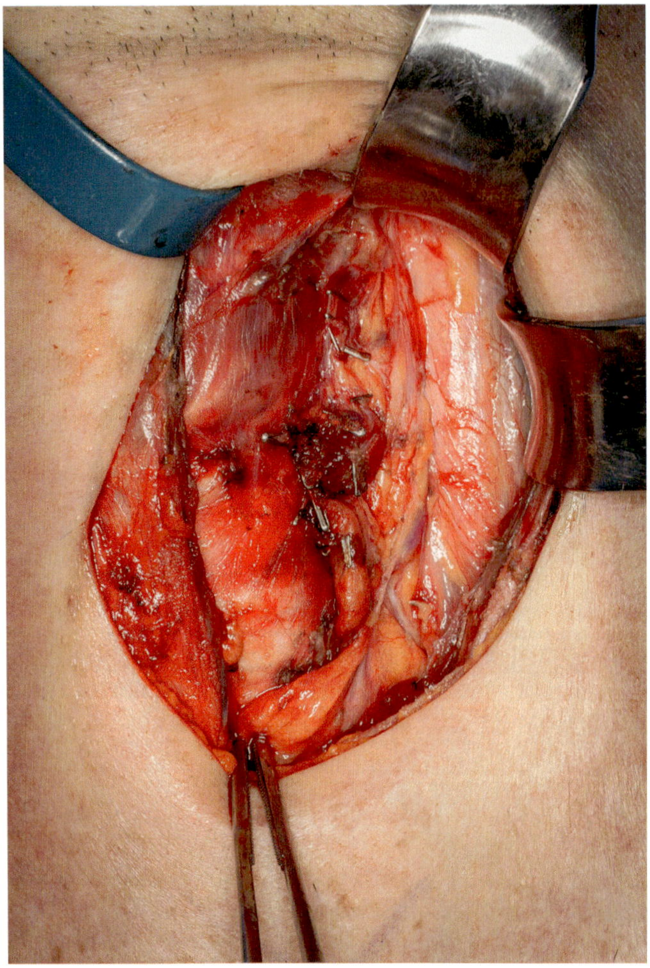

Fig. 3.19 The operative field is inspected for hemostasis

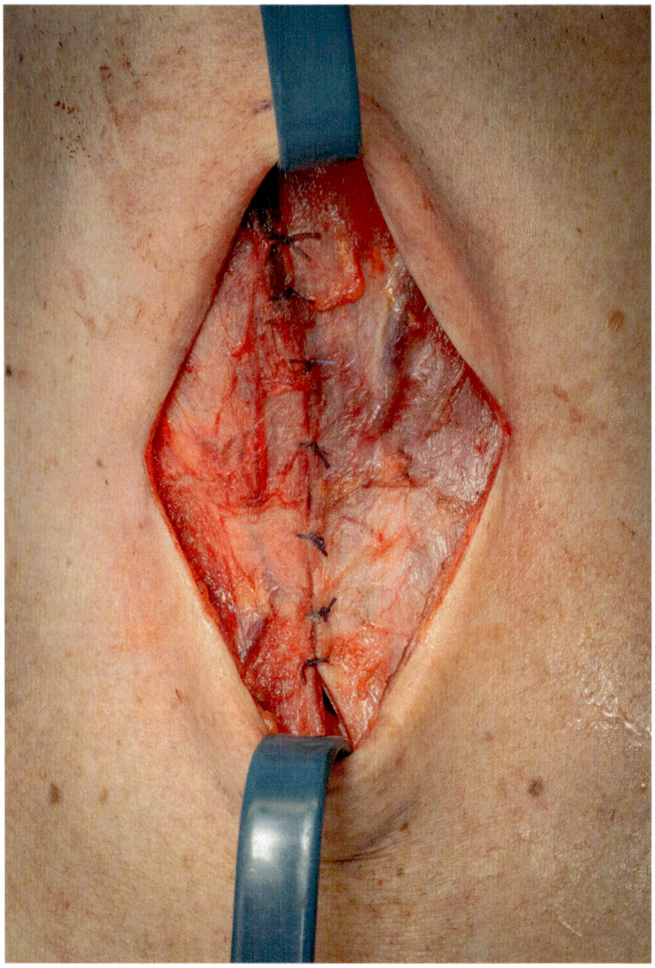

Fig. 3.20 The midline between strap muscles is closed with suture, leaving a small opening at the inferior most aspect

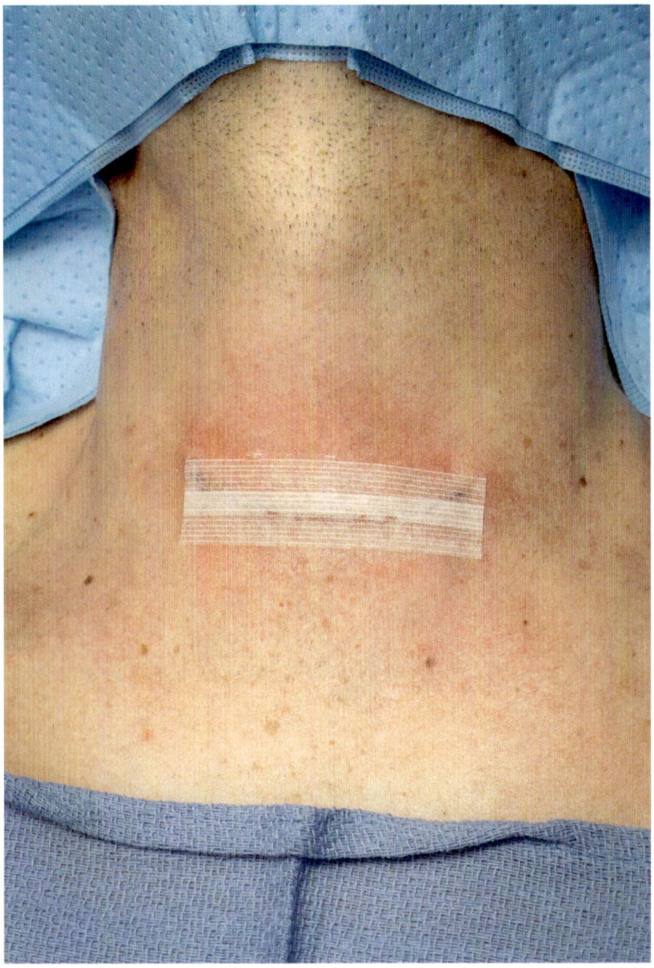

Fig. 3.21 The platysma and skin layers are closed, and the surgical site is then covered with Steri-Strip™

Reference

1. Haugen BR, Alexander EK, Bible KC, Doherty GM, Mandel SJ, Nikiforov YE, et al. 2015 American Thyroid Association Management Guidelines for adult patients with thyroid nodules and differentiated thyroid cancer: the American Thyroid Association Guidelines Task Force on Thyroid Nodules and Differentiated Thyroid Cancer. Thyroid. 2016;26(1):1–133.

Left Thyroid Lobectomy

4

Caitlin T. Yeo, Adrian Harvey, and Janice L. Pasieka

Case Description

The patient is a 40-year-old female with a history of a palpable left thyroid nodule measuring 3.6 cm. She is clinically euthyroid, and her thyroid-stimulating hormone (TSH) is 1.6 mlU/L (normal range: 0.2–4.0 mlU/L). An ultrasound is performed, which shows a hypoechoic nodule, and fine-needle aspirate reveals mildly enlarged, atypical, overlapping follicular cells in a microfollicular arrangement, which is classified as suspicious for follicular neoplasm (Bethesda IV). After a careful discussion with her surgeon, she is consented for a left thyroid lobectomy, given the 10–40% risk of malignancy.

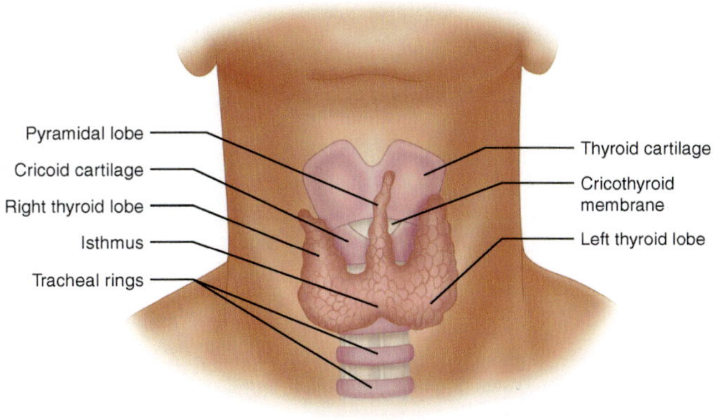

Fig. 4.1 Thyroid anatomy

Introduction

The thyroid gland is the first of the endocrine organs to develop and is critical in fetal brain development. It regulates the metabolic processes throughout the body through the production and release of the thyroid hormones thyroxine (T4) and triiodothyronine (T3) [1, 2]. The thyroid gland is located centrally in the lower neck, anterior to the trachea. It is composed of a left and right lobe, an isthmus, and a pyramidal lobe – a remnant from its embryologic descent (Fig. 4.1) [3]. The parathyroid glands, recurrent laryngeal nerves (RLN), and external branches of the superior laryngeal nerves (EBSLN) lie in close proximity, and care must be given to preserve these structures during dissection. Thyroid lobectomy is performed for diagnostic or therapeutic purposes. Diagnostic purposes include repeated fine-needle aspirate, which describe follicular lesion/atypia of unknown significance (Bethesda III) or follicular neoplasm (Bethesda IV), as these have a 5–18% and 10–40% risk of malignancy respectively [4]. Therapeutic purposes include low-risk unifocal suspicious (Bethesda V) or proven papillary thyroid cancer (Bethesda VI), solitary toxic nodule, unilateral retrosternal nodule or goiter, or clinical symptoms of compression.

Procedure

The left thyroid lobectomy is composed of several critical steps, outlined in the following chapter. During the lobectomy, it is also important to consider that a completion thyroidectomy may be required in the future. There are several steps that should always be done that will make a completion thyroidectomy safer (Table 4.1, Video 4.1).

Supplementary Information The online version contains supplementary material available at [https://doi.org/10.1007/978-3-030-93673-0_4].

C. T. Yeo
Section of General Surgery and Oncology, Department of Surgery, Cumming School of Medicine, University of Calgary, Calgary, AB, Canada

A. Harvey
Section of General Surgery and Surgical Oncology, Department of Surgery, Faculty of Medicine, Foothills Medical Center, University of Calgary, Calgary, AB, Canada

J. L. Pasieka (✉)
Section of Surgical Oncology and General Surgery, Department of Surgery, University of Calgary, Cumming School of Medicine, Calgary, AB, Canada
e-mail: Janice.pasieka@ahs.ca

A. Shifrin (ed.), *Atlas of Thyroid Surgery*, https://doi.org/10.1007/978-3-030-93673-0_4

Positioning

Surgery is performed with the patient under general anesthesia, with both arms tucked in at the sides, protecting the ulnar nerve. Cervical extension is achieved using a shoulder roll placed at the level of the scapular spines. Slight reverse Trendelenburg with knee flexion reduces venous pressure.

Table 4.1 Minimize the risks of a completion thyroidectomy

1. Be consistent in your operative approach and document the status of the parathyroids, EBSLN, and RLN in the operative report.
2. Remove the pyramidal lobe and pretracheal nodal tissue during the initial operation as this plane will become scarred down and may prove to be more difficult to dissect at the second operation.
3. Resect thyroid lobe and isthmus over to the edge of the contralateral strap muscle, leaving the midline of the trachea free of thyroid tissue.
4. Assess/confirm parathyroid viability and transplant devascularized glands.
5. Do not explore the contralateral thyroid and be sure to leave the sternothyroid muscle on the contralateral thyroid lobe.
6. Reapproximate separately both the sternothyroid and sternohyoid strap muscles at the midline.

Obtaining Exposure

A cervical skin incision is created in the midline approximately 2 fingerbreadths above the collar bone and extending from the anterior border of one sternocleidomastoid muscle (SCM) to the other, ideally in a natural crease for cosmesis (Fig. 4.2). The skin, subcutaneous tissues, and platysma are divided sharply with the knife. Subplatysmal flaps are developed in an avascular plane from the thyroid cartilage superiorly, the sternal notch inferiorly, and the anterior borders of the SCM laterally (Fig. 4.3). A device such as a Gelpi retractor is placed within the incision to maintain exposure.

The midline between the strap muscles is divided from the thyroid cartilage to the sternal notch and down to the level of the thyroid gland (Fig. 4.4). The sternohyoid muscle is elevated off the sternothyroid muscle laterally to the jugular vein (Fig. 4.5). The sternothyroid muscle overtop the thyroid is assessed for evidence of cancer invasion, and en bloc resection of the sternothyroid is performed if required. If there is no sternothyroid invasion, this muscle is elevated off the thyroid lobe with cautery. The sternothyroid can be

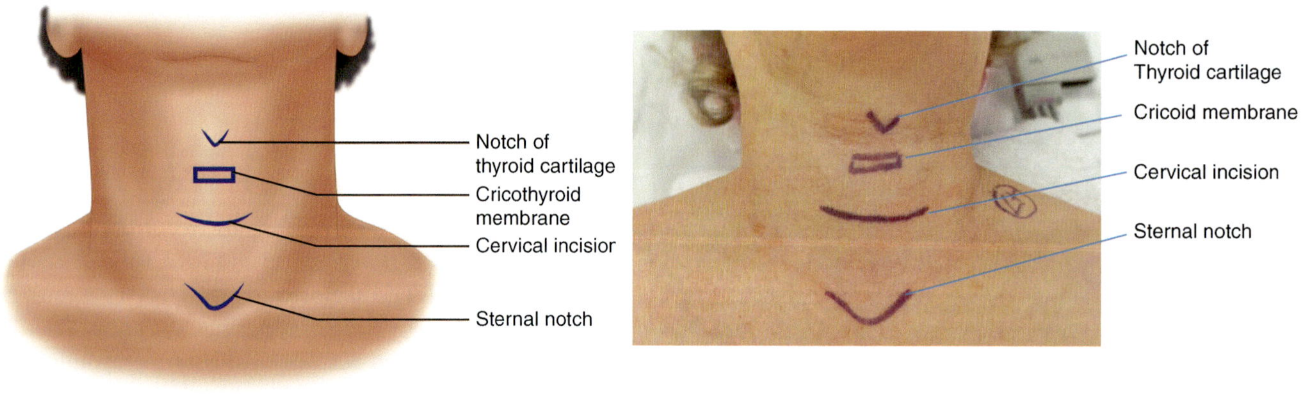

Fig. 4.2 Cervical incision and landmarks

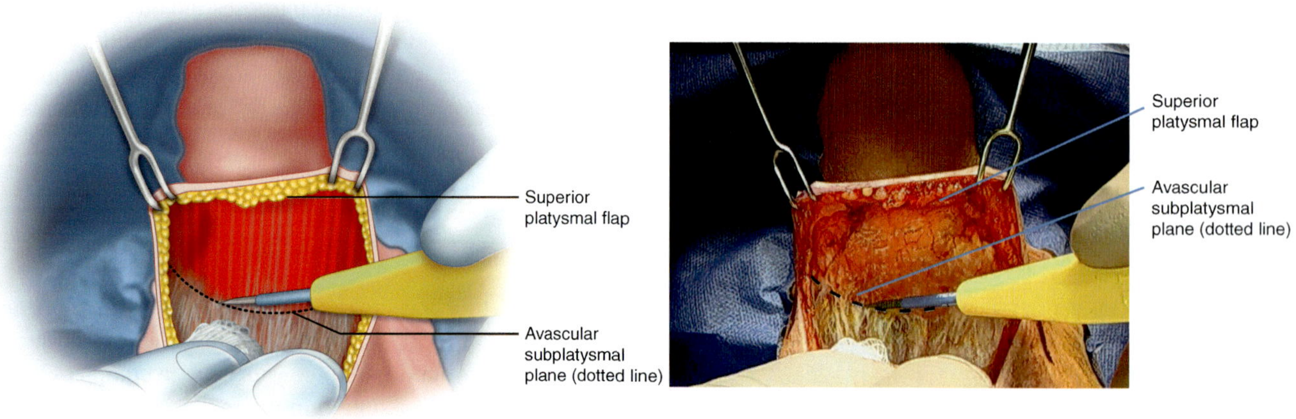

Fig. 4.3 Creation of superior subplatysmal flap

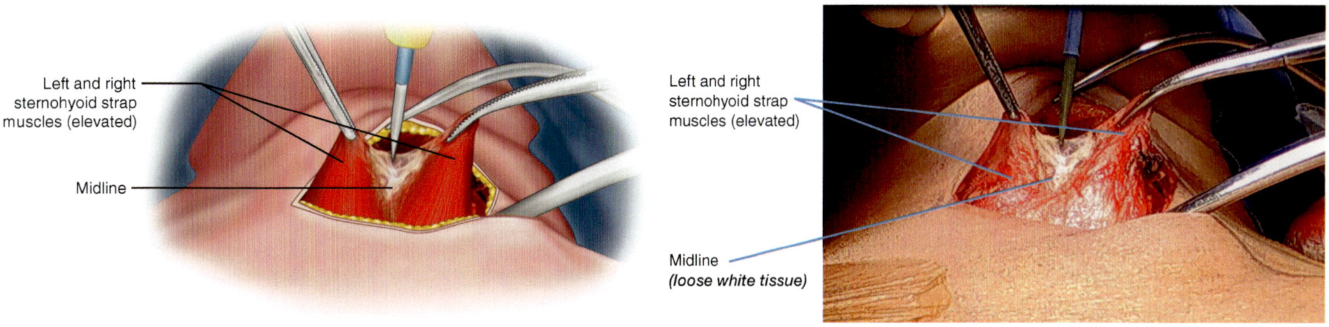

Fig. 4.4 Divide the strap muscles along the midline

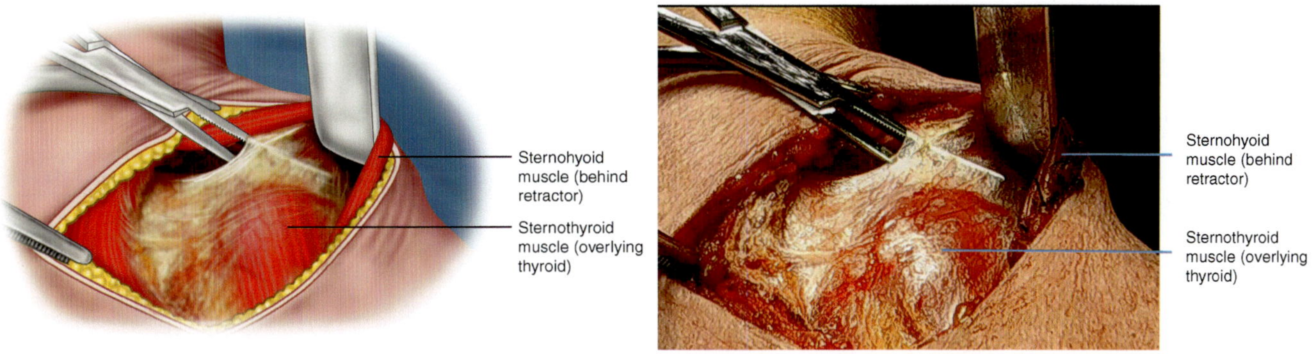

Fig. 4.5 Separate the sternohyoid from the sternothyroid muscles

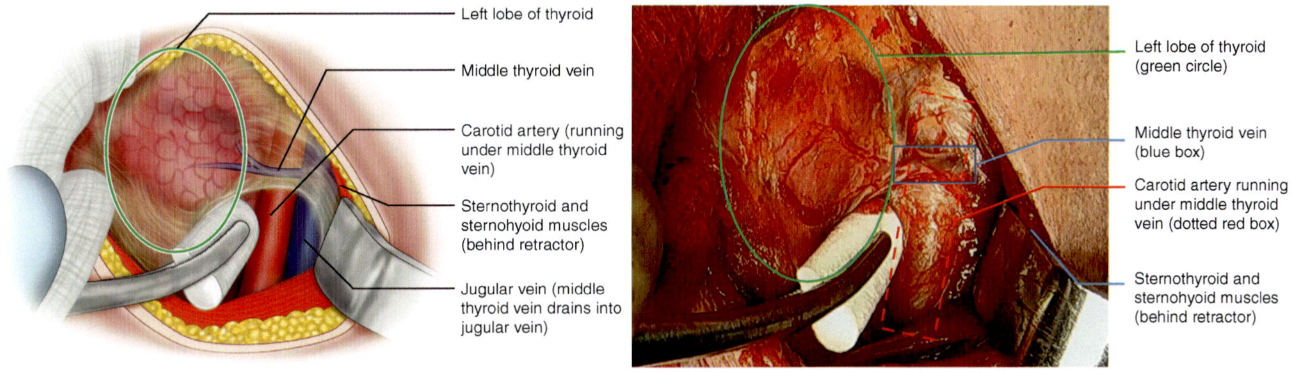

Fig. 4.6 Identify the middle thyroid vein crossing over the carotid artery

divided to improve access if the thyroid lobe or nodule is very large. The middle thyroid vein is then identified crossing over the carotid artery (Fig. 4.6), divided, and ligated.

Identification of the Recurrent Laryngeal Nerve

Once the middle thyroid vein is divided, the RLN should be identified. The RLN bisects the angle formed by the inferior thyroid artery entering the thyroid and the lateral edge of the trachea. The identification of these landmarks is helpful in finding the RLN (Fig. 4.7). The lack of RLN identification leads to a higher risk of injury, and thus it should be routinely identified [5].

Identification and Inclusion of Pyramidal Lobe

Retractors are positioned superiorly under the left and right sternohyoid muscles, and the pyramidal lobe and pretracheal nodal tissue between the thyrohyoid muscles are

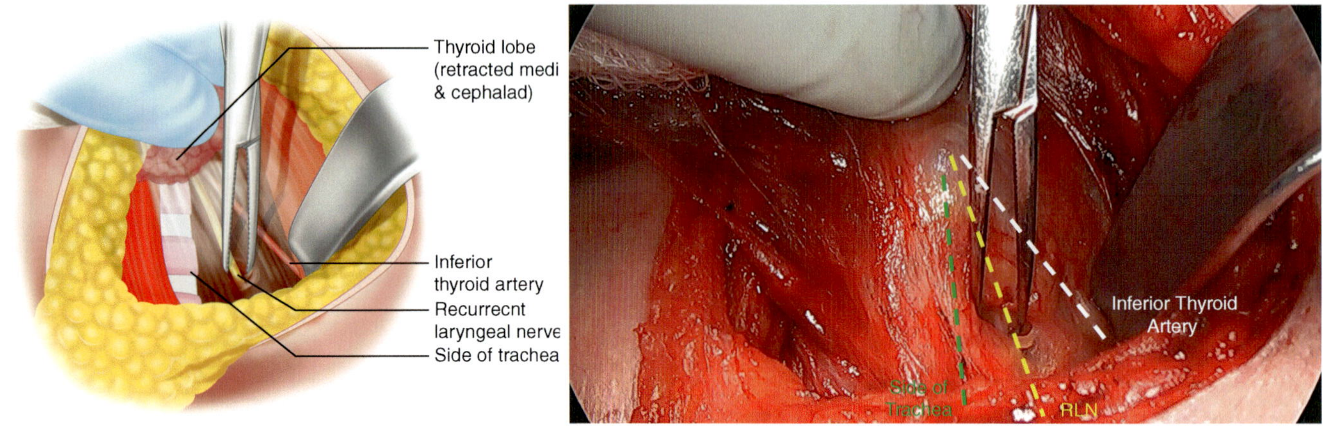

Fig. 4.7 Recurrent laryngeal nerve (RLN) bisecting the inferior thyroid artery and the side of the trachea

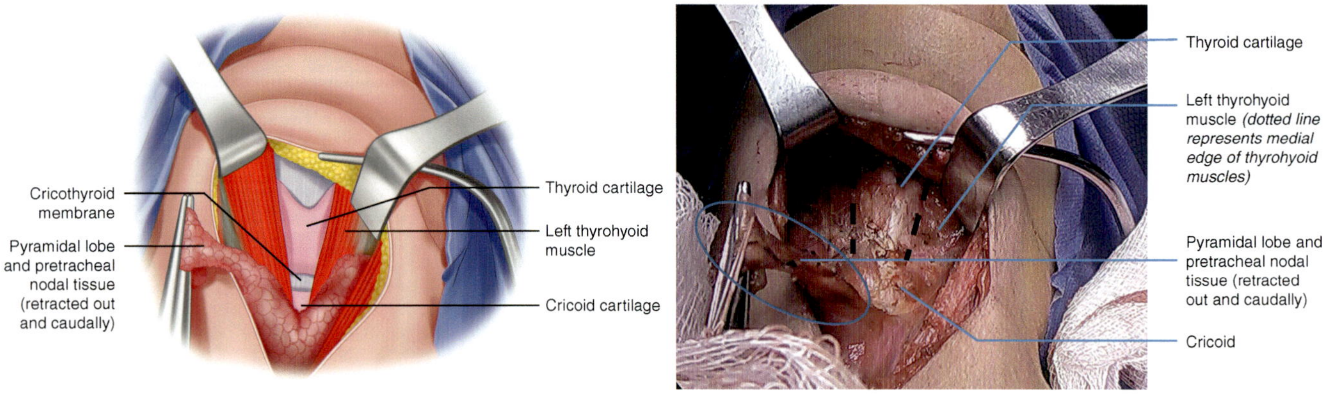

Fig. 4.8 Dissect out the pyramidal lobe and pretracheal nodal tissue

grasped and elevated. This tissue is dissected away from the thyrohyoid muscles and followed cephalad to the hyoid bone. The pyramidal lobe is ligated at the level of the hyoid bone. Then the pyramidal lobe and pretracheal nodal tissue are dissected off the tracheal cartilage and cricothyroid membrane down to the cricothyroid muscles, taking care not to injure the delicate cricothyroid membrane. The pyramidal lobe and pretracheal nodal tissue are included with the specimen (Fig. 4.8) and should be resected at the initial operation to improve reoperative exposure if completion of thyroidectomy is required.

Mobilization of the Superior Pole

Identify and open the avascular space of Reeves located between the superior pole of the thyroid and the cricothyroid muscles (Fig. 4.9). This assists with the traction of the superior pole into the surgical field. The maneuver also allows for the identification of the EBSLN as it enters the cricothyroid muscle. This nerve should be looked for, but unlike the RLN, it is not essential to identify it. The EBSLN is seen up to 70% of the time with careful dissection. Ligating the superior pole vessels as they enter the thyroid will help preserve the EBSLN, especially when it has not been visualized (Fig. 4.10) [6].

The investing fascia over the thyroid is divided to expose the lateral edge of the thyroid (Fig. 4.11). The lateral thyroid is mobilized using an extracapsular approach (remaining just outside the thyroid capsule), which facilitates the identification and preservation of the parathyroid glands contained within the adjacent fat pads. The superior parathyroid is typically located 1 cm around the inferior thyroid artery as it enters the thyroid and along the posterior aspect of the thyroid lobe (Fig. 4.12).

Mobilization of the Inferior Pole

The reidentification of the RLN is crucial prior to proceeding with the mobilization of the inferior pole. The inferior parathyroid can often be identified at this time, looking closely at the inferior pole of the thyroid and along the thyrothymic ligament (Fig. 4.13). Once these

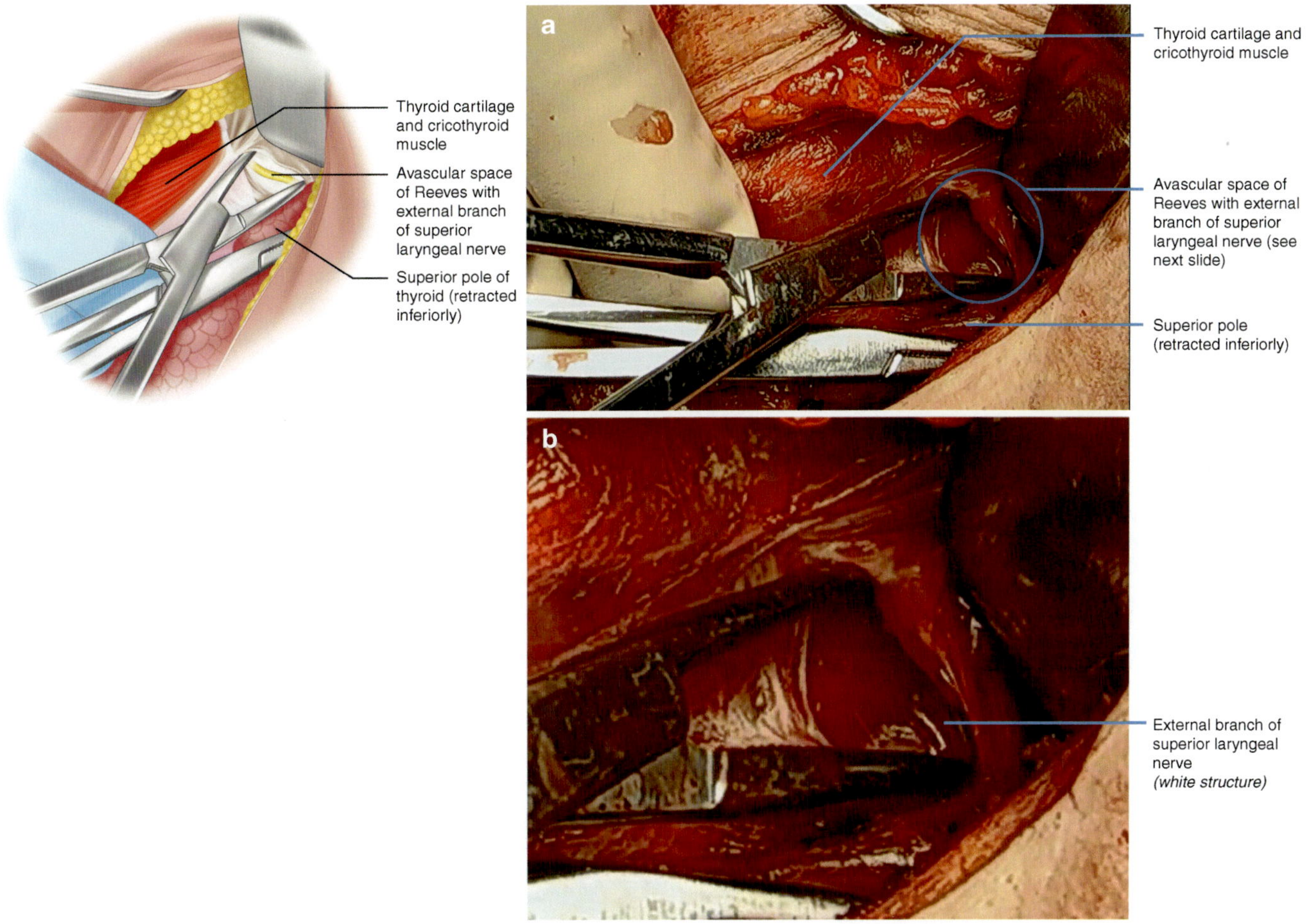

Fig. 4.9 (**a**, **b**) Develop the avascular space of Reeves and identify the external branch of the superior laryngeal nerve

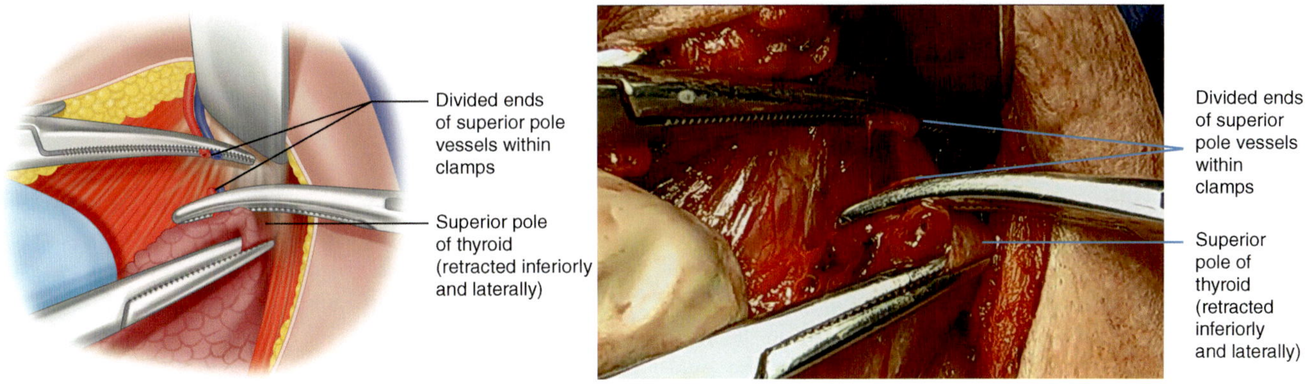

Fig. 4.10 Divide the superior pole vessels

structures are identified it is safe to dissect directly down onto the trachea at the midline and divide the inferior pole vessels. If pretracheal lymph nodes are required, then the level of dissection starts at the sternal notch. The vessels entering the inferior thyroid pole are divided using an extracapsular approach to protect the inferior parathyroid and RLN.

Medialization of the Thyroid

The RLN is at the highest risk during the part of the operation where it enters close to the cricothyroid muscle as it is tethered by the very vascular ligament of Berry. The dissection continues along the anterior surface of the RLN, dividing the branches of the inferior thyroid artery

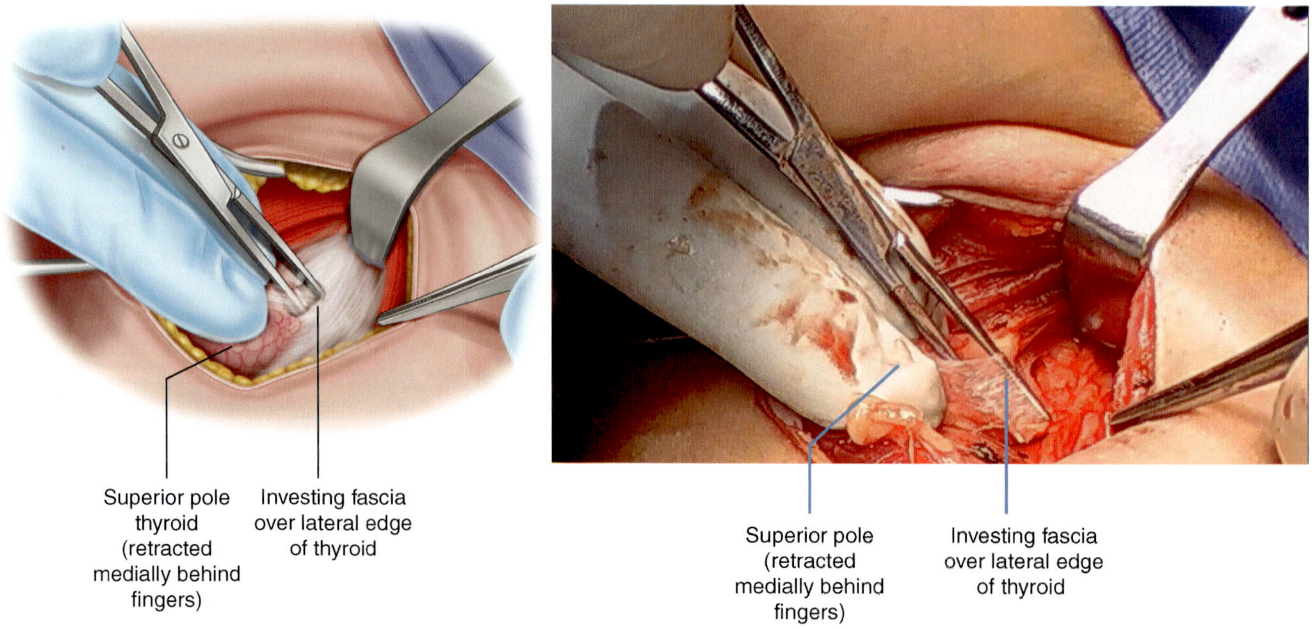

Fig. 4.11 Division of the investing fascia around the lateral edge of the superior pole

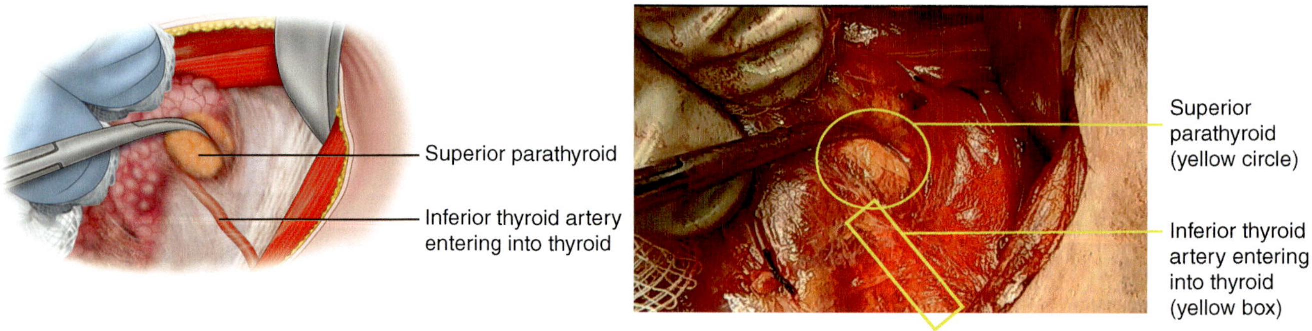

Fig. 4.12 Identify the superior parathyroid gland located within 1 cm radius superior to the insertion of inferior thyroid artery

that are crossing over the RLN into the thyroid. In 10–20% of patients, the RLN crosses over-top the inferior thyroid artery. The RLN frequently branches, and it is the medial branch that is usually responsible for vocal cord motor function [7]. The ligament of Berry is quite vascular, and the control of the vessels within the ligament should be performed using bipolar cautery or ties. Monopolar cautery and other energy devices should be avoided or utilized with caution in this area due to the proximity of the RLN. Once the ligament of Berry is detached, an avascular plane anterior to the trachea is encountered (Fig. 4.14). The thyroid and isthmus are elevated off the trachea over to the contralateral lobe. Be careful not to elevate the contralateral lobe off the trachea as you can injure the contralateral RLN at its insertion. The left lobe and isthmus are divided at the level of the contralateral strap muscles through various techniques such as using advanced hemostasis devices (i.e., Harmonic scalpel) or clamping and oversewing the cut edge with a running locking stitch.

Parathyroid Assessment and Transplantation

Once the thyroid lobe and isthmus are resected, the thyroid specimen should be inspected for devascularized parathyroid glands. It is important to assess the superior and inferior parathyroid glands to ensure viability. If in situ viability is uncertain, the surface of the parathyroid gland can be scored with a fresh sharp scalpel to look for arterial bleeding. If the parathyroid gland is completely devascularized, excise the gland and transplant it. If there is questionable viability, then

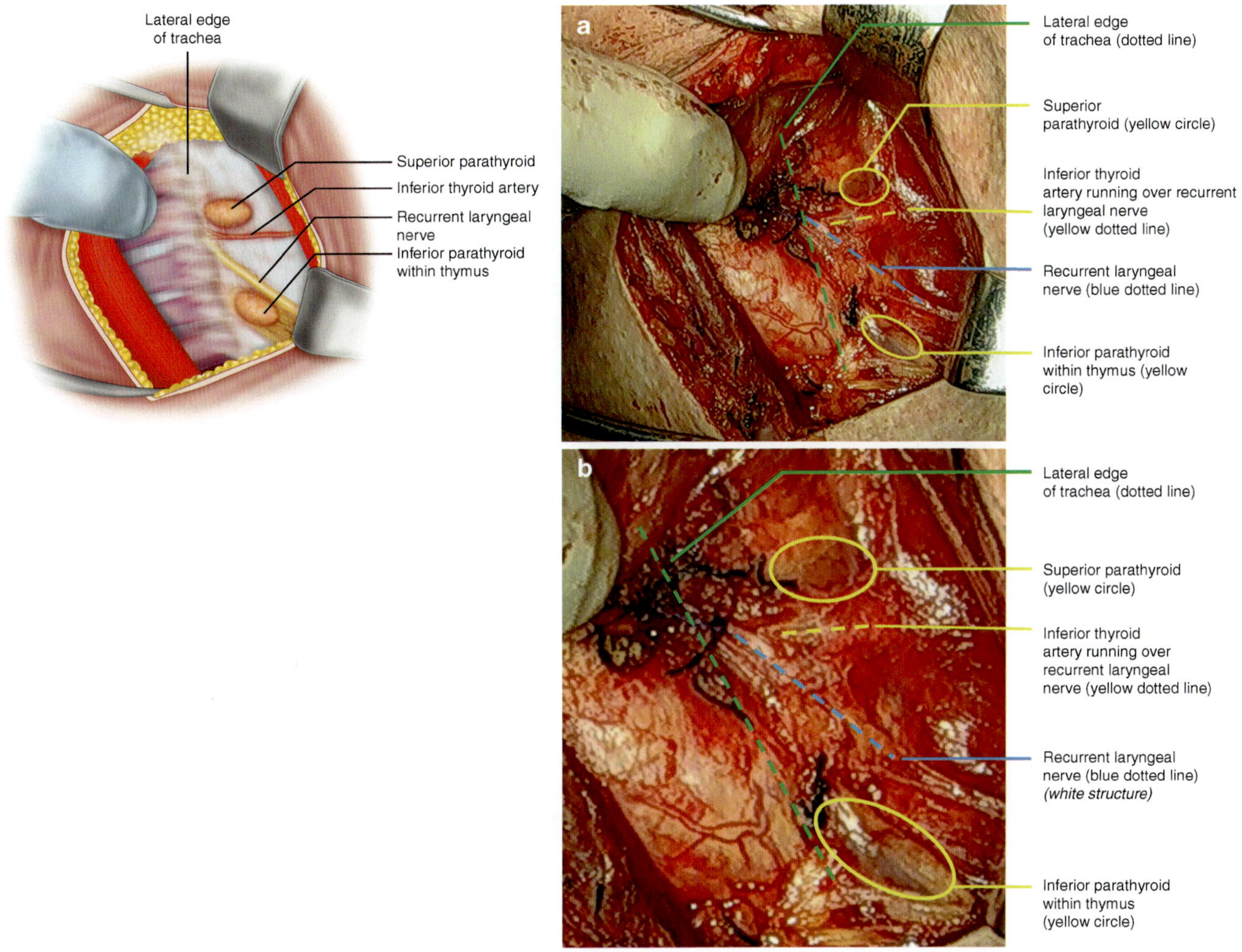

Fig. 4.13 (**a**, **b**) Location of RLN, superior and inferior parathyroid glands

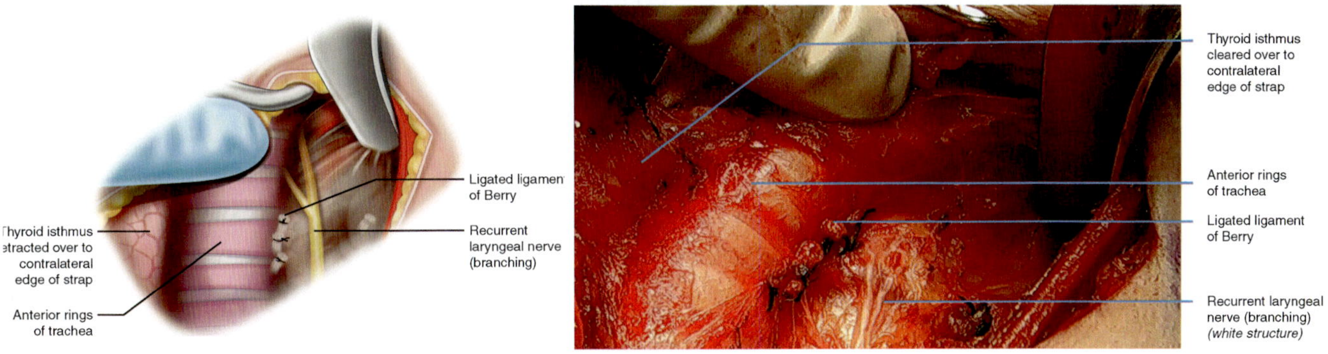

Fig. 4.14 Visualization of the RLN, ligated ligament of Berry, and anterior trachea

bisect the gland and transplant the excised portion while preserving the other half in situ, ensuring it is attached to the vascular pedicle. To transplant the parathyroid tissue, it should be emulsified. We prefer to use the sharp curved iris scissors on a piece of Telfa (Fig. 4.15). The emulsified parathyroid is drawn up in a saline-filled syringe (Fig. 4.16) and injected into the SCM (Fig. 4.17). Flush the needle with an additional 0.5 ml of saline into the muscle to ensure the needle is cleared of any parathyroid tissue. Prior to injecting the emulsified parathyroid, draw back on the syringe to ensure

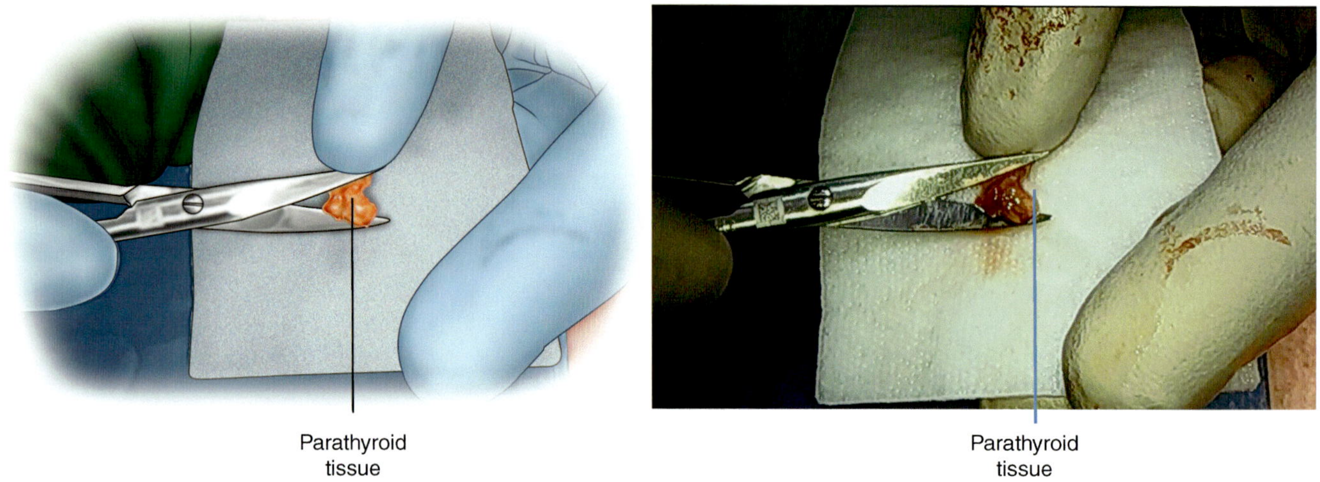

Fig. 4.15 Emulsify the parathyroid

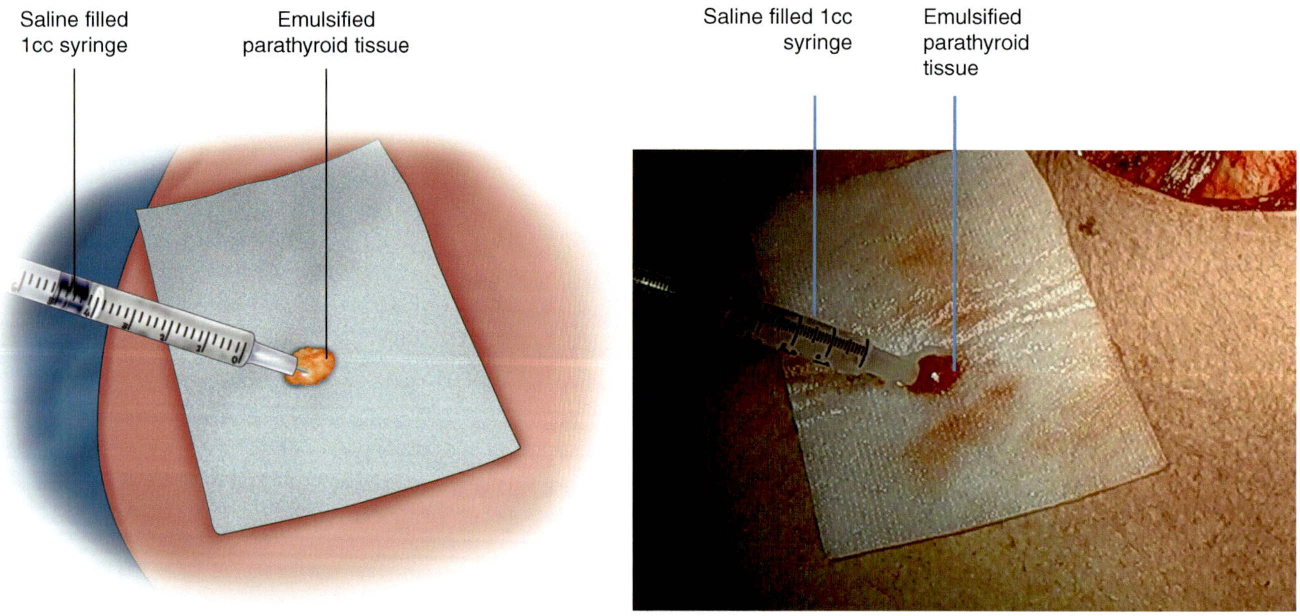

Fig. 4.16 Prepare the parathyroid for reimplantation

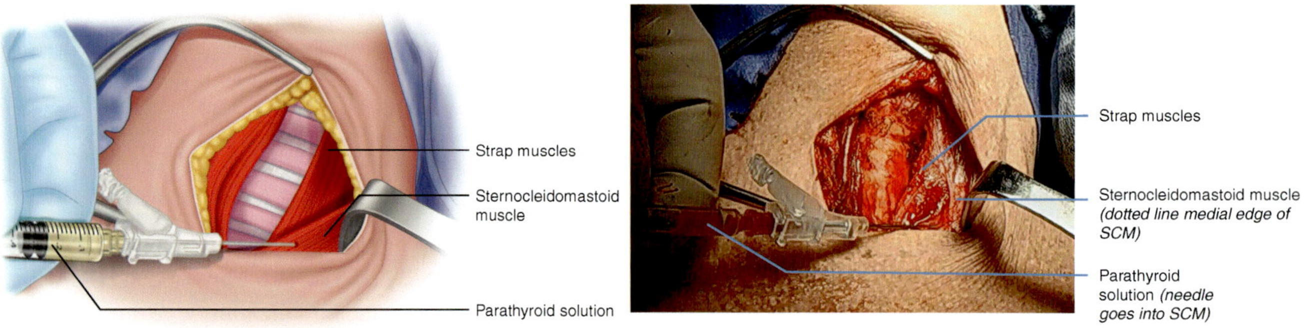

Fig. 4.17 Inject the parathyroid into the SCM

that it is not within the jugular vein. It is important to document the status of the parathyroids in the operative report.

Closure

Ensure good hemostasis prior to closure. The elevation of venous pressure (i.e., a Valsalva maneuver) or irrigation with sterile water may help identify small vessels at risk of bleeding [8]. Reapproximate both strap muscles individually at the midline, leaving a small gap inferiorly. Reapproximate the platysma in an interrupted fashion. Skin can be closed using a variety of techniques, including a dissolvable running subcuticular stitch or Dermabond.

Tips and Pitfalls

- A slightly longer incision in a skin crease leads to better cosmetic outcomes and less operative struggle than a shorter incision that is stretched to accommodate the surgery. Likewise developing broad flaps laterally will improve exposure and ease of surgery.
- Identifying and including the pyramidal lobe at the start of the case gives better tissue purchase, removes the pretracheal nodes, and prevents it from becoming the "forgotten lobe."
- Staying close to the thyroid in an extracapsular approach protects the critical structures (parathyroids, RLN, EBSLN). Watch for fat pads as the parathyroids are often contained within. Meticulous hemostasis prevents blood from staining the tissues and aids in the visualization of the parathyroid glands.
- The identification and protection of the RLN are critical to preventing injury. Occasionally, a near-total thyroid lobectomy (leaving a small cuff of the thyroid) adjacent to the RLN is necessary to avoid injury to the RLN and/or to protect the superior parathyroid. Using clips for hemostasis near the nerve may interfere with the ability to suture ligate bleeding from the ligament of Berry or distort postoperative imaging and therefore should be used sparingly in this area.
- Loop magnification aids in the identification of vital structures.

References

1. Stathatos N. Thyroid physiology. Med Clin. 2012;96(2):165–73.
2. Kester MH, Martinez de Mena R, Obregon MJ, Marinkovic D, Howatson A, Visser TJ, Hume R, Morreale de Escobar G. Iodothyronine levels in the human developing brain: major regulatory roles of iodothyronine deiodinases in different areas. J Clin Endocrinol Metab. 2004;89(7):3117–28.
3. Braun EM, Windisch G, Wolf G, Hausleitner L, Anderhuber F. The pyramidal lobe: clinical anatomy and its importance in thyroid surgery. Surg Radiol Anat. 2007;29(1):21–7.
4. Patel KN, Yip L, Lubitz CC, Grubbs EG, Miller BS, Shen W, Angelos P, Chen H, Doherty GM, Fahey TJ III, Kebebew E. The American Association of Endocrine Surgeons Guidelines for the definitive surgical management of thyroid disease in adults. Ann Surg. 2020;271(3):e21–93.
5. Hisham AN, Lukman MR. Recurrent laryngeal nerve in thyroid surgery: a critical appraisal. ANZ J Surg. 2002;72(12):887–9.
6. Potenza AS, Araujo Filho VJ, Cernea CR. Injury of the external branch of the superior laryngeal nerve in thyroid surgery. Gland Surg. 2017;6(5):552.
7. Makay O, Icoz G, Yilmaz M, Akyildiz M, Yetkin E. The recurrent laryngeal nerve and the inferior thyroid artery—anatomical variations during surgery. Langenbeck Arch Surg. 2008;393(5):681–5.
8. Edafe O, Cochrane E, Balasubramanian SP. Reoperation for bleeding after thyroid and parathyroid surgery: incidence, risk factors, prevention, and management. World J Surg. 2020;44(4):1156–62.

Total Thyroidectomy

5

Ujas S. Shah, Kristina J. Nicholson, and Sally E. Carty

Introduction

The patient presents with a single thyroid nodule that was positive for malignancy on biopsy, and with positive molecular testing, a total thyroidectomy was planned. The usual steps of this procedure are described, along with the potential pitfalls and key aspects of perioperative care.

The patient is placed supine with adequate anterior neck extension. A transverse incision is used, and the incision is carried through the platysma. Subplatysmal flaps are created, and the median raphe is widely incised. The strap muscles are then dissected off the thyroid lobe. The blood supply to the thyroid lobe is divided between fine ties, and the parathyroid glands are identified to be preserved in situ. The recurrent laryngeal nerve is identified and cleared, with avoidance of electrocautery or other injuries. As dissection progresses, the ligament of Berry is carefully ligated near the insertion of the recurrent laryngeal nerve, and then the thyroid is dissected off the trachea. The same steps are then used on the contralateral lobe, and the specimen is resected. Hemostasis must be ensured prior to the closure of the incision in layers.

Preoperative screening for concurrent primary hyperparathyroidism is routinely done, and vitamin D is repleted preoperatively if identified. We do not routinely use intraoperative nerve monitoring, but vocal cord assessment is performed in several ways. Postoperatively, monitoring for signs of cervical hematoma is important, as is the prevention of hypocalcemia.

Supplementary Information The online version contains supplementary material available at [https://doi.org/10.1007/978-3-030-93673-0_5].

U. S. Shah · S. E. Carty
Division of Endocrine Surgery, Department of Surgery, University of Pittsburgh School of Medicine, Pittsburgh, PA, USA

K. J. Nicholson (✉)
Department of Surgery, University of Pittsburgh School of Medicine, Pittsburgh, PA, USA
e-mail: nicholsonkj@upmc.edu

Case Description

The patient is an otherwise healthy 32-year-old male with a TIRADS 5, 1.7 cm right thyroid nodule without associated lymphadenopathy on cervical ultrasound. The nodule was positive for papillary thyroid cancer on fine-needle aspiration biopsy. After informed consent and under an institutional clinical trial, it was subjected to molecular testing with ThyroSeq® version 3 to determine the extent of initial thyroidectomy. Molecular results were positive for a BRAF V600E mutation, and total thyroidectomy was planned.

Procedure

The patient is positioned supine for the induction of anesthesia by endotracheal intubation. A rolled sheet is placed behind the scapulae, and a modified beach chair position is used to best expose the anterior neck. Care is taken to ensure that the patient has no history or features of cervical disk disease. After prepping and draping, a short transverse incision is marked within a natural skin crease, ideally 1–2 cm inferior to the cricoid cartilage, using concentric lateral hatch marks in case the incision should need to be extended. Here, the incision measured 4.8 cm. Local anesthesia with 0.5% bupivacaine with 1:200,000 epinephrine is infiltrated as a subcuticular wheal in the dermis, the skin is incised with a 15-blade scalpel, and the subcutaneous tissues and platysma are divided with electrocautery, taking care to preserve the anterior jugular veins. A Senn retractor is used to elevate the subplatysmal flaps superiorly and inferiorly using blunt dissection and electrocautery; this step facilitates excellent postoperative cosmesis (Figs. 5.1, 5.2, and 5.3).

The median raphe is then incised up to the thyroid cartilage and down to the sternal notch, and a self-retaining Weitlaner retractor is placed. It is preferable to begin the dissection on the side of the cancer, in this case the right side, but this is not mandatory in every setting. As the strap muscles are dissected off the lobe, care must be taken to widely

A. Shifrin (ed.), *Atlas of Thyroid Surgery*, https://doi.org/10.1007/978-3-030-93673-0_5

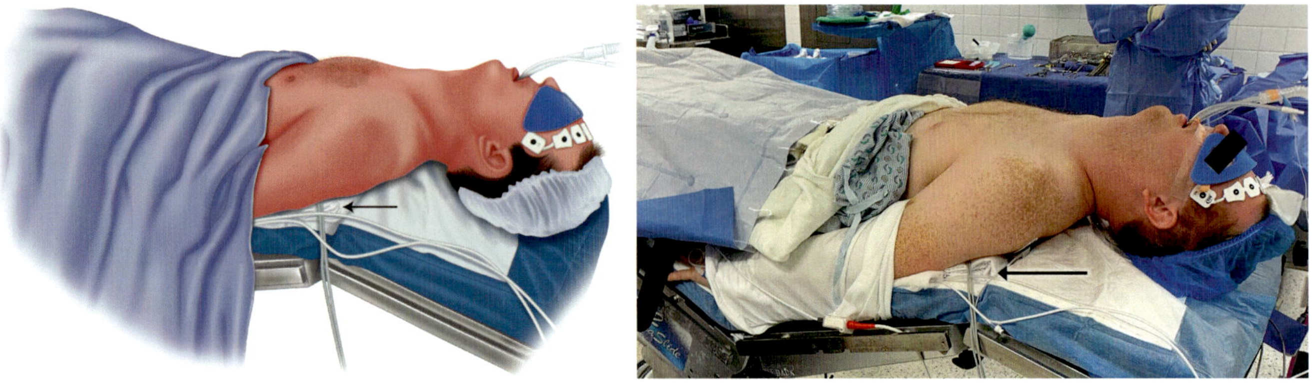

Fig. 5.1 Modified beach chair positioning with a rolled sheet as a shoulder roll (solid arrow) for adequate neck extension

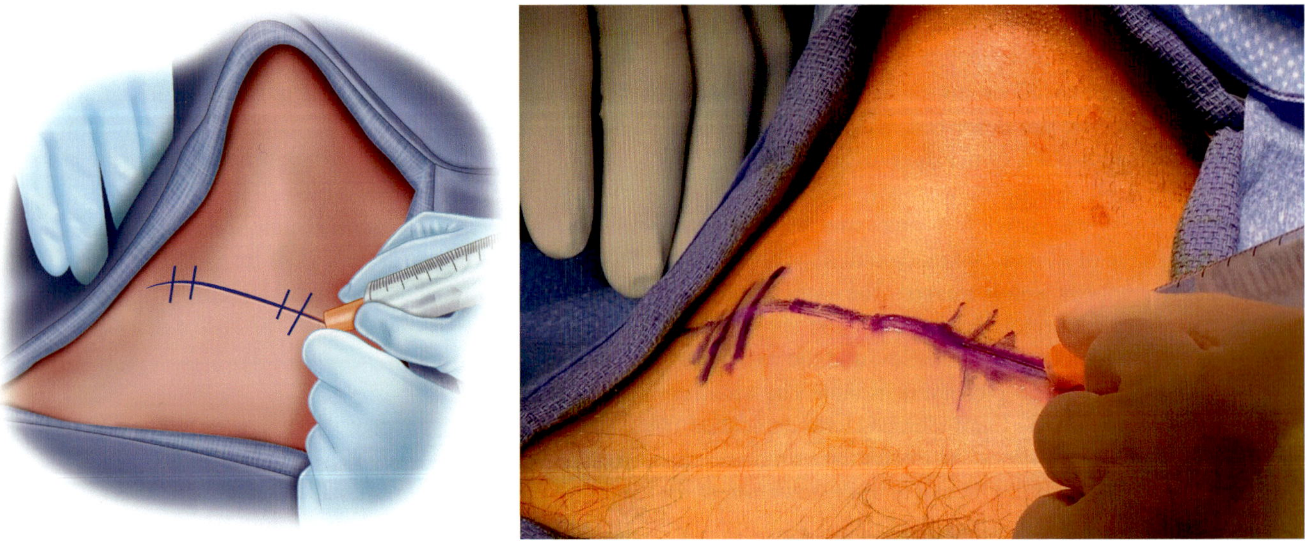

Fig. 5.2 Infiltration of subcuticular local anesthesia

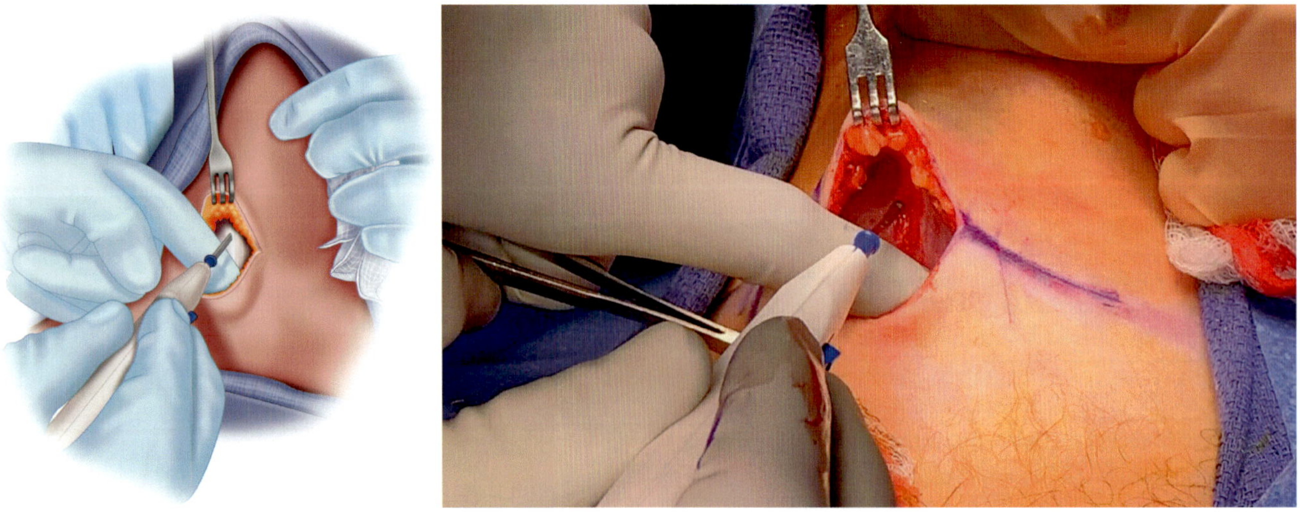

Fig. 5.3 Superior subplatysmal flap elevated with a combination of blunt dissection and electrocautery

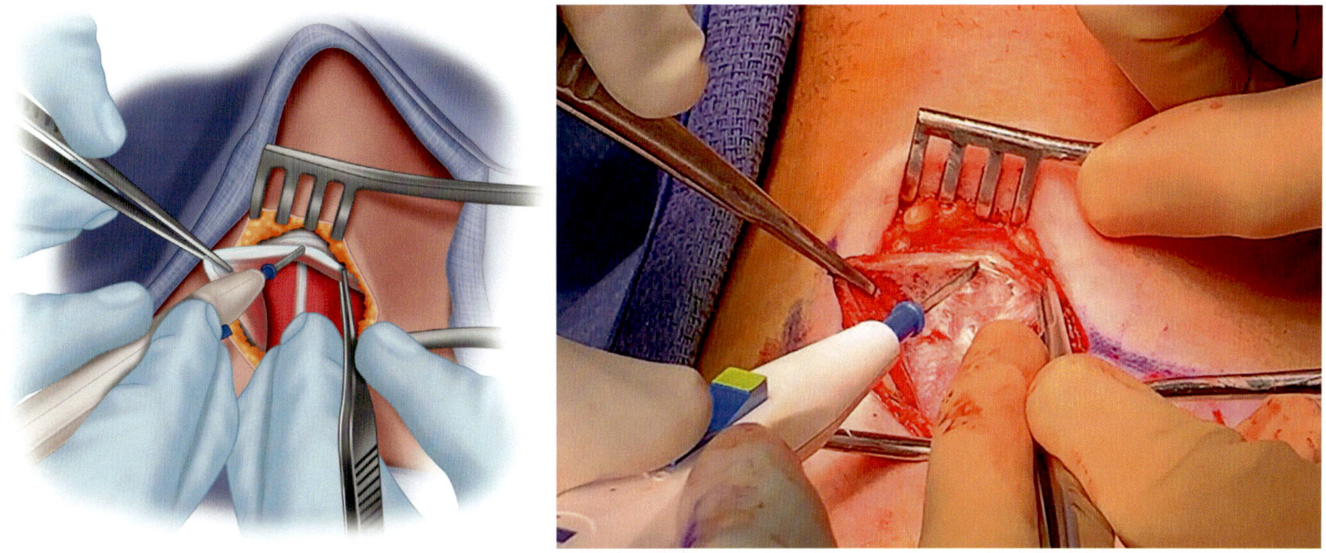

Fig. 5.4 Division of the median raphe superiorly toward the thyroid cartilage

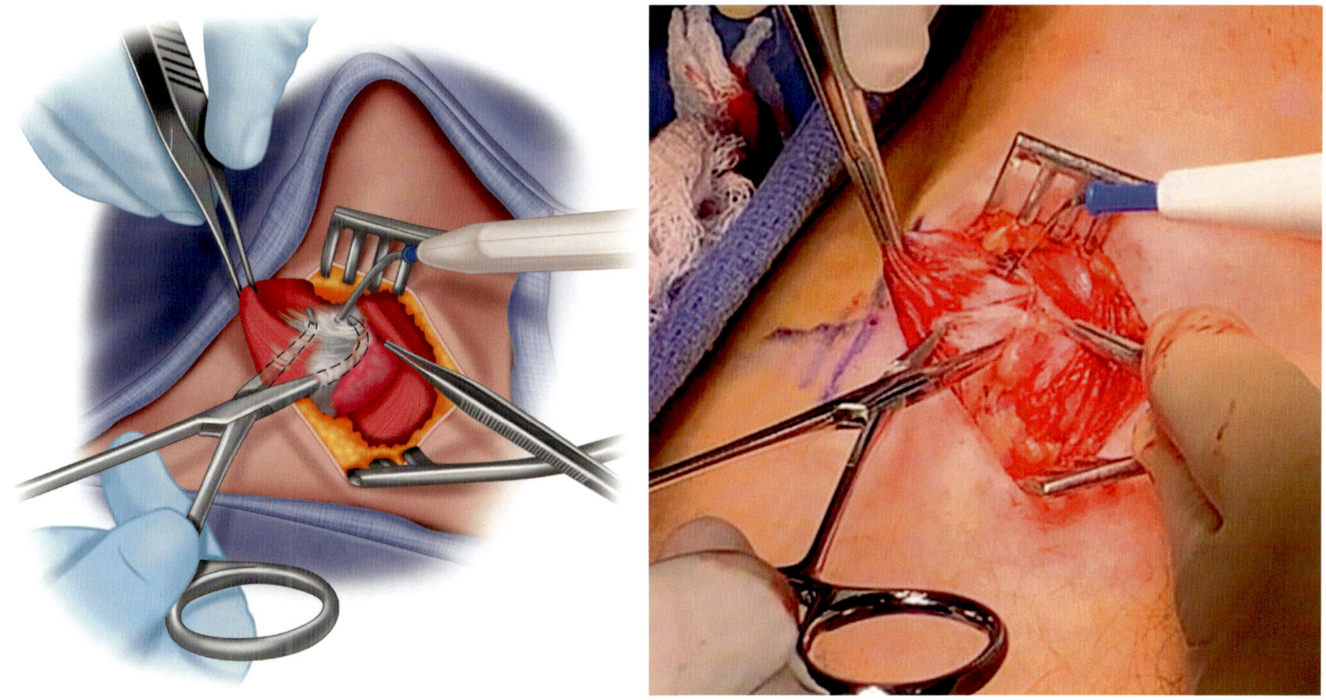

Fig. 5.5 Dissection of the right sternothyroid strap muscle from the thyroid gland

open the dissecting instrument (here a Mixter right-angle forceps) in order to prevent electrocautery arcing, which could potentially lead to thermal injury of the ipsilateral recurrent laryngeal nerve (RLN). When possible, lateral dissection should extend along the lateral strap muscle line to ensure that the surrounding lymphatic tissue remains with the thyroid specimen. This is called "opening the box" (Figs. 5.4 and 5.5).

During initial exposure of the lobe, (1) a manual Richardson retractor is placed laterally, (2) two Allis clamps are applied in parallel to facilitate medial rotation of the lobe while avoiding capsular disruption, and (3) the bed is tilted slightly to best bring the field into the light (i.e., the table is rotated slightly toward the contralateral lobe). As seen later in this video, with their nondominant hand, the assistant gradually everts the lobe while applying manual medial

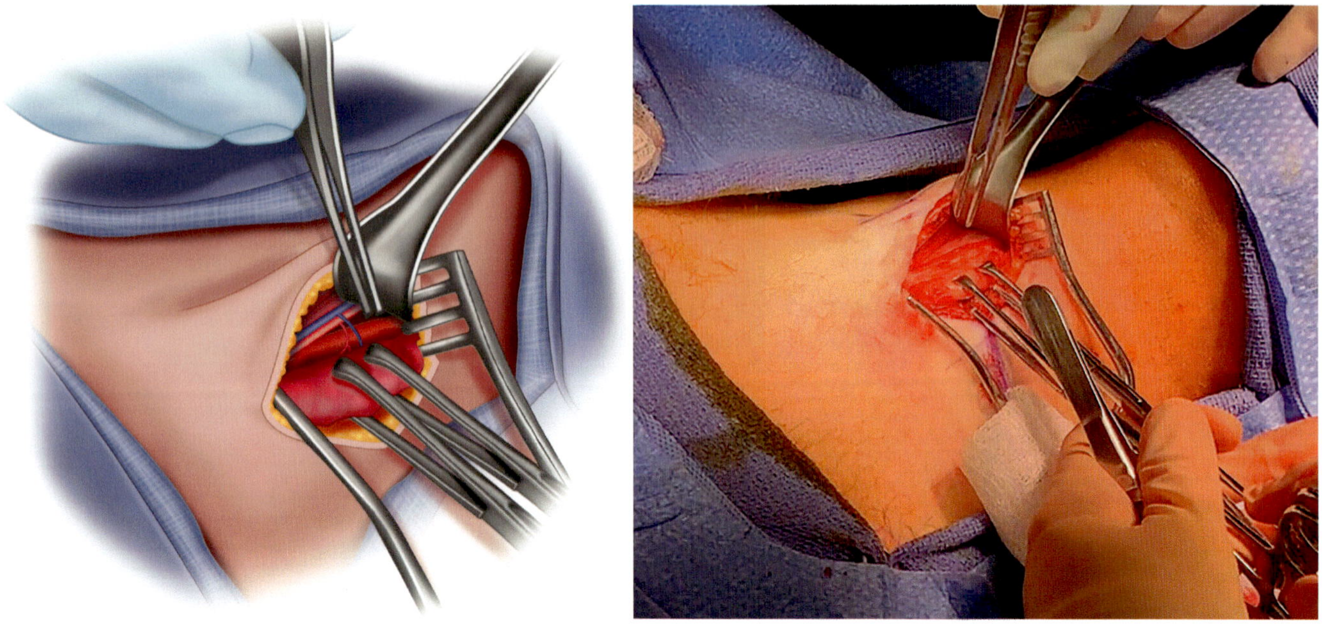

Fig. 5.6 Exposure of the right thyroid lobe with a lateral retraction of the strap muscle, medial retraction of the thyroid lobe, and tilt of the operating room table toward the left

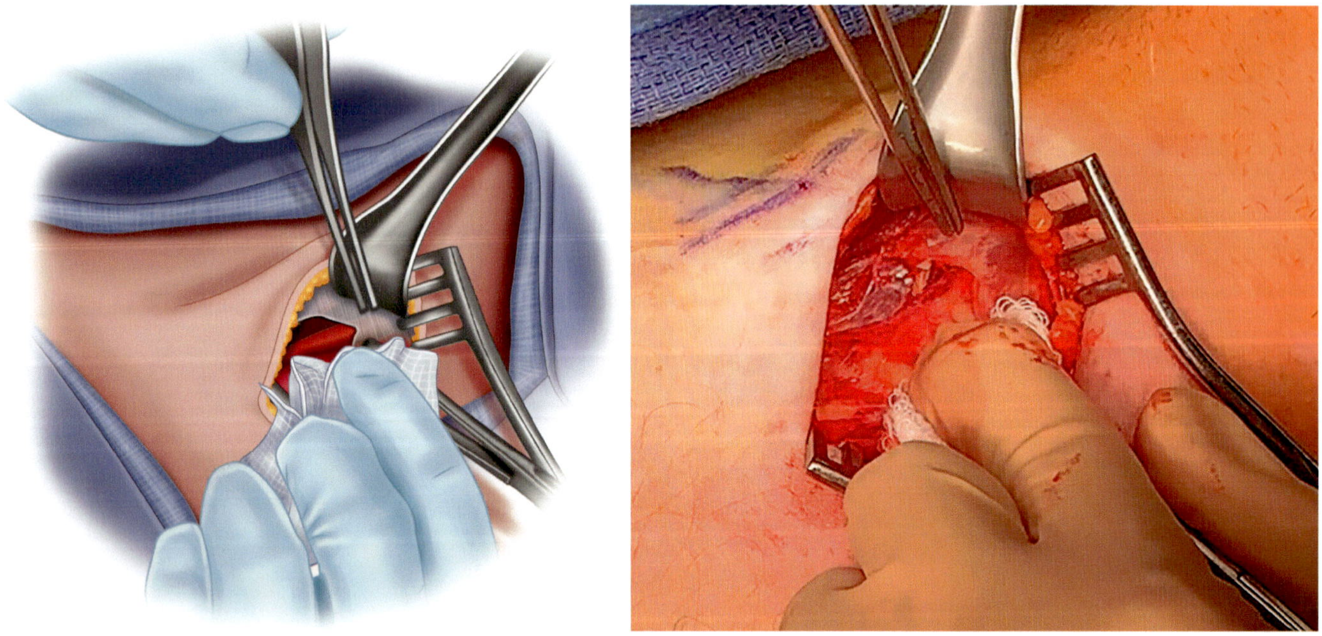

Fig. 5.7 Manual compression and eversion of the right thyroid lobe

compression, which works to improve both visualization and hemostasis (Figs. 5.6 and 5.7).

In general, as dissection progresses, the blood supply to the lobe is sequentially divided between fine ties, while the recurrent laryngeal nerve is delicately identified and cleared, and the ipsilateral parathyroid glands are recognized and preserved viably in situ. However, the specific thyroid lobe anatomy very much determines the order and conduct of these next steps—which can thus vary greatly. Often, the specific anatomy prompts early ligation of the middle thyroid vein between 4 and 0 absorbable ties, as seen here. The superior and inferior vascular pedicles are also early targets for division between ligatures. During dissection, manually thinning out the tissue helps the surgeon determine that a bite is safe to take. Electrocautery and energy devices should not be used within 1 cm of the course of the RLN. We do not use an

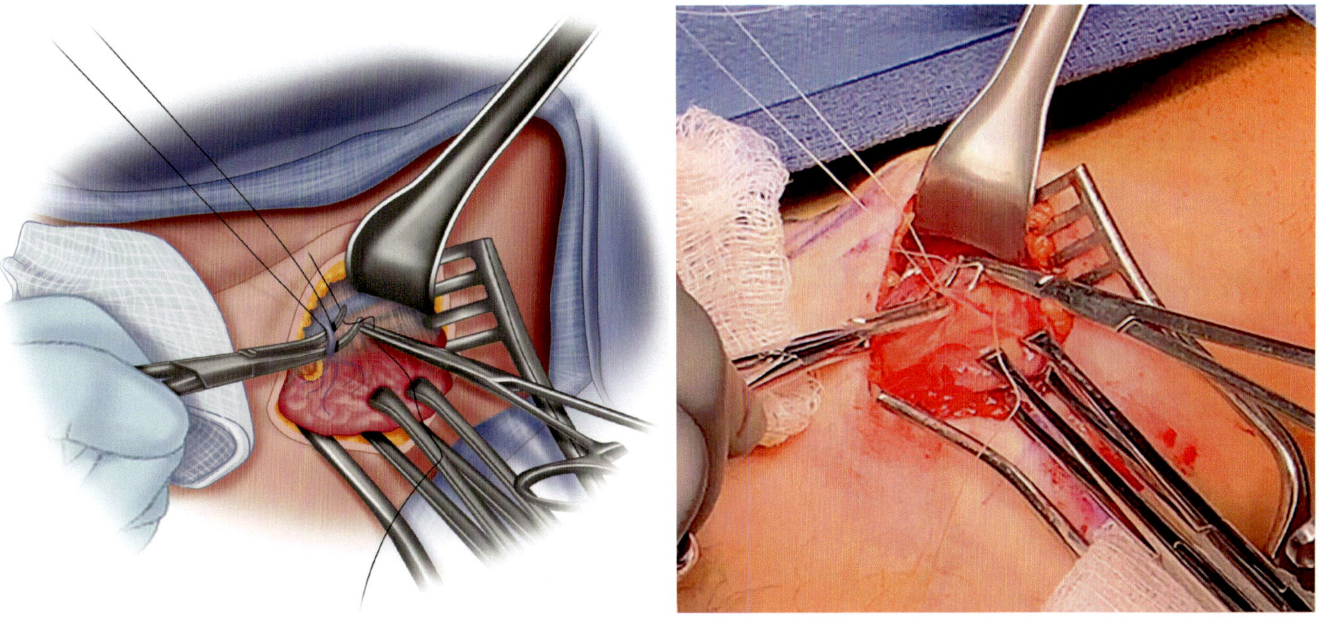

Fig. 5.8 Ligation of the middle thyroid vein between fine ties

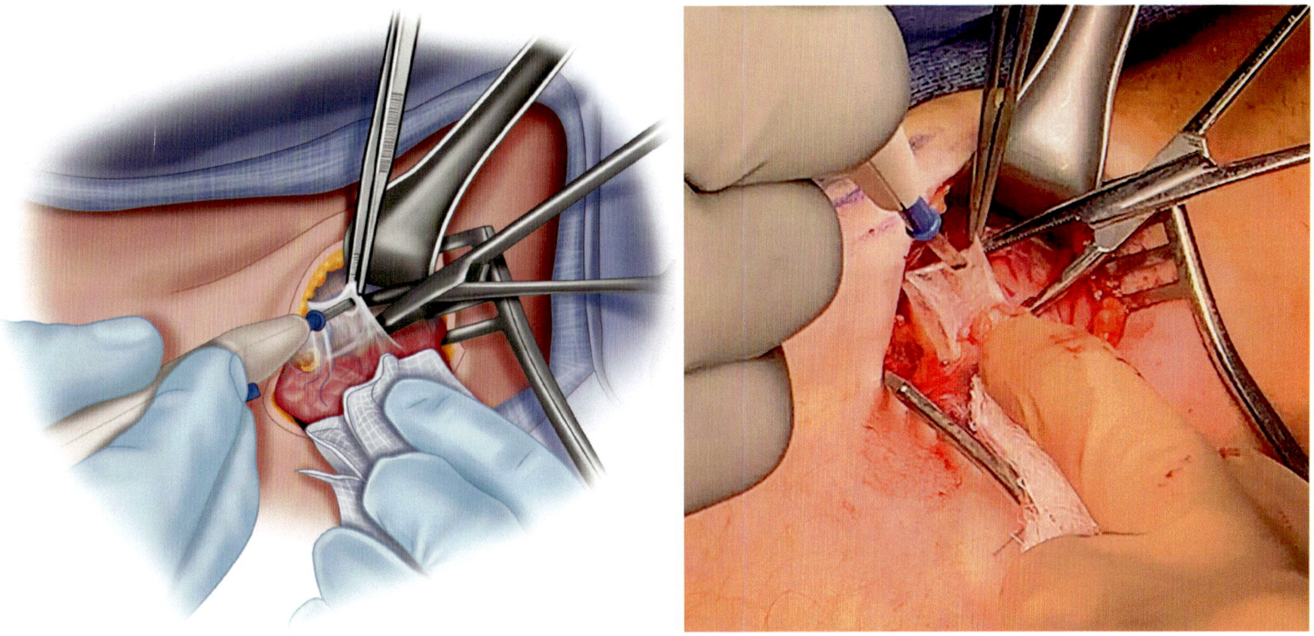

Fig. 5.9 Division of lateral attachments with electrocautery with a widely open dissector instrument to avoid thermal injury to nearby structures

energy device because of concerns of bleeding and iatrogenic injury, and we find that it does not save time as our average operative duration for a thyroid lobectomy is about 45 minutes (Figs. 5.8 and 5.9).

In this patient, the normal right inferior parathyroid gland is identified within the surrounding fat and preserved, while it was also marked with a titanium clip. This patient also has a superior thyroid pole that extends very cranially, almost to the angle of the mandible. The preservation of the external branch of the superior laryngeal nerve is routinely facilitated by dividing the superior vascular pedicle (and/or its arborizing branches) on the anterior surface of the superior thyroid pole. The estimated injury rate of the external branch of the superior laryngeal nerve is <4%. This patient also has a prominent tubercle of Zuckerkandl, which when present must be resected in full if safely possible. Here, the tubercle was rolled medially with finger traction to aid in mobilization (Figs. 5.10 and 5.11).

We can clearly see the two normal ipsilateral parathyroid glands, which are preserved and appear viable with

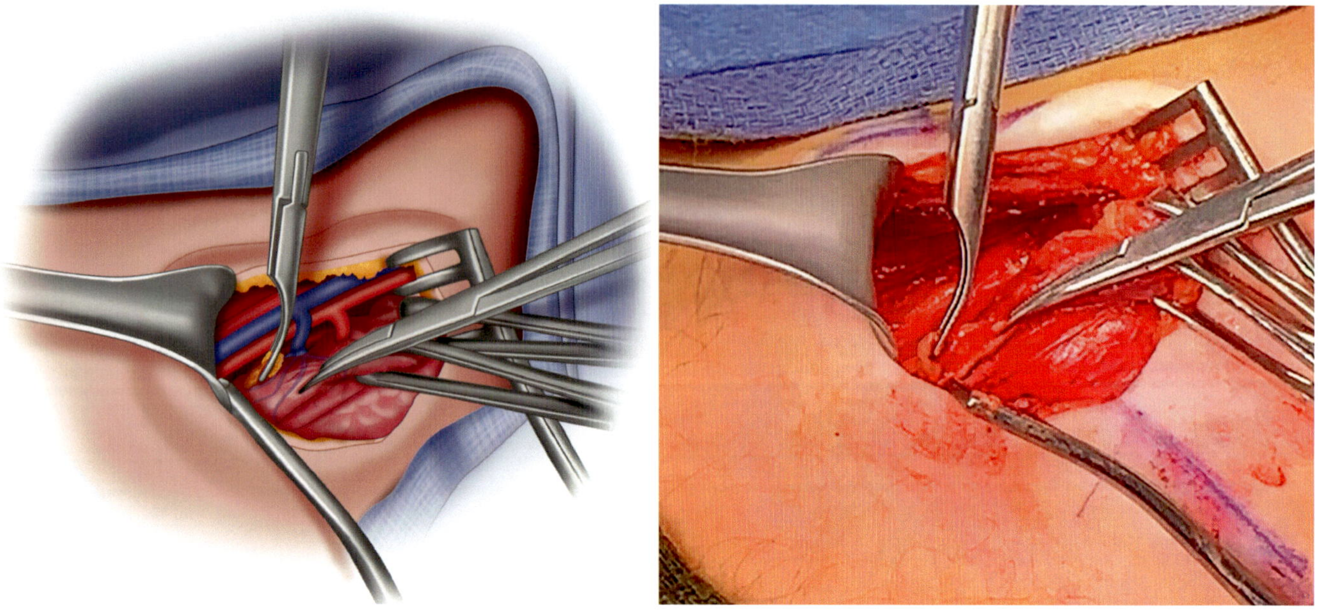

Fig. 5.10 The right inferior parathyroid gland is marked with a titanium clip

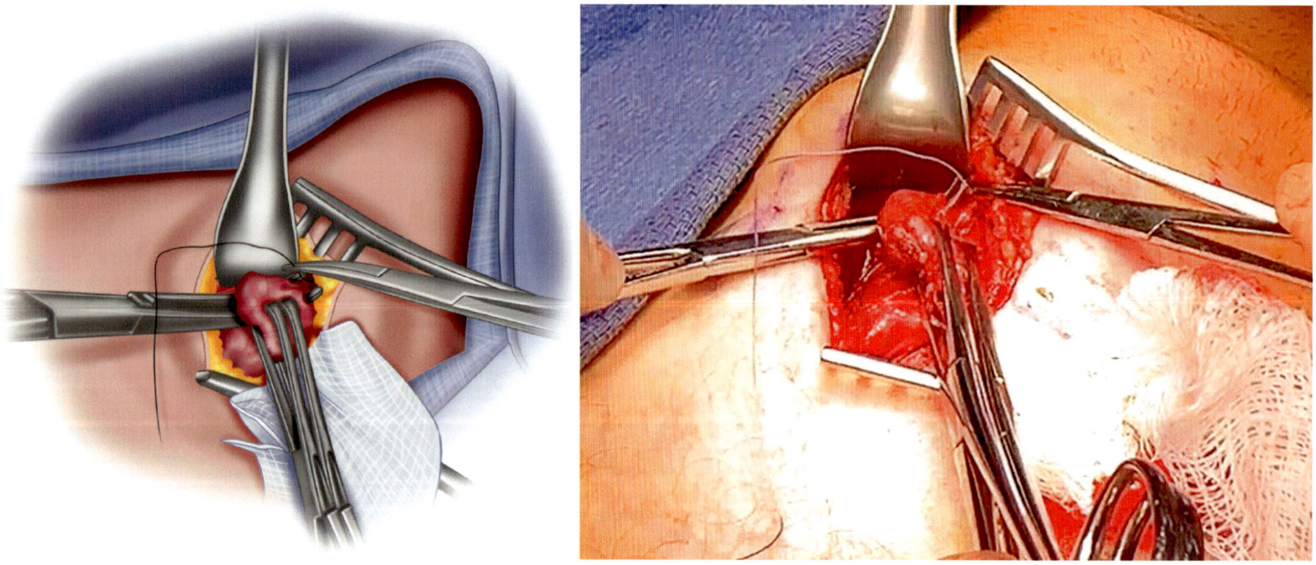

Fig. 5.11 A prominent tubercle of Zuckerkandl is carefully resected with the thyroid lobe

subtle differences in color and texture from the surrounding fat and lymph nodes. A normal parathyroid gland weighs about 20–50 mg. In general, an embryologic inferior gland is more anteriorly situated, often near the tip of the cervical thymus, while the superior parathyroid resides in a deeper plane and is often in or near the tracheoesophageal groove. If for any reason a normal parathyroid appears ischemic, it should be promptly harvested and minced sterilely into 1-mm fragments, with one fragment sent for frozen section to confirm tissue identity and the remainder autotransplanted into the ipsilateral strap or sternocleidomastoid muscle, marking that site with a permanent stitch. The likelihood of this being required in this program is <5%. The likelihood of permanent hypoparathyroidism with total thyroidectomy in this program is about 1 in 300 (Figs. 5.12, 5.13, 5.14, and 5.15).

As dissection progresses, atraumatic preservation of the RLN is facilitated by tracing its course from near the thoracic inlet into the larynx at the ligament of Berry. Here, we can see that the nerve has anterior and posterior branches. Studies have documented that it is the anterior branch that has a motor function; thus, it is imperative to preserve both branches

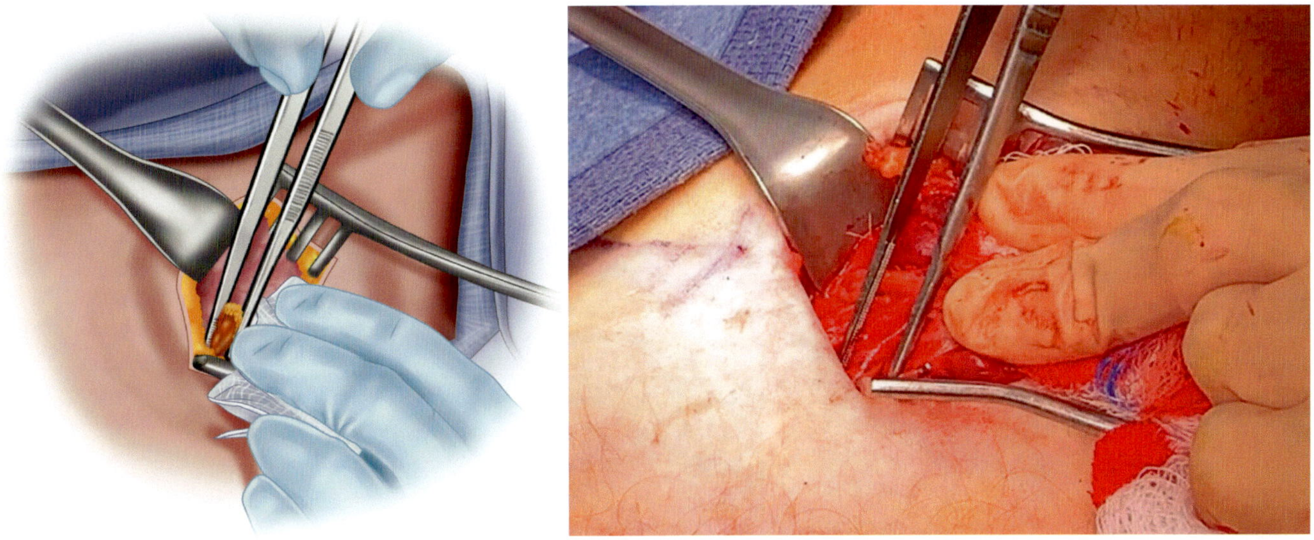

Fig. 5.12 Identification of the right inferior parathyroid gland

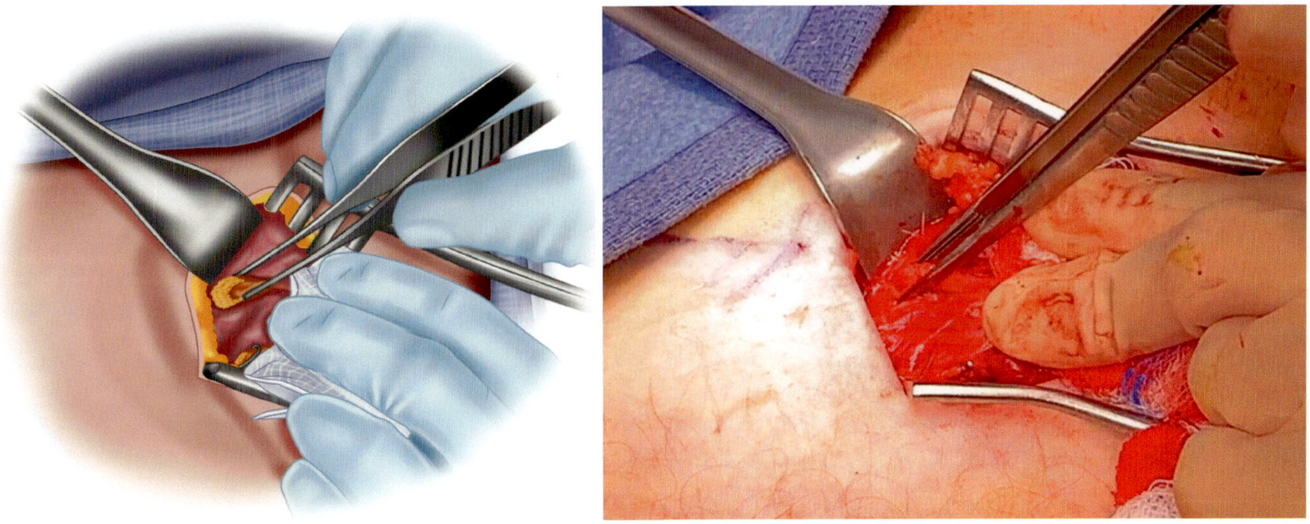

Fig. 5.13 Identification of the right superior parathyroid gland

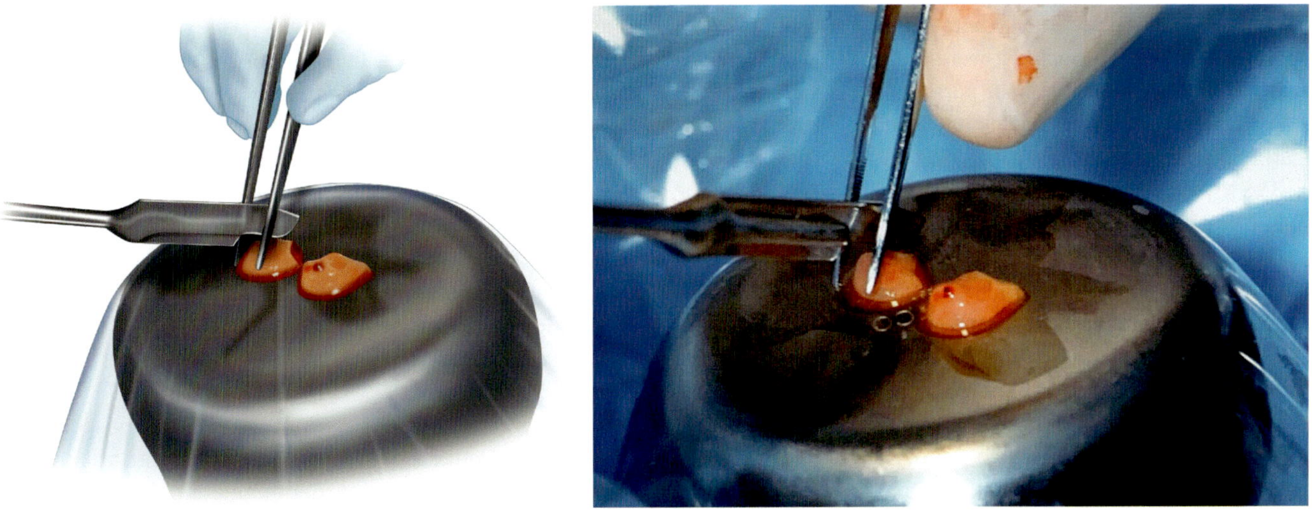

Fig. 5.14 A harvested parathyroid gland, with one fragment sent to pathology to confirm identity

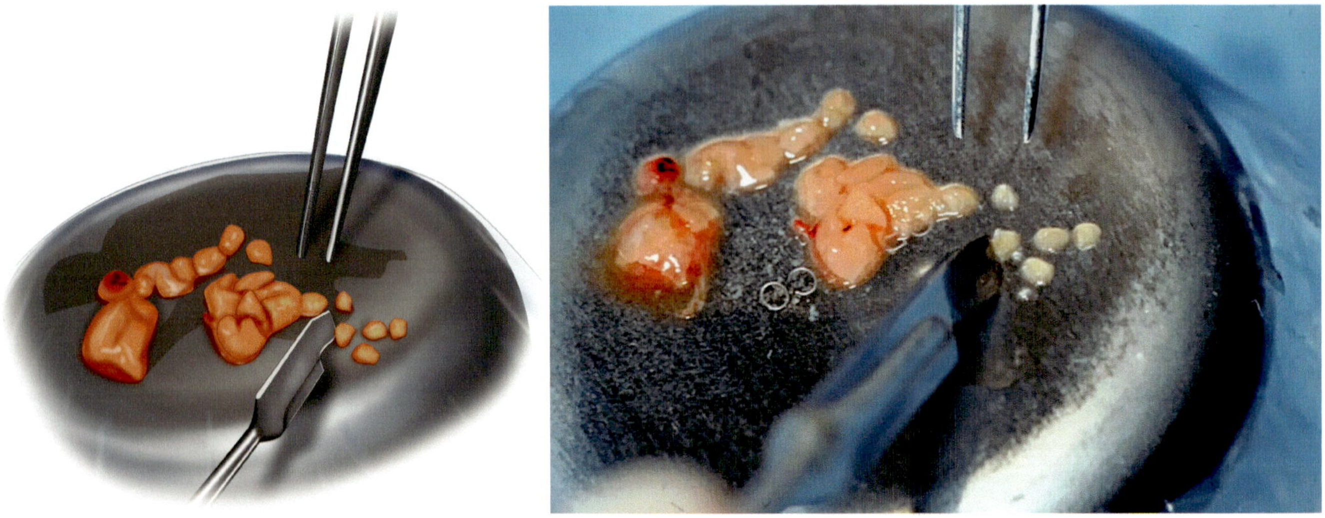

Fig. 5.15 The minced parathyroid gland prior to reimplantation

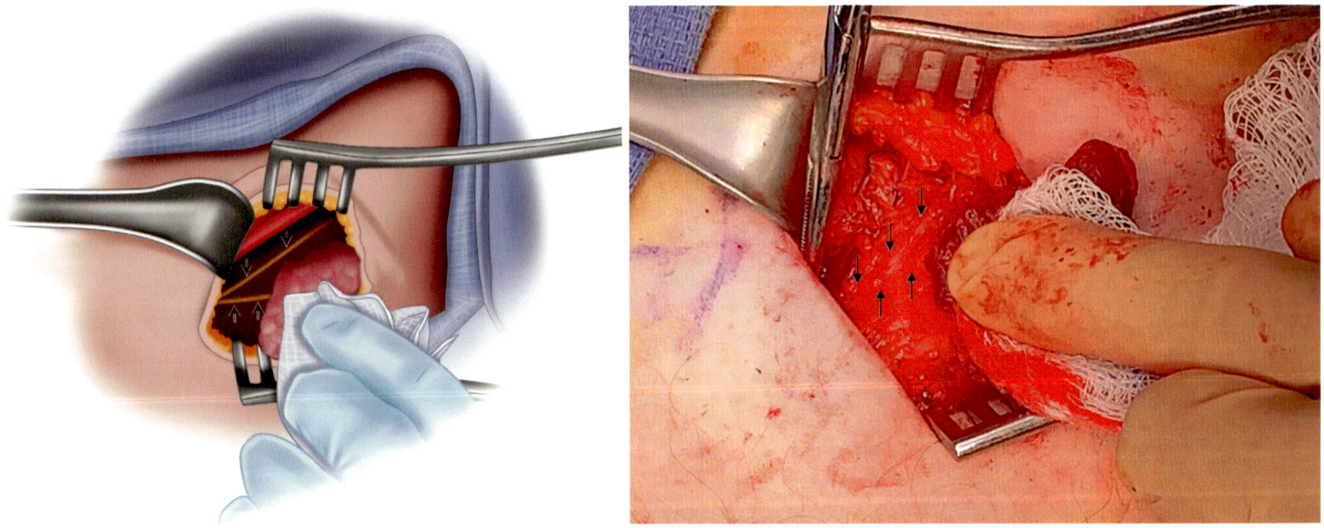

Fig. 5.16 The right recurrent laryngeal nerve is identified, and its two branches are traced (black arrows)

when branching is present. When dividing the ligament of Berry, the Mixter is directed toward the feet to avoid the cricoid membrane and to remain parallel to the course of the RLN. Once ligated, the ligament of Berry is often divided sharply for precision (Figs. 5.16, 5.17, and 5.18).

The thyroid isthmus is then dissected off the trachea in the avascular plane. If a pyramidal lobe is present (which is often bilobed and can even be trilobed), this tissue is resected entirely and in continuity with the isthmus; a pyramidal lobe typically has paired vascular pedicles that should be individually managed. Once mobilization is well away from the RLN, one can return to using electrocautery. Any thyroidea ima vessels near the isthmus are ligated and divided. When performing lobectomy, the junction of the isthmus and contralateral thyroid lobe represents the surgical margin and is transected and oversewn. At this point, a review of the exposed anatomy shows the inferior parathyroid gland, the recurrent laryngeal nerve, and the superior parathyroid gland, and the thyroid cancer can be seen near the inferior pole (Figs. 5.19, 5.20, 5.21, and 5.22).

For total thyroidectomy, attention is next turned to the contralateral lobe, and the same steps are used to expose, mobilize, and resect it. On the left side in this patient, a tiny but often present vascular bundle (termed here the "vein of doom") tethers the recurrent laryngeal nerve to the ligament of Berry, requiring delicate division to protect the nerve (Figs. 5.23, 5.24, and 5.25).

Once the specimen is resected, it must be inspected to assess for any attached parathyroid glands and oriented for pathology. At all layers of depth, the field is repeatedly

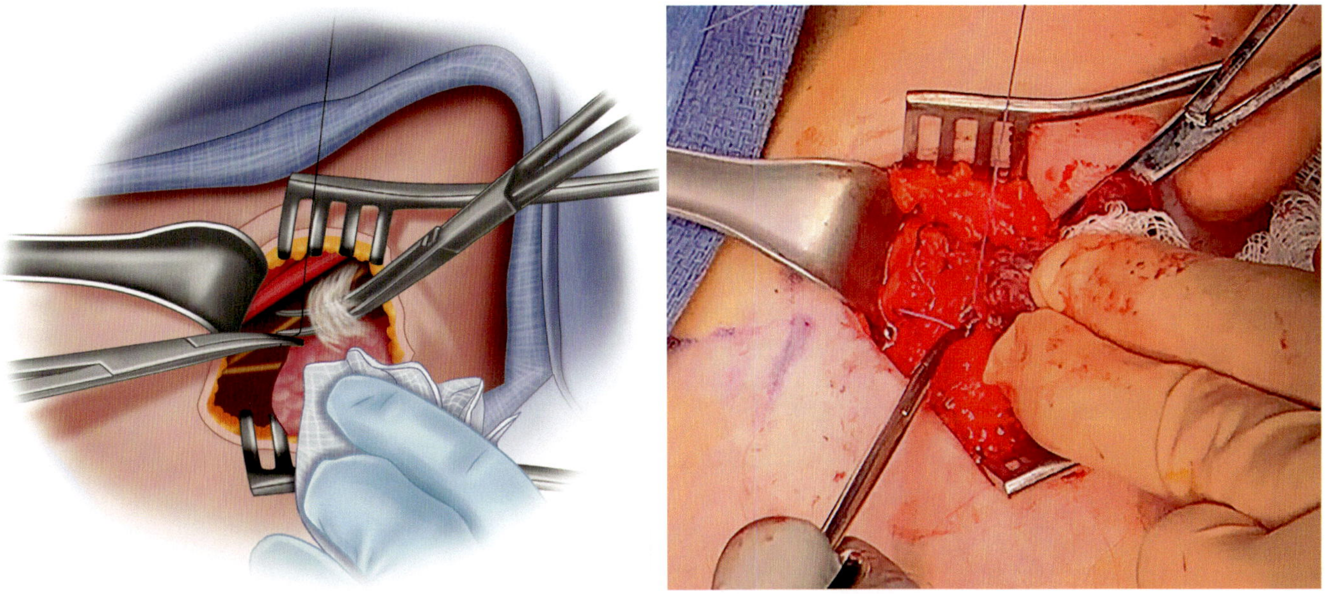

Fig. 5.17 Dissection of the ligament of Berry parallel and medial to the recurrent laryngeal nerve

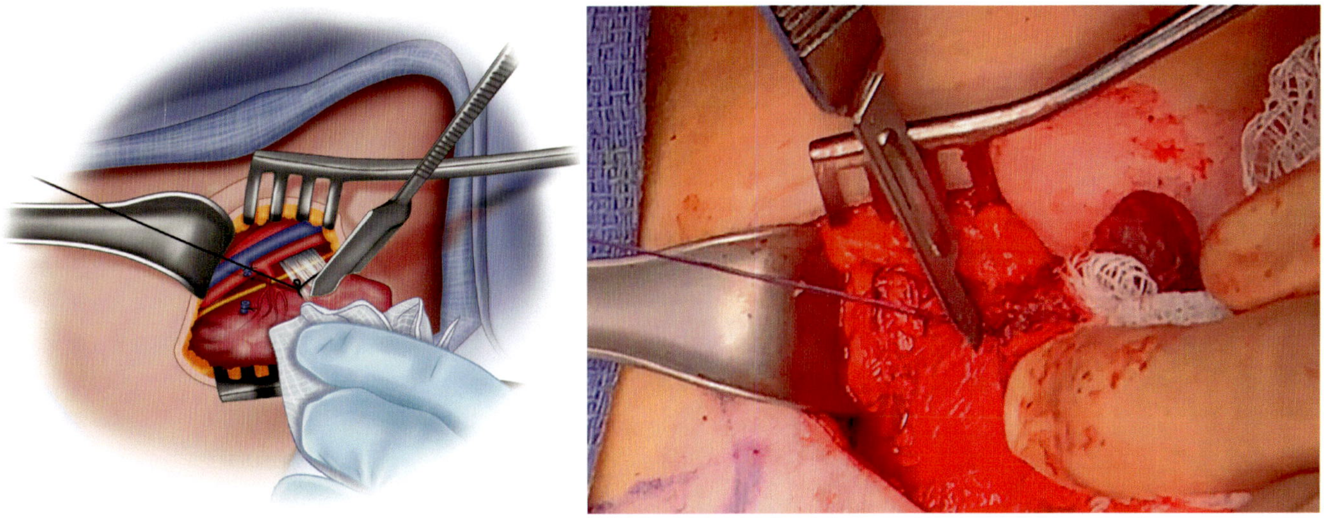

Fig. 5.18 Sharp division of the ligament of Berry

inspected to identify and manage any oozing and ensure meticulous hemostasis. Hemostatic agents are not routinely used. Closure is accomplished in three layers using running 3-0 absorbable suture to close the median raphe in the midline, inverted interrupted 3-0 absorbable to close the platysma, and subcuticular 5-0 absorbable monofilament for the skin. As incisions often stretch out during surgery, they often measure larger at the conclusion of the operation as this incision now measures 5.5 cm. We then place wound closure strips or topical skin adhesive over the incision (Figs. 5.26, 5.27, 5.28, 5.29, and 5.30).

At this high-volume thyroid center, we routinely screen for concurrent primary hyperparathyroidism, which is present in ~5% of patients and can greatly alter the conduct or extent of surgery. This patient had normal calcium, parathormone (PTH), and vitamin D levels preoperatively; vitamin D deficiency is quite common in our region, and vitamin D is routinely repleted preoperatively, which greatly reduces the likelihood and severity of postoperative hypocalcemia and paresthesias. This program also does not routinely use intraoperative nerve monitoring during initial surgery as multiple studies have not been able to demonstrate a benefit; however, we employ this adjunct for selected high-risk patients and often use it in reoperative thyroidectomy. This program does not use direct laryngoscopy for the initial surgery of patients who are assessed by the surgeon to have

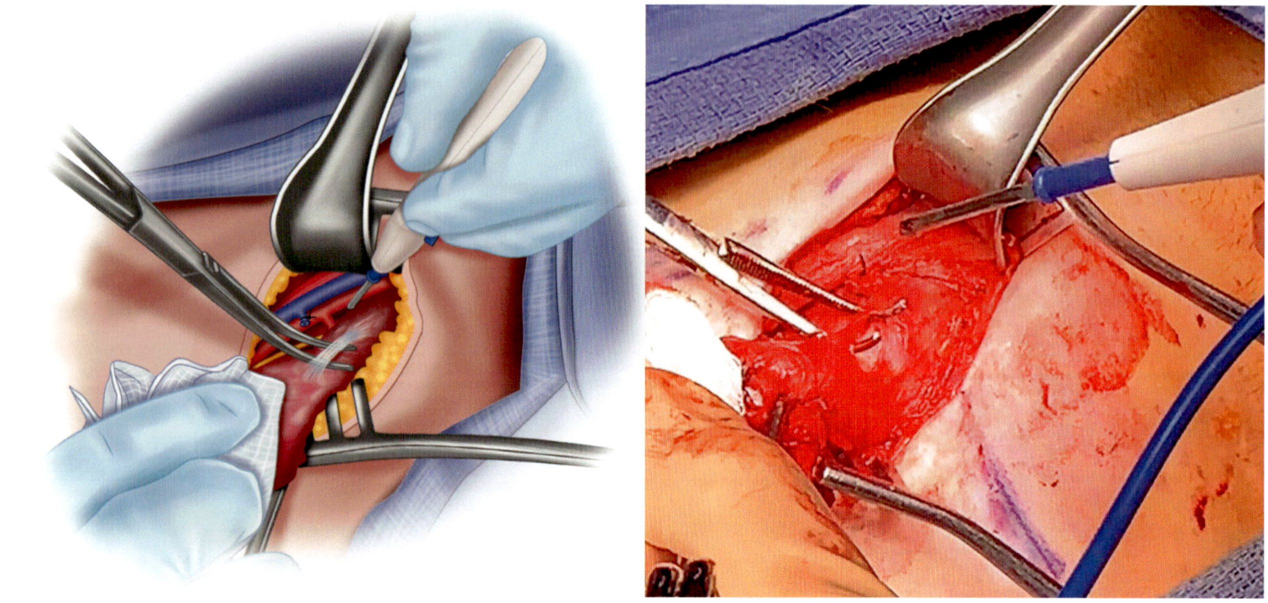

Fig. 5.19 Division of attachments to the pyramidal lobe

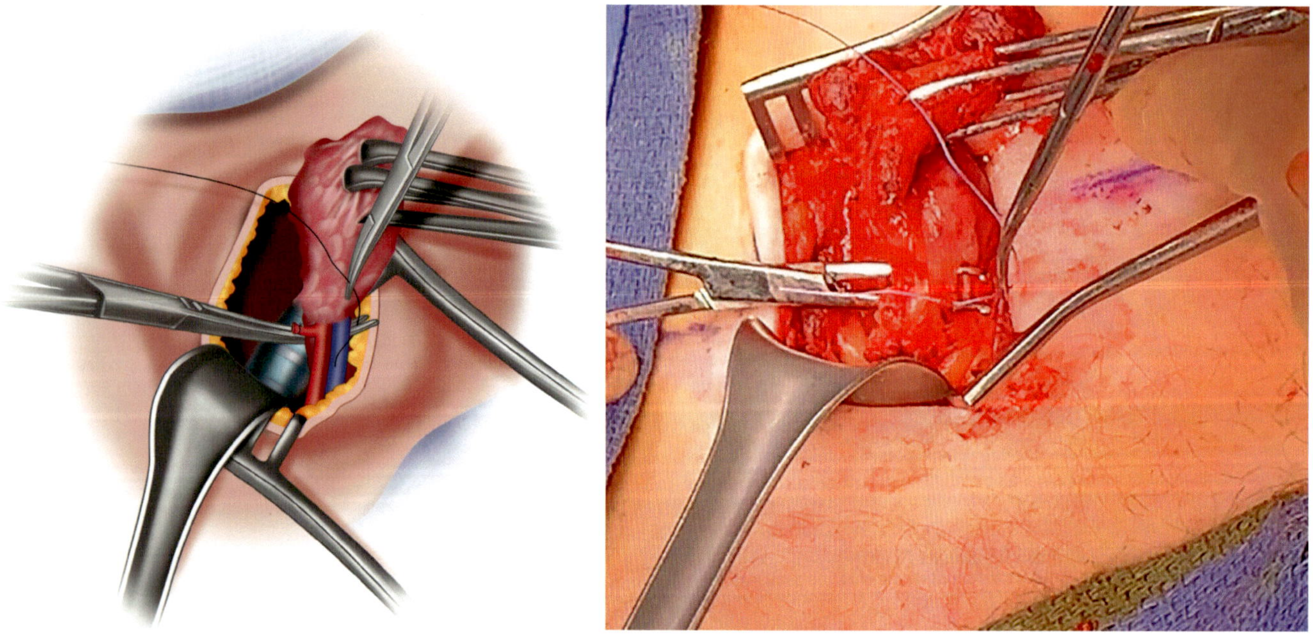

Fig. 5.20 Ligation of thyroidea ima vessels at the anterior surface of the trachea

normal vocal fold function, often employs vocal cord ultrasonography (VCUS) performed by the surgical team as a screening tool, and obtains preoperative laryngoscopy for all reoperative patients. If postoperative VCUS is abnormal, the patient is referred for laryngology evaluation and management, which in the immediate postoperative setting often includes nimodipine, an agent that can increase the likelihood of vocal fold recovery and decrease the interval to recovery. The rate of permanent vocal fold paralysis at this program is <1%.

Postoperatively, patients are monitored in the hospital for a minimum of 6 hours after a thyroid lobectomy and overnight after a total or completion thyroidectomy. An initial postoperative evaluation by the surgeon at 6 hours must evaluate for a cervical hematoma that would require operative evacuation. The incidence of a postoperative hematoma requiring evacua-

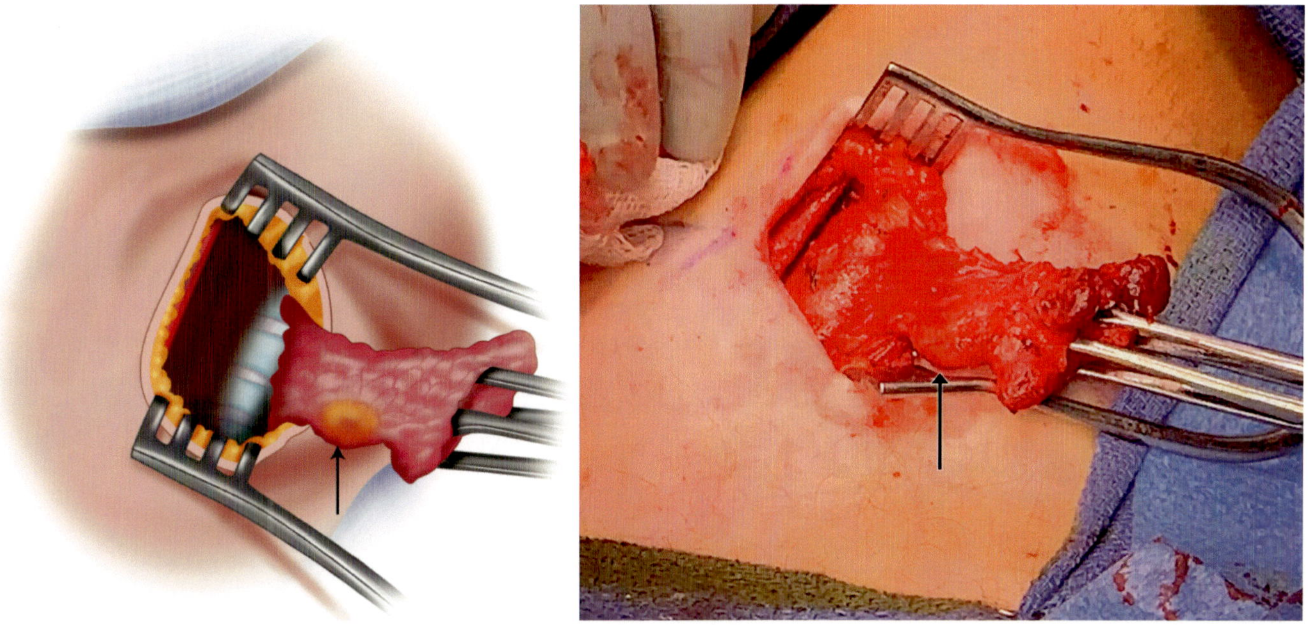

Fig. 5.21 Dissection carried along the anterior surface of the trachea to the junction of the thyroid isthmus and the left thyroid lobe. The cancerous nodule can be seen near the inferior pole of the right lobe (arrow)

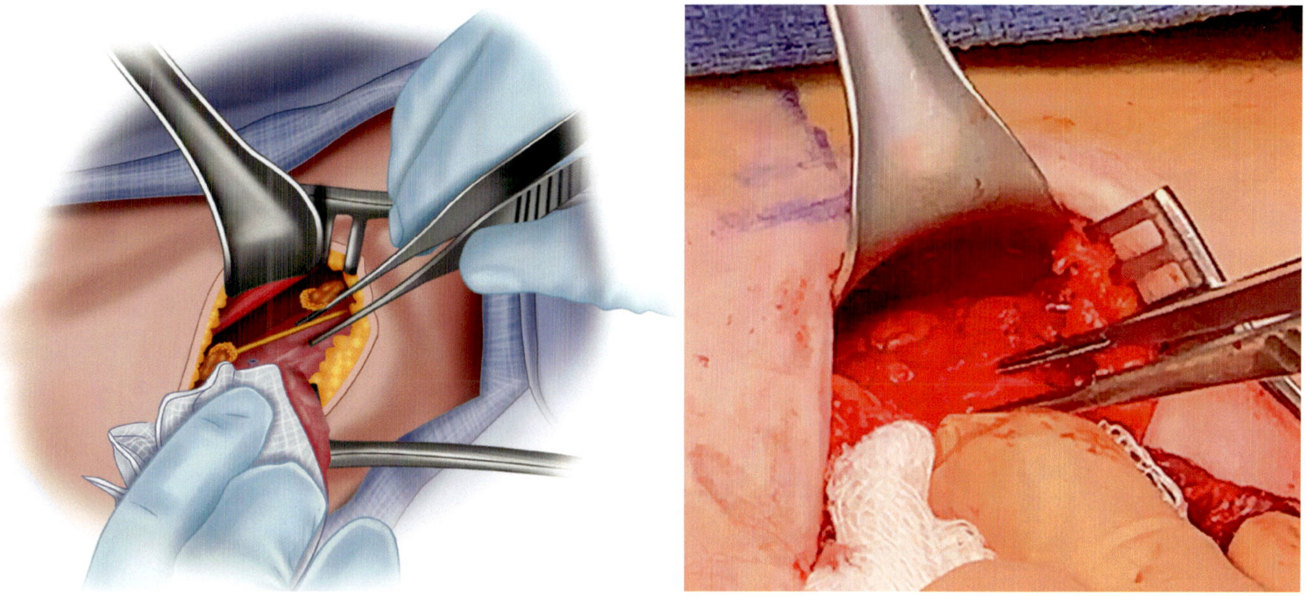

Fig. 5.22 Identification of the right recurrent laryngeal nerve, as well as the inferior parathyroid gland anteriorly and the superior parathyroid gland posteriorly

tion is about 1 in 300. Preoperative antibiotics are not routinely administered for thyroidectomy, and our wound infection rate is <1%. Thyroid lobectomy patients do not have postoperative labs checked and are not placed on oral calcium supplementation. After a total or completion thyroidectomy, a morning calcium level is checked, and patients are empirically placed on 2 g of calcium carbonate twice a day. If these patients have symptomatic hypocalcemia or an abnormally low morning calcium level, the frequency is increased to three times a day. All patients are given a standard postoperative instruction sheet that includes postoperative expectations, wound care, activity restrictions, and indications for calling the emergency contact number (Video 5.1).

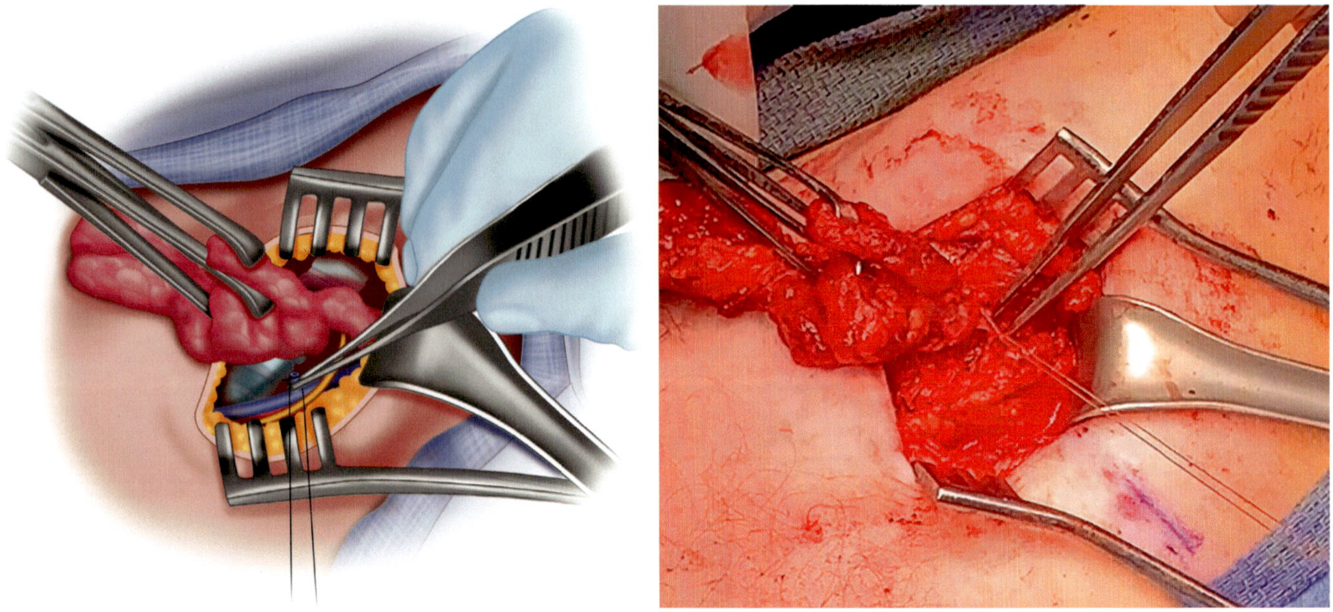

Fig. 5.23 The left "vein of doom" is carefully ligated near the insertion of the recurrent laryngeal nerve

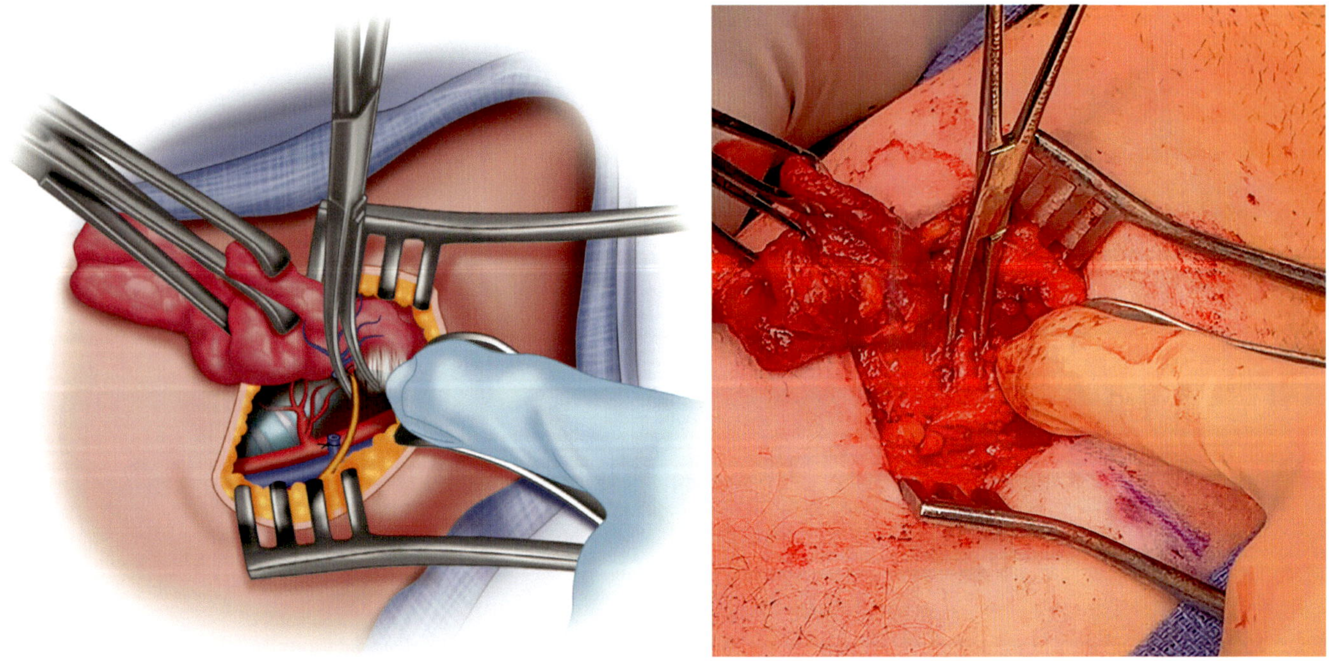

Fig. 5.24 Identification of the left recurrent laryngeal nerve

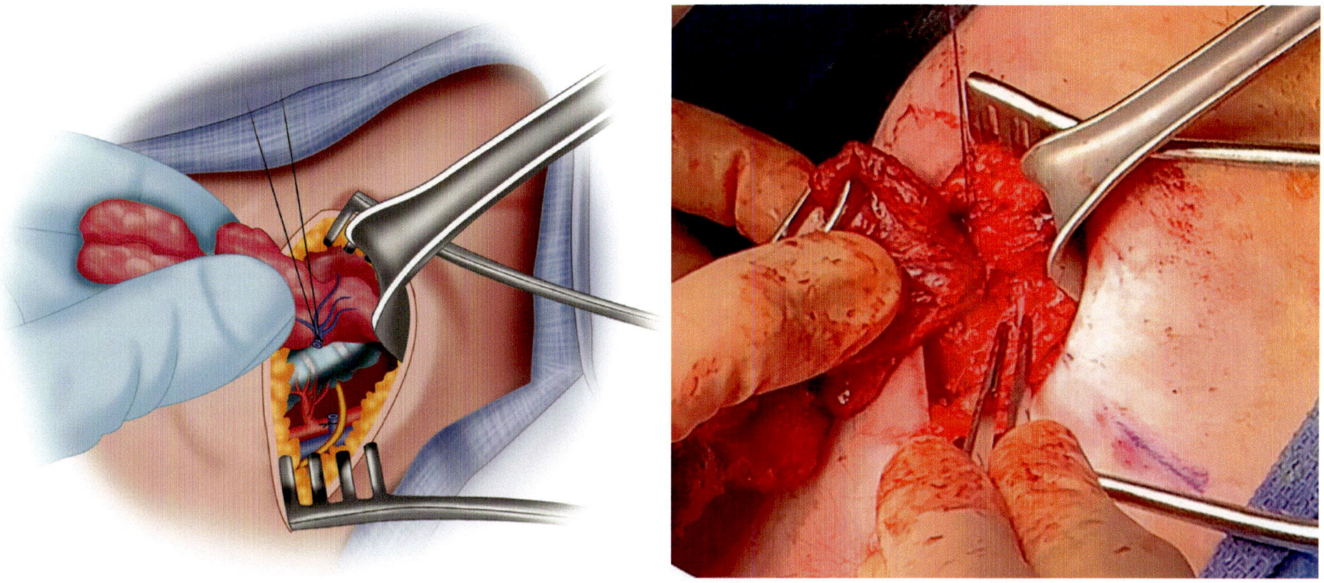

Fig. 5.25 Ligation of the left ligament of Berry while protecting the recurrent laryngeal nerve

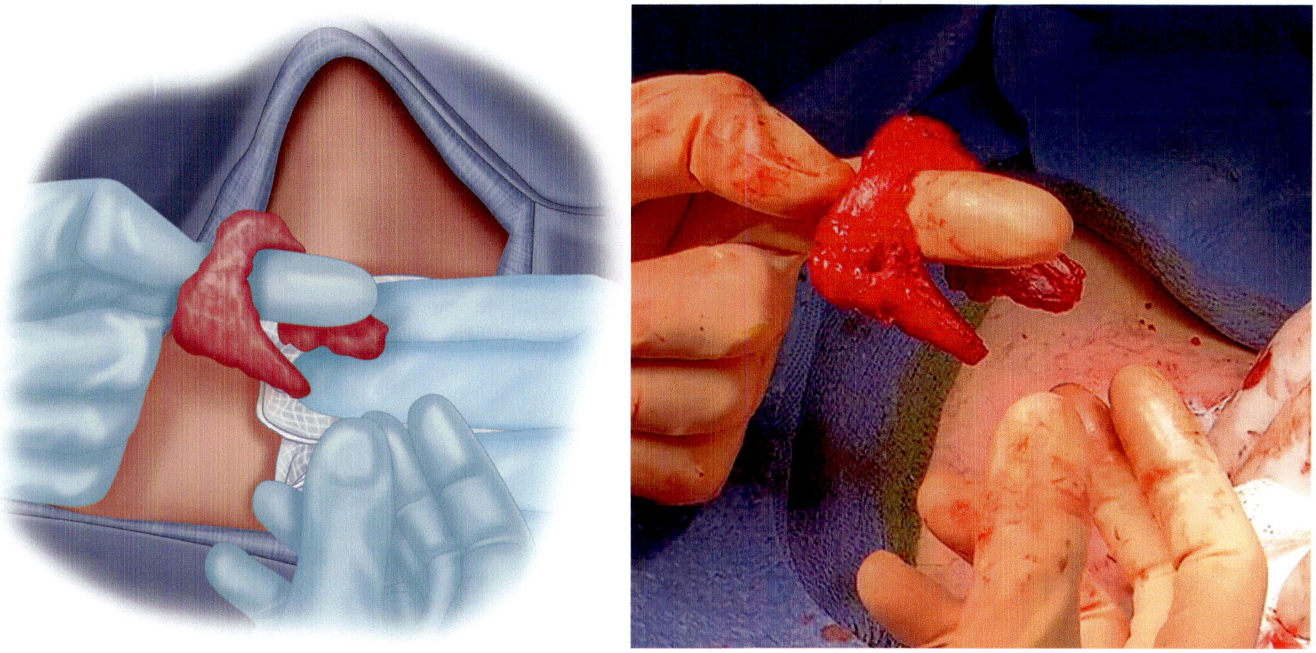

Fig. 5.26 Inspection of the resected thyroid gland for any attached parathyroid glands, with none identified here

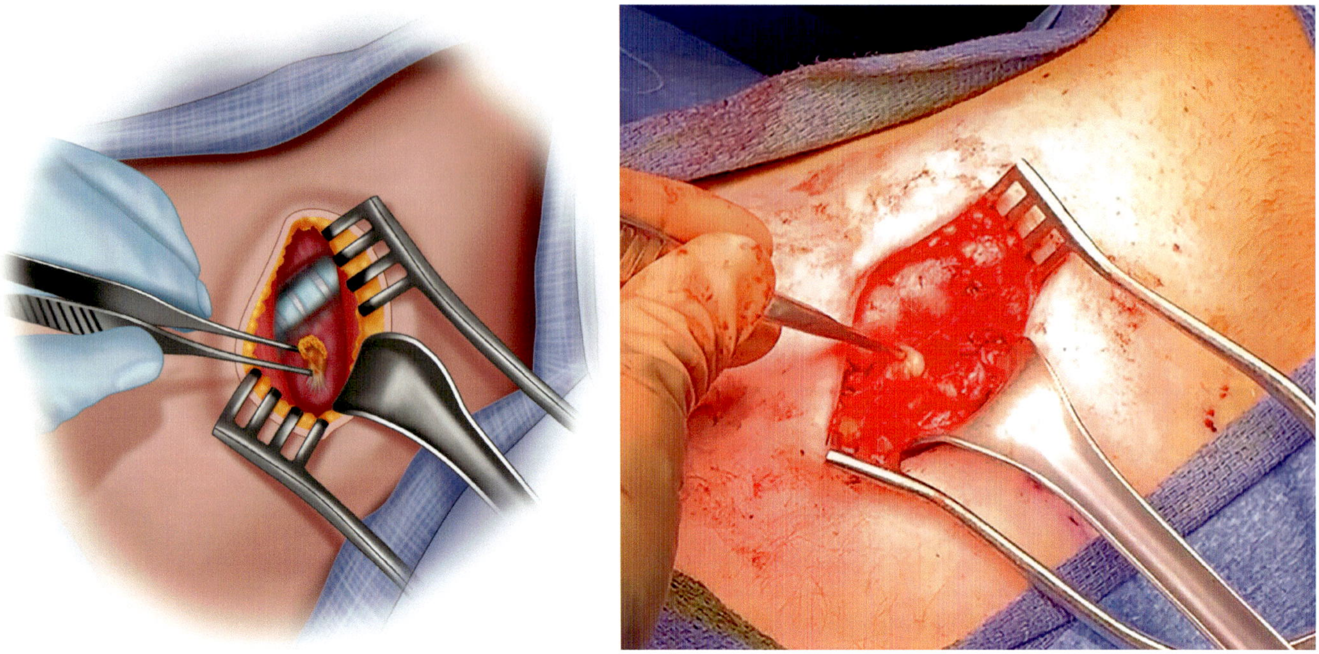

Fig. 5.27 Inspection for hemostasis, while the left inferior parathyroid gland is identified and appears viable

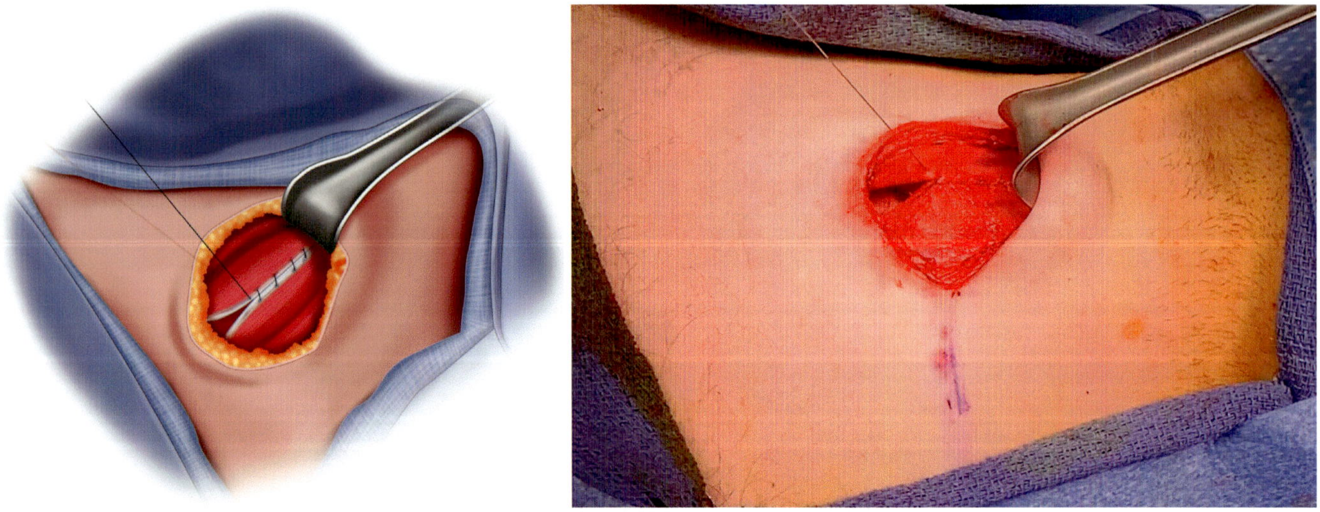

Fig. 5.28 Closure of the median raphe with a running suture

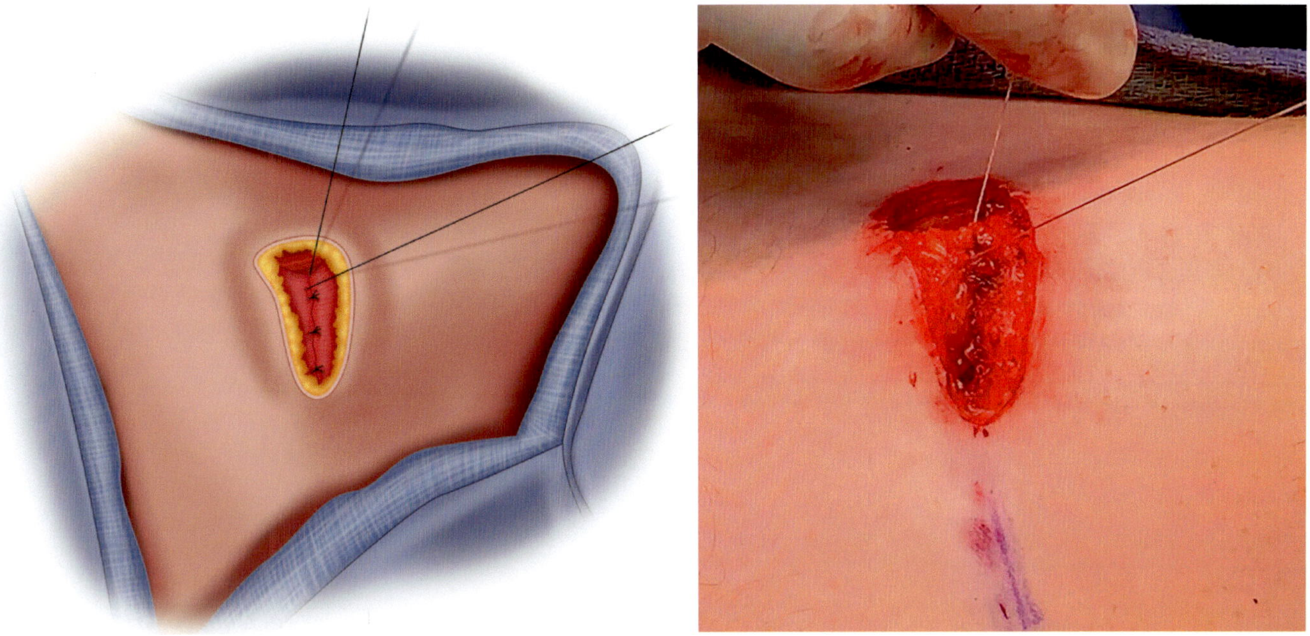

Fig. 5.29 Closure of the platysma with interrupted sutures

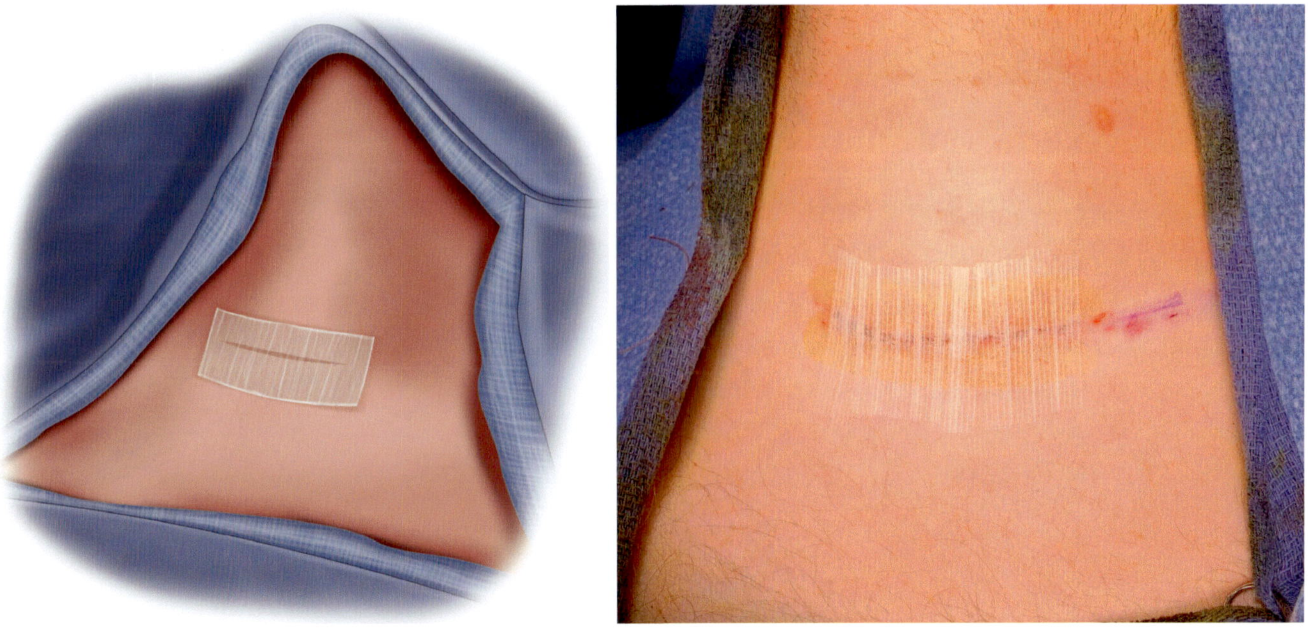

Fig. 5.30 Closed wound after application of wound closure strips

Suggested Reading

Patel KN, Yip L, Lubitz CC, Grubbs EG, Miller BS, Shen W, et al. The American Association of Endocrine Surgeons guidelines for the definitive surgical management of thyroid disease in adults. Ann Surg. 2020;271(3):e21–93.

Wang T, Lyden M, Sosa JA. Thyroidectomy. In: Chen W, editor. UpToDate. Waltham: UpToDate. Accessed 22 Dec 2020.

Total Thyroidectomy for Substernal Goiter

6

Benzon M. Dy and Melanie L. Lyden

Introduction

The removal of the thyroid for symptomatic goiters has been the treatment of choice for enlarging thyroid glands that result in compression with shortness of breath, dysphagia, or dysphonia. Other symptoms may include a globus sensation and an undesirable cosmetic appearance due to growth. There may be enlarged nodules that have suspicious features for cancer or those that cannot be appropriately assessed with ultrasound and a fine-needle aspiration (FNA) biopsy. In patients with large substernal components, provocative maneuvers such as raising of the arms can lead to the compression of the thoracic inlet and venous drainage, eponymously known as Pemberton's sign, leading to facial congestion and plethora (Hamidi et al., 2018). Although new technologies such as radiofrequency ablation may help with controlling the size of large goiters, the tissue cannot be examined after treatment and substernal components may be difficult to address (Haugen et al., 2016). Radioactive iodine treatment can also be used to arrest growth or to shrink goiters, but the initial phase of treatment may cause the swelling of the gland, increasing symptoms, and the overall decline in size averages about 20% of the gland size, which may not be sufficient treatment for diffusely enlarged goiters.

There are several important factors to consider prior to thyroidectomy for enlarged thyroids. Although iodine deficiency is rare in the United States, with iodine supplementation in salt readily available, patients may come from iodine-deficient areas, which can contribute to goiter formation. A thorough history and a physical exam are important in stratifying the risk of malignancy. Factors such as radiation exposure, family history, and duration of the symptoms are important factors to consider. Rapid growth can be caused by rare entities such as anaplastic thyroid cancer or intrathyroidal spontaneous hemorrhage, and either FNA or core biopsy for anaplastic lesions can help rule out aggressive malignancy. Preoperative imaging including ultrasound and cross-sectional imaging such as computed tomography (CT) scan will demonstrate the extent of growth of the thyroid and identify any suspicious nodules or adenopathy that should be evaluated prior to surgical resection (Patel et al., 2020; Pemberton, 1946). In addition, the use of a CT scan to identify the extent of substernal extension is significant in the preparation of a possible sternotomy to safely excise the thyroid, especially if it extends below the innominate vessels.

Procedure

A 57-year-old African American woman presented to her endocrinologist with an enlarged thyroid that had been monitored for 2 years with periodic ultrasound and benign biopsies of enlarged thyroid nodules. She noted recent growth with increasing dysphagia and intermittent shortness of breath with exertion (Fig. 6.1). She has no family or personal history of thyroid cancer and is currently euthyroid on both history and biochemical evaluation without the need for thyroid hormone supplementation. Ultrasound demonstrated diffuse enlargement of the thyroid gland with bilateral extension below the clavicles (Fig. 6.2). The CT scan demonstrated an 8-cm right thyroid lobe in its greatest dimension and a 7-cm left thyroid lobe with substernal extension extending down to the innominate artery with no significant narrowing of her trachea present down to the bifurcation (Fig. 6.3).

Under general endotracheal anesthesia, the patient is positioned supine in a beach chair position, flexing at the hips and knees and extending the neck (Fig. 6.4). The head is appropriately padded to ensure that the patient is resting comfortably on the operating room (OR) table and not in a suspended position. The patient is positioned with the arms adducted to her sides with appropriate padding to allow both the surgeon and assistant to stand adjacent to the patient. Our standard practice is to perform neuromonitoring of the recurrent laryngeal nerve with a Medtronic NIMS system

B. M. Dy (✉) · M. L. Lyden
Division of Endocrine and Metabolic Surgery, Mayo Clinic, Rochester, MN, USA
e-mail: Dy.Benzon@mayo.edu

A. Shifrin (ed.), *Atlas of Thyroid Surgery*, https://doi.org/10.1007/978-3-030-93673-0_6

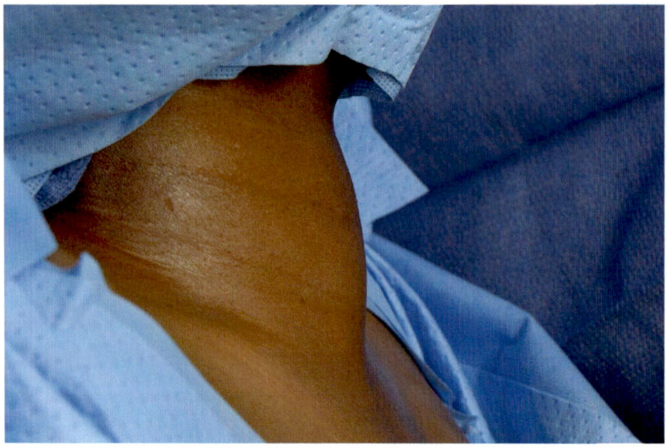

Fig. 6.1 Increasing fullness present within the neck displays the enlargement of the patient's thyroid, although the substernal component is not evident on visual examination

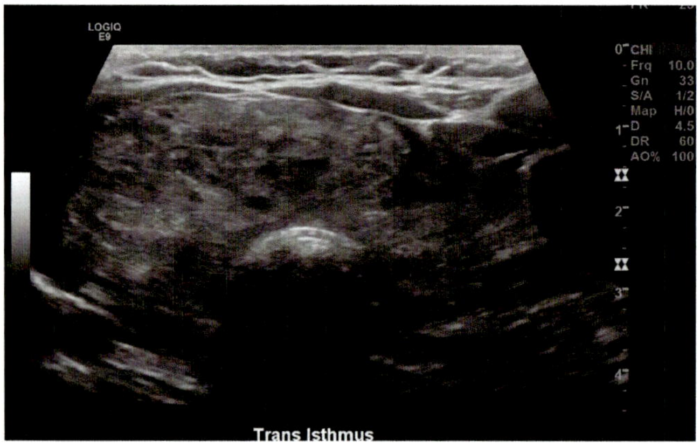

Fig. 6.2 Ultrasound image of bilateral diffuse enlargement of the thyroid. A US can be inadequate for imaging when there is significant extension of the thyroid into the thoracic inlet

incorporated into the endotracheal tube as an adjunct to the anatomic visualization of the nerve (Fig. 6.5). Often, anesthesia will use a fiber optic laryngoscope to ensure that the endotracheal tube is appropriately positioned at the time of the surgery.

A transverse Kocher incision is made one fingerbreadth below the cricoid cartilage with generous extension just medial to each sternocleidomastoid muscle (Fig. 6.6). A Superior and inferior subplatysmal flaps are created extending to the thyroid cartilage cephalad and down to the clavicles inferiorly (Fig. 6.7). The strap muscles are then separated in the avascular midline and retracted laterally (Fig. 6.8). In patients with large cervical components of the goiter, the sternothyroid muscle can be divided to improve exposure (Fig. 6.9). The superior pole is divided to allow for medial rotation of the thyroid and to ligate the superior thyroid vessels (Fig. 6.10). It is important to ensure that the caudal dissection is performed up to the interclavicular ligament to allow for the exposure of the

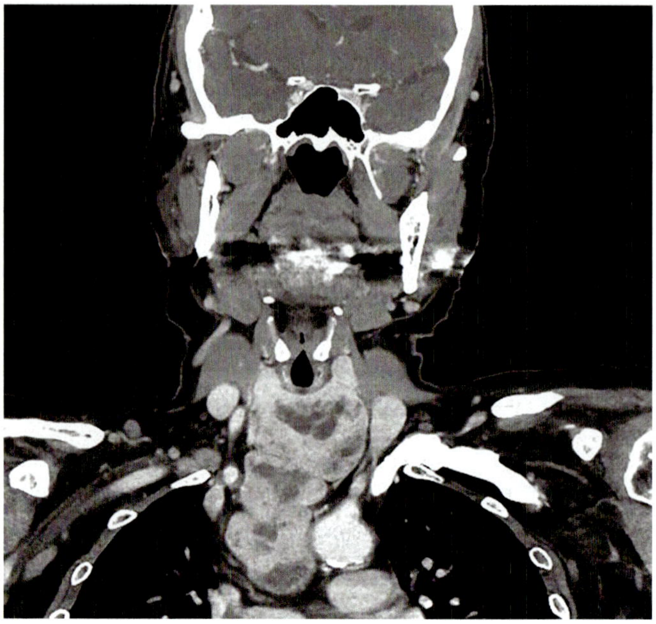

Fig. 6.3 Coronal section of a patient with a large substernal goiter with bilateral lobe involvement and substernal displacement of the innominate vessels

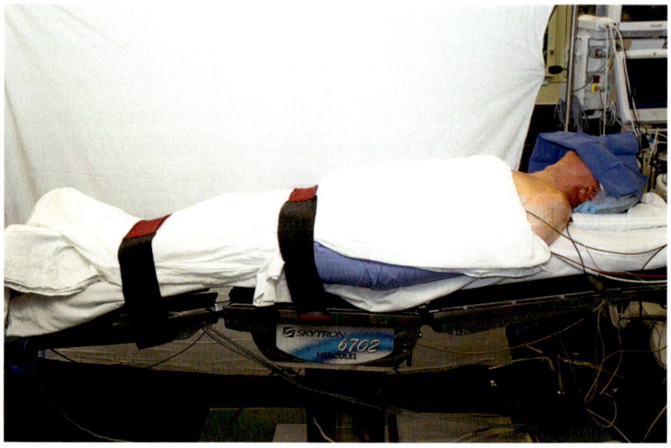

Fig. 6.4 Patient in beach chair position, which allows for gentle extension of the neck and elevation of the patient in reverse Trendelenburg position

mediastinum and to aid in the delivery of the thyroid into the cervical region (Fig. 6.11). Oftentimes, blunt dissection along the capsule of the thyroid may aid in mobilizing the thyroid within the cervical neck. Other options include the placement of Kocher clamps on the thyroid capsule to gently retract the thyroid cephalad. Once the thyroid is delivered into the neck, the recurrent laryngeal nerve is carefully protected throughout the process, along with the parathyroid glands (Fig. 6.12). Autotransplantation may be needed if the parathyroid and its vasculature are displaced by the inferior goiter.

The thyroid is examined grossly to confirm a complete resection of the thyroid gland and ensure that the specimen is

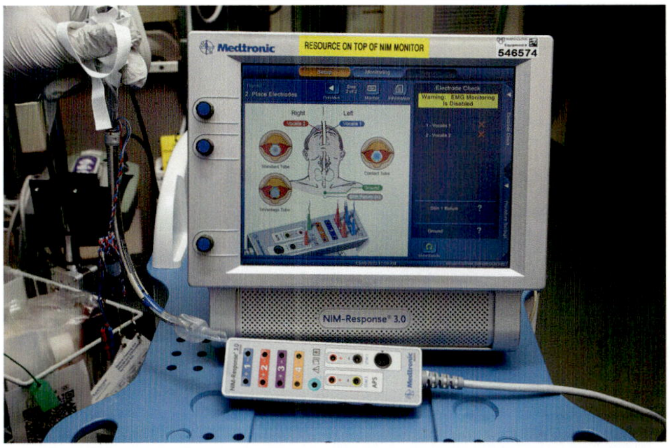

Fig. 6.5 The NIMS endotracheal tube and monitor allow for immediate feedback of the neuromonitoring of the recurrent laryngeal nerve throughout the course of surgery. Loss of signal may indicate traction, injury, or transection of the nerve

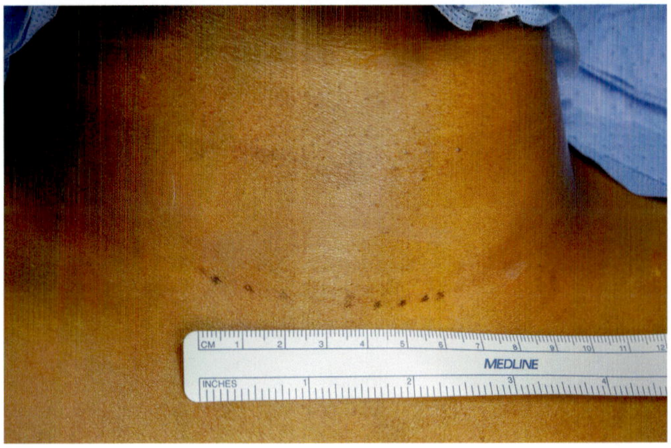

Fig. 6.6 A transverse Kocher incision is measured and marked prior to incision to ensure symmetry and placement in a natural skin crease to minimize scar formation

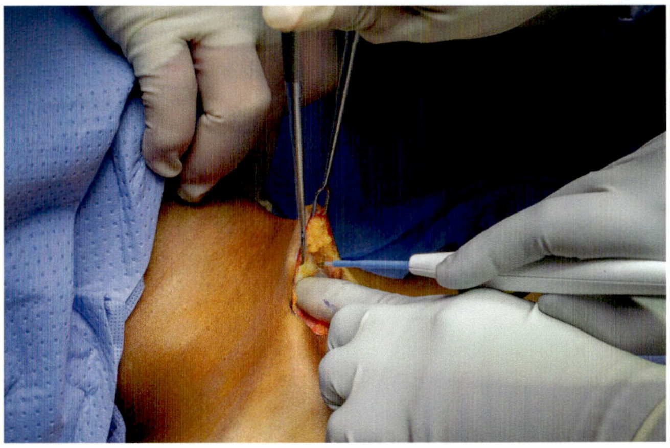

Fig. 6.7 Superior and inferior flaps created just deep into the platysma

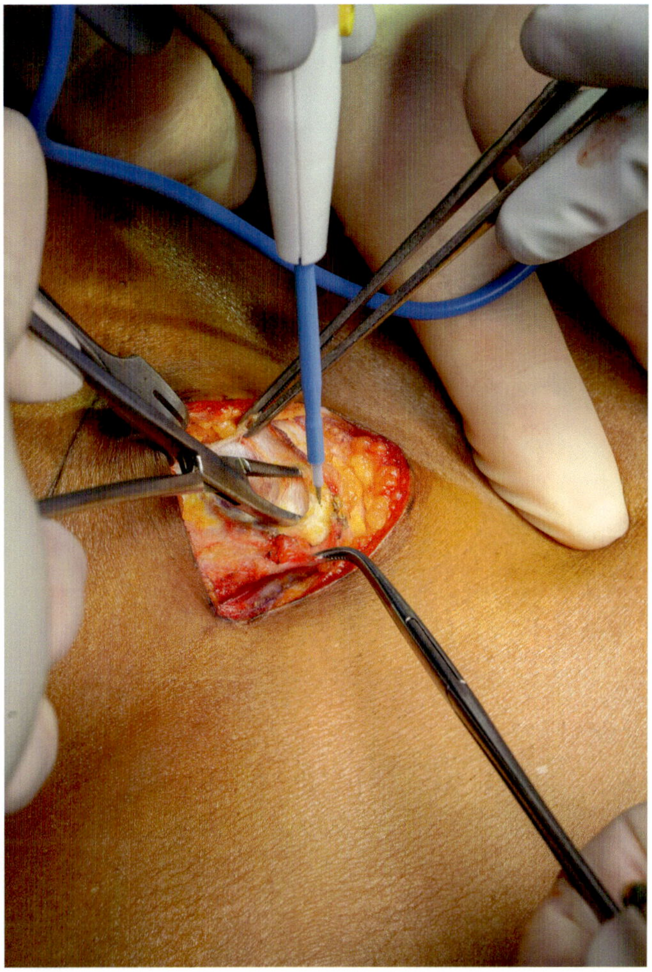

Fig. 6.8 Using electrocautery, the midline is identifiable with an avascular plane where the left and right sternohyoid muscles meet in the center of the neck. This can be occasionally displaced due to asymmetric growth of the thyroid

consistent with the preoperative imaging so that no portion of the thyroid is left within the substernal space (Fig. 6.13).

The neck is closed in the standard fashion with subcutaneous Vicryl sutures and a subcuticular 4-0 Monocryl closure (Fig. 6.14). Most often, a drain is not required post-operatively. However, if there is a large potential space, it may be prudent to place a drain either to avoid a seroma or if there is a concern regarding the disruption of the thoracic duct in very large substernal goiters.

Postoperatively, patients are observed overnight in the hospital for signs of bleeding, infection, or hypocalcemia. Patients are also cautioned of the risk of mild swelling in the subcutaneous space where the previous goiter was present, resulting in a temporary seroma. Bruising in the chest can result from drainage and gravity in the postoperative period. Today, sternotomy is rarely performed to deliver substernal glands unless there is a high preoperative risk of malignancy.

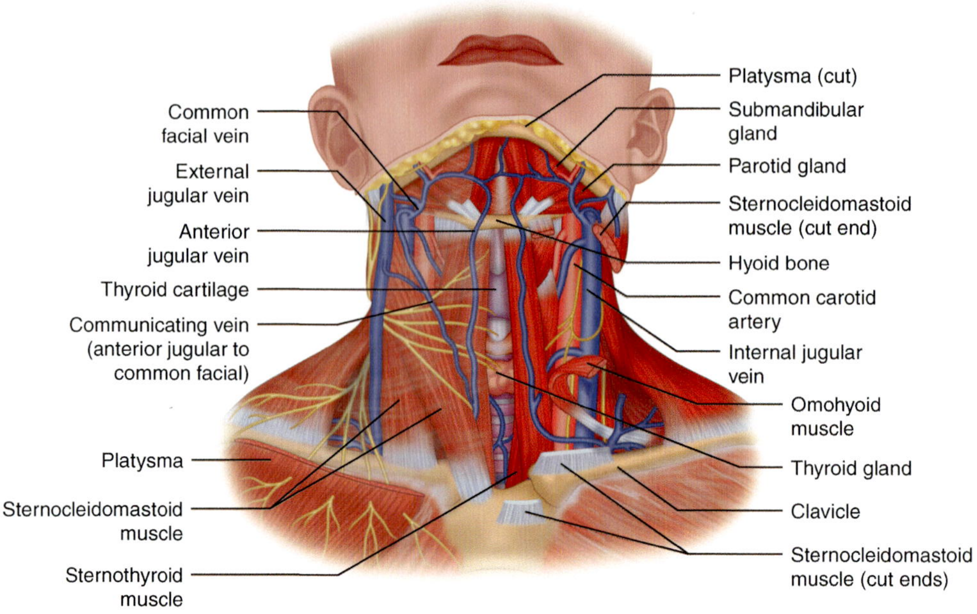

Fig. 6.9 The sternohyoid muscles are retracted laterally to expose the underlying thyroid

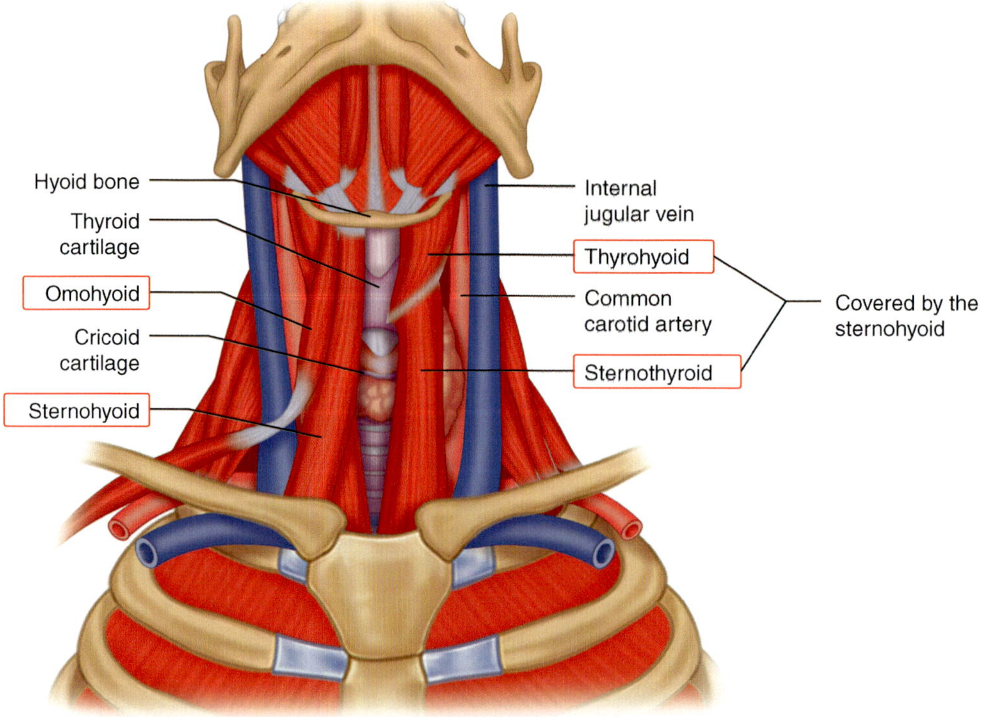

Fig. 6.10 The sternothyroid is one of the four strap muscles and is positioned adjacent to the thyroid. Although it is often stretched when a goiter is present, dividing the sternothyroid can often improve mobilization and visualization of the lateral aspect of the thyroid and provides space to rotate the gland medially

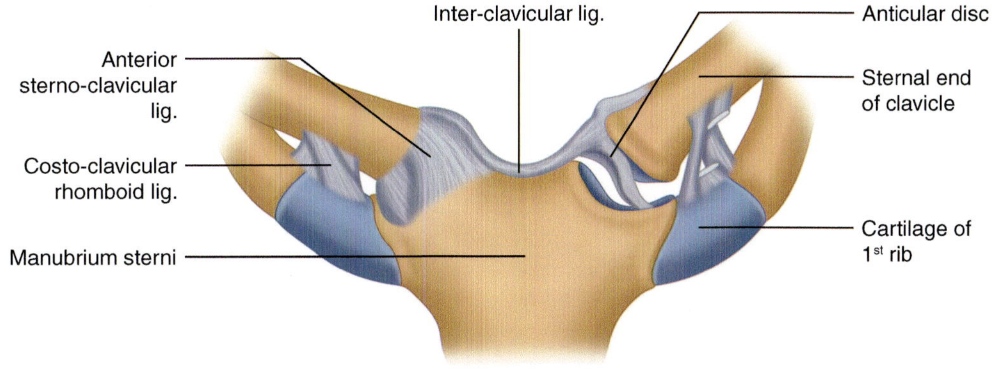

Fig. 6.11 The division of the interclavicular ligament aids in widening the space just cephalad to the manubrium to allow for the delivery of the substernal portion of the thyroid

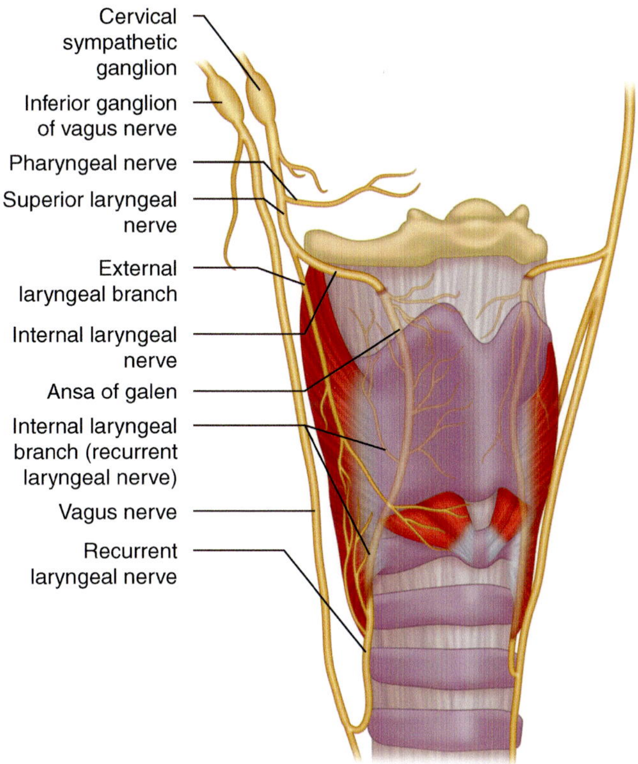

Fig. 6.12 The recurrent laryngeal nerve courses along the tracheo-esophageal groove. Care must be taken in cases of enlarged thyroids and goiters as these may be displaced and draped over enlarged thyroid tissue or stretched with an altered anatomic course

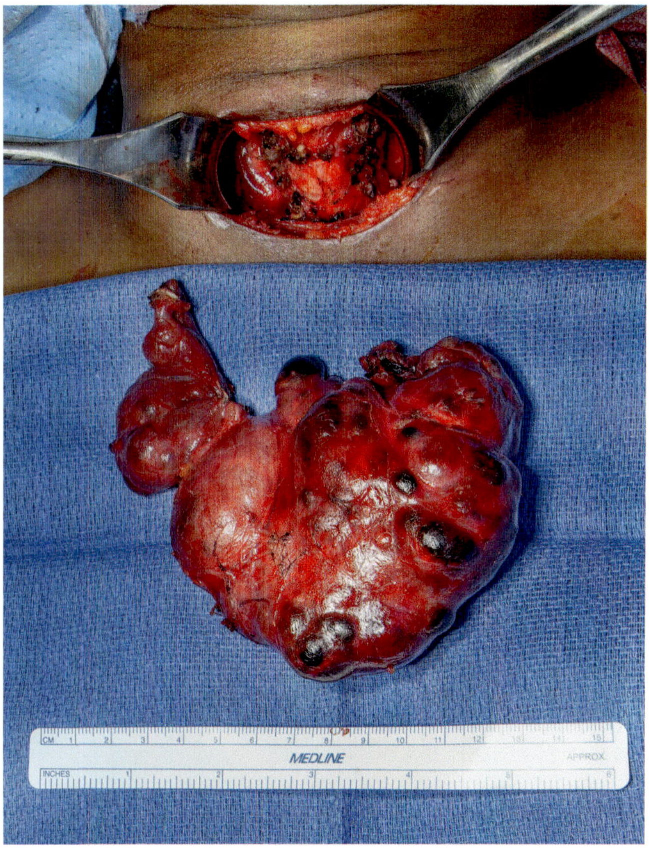

Fig. 6.13 The specimen is reviewed to ensure the parathyroid glands have not been inadvertently removed and the thyroid gland is intact

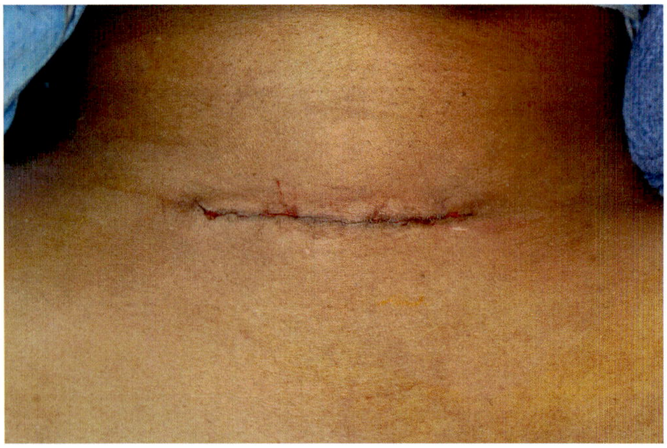

Fig. 6.14 Subcuticular sutures are most commonly utilized due to the excellent cosmetic outcome achieved with the closure

Suggested Reading

Hamidi O, Callstrom MR, Lee RA, Dean D, Castro MR, Morris JC, et al. Outcomes of radiofrequency ablation therapy for large benign thyroid nodules: a Mayo Clinic case series. Mayo Clin Proc. 2018;93(8):1018–25.

Haugen BR, Alexander EK, Bible KC, Doherty GM, Mandel SJ, Nikiforov YE, et al. 2015 American Thyroid Association Management Guidelines for adult patients with thyroid nodules and differentiated thyroid cancer: the American Thyroid Association Guidelines Task Force on Thyroid Nodules and Differentiated Thyroid Cancer. Thyroid. 2016;26(1):1–133.

Patel KN, Yip L, Lubitz CC, Grubbs EG, Miller BS, Shen W, et al. The American Association of Endocrine Surgeons Guidelines for the definitive surgical management of thyroid disease in adults. Ann Surg. 2020;271(3):e21–93.

Pemberton HS. Sign of submerged goitre [Letter]. Lancet. 1946;251:509.

Left Thyroid Lobectomy as Completion of Total Thyroidectomy with Central Neck Lymph Node Dissection on the Left

7

Alexander Shifrin

Introduction

Left thyroid lobectomy (also known as hemithyroidectomy) is the removal of the left thyroid lobe. When this procedure follows a previous right thyroid lobectomy, it is considered a completion of total thyroidectomy. Meticulous surgical technique and attention to detail are pertinent in performing a successful thyroidectomy. The main goal of thyroid surgery is not only to remove the diseased thyroid gland or lobe but also to prevent complications, such as RLN injury and hypoparathyroidism due to devascularization or incidental removal of the parathyroid glands. The complications of thyroidectomy by themselves could be more devastating than the disease that it was intended to cure. Therefore, the procedure of completion of total thyroidectomy, or thyroid lobectomy, involves, first, the identification, full exposure, and safe dissection of the RLN, then the identification and preservation of all parathyroid glands, followed by an indicated removal of the thyroid gland or lobe [1, 2]. Scarring and adhesions from prior surgery may complicate the dissection and make the anatomy very difficult to appreciate. The prevalence of RLN injury is higher in redo surgery than in primary thyroid operations, and it has been reported as high as 12.5% for transient RLN injury and 3.8% for permanent RLN injury [3]. Therefore, performing one side surgery (lobectomy) should not involve a "routine intraoperative assessment or evaluation" of the opposite normal thyroid lobe unless it is clinically indicated (which is almost never) and the surgeon intends to remove it. Therefore, coming back for the completion of total thyroidectomy will be much easier on the opposite side when there are no adhesions developed and the risk of complications, such as RLN and/or parathyroid gland injury, will be significantly lower. From a surgical safety standpoint, in order to reduce complications, the optimal timing for the completion of total thyroidectomy after a previous thyroid lobectomy is about 3 months. Considerations regarding the timing for the completion procedure should be made for patients with differentiated thyroid carcinoma who have indications for the administration of radioactive iodine (RAI). Since RAI is given in approximately 6–8 weeks after the surgery, the second (completion) procedure will delay the administration of RAI to 6–8 weeks after the second surgery [4].

The level VI central neck lymph node (CNLN) compartment anatomically is defined by hyoid bone superiorly, suprasternal notch and innominate (brachiocephalic) artery inferiorly, carotid artery laterally, and the superficial layer of the deep cervical fascia posteriorly. CNLN compartment in addition to paratracheal lymph nodes also includes pretracheal and prelaryngeal (or Delphian) lymph nodes. It is important to perform the dissection not only anteriorly but also posteriorly to the RLN (especially on the right side, where the RLN is positioned more laterally in the inferior part of the neck compared to the left side RLN). The number of lymph nodes contained within the central neck varies greatly between patients. CNLND should consist of the removal of the prelaryngeal, pretracheal, and paratracheal lymph nodes. CNLND may be therapeutic or prophylactic, unilateral or bilateral. Therapeutic CNLND is performed when there are obvious metastatic lymph nodes detected in the CNLN compartment on preoperative imaging studies or during the thyroidectomy. Prophylactic CNLND is performed when there are no findings or knowledge of enlarged or metastatic lymph nodes in the CNLN compartment either on preoperative imaging studies or during an intraoperative assessment. Prophylactic CNLND consists of the removal of all fibroadipose tissues (with presumptive lymph nodes) from the CNLN compartment prophylactically [5–8].

Almost all our thyroidectomies are performed as outpatient procedures with a 5-hour observation stay for lobectomy and 6 hours for total thyroidectomy [9–14]. Patients

Supplementary Information The online version contains supplementary material available at [https://doi.org/10.1007/978-3-030-93673-0_7].

A. Shifrin (✉)
Atlantic Health Oncology Service and Department of Surgery, CentraState Health System, Atlantic Health Partner, Freehold, NJ, USA

A. Shifrin (ed.), *Atlas of Thyroid Surgery*, https://doi.org/10.1007/978-3-030-93673-0_7

with severe medical comorbidities, those that travel from out of state or from a distance, as well as those who require modified radical neck dissection or sternotomy are staying overnight for observation (patients with sternotomy may stay longer until the chest tube is removed). All patients are evaluated with an assessment of the vocal cord function by flexible laryngoscopy prior to and right after the procedure. Intraoperative RLN monitoring (IONM) has gained widespread acceptance as an adjunct to the gold standard of identification and visualization of the RLN [13–16]. We perform IONM for all thyroidectomy and parathyroidectomy procedures in our practice. In addition, an external branch of the superior laryngeal nerve (EBSLN) monitoring is performed for all patients who require extra attention to their voice, such as singers, teachers, public speakers, and so on. Thyroidectomy and CNLND are considered clean surgical procedures, and no preoperative antibiotics are required. For extra precaution, we do give preoperative antibiotics only to patients with implantable metal devices, immunosuppressed patients, and patients who require sternotomy or a prolonged (over 4 hours) procedure, such as total thyroidectomy with modified radical neck dissection.

Please see "Anatomical Considerations" related to the anatomy of the RLN, inferior thyroid artery (ITA), tubercle of Zuckerkandl, and parathyroid glands in Chap. 1 of this Atlas.

Regarding the difference in the anatomy of the RLN, the left RLN is located more medially and anteriorly on the trachea and in the tracheoesophageal groove compared to the right RLN, where it is ascending more laterally (Fig. 7.1). It is almost imperative to assume that the left RLN is so medially and anteriorly located that if the thyroid lobe is retracted, the RLN will be immediately under the lobe and, most of the time, attached to the thyroid lobe posteriorly (Video 7.1).

Instruments (See Chap. 1, Fig. 7.3)

Case

A 27-year-old female was presented with incidental findings of a 3.6-cm right thyroid nodule, with no significant symptoms, no history of radiation exposure, and no significant family history. An ultrasound-guided fine-needle aspiration biopsy of a nodule showed findings suspicious for follicular neoplasm (Bethesda category 4). She underwent a right thyroid lobectomy. The final pathological diagnosis was consistent with a 3.6-cm follicular variant of papillary thyroid carcinoma with multiple foci of angioinvasion. At a multidisciplinary tumor board discussion, the left thyroid lobectomy as completion of a total thyroidectomy with prophylactic central neck lymph node dissection was recommended. She has also developed a hypertrophic scar after her previous right thyroid lobectomy, and scar excision was planned. She was consented for surgery and presented for the procedure with the understanding that she will require a lifetime commitment for the thyroid hormone replacement therapy.

Procedure Step By Step

1. Patient position, old scar excision, muscle incision, and access to the thyroid lobe
2. Lateral mobilization of the left thyroid lobe with division of the middle thyroid vein
3. Mobilization and transection of the superior pole vessels with identification and preservation of the external branch of the superior laryngeal nerve (EBSLN)

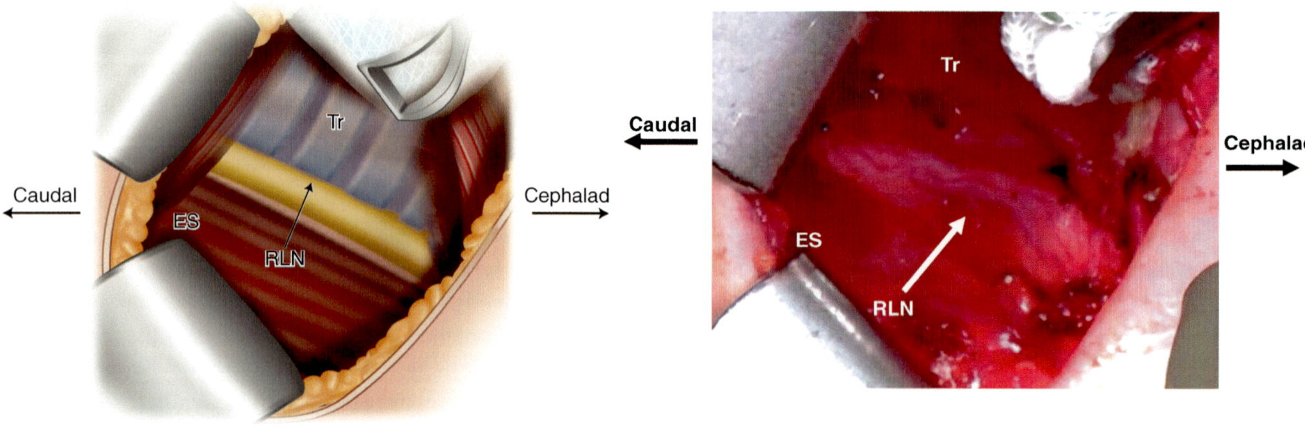

Fig. 7.1 Anatomical location of the left recurrent laryngeal nerve (RLN). Left RLN (arrow) is located in the tracheoesophageal groove. Tr – trachea; Es – esophagus; RLN – recurrent laryngeal nerve

4. Identification of the left recurrent laryngeal nerve (RLN)
5. Identification and preservation of the left inferior parathyroid gland
6. Identification and dissection of the left recurrent laryngeal nerve and the left superior parathyroid gland
7. Transection of Berry's ligament
8. Dissecting the thyroid lobe off the trachea
9. Central neck lymph node dissection
10. Irrigation, followed by muscle and skin closure

Patient Position, Old Scar Excision, Muscle Incision, and Access to the Thyroid Lobe

The patient is taken to the operating room and placed in a supine position. Sequential compression devices are placed on lower extremities bilaterally for deep venous thrombosis prophylaxis. General anesthesia is administered, and the patient is intubated using a 7.0 endotracheal tube (ET tube) with the electrodes for IONM. Both arms are tucked at the patient's sides, ensuring the padding of pressure points is given close attention to mitigate brachial and ulnar nerve injury. A shoulder roll is placed under the shoulders for neck hyperextension to promote the visibility of the surgical site; however, it should not be hanging. The head is placed in a foam head cradle (Fig. 7.2). Then flexible laryngoscopy is performed to position the ET tube IONM electrode over the vocal cords, the ET balloon is inflated, and the ET tube is secured in place. A ground electrode for IONM is placed subcuticularly into the left shoulder. The placement of an esophageal probe is important not only for intraoperative temperature monitoring but

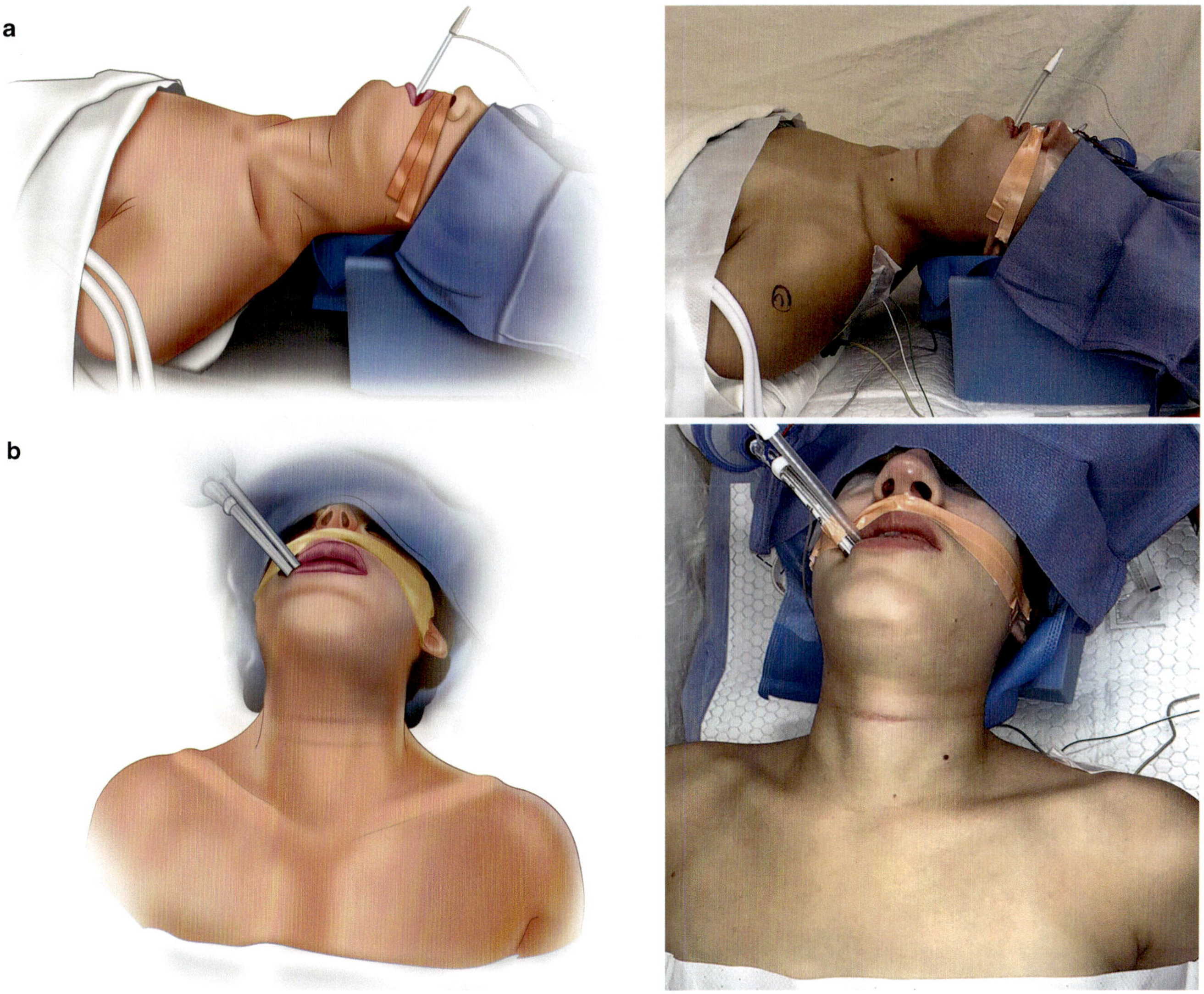

Fig. 7.2 (**a**, **b**). Patient's position. Patient is positioned supine with a shoulder roll, the head is positioned on a foam cradle and hyperextended. (**a**) Lateral view, (**b**) Anterior view

also for the identification of the esophagus in case of difficult dissection.

You can appreciate the appearance of a mildly hypertrophic scar from the previous right thyroid lobectomy in Fig. 7.2b. The patient is prepped with chlorhexidine surgical skin prep and draped with blue sterile paper drape towels and strips of an IOBAN antimicrobial adhesive drape to box off the paper drapes for a tight seal of the field. This is done to prevent accidental gas leaks from the anesthesia ventilation (to avoid fire hazards from using a Bovie cautery in the presence of oxygen) and for sterility of the field. Preoperative antibiotics are not usually given unless the patient is immunosuppressed or has metal implantable devices (joint replacements, heart valves, defibrillator, and so on), or other risk factors for infection, and in the presence of a large substernal goiter.

Skin is marked around the scar (Fig. 7.3a), and the scar is excised using a #15 blade (Fig. 7.3b). The platysma muscle is separated at the midline using Bovie cautery (Fig. 7.4). Adson tonsil forceps are placed under the plain of the platysma muscle to facilitate the dissection and prevent injury to the anterior jugular veins.

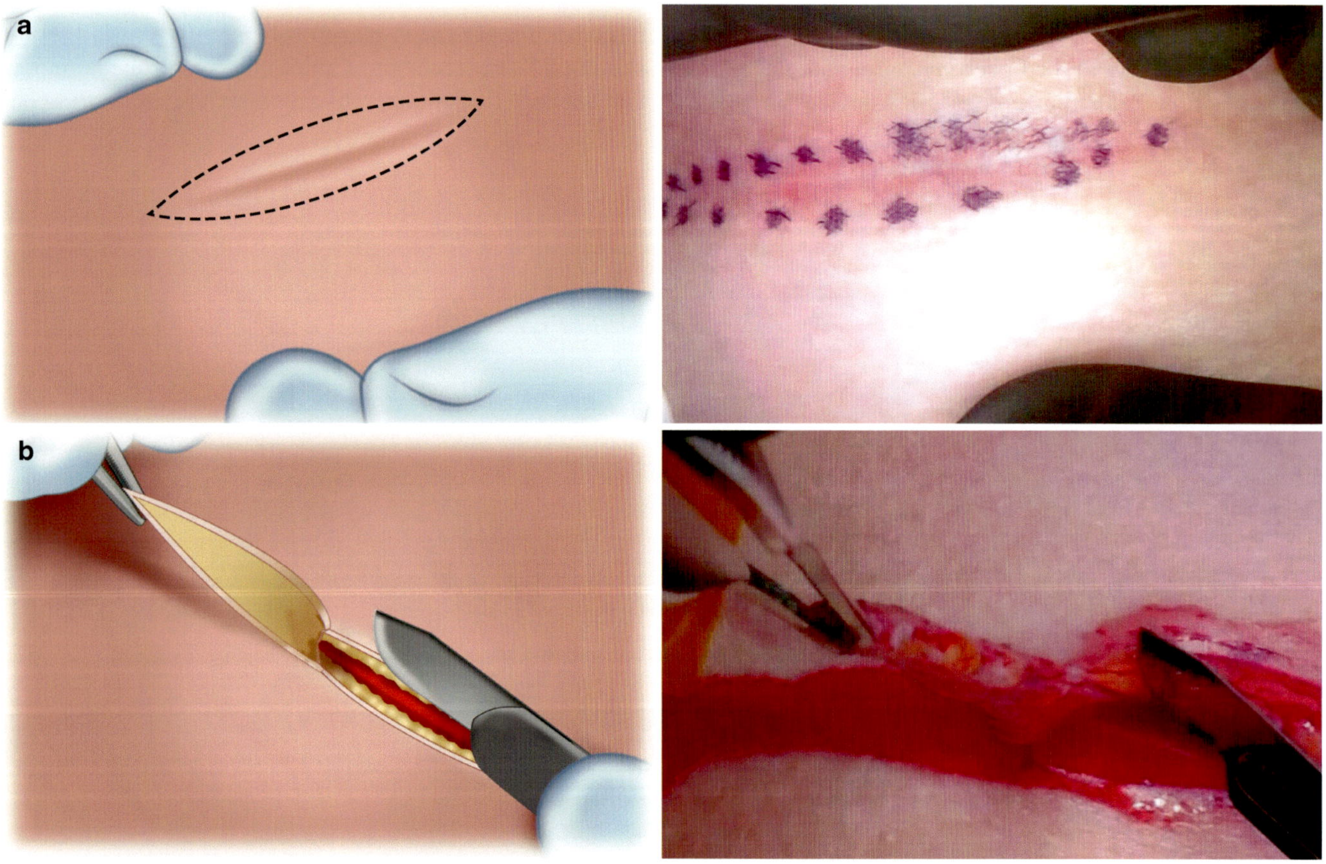

Fig. 7.3 (**a**, **b**). Skin marking and scar excision. Skin scar is marked and excised using #15 blade

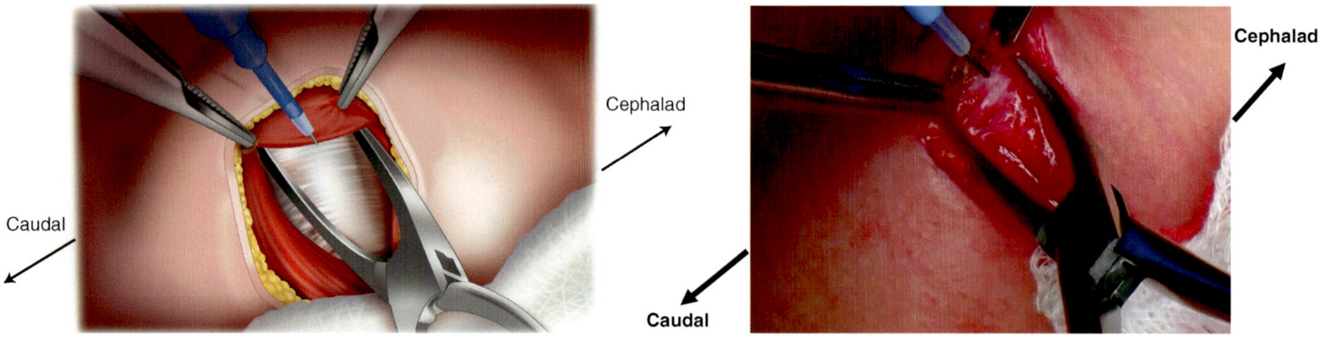

Fig. 7.4 Incision of the platysma muscle. The platysma is separated at midline using Bovie cautery

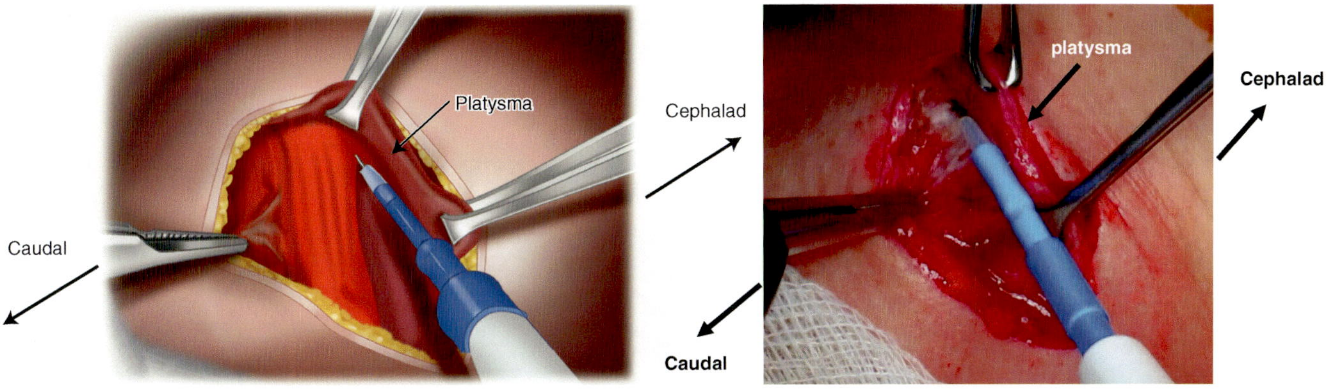

Fig. 7.5 Creation of subplatysmal flaps. Holding the platysma muscle with Allis clamps, subplatysmal flaps are created superiorly by using Bovie cautery

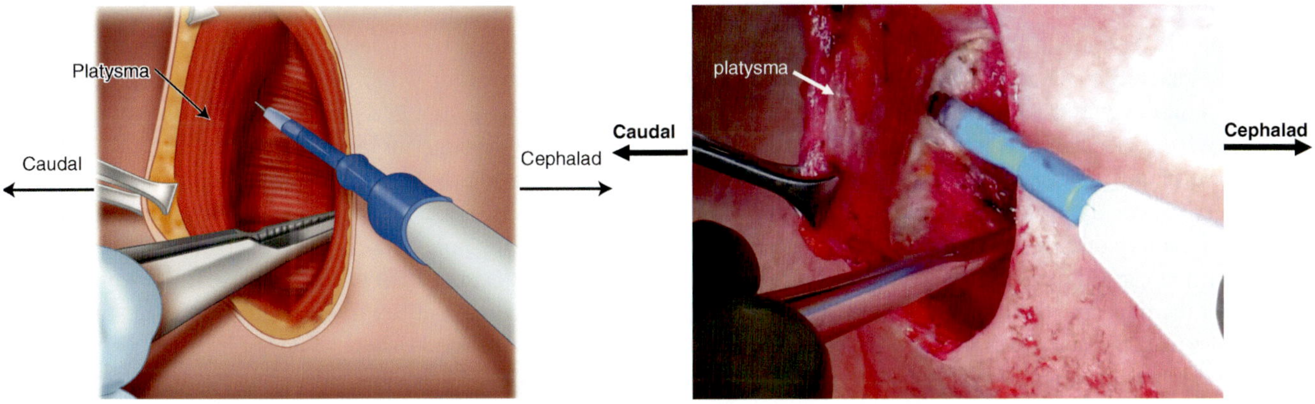

Fig. 7.6 Creation of subplatysmal flaps. Holding the platysma muscle with Allis clamps, subplatysmal flaps are created inferiorly by using Bovie cautery

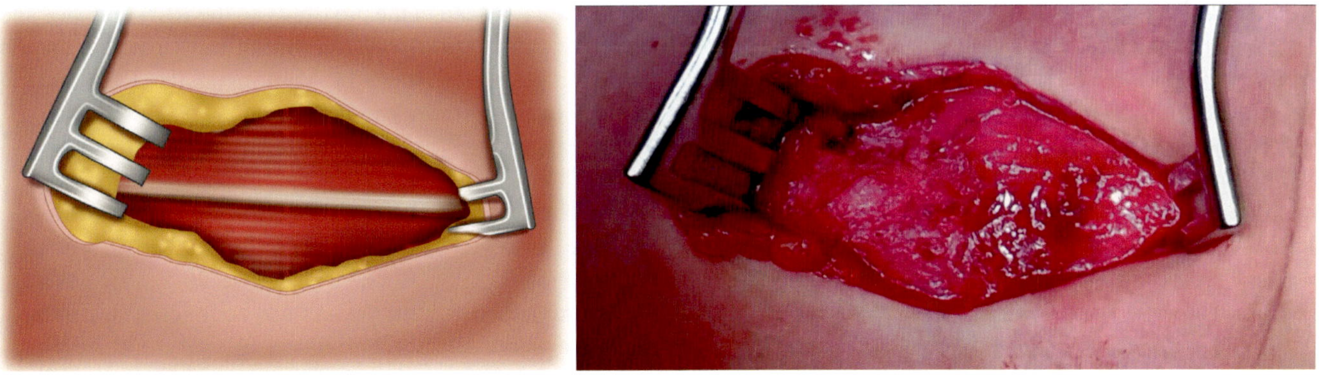

Fig. 7.7 Retraction of the platysmal flaps and exposure of the strap muscles at midline. Weitlaner self-retaining retractors are used to spread the skin and the platysma muscle edges to expose strap muscles at midline

Holding the platysma with two Allis clamps, subplatysmal flaps are created superiorly (Fig. 7.5) and inferiorly (Fig. 7.6) by using Bovie cautery. The superior flap should be smaller than the inferior flap in order to avoid denervation of the superior skin flap, which could present as postoperative skin numbness at the level of the lower chin. Weitlaner self-retaining retractors are used to spread the skin and the platysma muscle edges to expose strap muscles at the midline (Fig. 7.7). By using Adson forceps the, a space is created under the strap muscles. Then by using the Bovie cautery, strap muscles are split at the midline along the *linea alba* (Fig. 7.8).

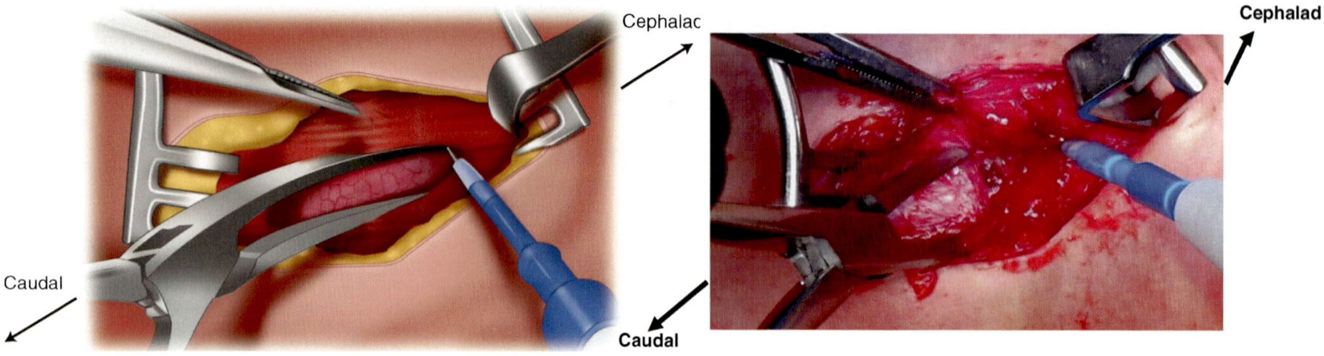

Fig. 7.8 Incision of the strap muscle. Strap muscles are split at midline along the *linea alba*

Lateral Mobilization of the Left Thyroid Lobe with Division of the Middle Thyroid Vein

The next step is the mobilization of the thyroid lobe off the strap muscles laterally. Two army/navy retractors are placed to retract the skin, the platysma, and strap muscles laterally and inferiorly. When performing lateral retraction by army/navy, be very careful not to cause significant pressure over the carotid artery, especially in elderly patients or those with a history of carotid artery disease (calcifications and occlusion), to avoid accidental carotid plug dislodgement, which can cause liberation of the plug into the circulation, which can, in turn, result in a stroke. By using Adson forceps with peanut, the thyroid lobe is retracted medially. Army/navy retractors are used to pull strap muscles and the skin laterally to create contra tension, while Debakey forceps are used to pull some of the muscle fibers off the thyroid lobe laterally to under the army/navy retractors (Fig. 7.9a). The middle thyroid vein is mobilized circumferentially with Adson forceps. It is important to dissect the vein off the underlying carotid artery and jugular vein to prevent injuries to them. When the vein is mobilized, the small Gemini right angle forceps are inserted under the middle thyroid vein to elevate it off the carotid sheet. Then the middle thyroid vein is transected in between the jaws of the small Gemini right angle forceps by using the Harmonic focus device. It is always important to keep the mid thyroid vein elevated up and away from the carotid sheet with the small Gemini right angle forceps during this maneuver (Fig. 7.9b).

Mobilization and Transection of the Superior Pole Vessels with Identification and Preservation of the External Branch of the Superior Laryngeal Nerve (EBSLN)

After the middle thyroid vein is transected, two army/navy retractors are moved superiorly. The first army/navy retractor is placed lateral to the superior pole with the deep end in, and the second is medial to the superior pole with the short end in. By holding the superior pole with Debakey forceps, it is grabbed with an Allis clamp and pulled inferiorly (Fig. 7.10). By using Adson forceps (Adson hemostatic clamp), the avascular space of Reeve (SR) is entered and dissected to separate the superior pole vessels from the cricothyroid muscles (Fig. 7.11). Keeping this space dry is crucial for the safe dissection and prevention of injury to the external branch of the superior laryngeal nerve (EBSLN). EBSLN usually lies medially on or in between the fibers of the cricothyroid muscle. By using small Gemini right angle forceps, several superior pole vessels are dissected and elevated up (Fig. 7.12). It is important to stay as close to the thyroid lobe as possible to avoid injury to the EBSLN. Nerve stimulation (NS) can also be used to determine the location and integrity of the EBSLN. Then superior pole vessels are transacted using the Harmonic Focus device in between the jaws of the Gemini right angle forceps (Fig. 7.13). These steps are repeated until all superior pole vessels are transected. To avoid incidental injury to the RLN, dissection should not be conducted too deep in the proximity to the RLN entrance site into the cricothyroid muscle. Significant traction on the superior pole may result in traction on the RLN, neural stretch, and temporary paralysis.

Identification of the Left Recurrent Laryngeal Nerve

After the superior pole vessels are completely transacted, army/navy retractors are replaced laterally and inferiorly (Fig. 7.14). Keeping the superior Allis clamp on the superior pole of the left thyroid lobe, the second Allis clamp is placed on the inferior pole of the left thyroid lobe. Be careful to not accidentally grab the inferior parathyroid gland during the placement of the lower Allis clamp on the inferior pole. The left thyroid lobe is retracted medially and anteriorly by pooling on two Allis clamps. Debakey forceps are used to pull the fibrous tissue overlying the area laterally. The RLN is identified by dissecting these tissues with a mosquito clamp along the area of the presumptive course of the RLN directed inferiorly (Fig. 7.15a). A nerve stimu-

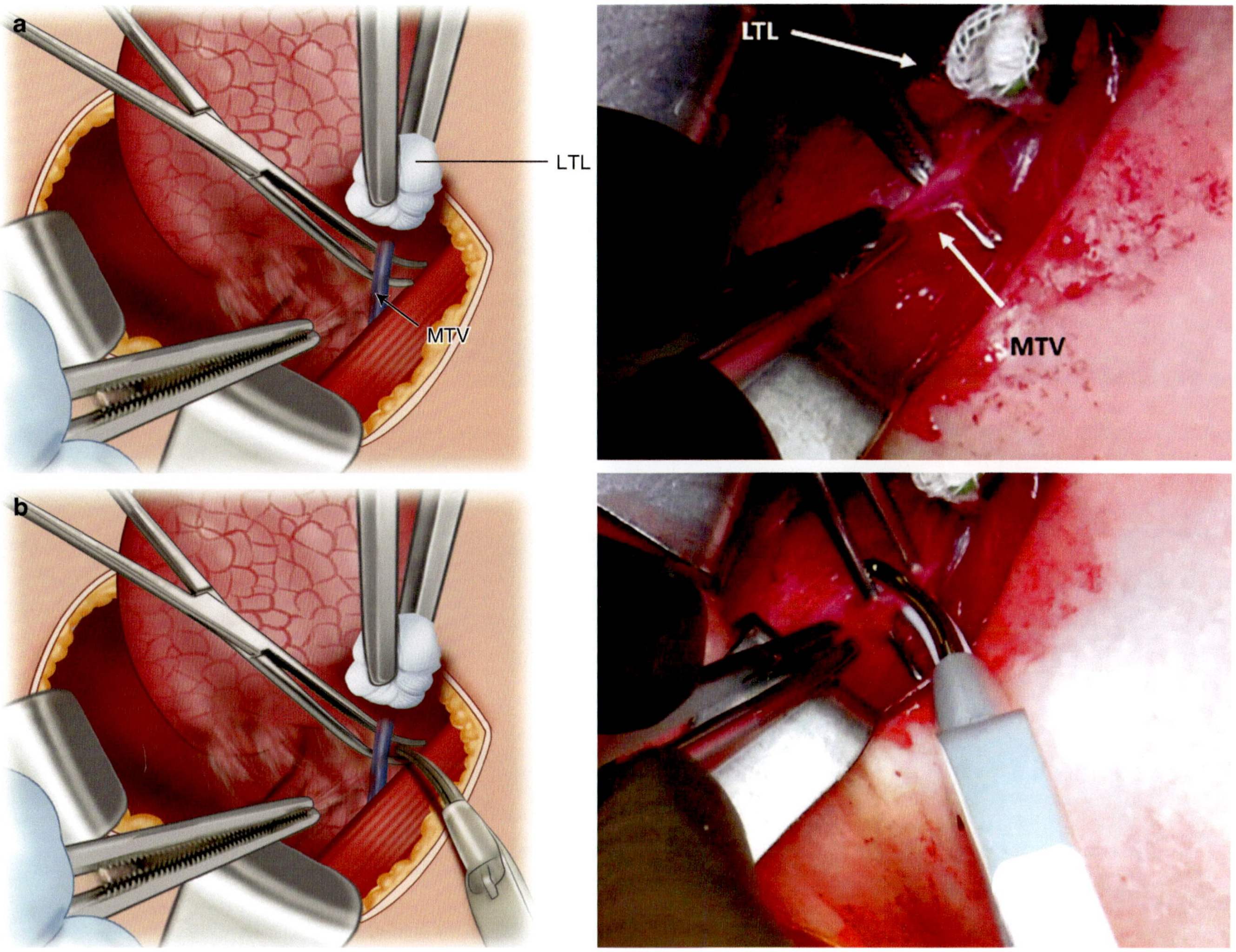

Fig. 7.9 (**a**, **b**). Lateral mobilization of the left thyroid lobe with division of the middle thyroid vein. Two army/navy retractors are placed to retract the skin, the platysma, and strap muscles laterally and inferiorly. By using Adson hemostatic forceps with peanut, the thyroid lobe is retracted medially. Army/navy retractors are used to pull the strap muscles and skin laterally to create contra tension, while Debakey forceps are used to pull some of the muscle fibers off the thyroid lobe laterally to under the army/navy retractors. The middle thyroid vein is mobilized with Adson hemostatic forceps, then with right angle (**a**) and transected by using the Harmonic Focus device (**b**). MTV – middle thyroid vein; LTL – right thyroid lobe

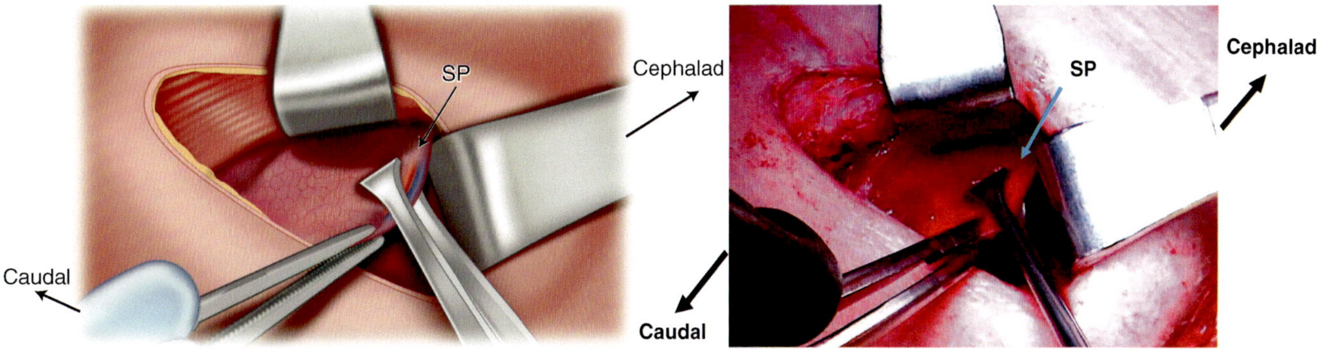

Fig. 7.10 Mobilization of the superior pole vessels. By holding the superior pole with Debakey forceps, it is grabbed with an Allis clamp and pulled inferiorly. Arrow is pointing at the superior pole vessels. SP – superior pole

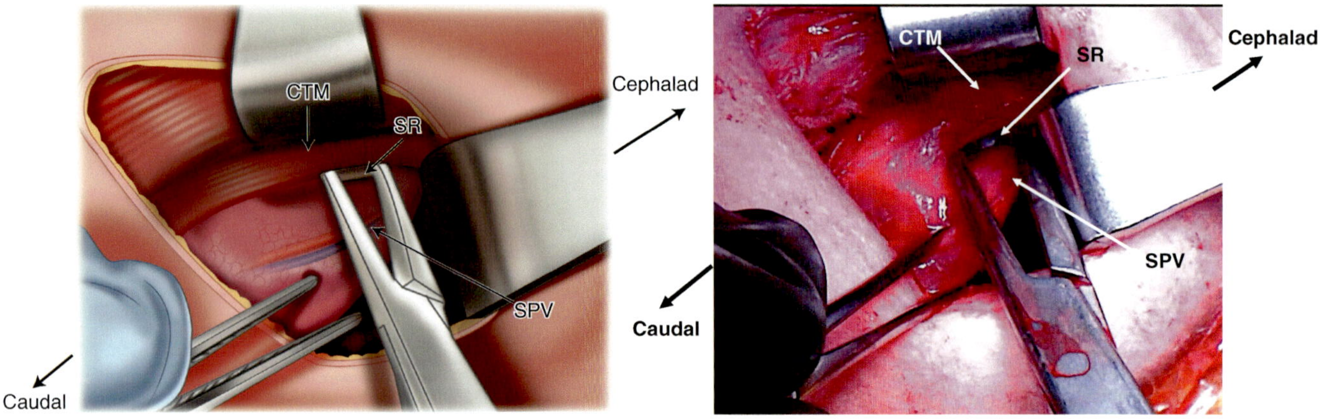

Fig. 7.11 Mobilization of the superior pole vessels. Avascular space of Reeve (SR) is entered and dissected to separate the superior pole vessels (SPV) from the cricothyroid muscles (CTM)

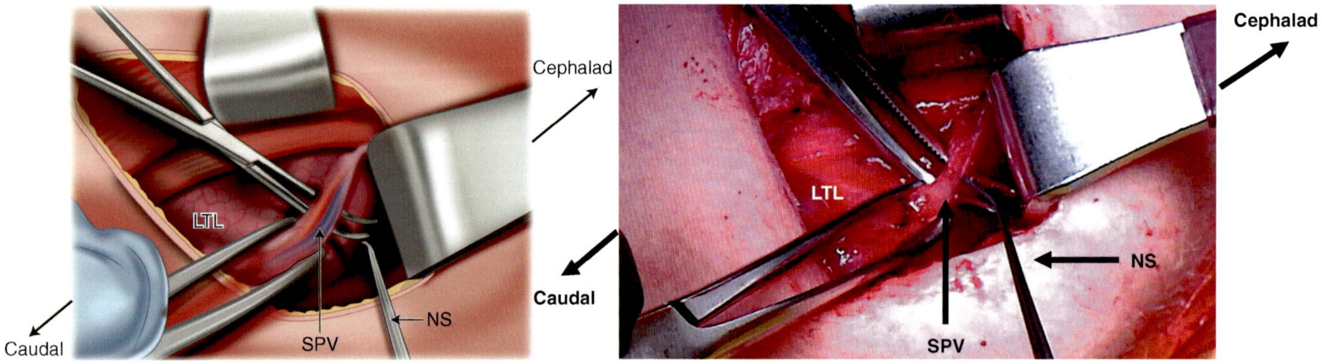

Fig. 7.12 Mobilization of the superior pole vessels. Gemini right angle forceps are used to dissect and elevate superior pole vessels. External branch of the superior laryngeal nerve (EBSLN) monitoring is used to determine the location and integrity of the EBSLN. SPV – superior pole vessels of the right thyroid lobe, LTL – left thyroid lobe; NS – nerve stimulator probe

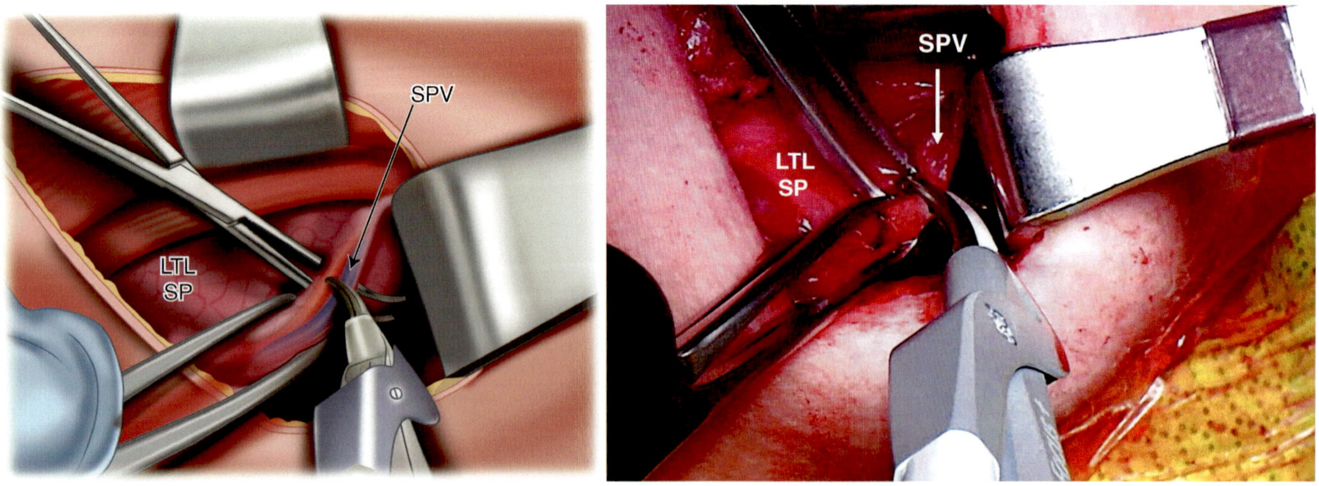

Fig. 7.13 Transection of the superior pole vessels. Superior pole vessels are transected with the use of the Harmonic Focus device. SPV – superior pole vessels of the right thyroid lobe; LTL – left thyroid lobe; SP – superior pole

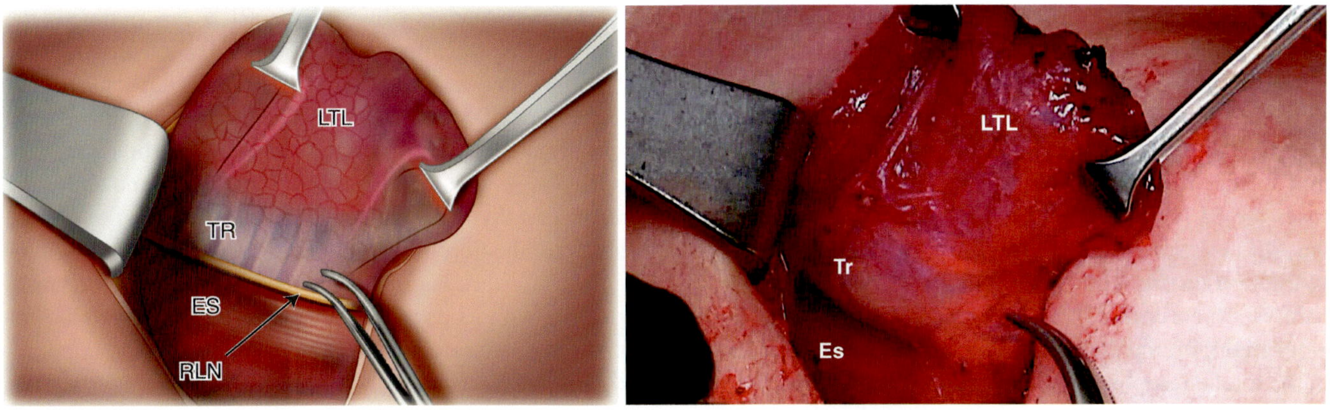

Fig. 7.14 Identification of the left recurrent laryngeal nerve. Keeping the superior Allis clamp on the superior pole (SP) of the thyroid lobe, the second Allis clamp is placed on the inferior pole (IP) of the right thyroid lobe to retract the thyroid lobe medially. In order to identify the RLN, the dissection starts along the course of the RLN with mosquito clamps going from the cephalad to the caudal direction. LTL – left thyroid lobe; Tr – trachea; Es – esophagus

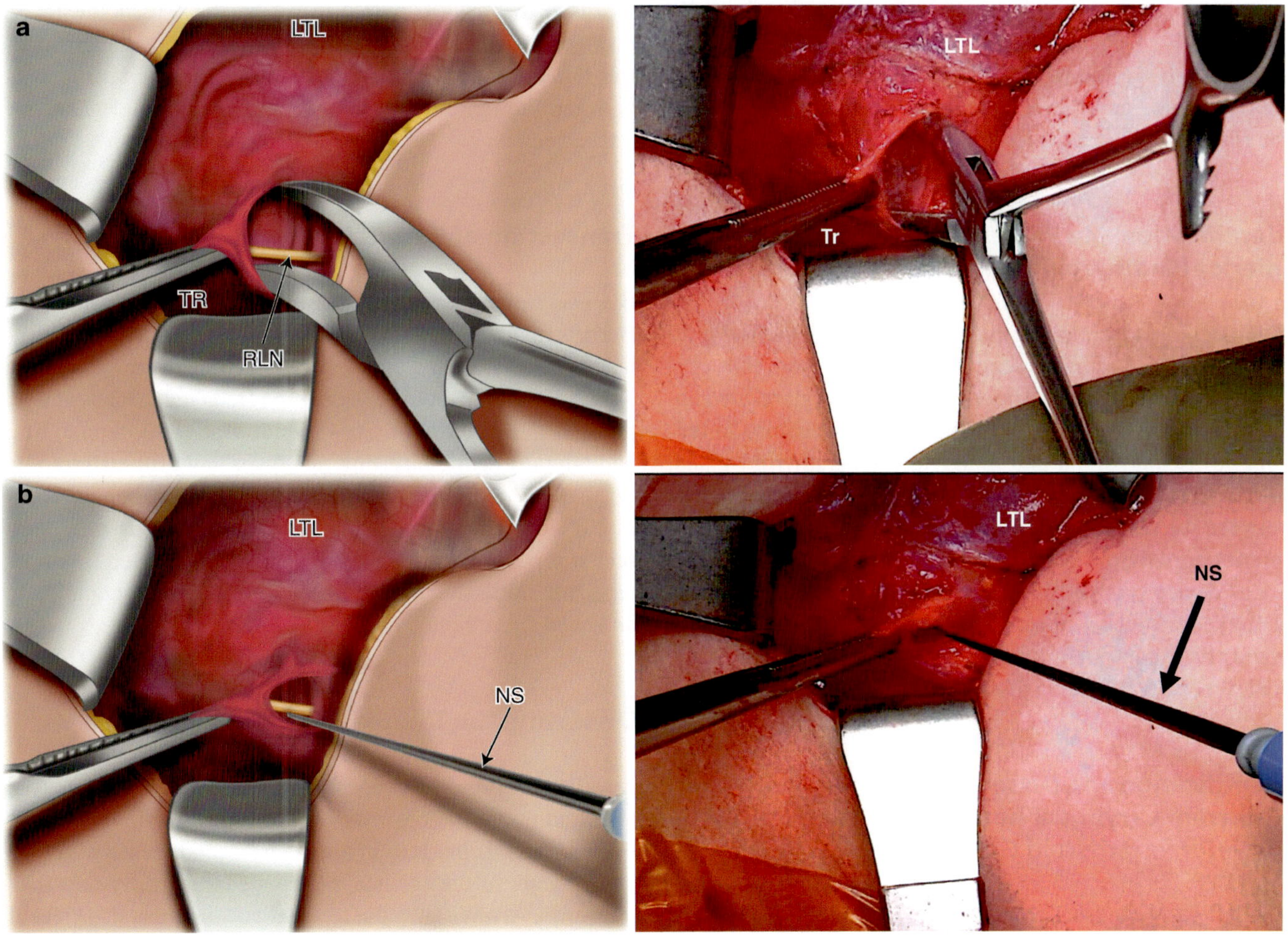

Fig. 7.15 (**a**, **b**). Identification of the left recurrent laryngeal nerve. Holding the tissue, overlapping the area of the presumptive location of the RLN under the thyroid with Debakey forceps and spreading with mosquito clamp, the RLN is identified (**a**). Nerve stimulator (NS) is used to confirm the integrity of the RLN. IONM also can be used to identify the location of the RLN if it is not immediately visualized (**b**) and to confirm the integrity of the nerve to prevent extensive traction on the nerve that could result in neuropraxia. LTL – left thyroid lobe; Tr – trachea; NS – nerve stimulator

lator (NS) is used to ensure that RLN is intact. IONM also can be used to identify the location of the RLN if it is not immediately visualized (Fig. 7.15b). Meticulous dissection and magnification with surgical loupes make it easier to identify the position of the RLN and its branches, in relation to the inferior thyroid artery (ITA), since in 24% of cases the RLN runs anterior to ITA. Significant traction on the Allis clamps while holding the thyroid lobe may result in traction on the RLN with neural stretch and temporary paralysis (neuropraxia). The left recurrent laryngeal nerve is located more medially and anteriorly on the trachea and in the tracheoesophageal groove compared to the right side RLN, where it is ascending more laterally. It is almost imperative to assume that most of the time the left RLN is positioned so medially and anteriorly that if the thyroid lobe is retracted, the RLN will be immediately under the thyroid lobe and attached to it posteriorly. If you can't find it right away, it is right under the left thyroid lobe and attached to the thyroid lobe posteriorly, rather than laterally or inferiorly! Debakey forceps are used to pull the fibrous tissue overlying the RLN and the ITA laterally, then both (fibrous tissue and the ITA) are transected with the use of the Harmonic Focus device.

Identification and Preservation of the Left Inferior Parathyroid Gland

After the exact location of the RLN is defined, the left inferior parathyroid gland is identified.

Attachments to the left inferior parathyroid gland are gently held and pulled inferiorly with Debakey forceps. To prevent devascularization and injury to the parathyroid gland, the traction should be very gentle. Then inferior attachments between the inferior pole of the left thyroid lobe and the left inferior parathyroid gland are transected with the Harmonic Focus device (Fig. 7.16a). The parathyroid gland's location is marked with the 5-mm clip (placed on the tissue above the gland) for future identification and preservation during the central neck lymph node dissection (Fig. 7.16b, c).

Identification and Dissection of the Left Recurrent Laryngeal Nerve and the Left Superior Parathyroid Gland

The left RLN is visualized along the left side of the trachea ascending from the tracheoesophageal groove toward Berry's ligament (Fig. 7.17). It is dissected up toward Berry's ligament and to its insertion side into the cricothyroid muscle with a mosquito clamp. The left superior parathyroid gland is identified below and anteriorly to Berry's ligament (Fig. 7.18). The RLN was located right under it and medially. When the exact location and position of the RLN are outlined, the attachments between the inferior pole of the left thyroid lobe and the trachea are transected using the Harmonic Focus device (Fig. 7.19). This step in the mobilization of the thyroid lobe will help in performing the next steps of the dissection. The RLN is seen going under Berry's ligament and above the superior parathyroid gland (Fig. 7.20a). Debakey forceps are used to pull the fibrous tissue overlying the RLN and the inferior thyroid artery laterally. The pair of mosquito forceps is placed flat with its back curved side on the RLN, and dissection is directed up toward its insertion site into the cricothyroid muscle. Tissues overlying the RLN, including the ITA, are transected using the Harmonic Focus device. If the RLN is branched out, the most medial and anterior branch would be the motor branch. The integrity of the RLN is confirmed by the nerve stimulator with every step of the dissection to avoid extensive pulling on the thyroid, which can cause tension on the RLN, resulting in neuropraxia. Mosquito forceps are used to create a tunnel space on the top of the RLN, between the RLN, and under the attachments to the left superior parathyroid gland (Fig. 7.20a, b). Then the attachments between the thyroid and left superior parathyroid gland are transected using the Harmonic Focus device (Fig. 7.21).

Transection of Berry's Ligament

By using the Debakey forceps, fibrous tissues attaching Berry's ligament to the trachea are retracted laterally. A tunneled space is created under these attachments by using mosquito forceps. Without replacing the Debakey forceps and by holding these fibrous tissues, gentle traction is applied up and laterally while inserting the lower jaw of the Harmonic Focus device into the tunneled space. Always keep the RLN in full view. The superficial layer of this fibrous tissue is transected opening the tunneled space. These steps can be repeated until the entire Berry's ligament is completely detached from the trachea (Fig. 7.22).

Dissecting the Thyroid Lobe Off the Trachea

By using mosquito forceps, a space in between the thyroid lobe and trachea is created. The lower jaw of the Harmonic Focus device is inserted into that space, and the thyroid lobe attachments to the trachea are divided superiorly and then inferiorly. Always keep the top "active" (non isolated) jaw of the Harmonic Focus device away from the trachea to avoid an accidental burning injury to it or to prevent tracheal penetration. The scar from the previous removal of the right thyroid lobe at the midline and the left thyroid lobe is transected using the Harmonic Focus device (Fig. 7.23a, b).

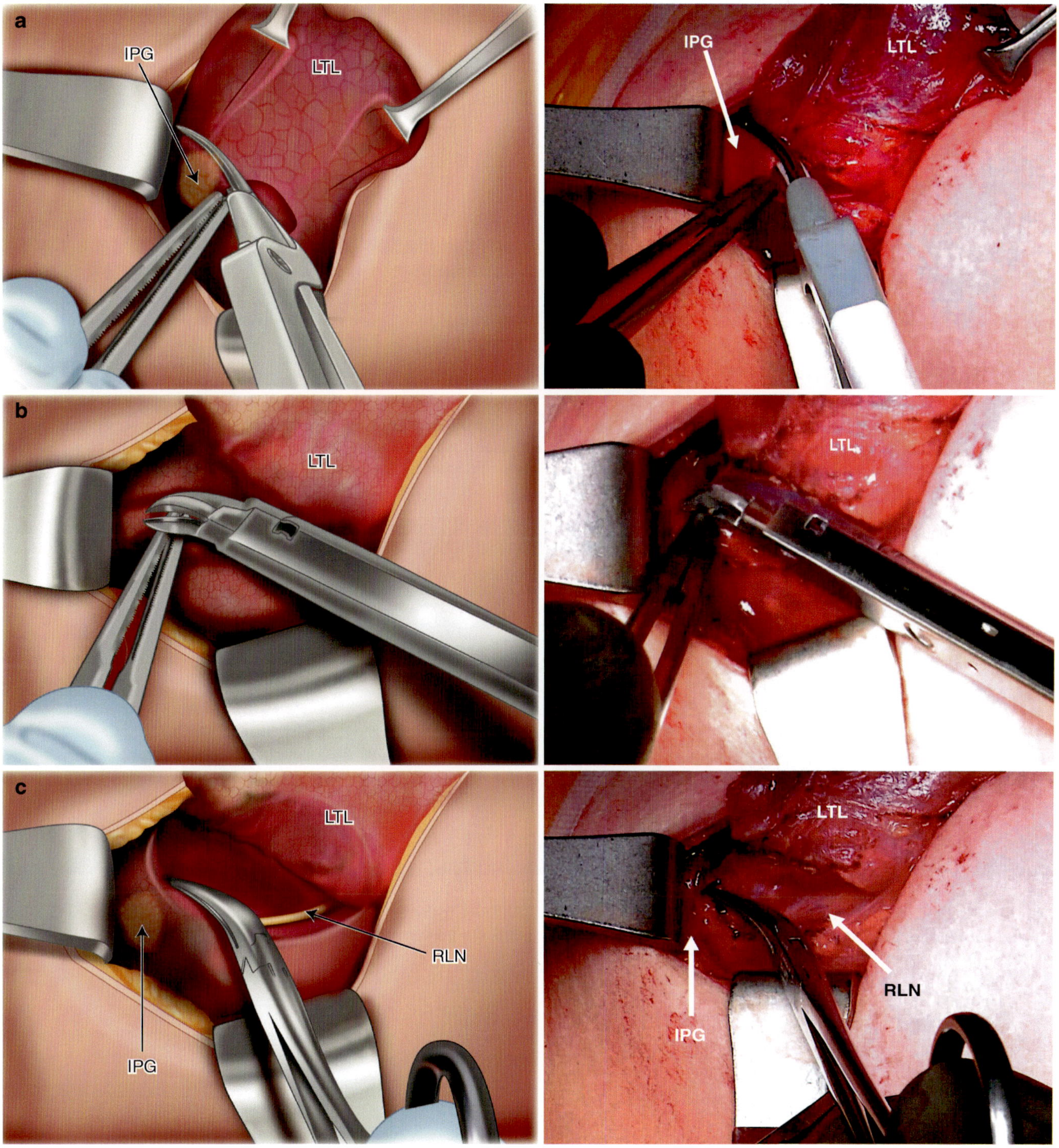

Fig. 7.16 (**a**–**c**). Identification and preservation of the left inferior parathyroid gland. After the exact location of the RLN is defined, the left inferior parathyroid gland is identified and inferior attachments between the inferior pole of the left thyroid lobe and the left inferior parathyroid gland are transected with the Harmonic Focus device (**a**). The parathyroid gland location is marked with the 5-mm clip (placed on the tissue above the gland) for future identification and preservation during the central neck lymph node dissection (**b**). Mosquito clamp is pointing at the attachments toward the top portion of the left inferior parathyroid gland that is marked with the 5-mm clip (**c**). LTL – left thyroid lobe; IPG – left inferior parathyroid gland; RLN – recurrent laryngeal nerve

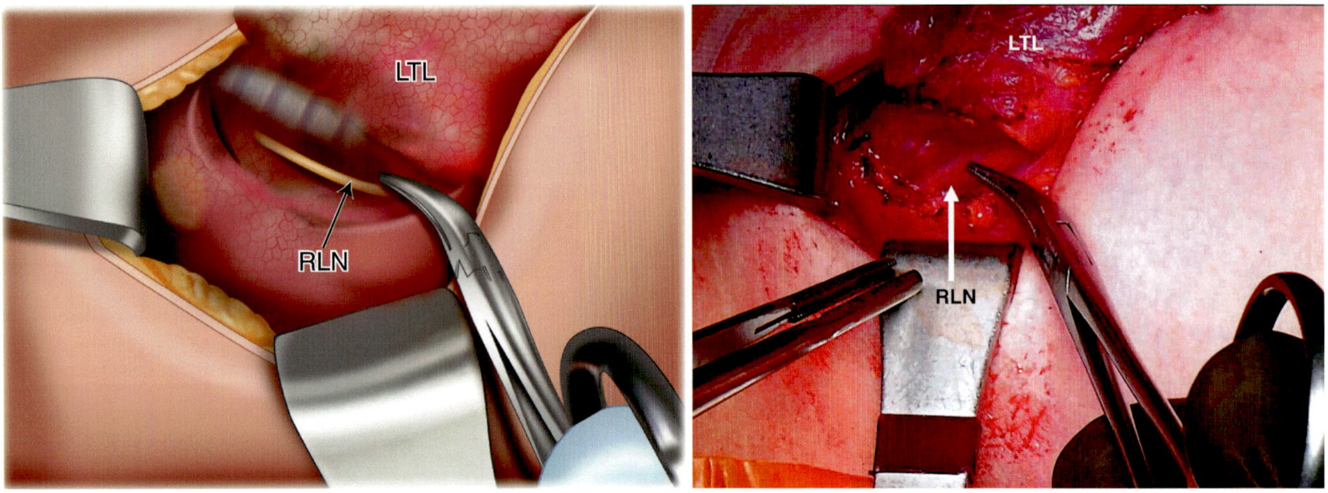

Fig. 7.17 Identification and dissection of the left recurrent laryngeal nerve. The left RLN is visualized along the left side of the trachea ascending from the tracheoesophageal groove toward Berry's ligament. It has been dissected with mosquito clamps in a superior direction toward its insertion site. Mosquito is pointing at the RLN. LTL – left thyroid lobe; RLN – recurrent laryngeal nerve

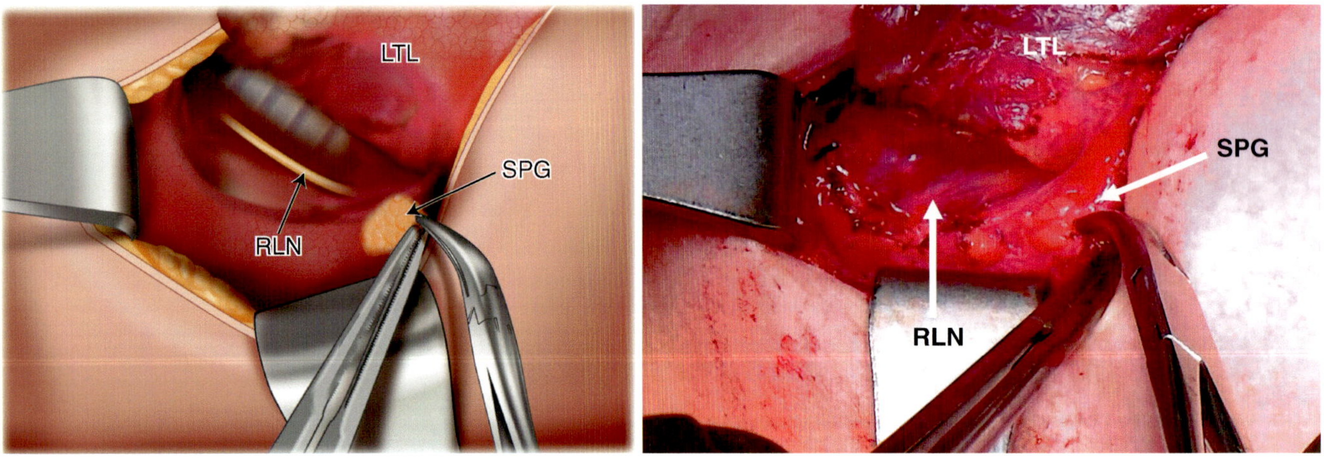

Fig. 7.18 Identification of the left superior parathyroid gland. Left superior parathyroid gland is identified below and anteriorly to Berry's ligament (mosquito is pointing at the left superior parathyroid gland). LTL – left thyroid lobe; RLN – recurrent laryngeal nerve; SPG – left superior parathyroid gland

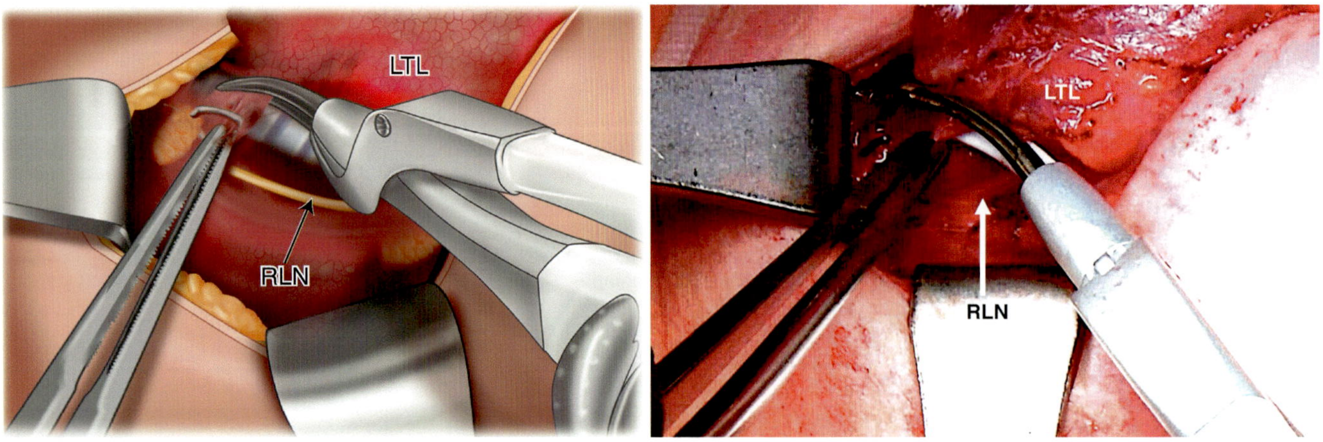

Fig. 7.19 Transection of attachments between the inferior pole of the left thyroid lobe and the trachea. The attachments between the inferior pole of the left thyroid lobe and the trachea are transected using the Harmonic Focus device. This step will help in performing the following dissection of the RLN. Arrow is pointing at the RLN. RLN – recurrent laryngeal nerve, LTL – left thyroid lobe; RLN – recurrent laryngeal nerve

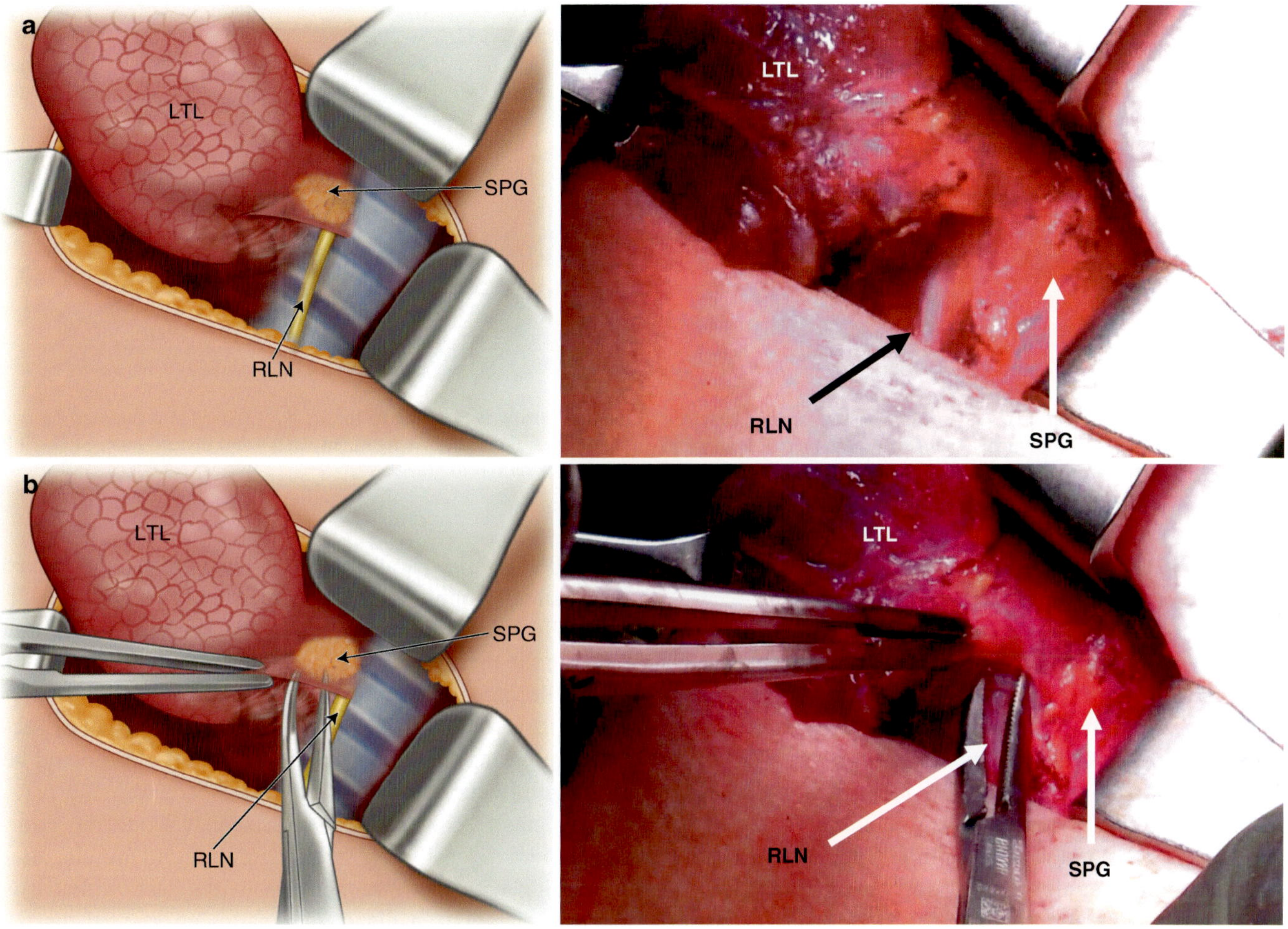

Fig. 7.20 (**a**, **b**). Dissection and preservation of the left superior parathyroid gland. Mosquito forceps are used to create a tunnel space on the top of the RLN, in between the nerve, and under the attachments to the left superior parathyroid gland. SPG – left superior parathyroid gland, LTL – left thyroid lobe; RLN – recurrent laryngeal nerve

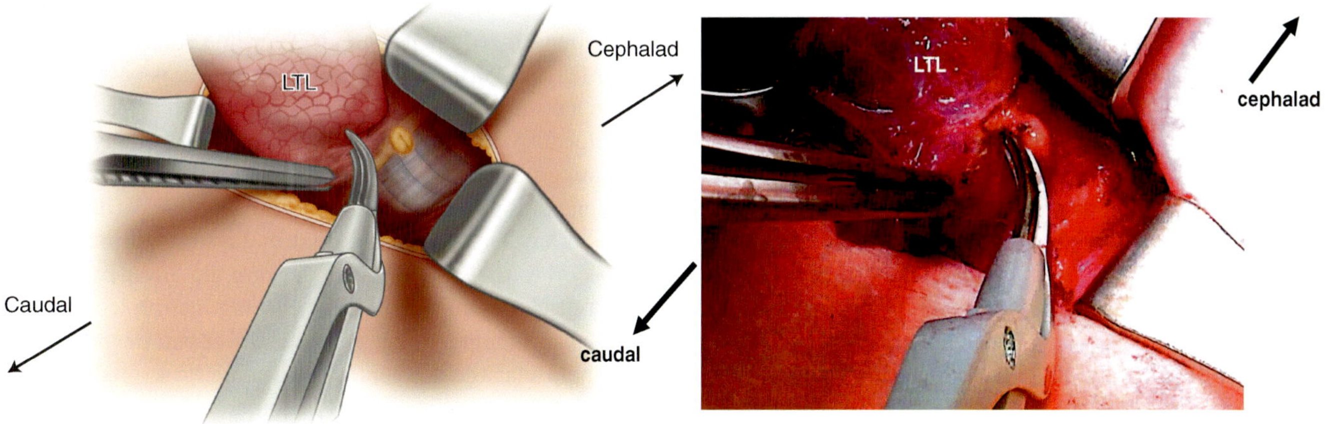

Fig. 7.21 Dissection and preservation of the left superior parathyroid gland. Attachments between the thyroid and left superior parathyroid gland are transected using the Harmonic Focus device. LTL – left thyroid lobe

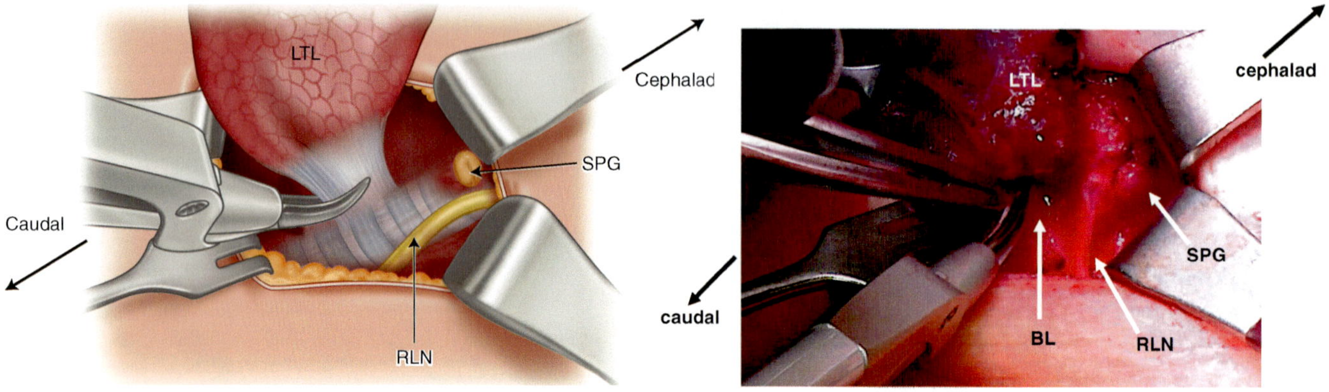

Fig. 7.22 Transection of Berry's ligament. Space is created between the Berry's ligament and the trachea using mosquito clamp. Harmonic Focus device is used to transect attachments of Berry's ligament to the trachea. Arrow is pointing to the RLN, which is also outlined by two white lines; BL – Berry's ligament; LTL – left thyroid lobe; SPG – left superior parathyroid gland

Central Neck Lymph Nodes Dissection

In our case, there were no positive or enlarged lymph nodes identified, and prophylactic CNLND dissection on the left was performed. Prelaryngeal lymph nodes (including Delphian) were removed, together with the pyramidal lobe, during the previous right thyroid lobectomy.

The exact location of the RLN is identified (including all branches if present) from its insertion site at the cricothyroid muscle down to the thoracic inlet (Fig. 7.24a). The left RLN lies more medially and anteriorly in the tracheoesophageal groove, compared to the right RLN. Using an Adson (or tonsil) clamp, the RLN is dissected off the fibroadipose tissues overlying it anteriorly and laterally (Fig. 7.24b). By gently grabbing the fibroadipose tissues overlying the RLN with Debakey forceps and applying gentle traction anteriorly and superiorly, the Adson (or tonsil) clamp is used to dissect the fibroadipose tissues with lymph nodes off the nerve while trying to maintain an *en bloc* technique (Fig. 7.25a). The Harmonic Focus device is used to transect medial attachments of the fibroadipose tissues with lymph nodes to the trachea, keeping the RLN in full view (Fig. 7.25b).

Then with the Debakey forceps and applying gentle traction anteriorly and superiorly, the fibroadipose tissues with lymph nodes are dissected using the Adson (or tonsil) clamp down into the thoracic inlet and anteriorly over the trachea (inferior pretracheal lymph nodes above the sternal notch), dissecting them off the RLN on the left and trying to maintain an *en bloc* technique (Fig. 7.26a). A nerve stimulator is used to confirm the integrity of the RLN in each step of the dissection (Fig. 7.26b). The Harmonic Focus device is used to transect inferior attachments of the fibroadipose tissues with lymph nodes, keeping the RLN in full view (Fig. 7.27).

When doing inferior dissection, be careful not to injure the thoracic duct.

The left inferior parathyroid gland was previously marked with a small 5-mm titanium clip and should be preserved. It is usually located more anteriorly and laterally, most often found in the thyrothymic tract. Freeing up the gland from its medial fibroareolar attachments helps in to moving it laterally on its vascular pedicle and away from the area of dissection. Preserving the left inferior parathyroid gland could be challenging with bulky central lymphadenopathy. If a parathyroid gland becomes devascularized, it should be reimplanted into the ipsilateral sternocleidomastoid muscle, after confirming with the intraoperative frozen section that it is indeed a parathyroid gland. Compartment-oriented dissection is critical, and no "berry picking" should be performed.

Irrigation, Followed by Muscle and Skin Closure

The wound is irrigated with sterile saline solution or sterile water (Fig. 7.28a), then a Valsalva maneuver is performed to create a positive intrathoracic pressure, which helps visualize any bleeding vessels and confirm the absence of any air leak indicating tracheal injury. Fibrillar, a hemostatic and bactericidal agent, is placed in the cavity (Fig. 7.28b). We do not use drains. Then the wound is closed by layers with interrupted 3.0 Vicryl to the strap muscles, leaving the lower part of the strap muscles open (Fig. 7.29a). Placing interrupted sutures, rather than running, and leaving the lower part of the muscle open help manage a potential hematoma or seroma without opening the entire incision. This could be done in the office without going to the operating room. Then the platysma muscle is closed with interrupted 4.0 Vicryl (Fig. 7.29b). The skin is closed with a single running 5.0 Monocryl (Fig. 7.30a), leaving the ends of the stitch on both sides of the incision without nodes. Dermabond is placed on the wound, and the

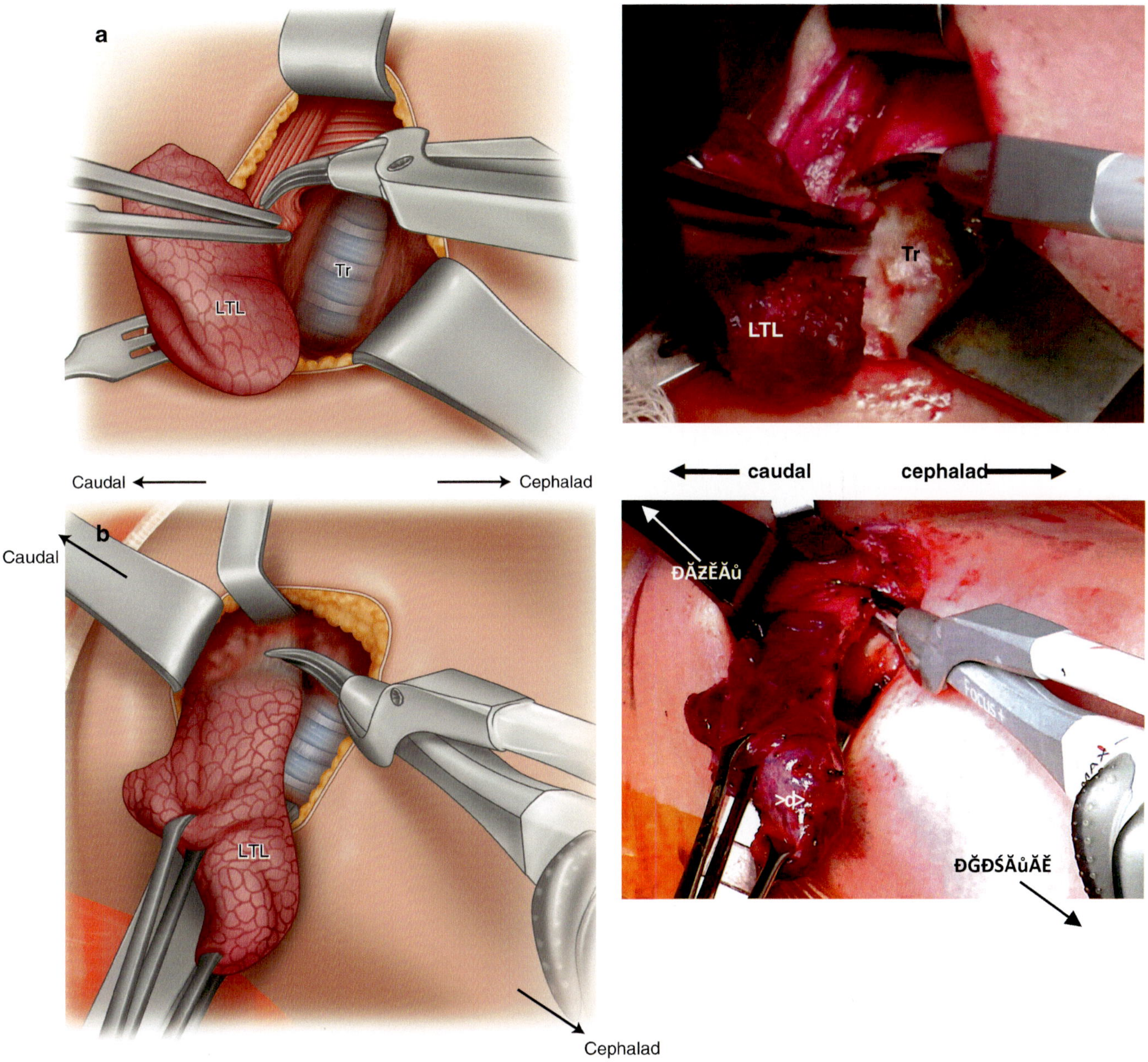

Fig. 7.23 (**a**, **b**). Dissecting the thyroid lobe off the trachea. The remaining attachments between the trachea and left thyroid lobe (**a**) and the scar from previous removal of the right thyroid lobe at midline (**b**) are transected using the Harmonic Focus device. LTL – left thyroid lobe; Tr – trachea

ends of the Monocryl stitch are cut at the level of the skin without leaving any nodes. (Fig. 7.30b).

After the patient is extubated, a flexible laryngoscopy is performed to confirm the normal function of the vocal cords. An ice pack is placed on the neck over a towel in the recovery room. The patient is observed for approximately 5–6 hours in an outpatient recovery unit and monitored to make sure there are no hematoma developments. Approximately 2 weeks later, the patient follows up in the office for a postoperative wound check and to review pathology results.

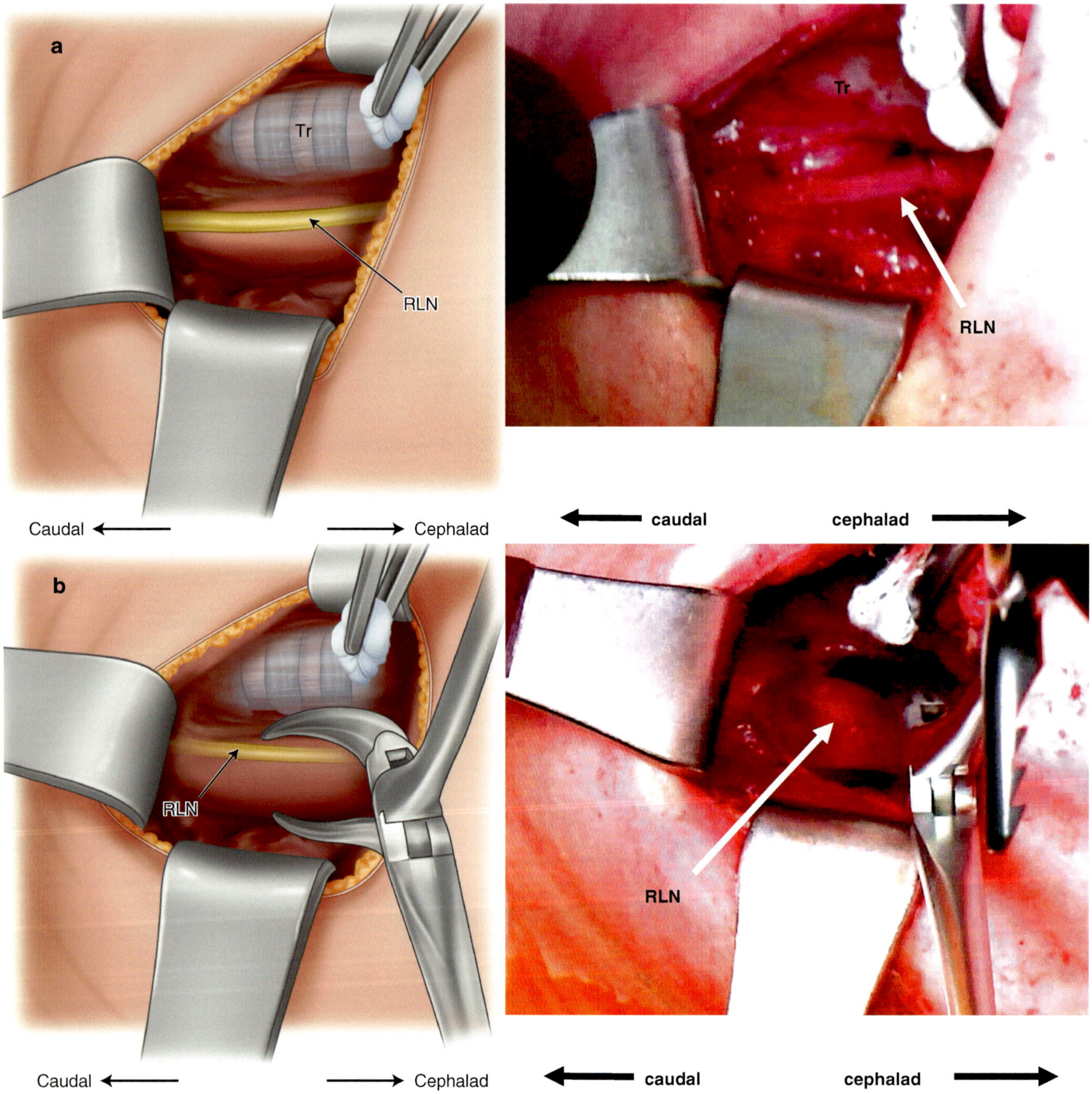

Fig. 7.24 (**a**, **b**). Central neck lymph node dissection. Trachea is retracted with the peanut, exposing the CNLN compartment (**a**). Dissection is carried out with Adson clamp on the top of the RLN (**b**). Tr – trachea; RLN – recurrent laryngeal nerve

Surgical Pearls and Management of Complications

Please see Chap. 1 for "*Surgical Pearls,*" the management of *postoperative hematoma*, *postoperative hypocalcemia*, and *RLN injury*.

Thoracic Duct Injury

If a chyle leak is detected during the surgery (white milky fluid is coming out from the inferior part of the wound), a thoracic duct injury should be suspected. Since in most cases the duct itself will not be visualized, all attempts should be

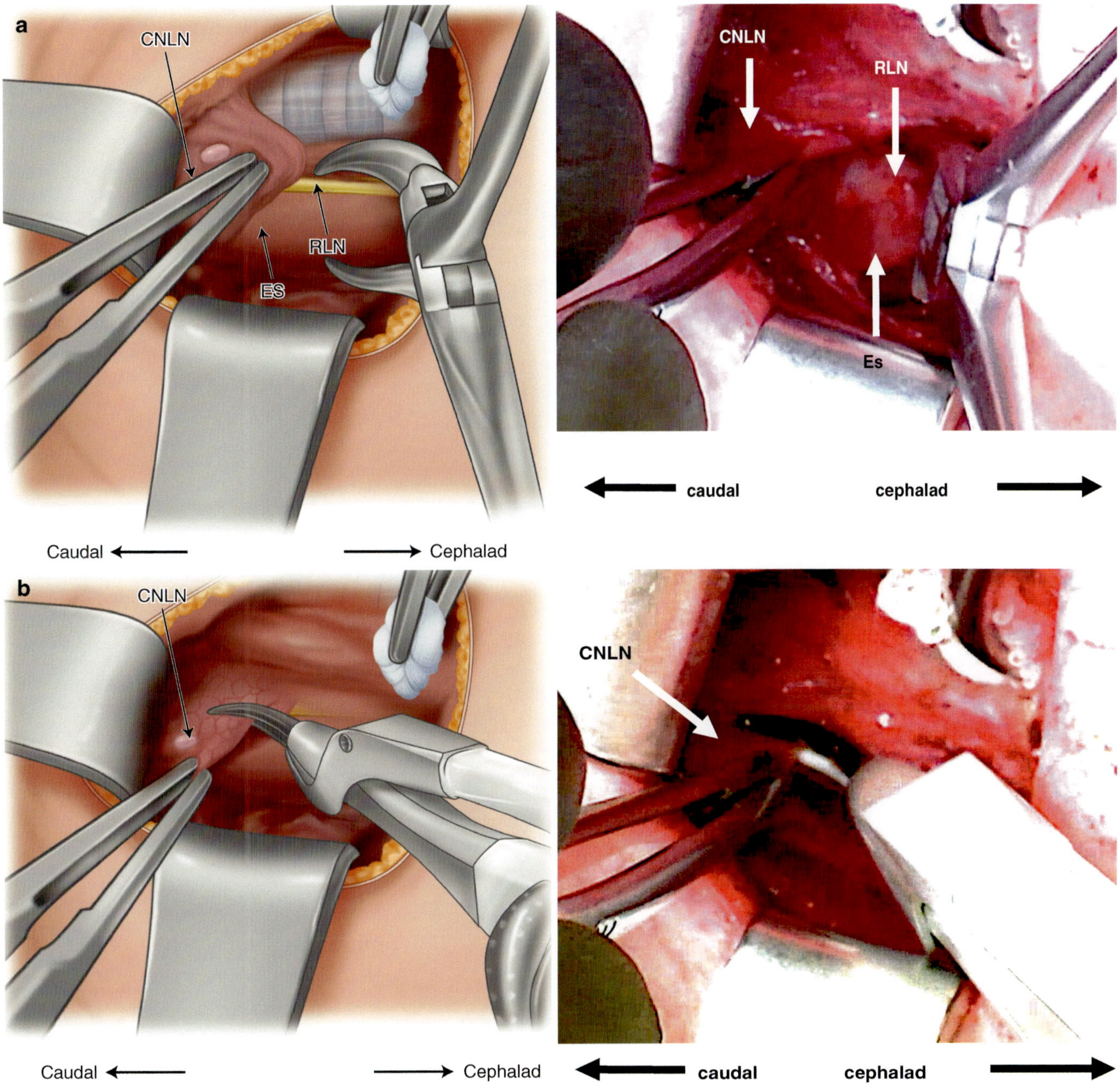

Fig. 7.25 (**a**, **b**). Central neck lymph node dissection. By holding with Debakey forceps the fibroadipose tissues with lymph nodes, the underlying left RLN is dissected off (**a**). The Harmonic Focus device is used to transect medial tracheal attachments of fibroadipose tissues with lymph nodes (**b**). RLN – recurrent laryngeal nerve, CNLN – central neck lymph node specimen, Es – esophagus

made to either put a large clip on the area of a leak or ligate the area of the leak even without identifying the thoracic duct itself. It can be achieved by gently grabbing the area of a leak with the Debakey forceps and placing the large clip on a fibrous tissue under the Debakey forceps. Creating an increased intrathoracic pressure by performing a Valsalva maneuver or giving a methylene blue dye intravenously or giving a dose of propofol will help identify the area of the leak and confirm the seal after the ligation or clip placement. Be careful not to put a clip on or ligate the subclavian vein or internal jugular vein since the thoracic duct enters at the confluence of those veins.

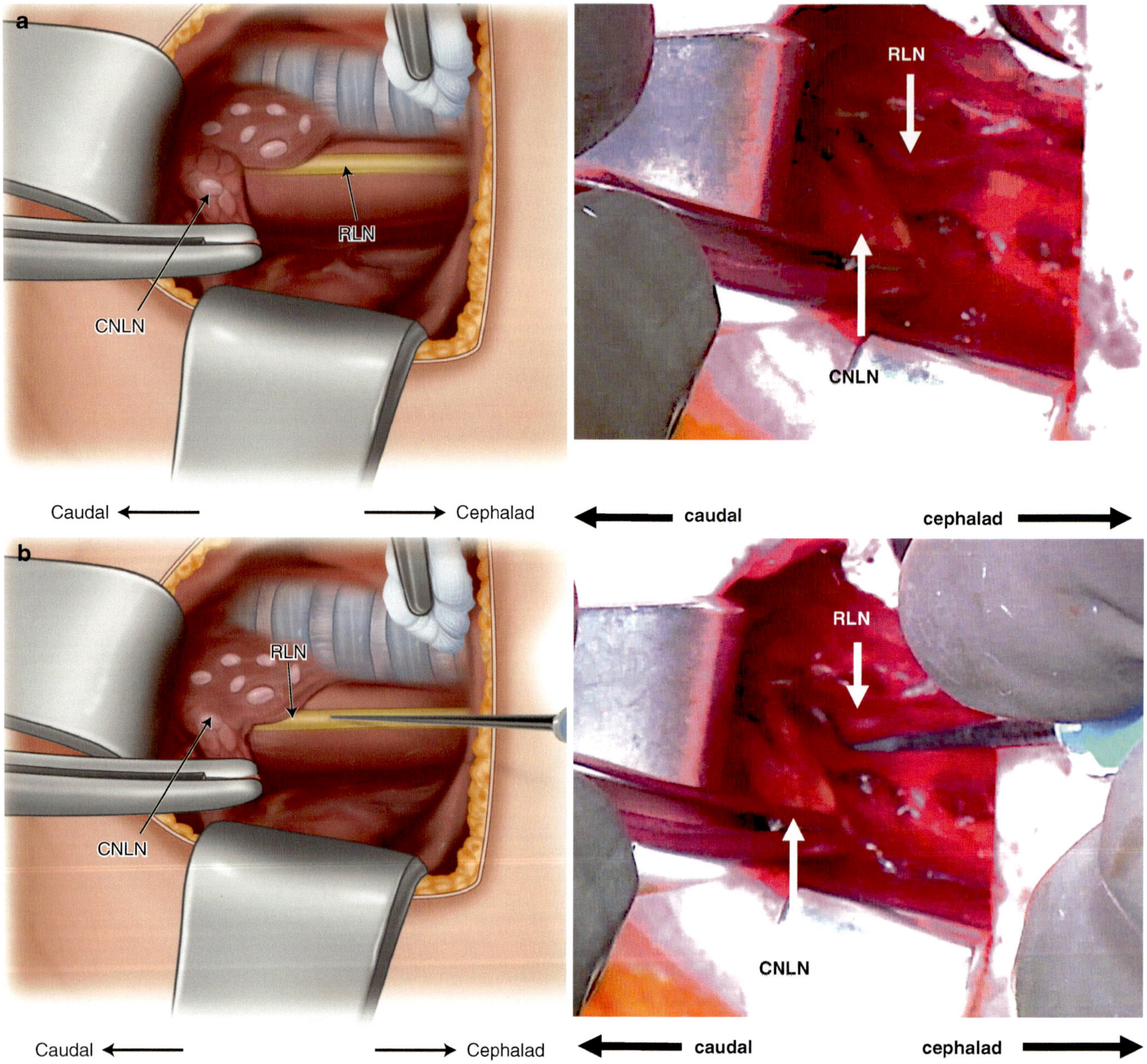

Fig. 7.26 Central neck lymph node dissection (paratracheal). Paratracheal fibroadipose tissues with lymph nodes are dissected using Adson clamp down into the thoracic inlet and anteriorly over the RLN (**a**); nerve stimulator is used to confirm integrity of the RLN with each step of the dissection (**b**). RLN – recurrent laryngeal nerve, CNLN – central neck lymph node specimen

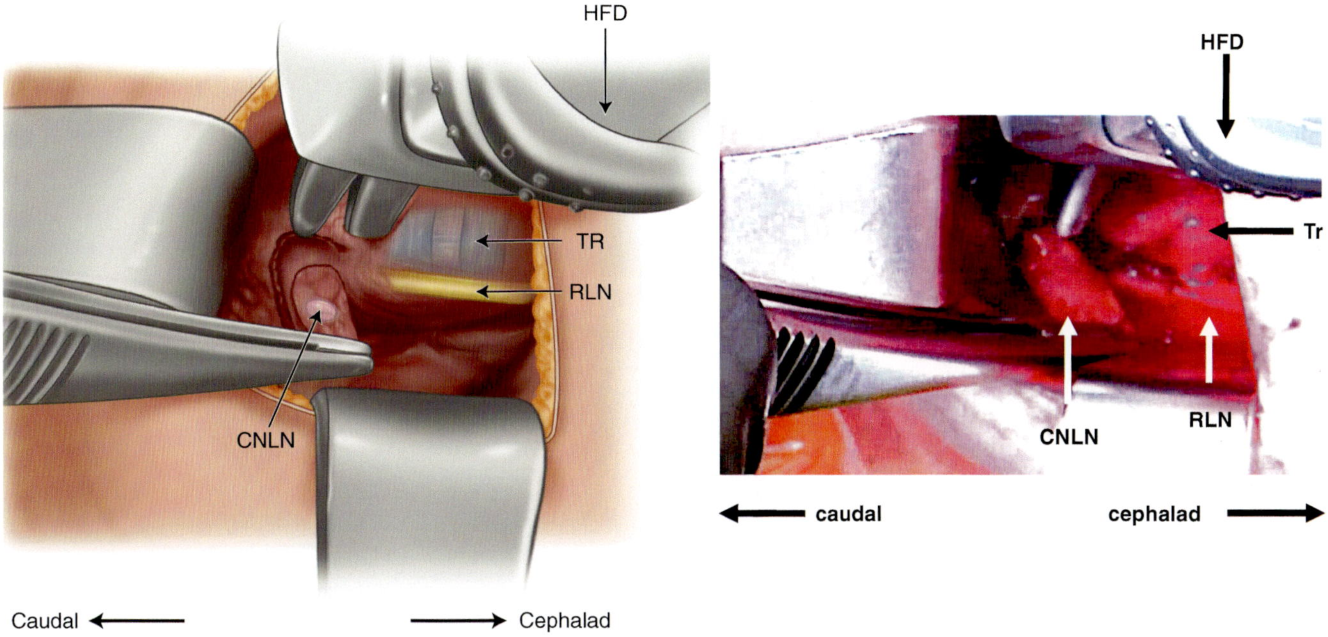

Fig. 7.27 Central neck lymph node dissection (pretracheal). The Harmonic Focus device is used to transect inferior pretracheal attachments of fibroadipose tissues with lymph nodes, keeping the RLN in full view. Tr –trachea, RLN – recurrent laryngeal nerve, CNLN – central neck lymph nodes specimen, HFD – Harmonic Focus device

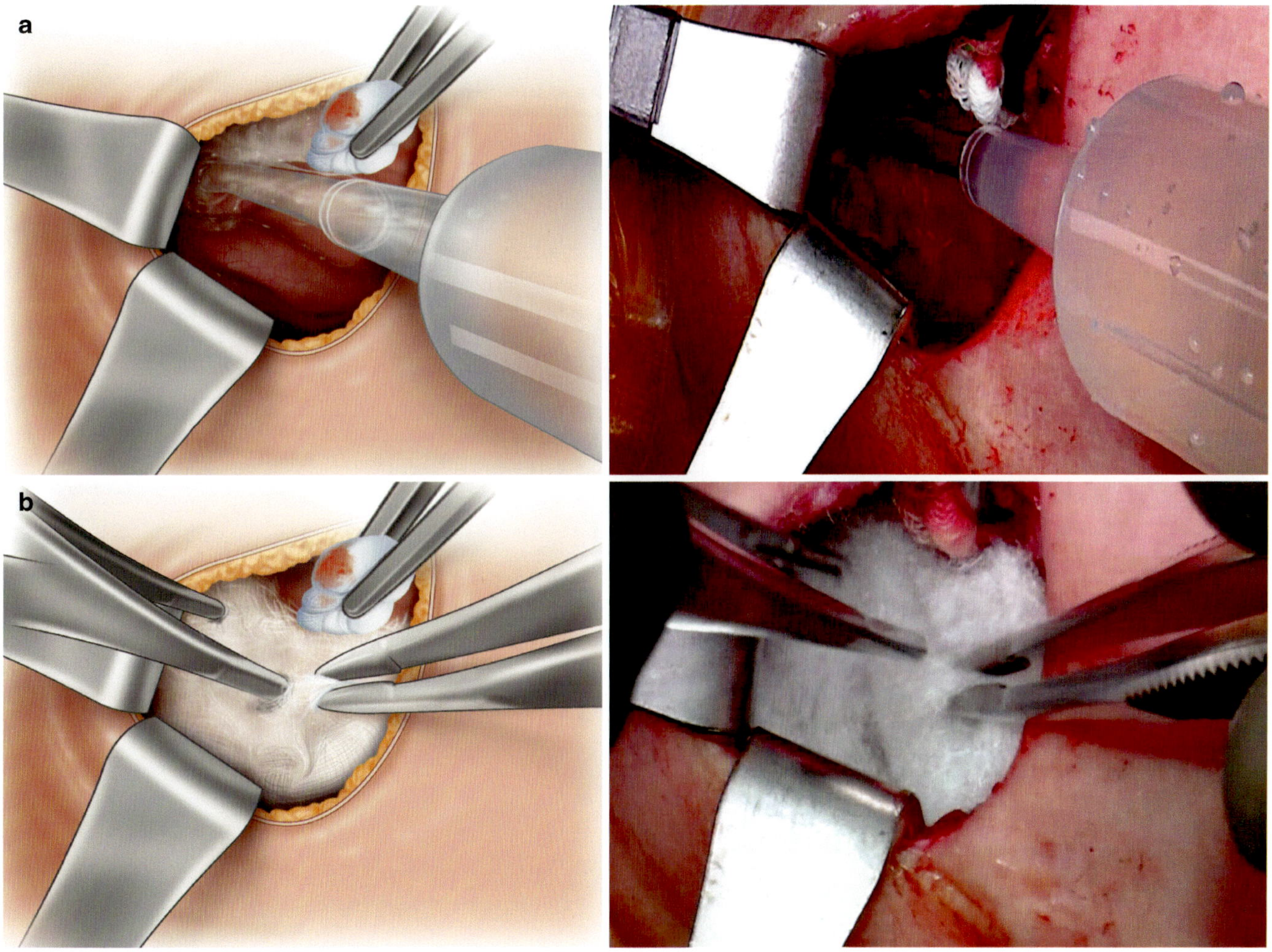

Fig. 7.28 (**a**, **b**). The wound is irrigated (**a**), and the Valsalva maneuver is performed. Then Fibrillar is placed into the wound (**b**)

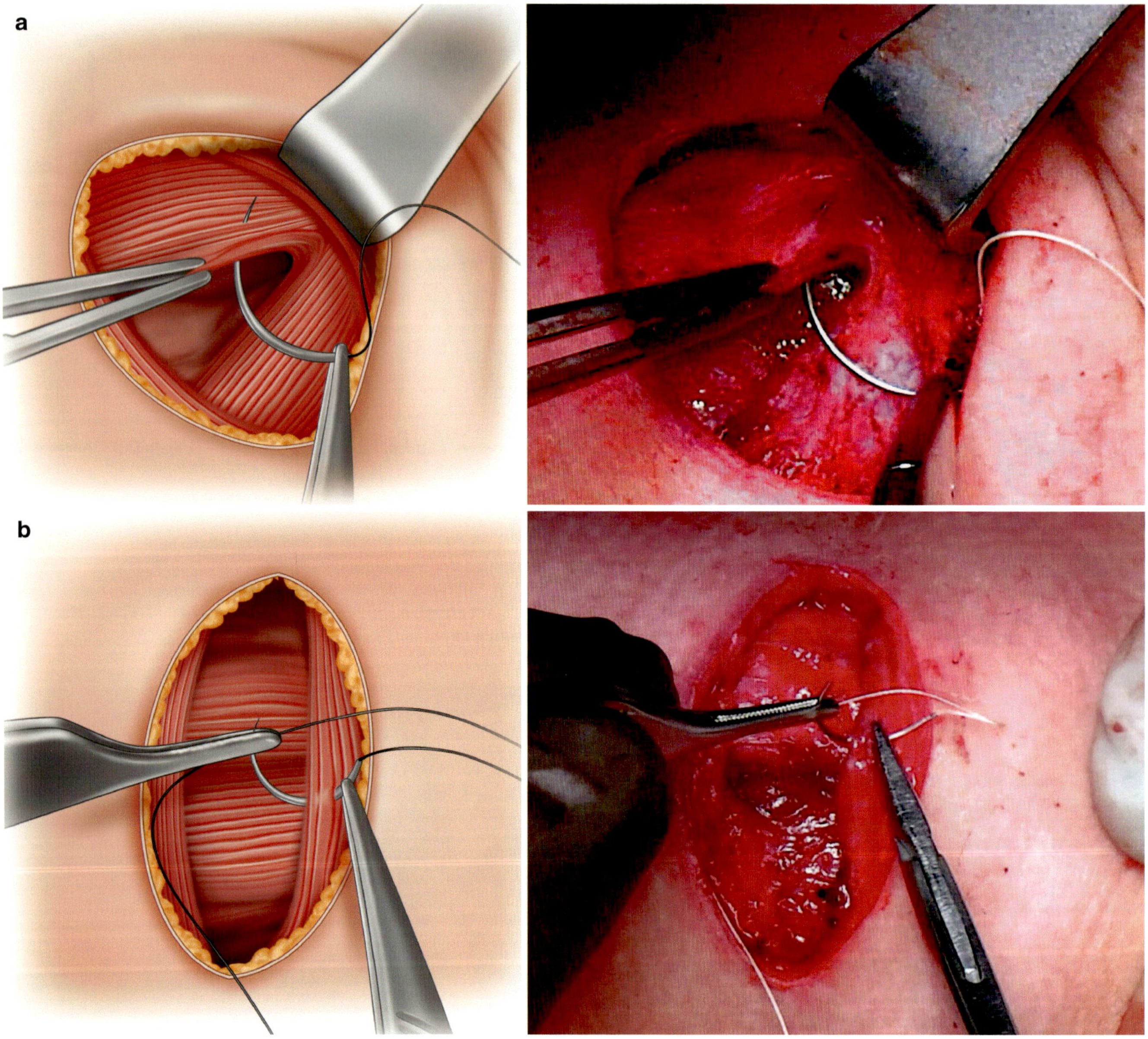

Fig. 7.29 (**a**, **b**). Wound closure. The strap muscles are approximated with interrupted 3.0 Vicryl (**a**), leaving the lower part of the wound open. The platysma is closed with interrupted 4.0 Vicryl (**b**)

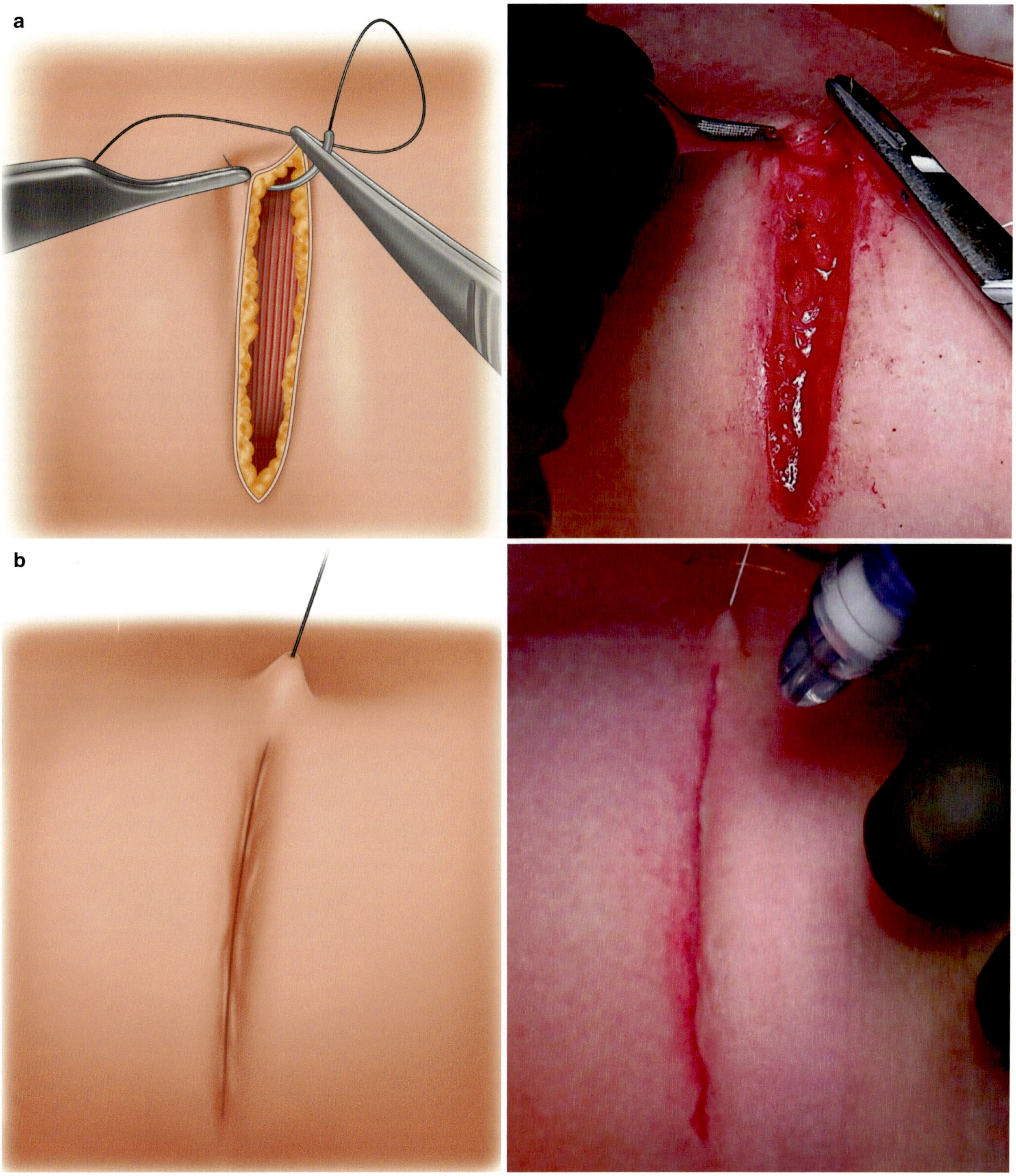

Fig. 7.30 (**a, b**) Wound closure. Skin is closed with a single running 5.0 Monocryl, leaving the ends of the stitch on both sides of the incision without nodes (**a**). Dermabond is placed on the wound, and the ends of the Monocryl stitch are cut at the level of the skin without leaving any nodes (**b**)

References

1. Randolph GW. Surgery of the thyroid and parathyroid glands. 2nd ed. Philadelphia: Elsevier; 2012.
2. Terris DJ, Duke W, editors. Thyroid and parathyroid diseases: medical and surgical management. 2nd ed. New York: Thieme; 2016.
3. Barczyński M, Konturek A, Pragacz K, Papier A, Stopa M, Nowak W. Intraoperative nerve monitoring can reduce prevalence of recurrent laryngeal nerve injury in thyroi reoperations: results of a retrospective cohort study. World J Surg. 2014;38(3):599–606.
4. Dueñas J, Duque C, Cristancho L, Méndez M. Completion thyroidectomy: is timing important for transcervical and remote access approaches? World J Otorhinolaryngol Head Neck Surg. 2020;6(3):165–70.
5. Carty S, Cooper D, Doherty G, Duh Q-Y, Kloos R, Mandel S, Randolph G, Stack B Jr, Steward D, Terris D, Thompson G, Tufano R, Tuttle RM, Udelsman R. Consensus Statement on the Terminology and Classification of Central Neck Dissection for Thyroid Cancer. The American Thyroid Association Surgery Working Group with Participation from the American Association of Endocrine Surgeons, American Academy of Otolaryngology—Head and Neck Surgery, and American Head and Neck Society. Thyroid. 2009;19(11):1153–8.
6. Machens A, Hauptmann S, Dralle H. Lymph node dissection in the lateral neck for completion in central node-positive papillary thyroid cancer. Surgery. 2009;145(2):176–81.
7. Hughes D, Rosen J, Evans D, Grubbs E, Wang T, Solórzano C. Prophylactic central compartment neck dissection in papillary thyroid cancer and effect on locoregional recurrence. Ann Surg Oncol. 2018;25(9):2526–34.
8. Giugliano G, Proh M, Gibelli B, Grosso E, Tagliabue M, De Fiori E, Maffini F, Chiesa F, Ansarin M. Central neck dissection in differentiated thyroid cancer: technical notes. Acta Otorhinolaryngol Ital. 2014;34(1):9–14.
9. Inabnet WB, Shifrin AL, Ahmed L, Sinha P. Safety of same day discharge in patients undergoing sutureless thyroidectomy: a comparison of local and general anesthesia. Thyroid. 2008;18(1):57–61.
10. Terris DJ, Snyder S, Carneiro-Pla D, et al. American thyroid association statement on outpatient thyroidectomy. Thyroid. 2013;23:1193–202.
11. Snyder SK, Hamid KS, Roberson CR, et al. Outpatient thyroidectomy is safe and reasonable: experience with more than 1,000 planned outpatient procedures. J Am Coll Surg. 2010;210:575–82, 582–4.
12. Terris DJ, Moister B, Seybt MW, et al. Outpatient thyroid surgery is safe and desirable. Otolaryngol Head Neck Surg. 2007;136:556–9.
13. Randolph GW, Dralle H, International Intraoperative Monitoring Study Group, Abdullah H, Barczynski M, Bellantone R, Brauckhoff M, Carnaille B, Cherenko S, Chiang FY, Dionigi G, Finck C, Hartl D, Kamani D, Lorenz K, Miccolli P, Mihai R, Miyauchi A, Orloff L, Perrier N, Poveda MD, Romanchishen A, Serpell J, Sitges-Serra A, Sloan T, Van Slycke S, Snyder S, Takami H, Volpi E, Woodson G. Electrophysiologic recurrent laryngeal nerve monitoring during thyroid and parathyroid surgery: international standards guideline statement. Laryngoscope. 2011;121 Suppl 1:S1–16.
14. Barczyński M, Randolph GW, Cernea CR, Dralle H, Dionigi G, Alesina PF, Mihai R, Finck C, Lombardi D, Hartl DM, Miyauchi A, Serpell J, Snyder S, Volpi E, Woodson G, Kraimps JL, Hisham AN, International Neural Monitoring Study Group. External branch of the superior laryngeal nerve monitoring during thyroid and parathyroid surgery: International Neural Monitoring Study Group standards guideline statement. Laryngoscope. 2013;123 Suppl 4:S1–14.
15. Phelan E, Potenza A, Slough C, Zurakowski D, Kamani D, Randolph G. Recurrent laryngeal nerve monitoring during thyroid surgery: normative vagal and recurrent laryngeal nerve electrophysiological data. Otolaryngol Head Neck Surg. 2012;147(4):640–6.
16. Randolph GW. The recurrent and superior laryngeal nerves. 1st ed. Switzerland: Springer International Publishing; 2016 edition.

Total Thyroidectomy

8

Rafael Humberto Pérez-Soto, Alicia Maybí Trolle-Silva, and Miguel F. Herrera

Introduction

Thyroid resection, either lobectomy or total thyroidectomy, is the most common surgical endocrine operation [1]. Although in the last decades new surgical approaches have been described, conventional open thyroidectomy remains the gold standard for the surgical treatment of both benign and malignant disorders [2–9] Since the refinement of this surgical procedure by the Nobel Prize awarded surgeon Theodore Kocher, advancements in surgical techniques and the development of ancillary tools such as surgical loupes, advanced energy devices, and intraoperative neuromonitoring (ioNM) systems have helped in diminishing operative time and procedure-associated complications. Although their use is not compulsory, it is recommended by the current scientific literature [10, 11–14]. In addition, the development of endocrine surgery training programs has significantly improved the outcomes of patients with thyroid-related disorders [15].

It is noteworthy to mention that in order to perform a thyroidectomy, it is important to have a deep knowledge of the neck's surgical anatomy and procedure indications. Before surgery, a complete clinical and biochemical patient assessment, as well as a joint discussion with the patient regarding the extent of the surgical procedure, potential complications, and expectations, is highly important [16].

Surgical Procedure

A 30-year-old woman presented to the endocrine surgery outpatient clinic with an incidentally diagnosed papillary thyroid microcarcinoma (mPTC). She was asymptomatic and biochemically euthyroid. She had an irrelevant familiar and past medical history. Using ultrasonography, a 1-cm lesion was observed near the posterior capsule of the left thyroid lobe. Fine-needle aspiration was performed, observing cytological findings consistent with papillary thyroid carcinoma. After a thorough discussion of the therapeutic alternatives, total thyroidectomy was elected.

The procedure is performed under general anesthesia using endotracheal tube for intraoperative nerve monitoring. The patient is placed in a supine position with a 30-degree chest elevation and slight cervical extension to enhance neck exposure. Both arms are tucked into the body (Fig. 8.1a, b). The neck is prepped, and anatomical references, such as the thyroid cartilage, sternal border, and incision site, are marked (Fig. 8.2). A 5-cm semi-collar skin incision is performed following Langer's skin tension lines (Fig. 8.3). Further in-depth dissection of the subcutaneous fat and transection of the platysma muscle is performed using monopolar cautery (Fig. 8.4). Myocutaneous (subplatysmal) flaps are created, first in the cephalad direction up to the upper edge of the thyroid cartilage (Fig. 8.5), followed by the cau-

Supplementary Information The online version contains supplementary material available at [https://doi.org/10.1007/978-3-030-93673-0_8].

R. H. Pérez-Soto · M. F. Herrera (✉)
Department of Surgery, Division of Endocrine and Advanced Laparoscopic Surgery, Instituto Nacional de Ciencias Médicas y Nutrición, Salvador Zubirán, Tlalpan, Mexico City, Mexico

A. M. Trolle-Silva
Department of Anatomical Pathology, National Institute of Medical Sciences and Nutrition Salvador Zubirán, Mexico City, Mexico

A. Shifrin (ed.), *Atlas of Thyroid Surgery*, https://doi.org/10.1007/978-3-030-93673-0_8

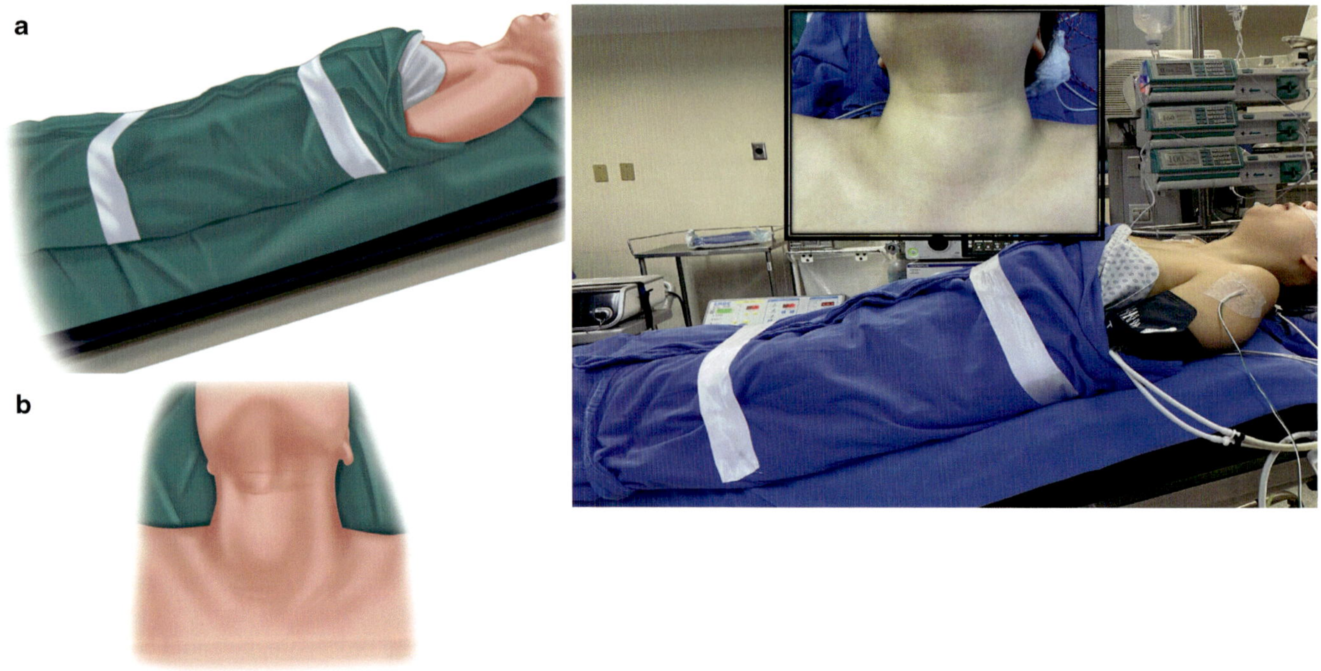

Fig. 8.1 Patient preparation. (**a**) Supine position with complete adduction of the arms and a 30-degree torso elevation. (**b**) Partial neck extension is used to improve cervical exposure

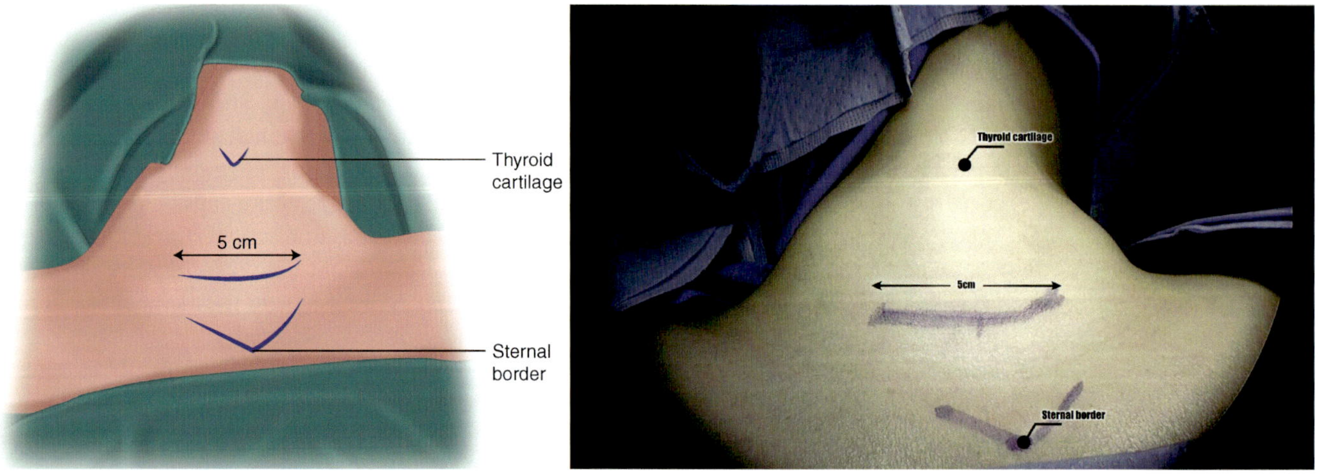

Fig. 8.2 Landmarks. Anatomical references are drawn with a surgical pen at the thyroid cartilage, superior sternal border, and incision site

dal flap up to the upper sternal border (Fig. 8.6). Special care must be taken to avoid anterior jugular vein injury. An automatic retractor is positioned. The strap muscles at the midline (*linea alba cervicalis*) are incised using ultrasonic advanced energy (Fig. 8.7).

The diseased thyroid lobe is initially approached, mobilizing the left strap muscles laterally (Fig. 8.8) until the left carotid sheath is exposed (Fig. 8.9). The left carotid sheath is opened and the vagus nerve is identified for an initial functional evaluation (V1) using the ioNM equipment (Fig. 8.10a, b). The plane between the medial aspect of the superior pole and the cricothyroid muscle (inter-cricothyroid space) is opened (Fig. 8.11), and the external branch of the superior laryngeal nerve (EBSLN) is identified both visually and functionally (S1) (Fig. 8.12a, b). The superior vascular pedicle is controlled using ultrasonic energy, ensuring that no

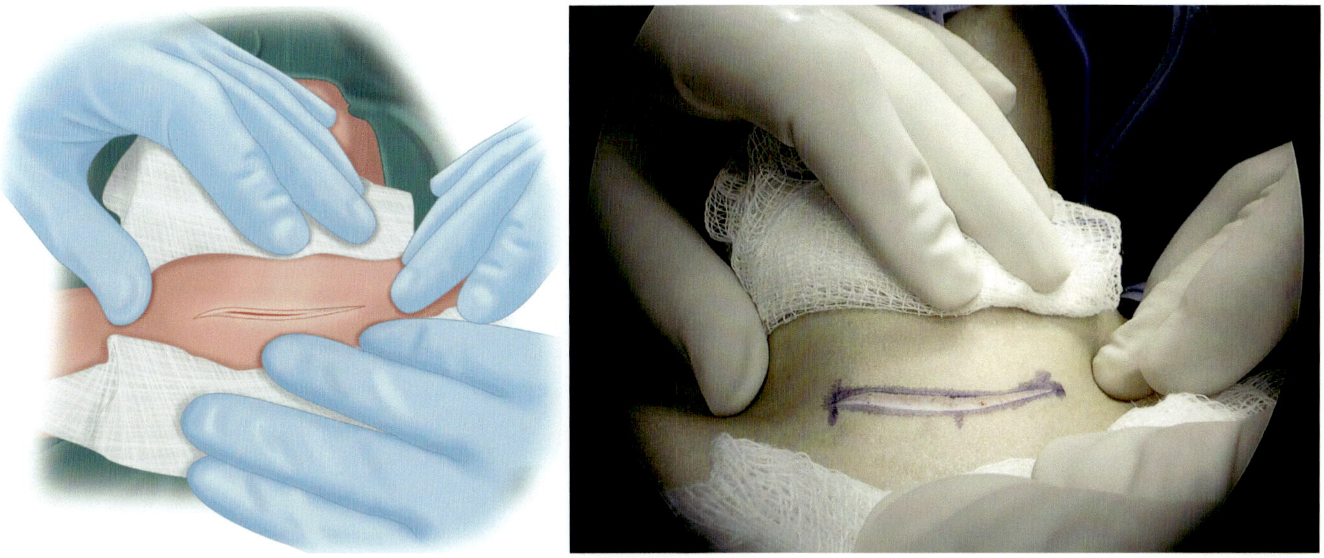

Fig. 8.3 Skin incision. A 5-cm low-collar incision following Langer's skin lines is performed using a #15 scalpel blade

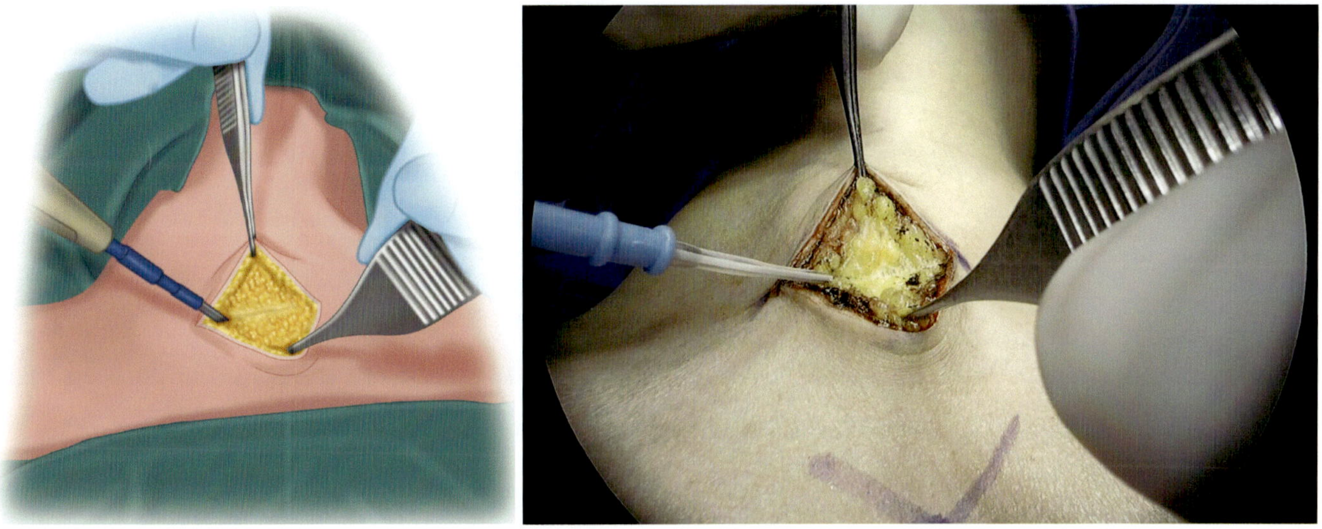

Fig. 8.4 In-depth dissection. Further in-depth dissection is carried out through subcutaneous fat tissue and platysma muscle transection using monopolar cautery

thyroid tissue is left behind and that the EBSLN is preserved (Fig. 8.13). Further lateral dissection of the upper thyroid lobe is carried out with identification and preservation of the superior parathyroid gland, along with its vascular supply (Fig. 8.14). The left recurrent laryngeal nerve (RLN) is identified visually (Fig. 8.15), and an initial functional evaluation (R1) is performed (Fig. 8.16a,b). The inferior pole of the left thyroid lobe is dissected, identifying and preserving the inferior parathyroid gland (Fig. 8.17). The branches of the inferior thyroid artery are transected, the thyroid lobe is retracted medially, and Berry's ligament is divided. Lobectomy is completed with the transection of the thyroid isthmus (Figs. 8.18 and 8.19).

The left thyroid lobe is inspected, identifying the tumor (Fig. 8.20). Postdissection functional evaluation of the left vagus nerve (V2), EBSLN (S2), and RLN (R2) is performed, as well as visual confirmation of the integrity and viability of the parathyroid glands (Fig. 8.21a–d). Right lobectomy is

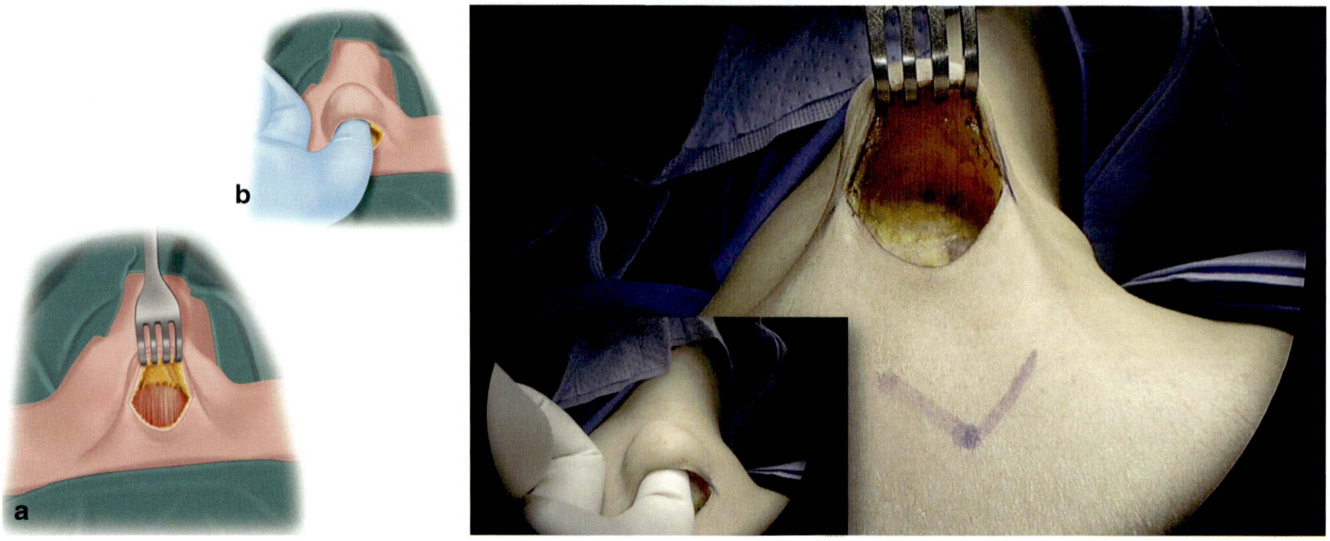

Fig. 8.5 Superior subplatysmal flap. (**a**) Cephalic dissection of a myocutaneous flap is performed using monopolar cautery and blunt dissection (**b**) until the thyroid cartilage is reached

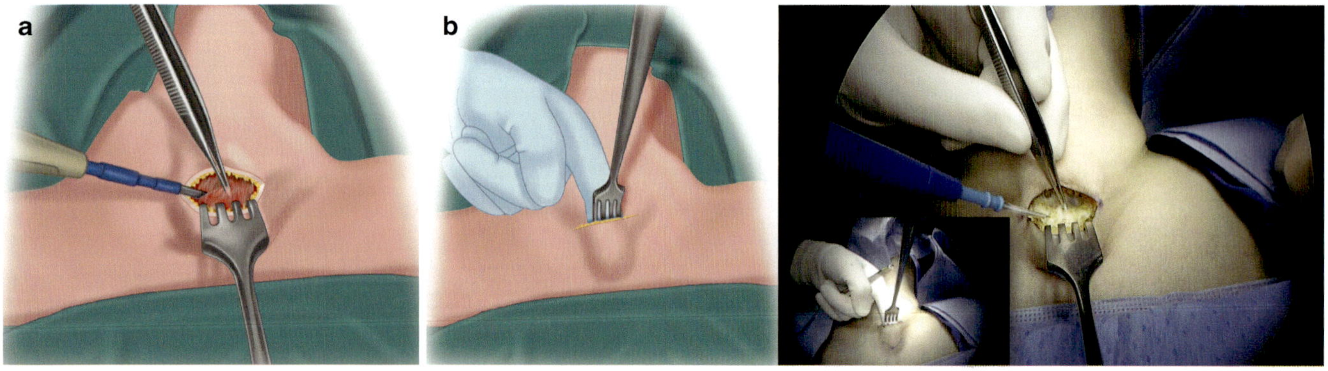

Fig. 8.6 Inferior subplatysmal flap. (**a**) Inferior myocutaneous flap is created (**b**) until the superior sternal border is identified

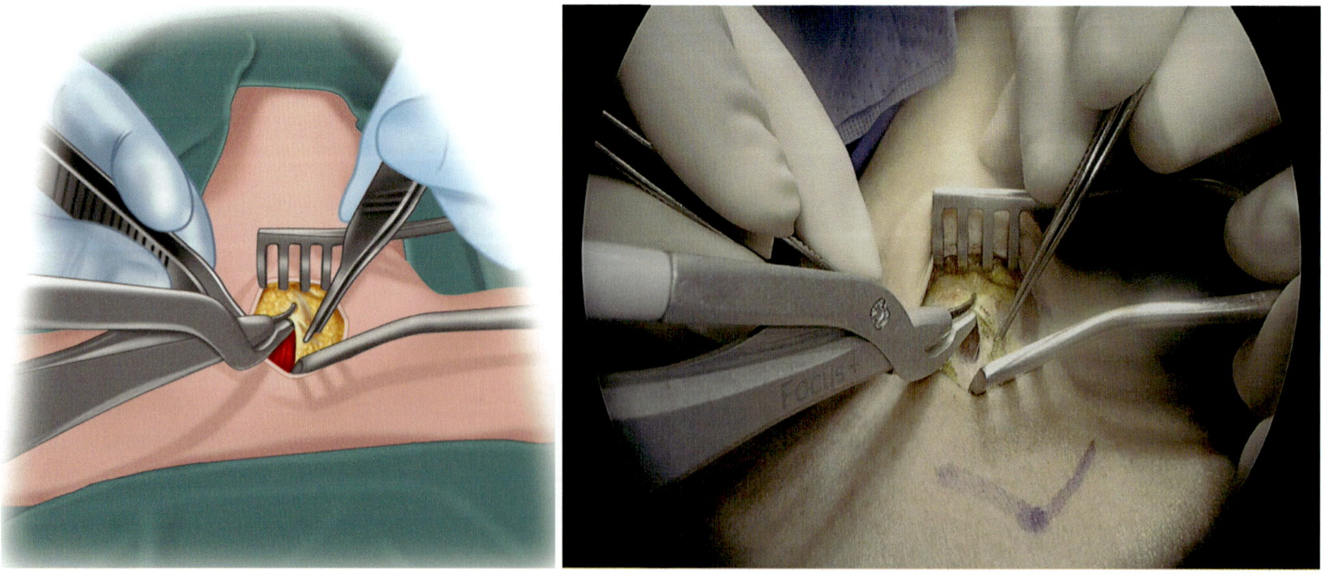

Fig. 8.7 Strap muscle midline incision. The strap muscles at the midline are identified and separated using an ultrasonic energy device

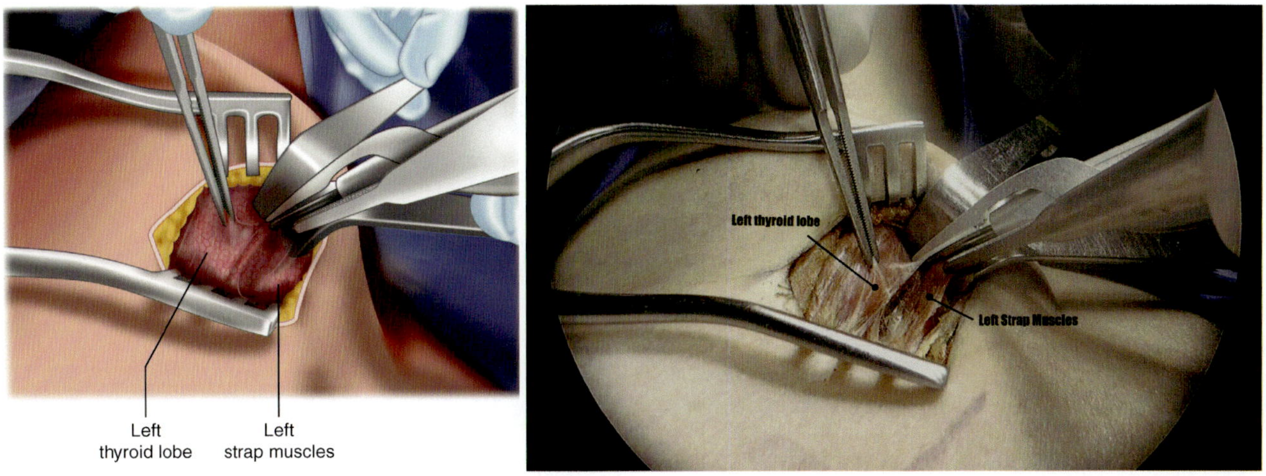

Fig. 8.8 Mobilization of strap muscles. Blunt dissection of the left strap muscles is performed to achieve their complete mobilization laterally and the exposure of the entire left thyroid lobe. Attachments of the strap muscles to the thyroid capsule are divided using an ultrasonic energy device

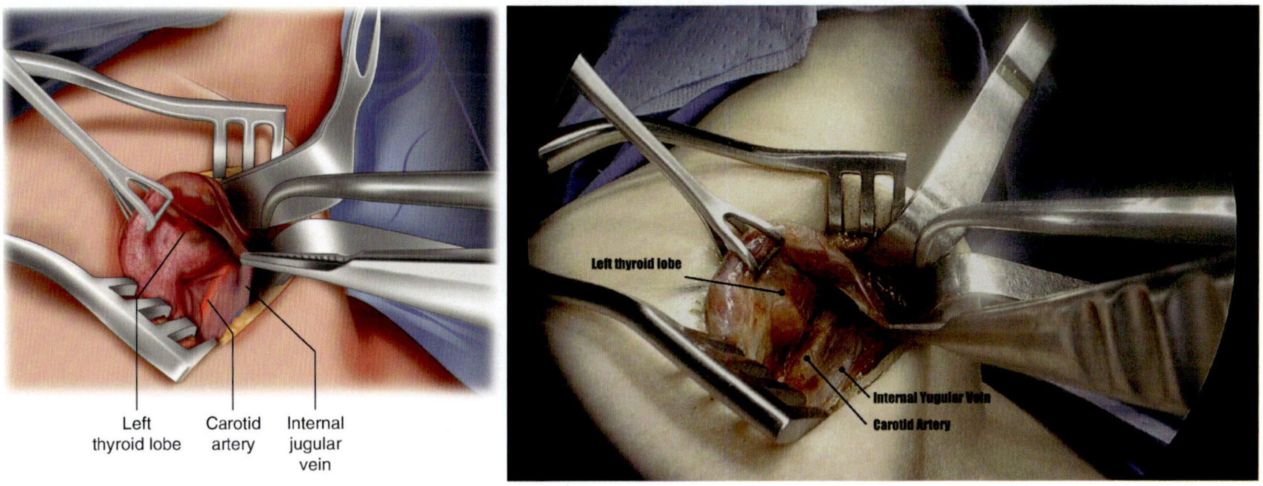

Fig. 8.9 Carotid sheath exposure. Lateral mobilization of strap muscles is continued until the carotid sheath is visualized

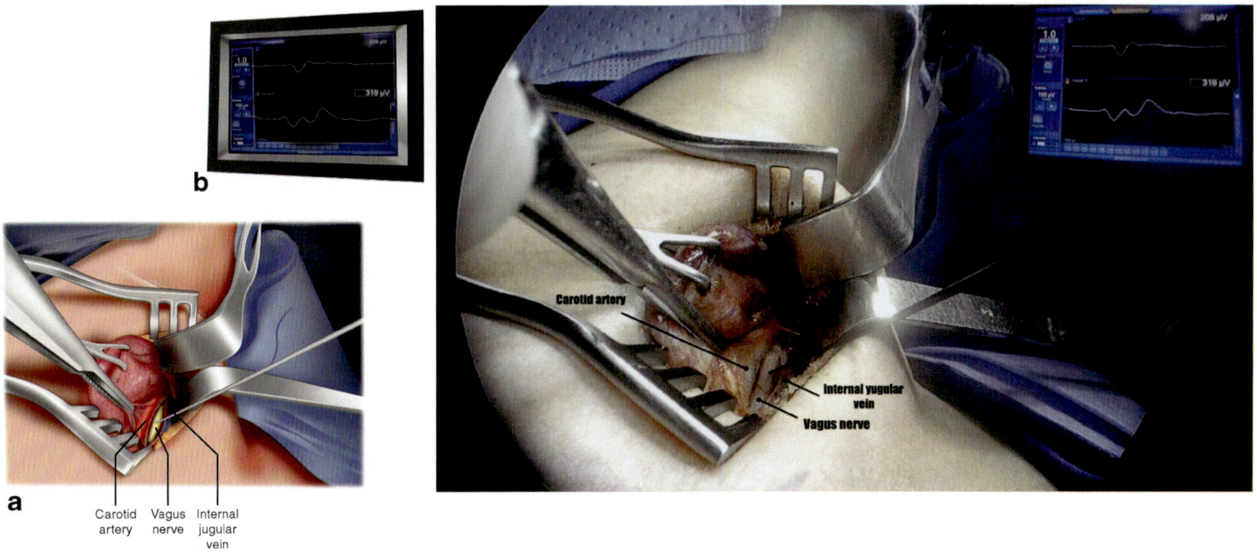

Fig. 8.10 Initial vagus nerve functional evaluation (V1). (**a**) The carotid sheath is opened through blunt dissection, and the vagus nerve is identified and exposed. (**b**) Functional evaluation is carried out with the stimulating probe of the ioNM equipment, and EMG signal is recorded in the ioNM monitor

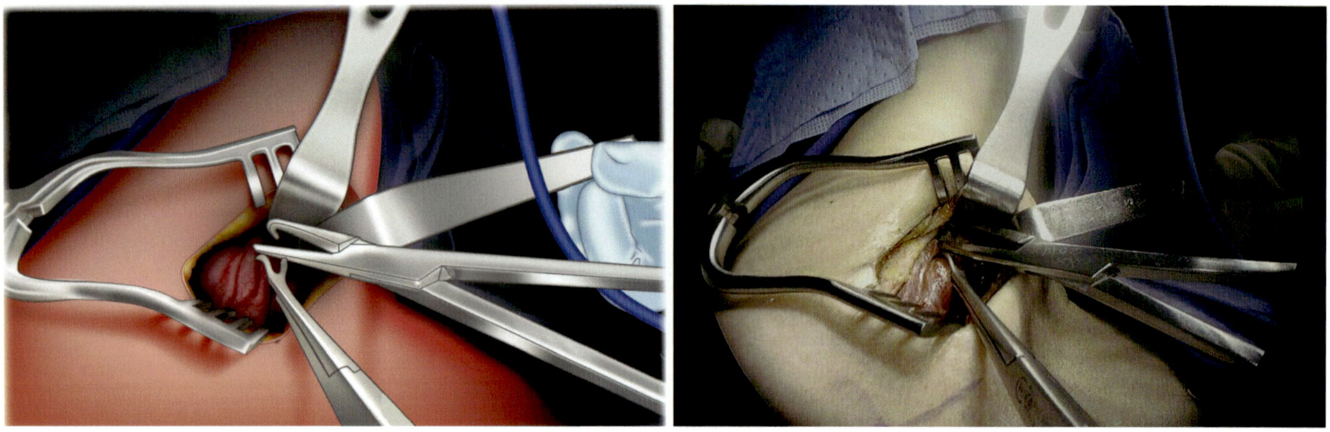

Fig. 8.11 Inter-cricothyroid space dissection. The avascular space between the upper thyroid lobe and the cricothyroid muscle is opened using blunt dissection

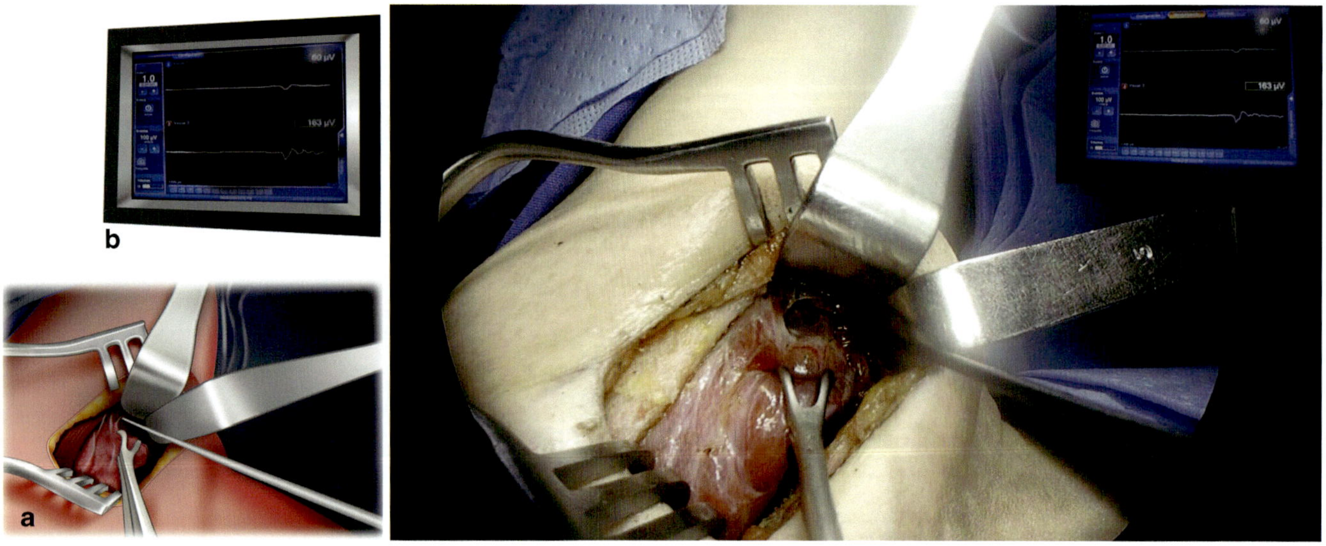

Fig. 8.12 Initial EBSLN functional evaluation (S1). (**a**) The EBSLN is identified within the inter-cricothyroid space, and (**b**) functional evaluation using the ioNM equipment is performed

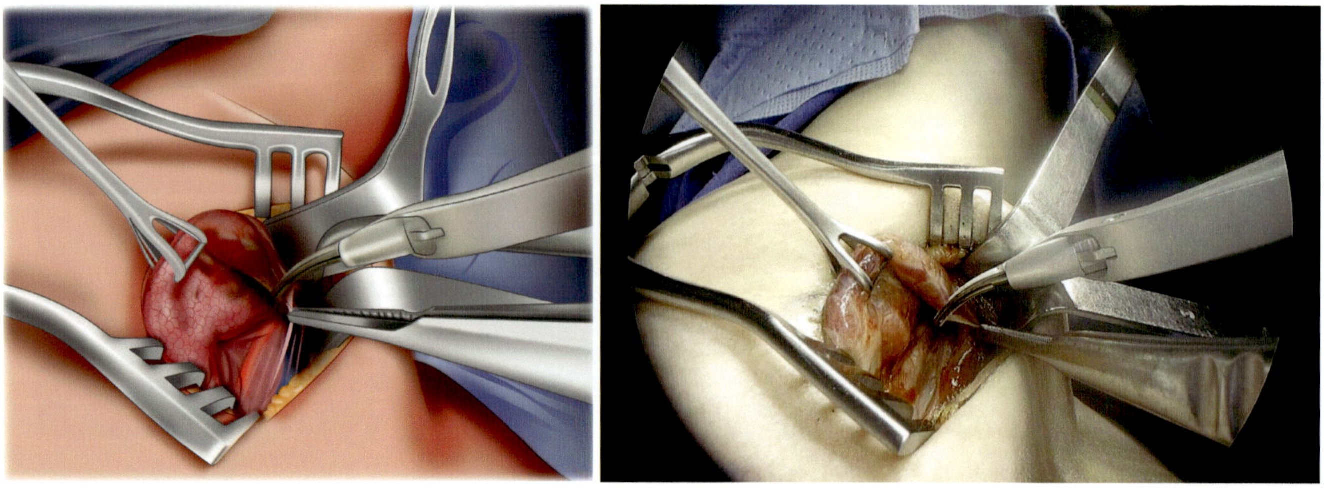

Fig. 8.13 Control of the superior vascular pedicle. Blunt dissection of the superior vascular pedicle is performed. Hemostasis and section of the superior thyroid vessels is achieved using the ultrasonic energy device

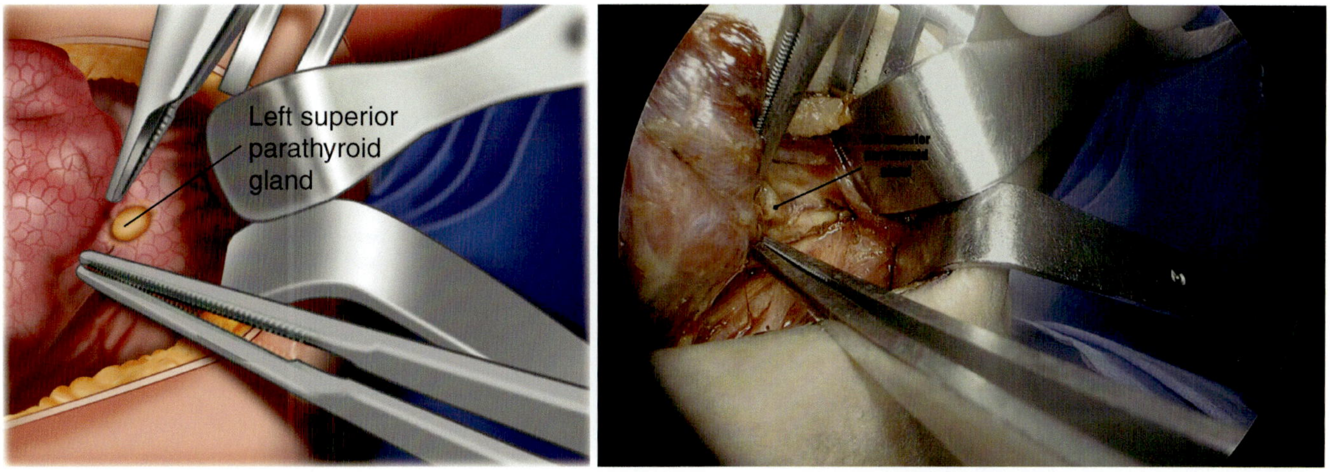

Fig. 8.14 Identification and preservation of the superior parathyroid gland. Further blunt dissection is carried out in the superior third of the thyroid lobe. Identification of the superior parathyroid gland is achieved, and careful dissection of its vascular supply is performed. The most common anatomical reference for superior parathyroid gland localization is a 1-cm distance above the intersection of the recurrent laryngeal nerve and the inferior thyroid artery

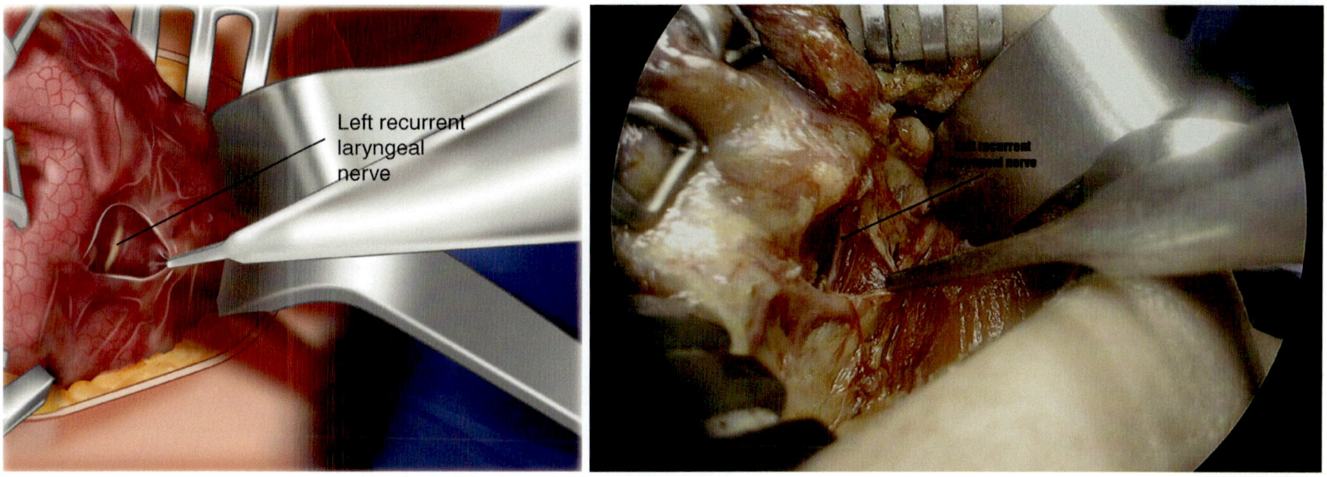

Fig. 8.15 Identification of the recurrent laryngeal nerve. Lateral blunt dissection is continued, and the RLN is identified in the tracheoesophageal groove

carried out in a similar fashion (Fig. 8.22a–f). The central neck compartment is inspected, looking for suspicious lymph nodes for metastatic disease that were absent. Hemostasis is assured, and the strap muscles are approximated using interrupted 4-0 absorbable sutures (Fig. 8.23). The platysma muscle and subcutaneous fat tissue are closed using inverted interrupted sutures with 4-0 absorbable material (Fig. 8.24). Finally, the skin is closed with a subcutaneous running 5-0 absorbable sutures (Fig. 8.25).

Biochemical workup the day after surgery showed an albumin-corrected calcium serum level of 9.0 mg/dL (normal range: 8.6–10.3 mg/dL), phosphorus serum level of 4.6 mg/dL (normal range: 2.5–5 mg/dL), and PTH serum level of 43.10 pg/mL (normal range: 12–88 pg/mL). The patient was then discharged uneventfully (Video 8.1).

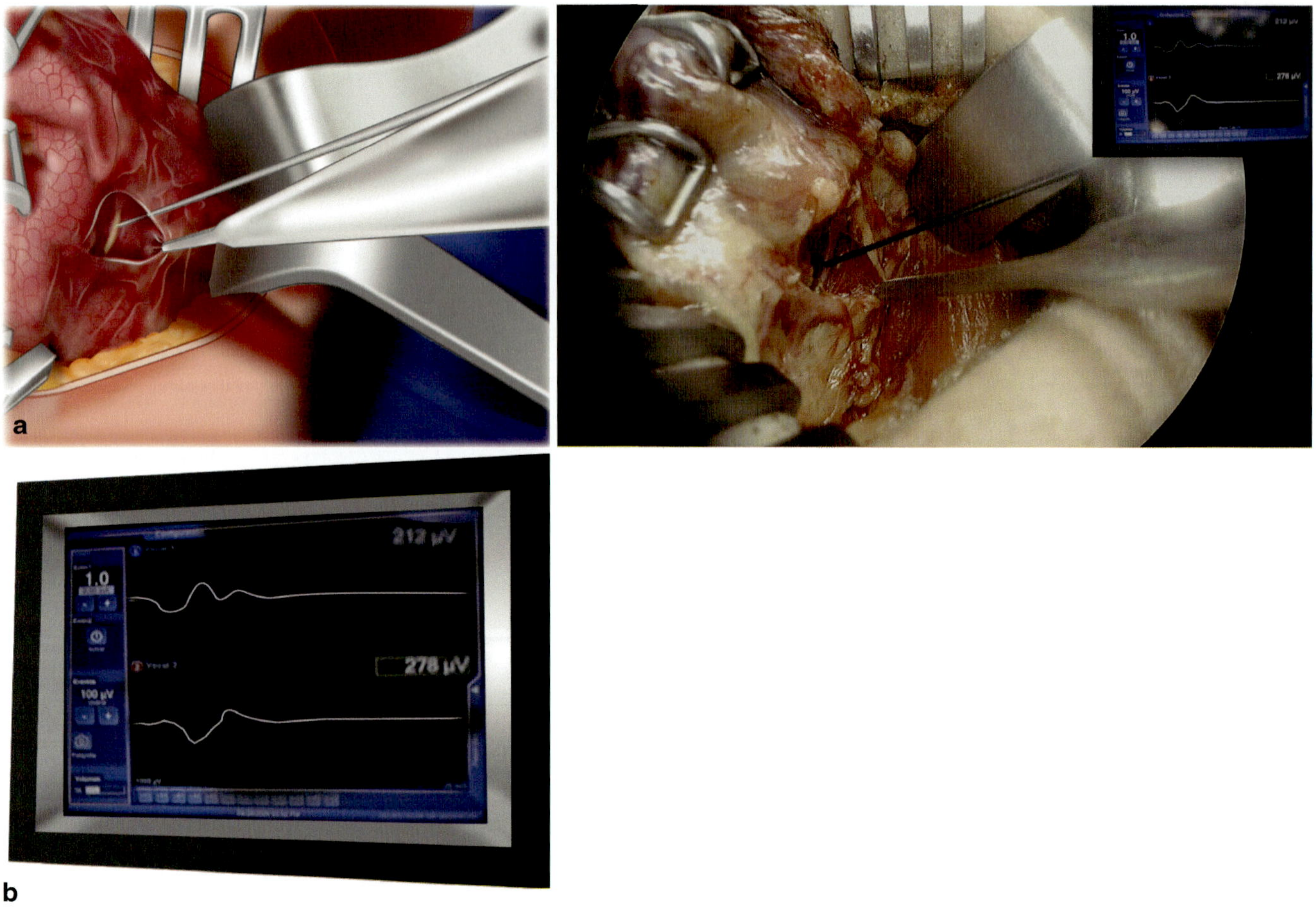

Fig. 8.16 Functional assessment of RLN. (**a**) The RLN is stimulated with ioNM probe, and (**b**) EMG signal is recorded in the ioNM equipment monitor

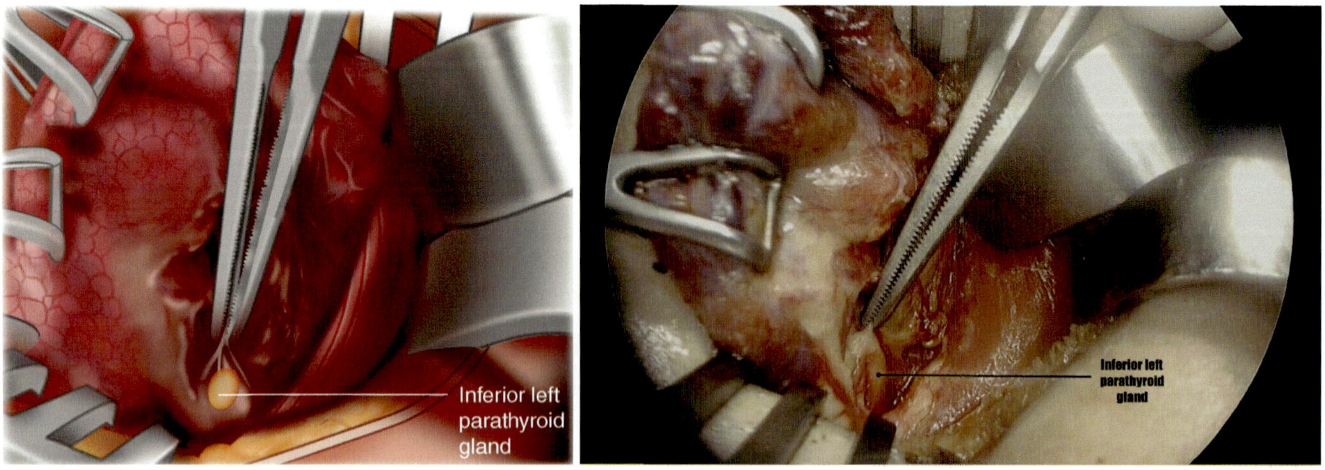

Fig. 8.17 Identification and preservation of the inferior parathyroid gland. Inferior thyroid pole is dissected, and inferior parathyroid gland identification is achieved. Subcapsular dissection prevents the injury to inferior thyroid artery branches supplying the parathyroid tissue

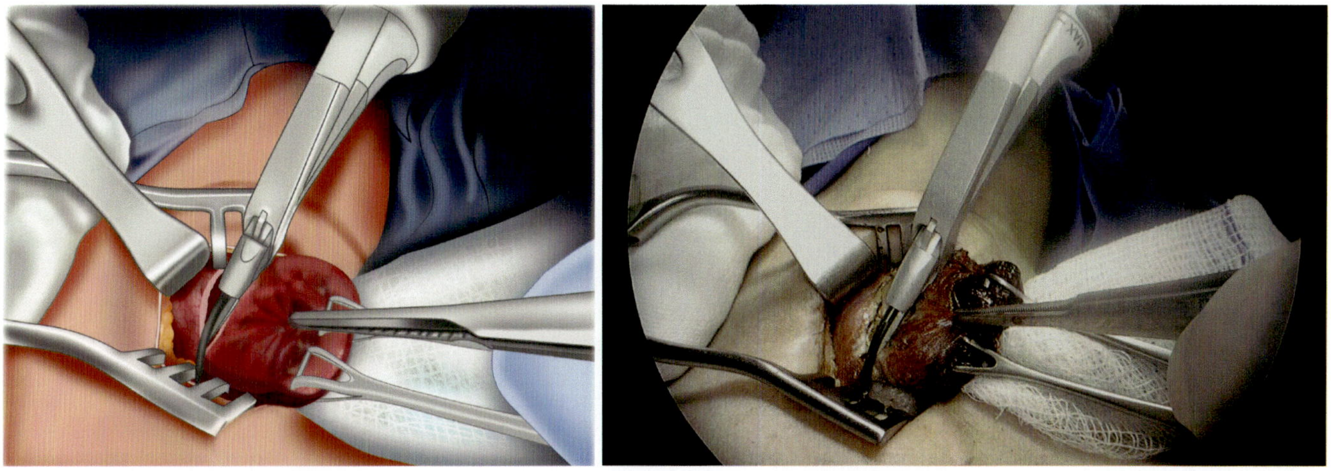

Fig. 8.18 Thyroid isthmus transection. The thyroid isthmus is transected using an ultrasonic energy device

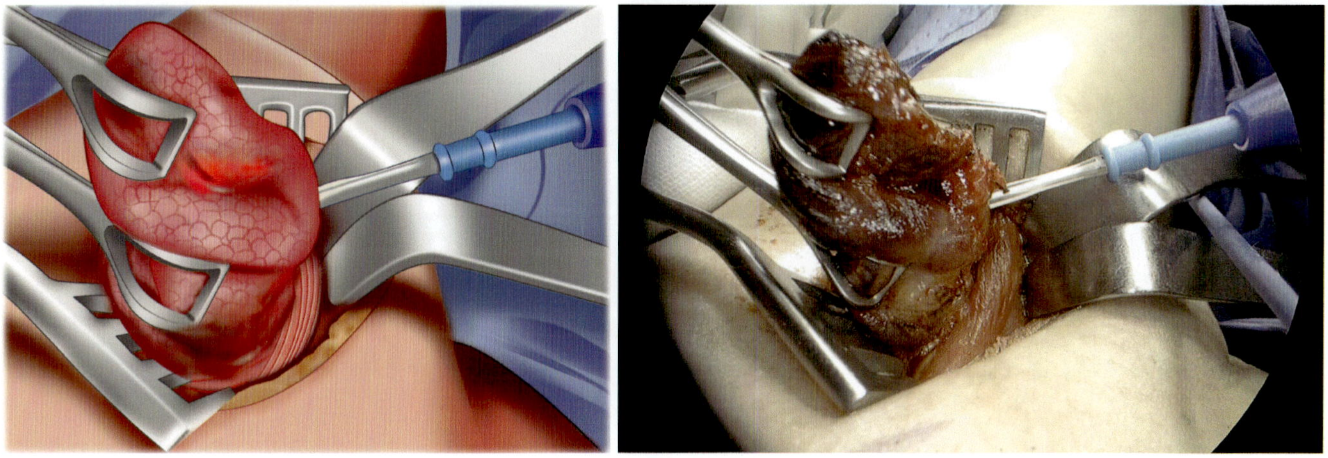

Fig. 8.19 Lobectomy. Attachments of the left thyroid lobe to the trachea are divided, assuring the safety of the RLN

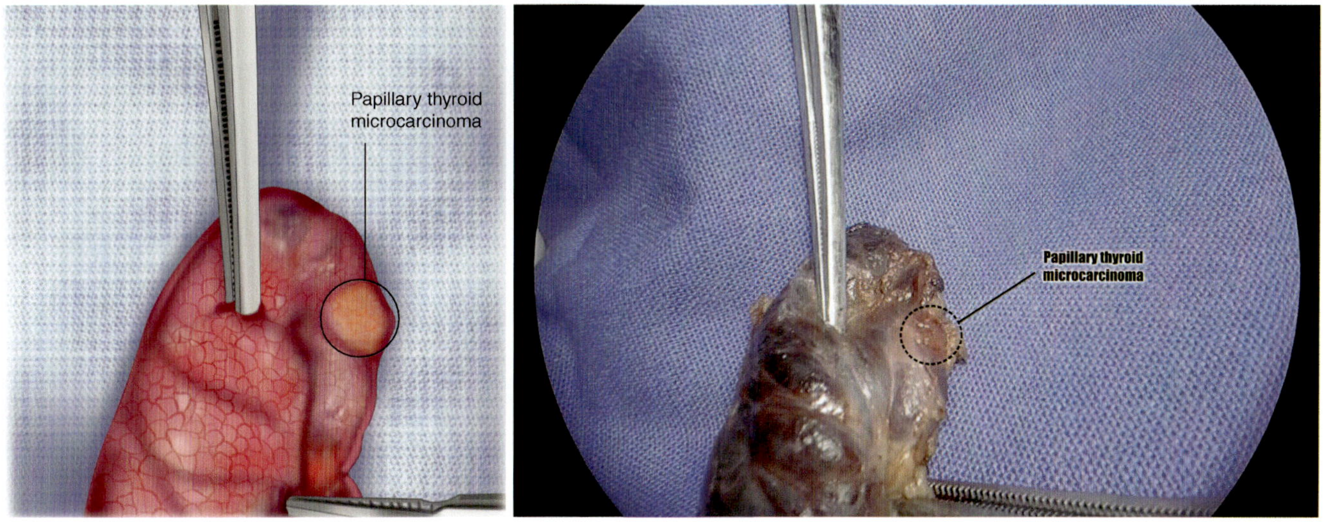

Fig. 8.20 Specimen assessment. The resected left thyroid lobe is inspected to identify the lesion and inadvertently removed parathyroid glands

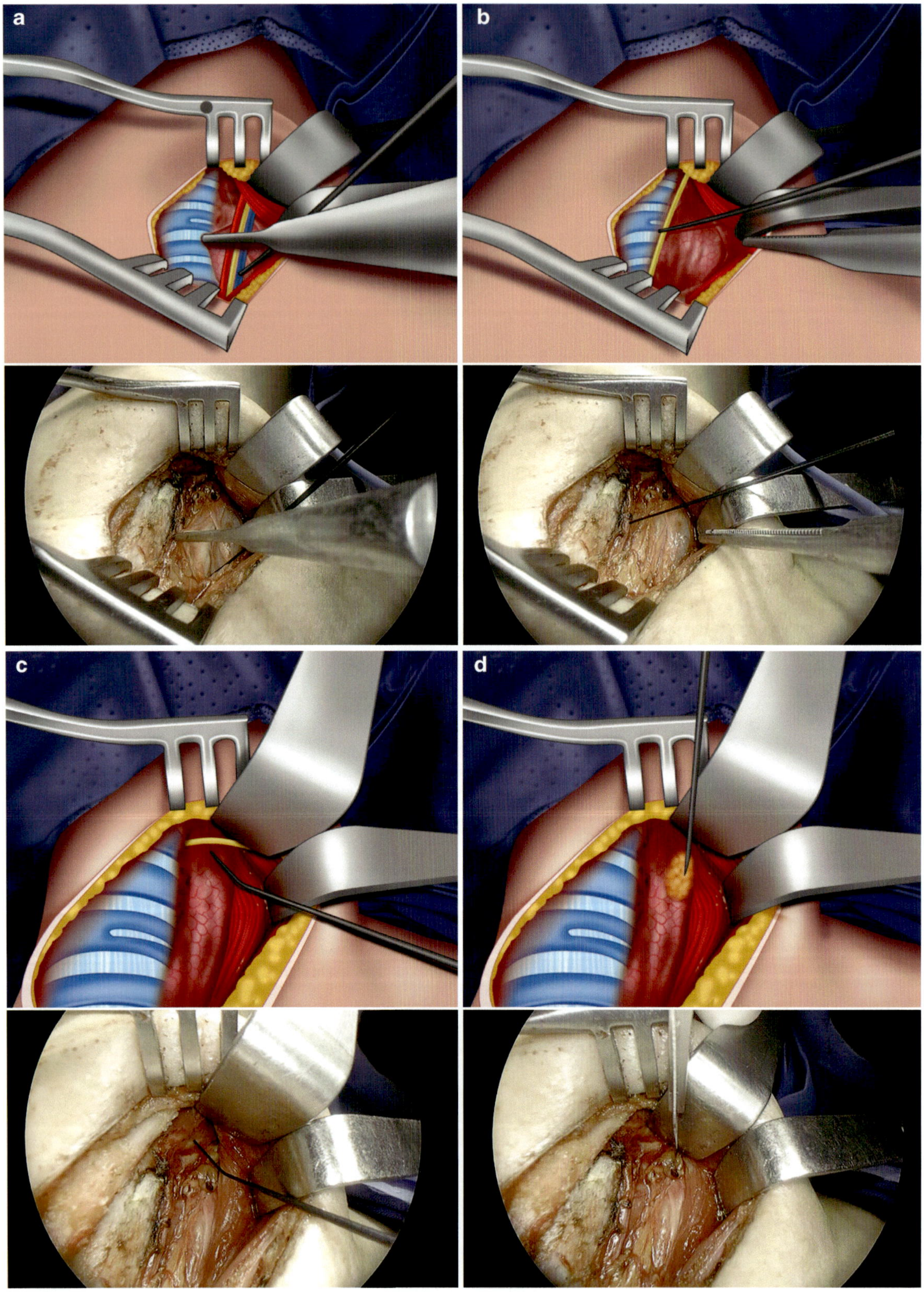

Fig. 8.21 Postlobectomy surgical field assessment. Before deciding to approach the contralateral lobe, functional evaluation of the (**a**) vagus nerve (V2), (**b**) RLN (R2), and (**c**) EBSLN (S2) is performed, followed by (**d**) parathyroid gland vascular supply assessment

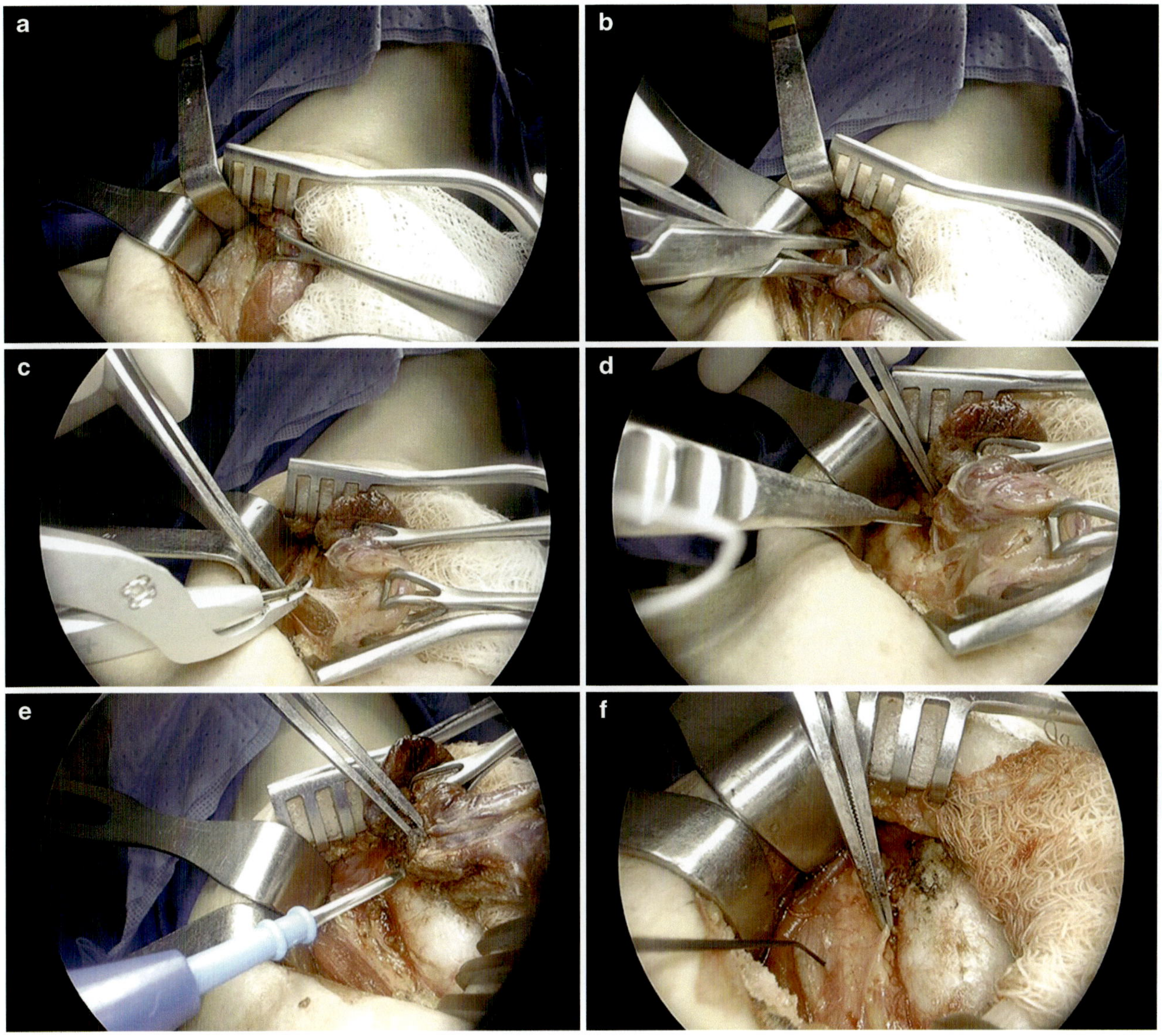

Fig. 8.22 Contralateral lobectomy. Contralateral thyroid lobe resection is carried out following the same steps. (**a**) Strap muscles mobilization, (**b**) inter-cricothyroid space dissection with EBSLN identification, (**c**) lateral blunt dissection of the thyroid lobe with identification of parathyroid gland tissue, (**d**) RNL identification, (**e**) transection of thyroid lobe attachments to the trachea, and (**f**) post-dissection nerve functional evaluation and parathyroid gland vascular supply

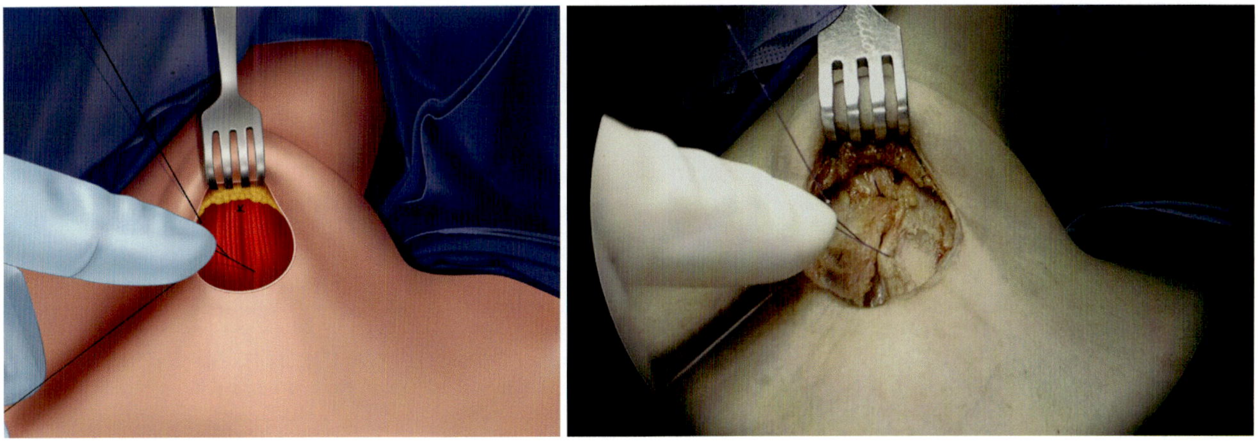

Fig. 8.23 Strap muscle approximation. The strap muscles at the midline are approximated using interrupted 4-0 absorbable sutures. Care must be taken to avoid injuries to the anterior jugular veins

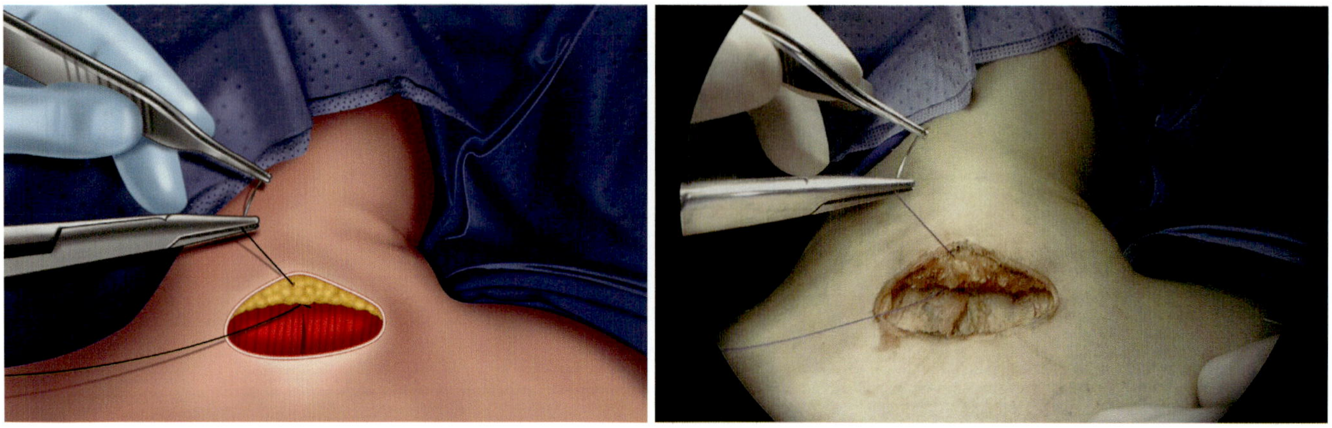

Fig. 8.24 Platysma muscle closure. The platysma and subcutaneous fat tissue are closed using inverted and interrupted 4-0 absorbable sutures

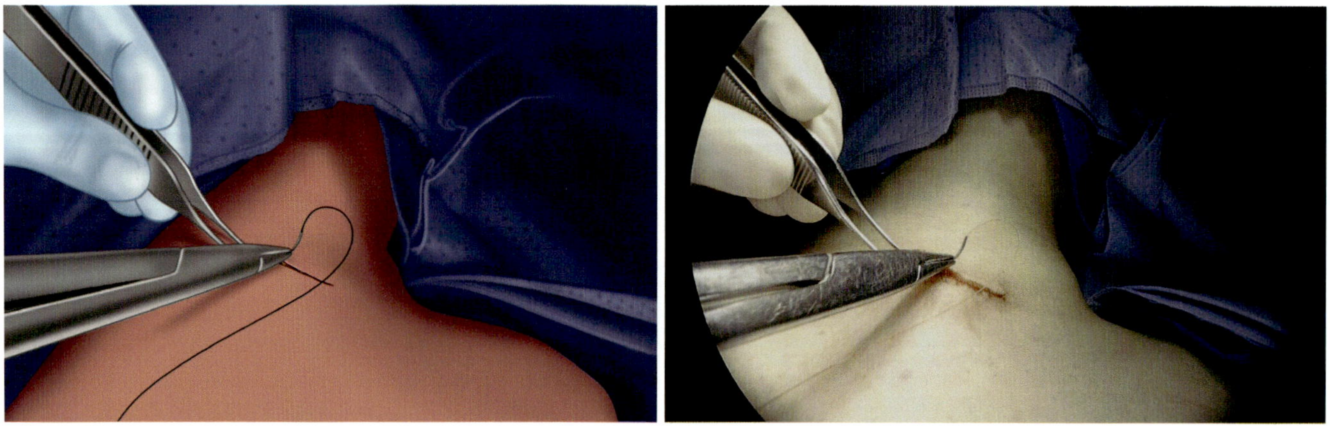

Fig. 8.25 Skin closure. A subcutaneous running 5-0 absorbable suture is used to close the skin incision

References

1. Oertli D. Technique of thyroidectomy. In: Oertli D, Udelsman R, editors. Surgery of the thyroid and parathyroid glands. Berlin, Heidelberg: Springer; 2007. https://doi.org/10.1007/978-3-540-68043-7_7.
2. Gosnell JE, Clark OH. Surgical approaches to thyroid tumors. Endocrinol Metab Clin N Am. 2008;37(2):437–55.
3. Ikeda Y, Takami H, Sasaki Y, Kans S, Niimi M. Endoscopic neck surgery by the axillary approach. J Am Coll Surg. 2000;191(3):336–40.
4. Ohgami M, Ishii S, Arisawa Y, Ohmori T, Noga K, Furukawa T, Kitajima M. Scarless endoscopic thyroidectomy: breast approach for better cosmesis. Surg Laparosc Endosc Percutan Tech. 2000;10(1):1–4.
5. Miccoli P, Berti P, Raffaelli M, Conte M, Materazzi G, Galleri D. Minimally invasive video-assisted thyroidectomy. Am J Surg. 2001;181:567–70.
6. Shimazu K, Shiba E, Tamaki Y, Takiguchi S, Taniguchi E, Ohashi S, Noguchi S. Endoscopic thyroid surgery through the axillo-bilateral-breast approach. Surg Laparosc Endosc Percutan Tech. 2003;13(3):196–201.
7. Choe JH, Kim SW, Chung KW, Park KS, Han W, Noh DY, Oh SK, Youn YK. Endoscopic thyroidectomy using a new bilateral axillo-breast approach. Word J Surg. 2007;31(3):601–6.
8. Terris DJ, Singer MC, Seybt MW. Robotic facelift thyroidectomy: patient selection and technical considerations. Surg Laparosc Endosc Percutan Tech. 2011;21(4):237–42.
9. Anuwong A. Transoral endoscopic thyroidectomy vestibular approach: a series of the first 60 human cases. World J Surg. 2016;40(3):491–7.
10. Duke WS, Chaung K, Terris DJ. Contemporary surgical techniques. Otolaryngol Clin N Am. 2014;47(4):529–44.
11. Cirocchi R, D'Ajello F, Trastulli S, Santoro A, Di Rocco G, Vendettuoli D, Rondelli F, Giannotti D, Sanguinetti A, Minelli L, Redler A, Basoli A, Avenia N. Meta-analysis of thyroidectomy with ultrasonic dissector versus conventional clamp and tie. World J Surg Oncol. 2010;8:112.
12. D'Orazi V, Panunzi A, Di Lorenzo E, Ortensi A, Cialini M, Anichini S, Ortensi A. Use of loupes magnification and microsurgical technique in thyroid surgery: ten years' experience in a single center. G Chir. 2016;37(3):101–7.
13. Smith RB, Coughlin A. Thyroidectomy hemostasis. Otolaryngol Clin N Am. 2016;49(3):727–48.
14. Schneider R, Machens A, Lorenz K, Dralle H. Intraoperative nerve monitoring in thyroid surgery-shifting current paradigms. Gland Surg. 2020;9(Suppl 2):S120–8.
15. Runkel N, Riede E, Mann B, Buhr HJ. Surgical training and vocal-cord paralysis in benign thyroid disease. Langenbeck's Arch Surg. 1998;383:240–2.
16. Yip L, Stang MT, Carty SE. Thyroid carcinoma: the surgeon's perspective. Radiol Clin N Am. 2011;49(3):463–71.

9 Left Thyroid Lobectomy and Isthmusectomy

Rajshri M. Gartland and Richard A. Hodin

Introduction

Open thyroidectomy remains the most common approach for the management of benign and malignant thyroid pathologies. While recurrent laryngeal nerve monitoring (RLNM) has become an increasingly popular adjunct in thyroid surgery over the past few decades, no large-scale multi-institutional studies have demonstrated a significant difference in RLN injury rates with its use, and many high-volume surgeons continue to rely solely on intraoperative visualization and knowledge of normal and variant anatomy to preserve RLN structure and function during thyroidectomy. In addition, novel hemostatic devices, such as electrothermal bipolar vessel sealers and ultrasonically activated shears, have become increasingly utilized in thyroid surgery; while these tools have been shown to be effective, they are also more expensive than traditional modes of effective hemostasis, such as knot tying, clips, and monopolar electrocautery. In this chapter, a safe, reliable, efficient, and low-cost technique for left thyroid lobectomy and isthmusectomy, without the use of RLNM or a vessel-sealing device, is described.

Description: Left Thyroid Lobectomy and Isthmusectomy

A 45-year-old man presented with a 1.2-cm left thyroid nodule, which was found to be suspicious for follicular neoplasm on a fine-needle aspiration biopsy. After a discussion of the risks, benefits, and alternatives to surgery, the patient opted to undergo a left thyroid lobectomy. He was brought to the operating room and positioned supine. After general endotracheal anesthesia was induced, the patient's neck was extended and prepared and draped in a sterile fashion.

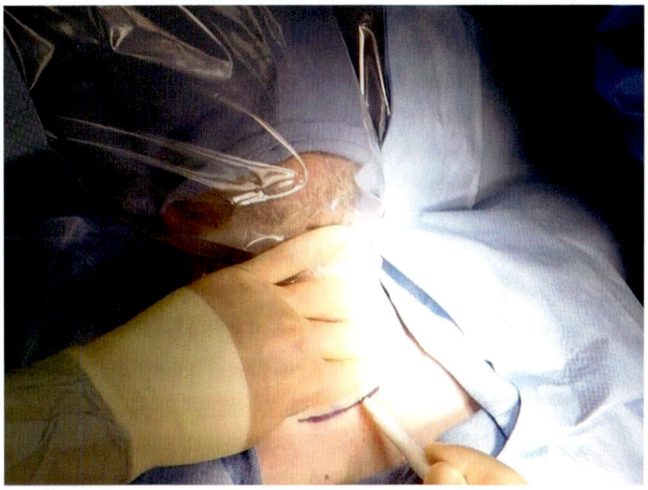

Fig. 9.1 A natural skin crease between the cricoid cartilage and sternal notch was marked in the preoperative area and remarked prior to skin incision

After a time-out was performed to verify patient, procedure, laterality, and other important case details, a standard skin incision was made in a natural skin crease, which was initially marked in the preoperative area (Fig. 9.1). The subcutaneous tissues and platysma were divided with electrocautery (Fig. 9.2). Subplatysmal flaps were raised superiorly and inferiorly (Fig. 9.3). After insertion of a self-retaining spring retractor (Fig. 9.4), the cervical fascia was incised in the midline. Electrocautery was used to expose the trachea at the inferior border of the isthmus (Fig. 9.5), and then the isthmus was divided with electrocautery at its junction with the right thyroid lobe (Fig. 9.6).

R. M. Gartland (✉) · R. A. Hodin
Department of Surgery, Massachusetts General Hospital, Boston, MA, USA

A. Shifrin (ed.), *Atlas of Thyroid Surgery*, https://doi.org/10.1007/978-3-030-93673-0_9

The left strap muscles were reflected laterally, and the left thyroid lobe was mobilized medially (Fig. 9.7). The thyroid lobe contained a palpable nodule, and no extracapsular extension or adenopathy was seen. Next, the superior pole vessels were exposed and ligated (Figs. 9.8, 9.9, 9.10, and 9.11). Care was taken to avoid injury to the external branch of the superior laryngeal nerve. The loose areolar tissue attached to the thyroid capsule was gently swept posteriorly, which enabled the preservation of both the superior and inferior parathyroid glands (Fig. 9.12). The recurrent laryngeal nerve was then identified close to its insertion in the larynx, and a right-angle dissector was used to trace the nerve inferiorly (Figs. 9.13 and 9.14). With the recurrent laryngeal nerve in view, the lower pole attachments were clipped close to the thyroid capsule and ligated with electrocautery down to the level of the trachea (Fig. 9.15). The thyroid lobe was dissected off the trachea using a combination of clips and electrocautery, leaving a tiny remnant in the adherent zone for safety reasons (Figs. 9.16 and 9.17). The isthmus and pyramidal lobe were removed with the specimen. Cautery was applied to the cut edge of the right thyroid lobe for hemostasis (Fig. 9.18).

The wound bed was irrigated, and hemostasis was tested in the Trendelenburg position with positive pressure. The wound was closed in layers using 4-0 silk stitches to approximate the strap muscles and platysma (Figs. 9.19 and 9.20). Absorbable sutures can be used instead of silk, but silk stitches are chosen to facilitate the identification of tissue layers if there is a need for a second operation (e.g., completion thyroidectomy). The skin was closed with a subcuticular stitch using 4-0 Monocryl, and the incision was covered with Steri-Strips (Fig. 9.21).

The patient tolerated the procedure well without complications. Total operative time, including the induction of anesthesia, was less than an hour. Perioperative steroids and ketorolac were administered to reduce perioperative pain and nausea. He was observed in the recovery room for 4 hours, where he remained hemodynamically stable with a soft neck and normal voice. His pain was controlled without the use of narcotics, and he was tolerating a diet. He was thus discharged home. His final pathology was notable for a 1.2-cm follicular adenoma.

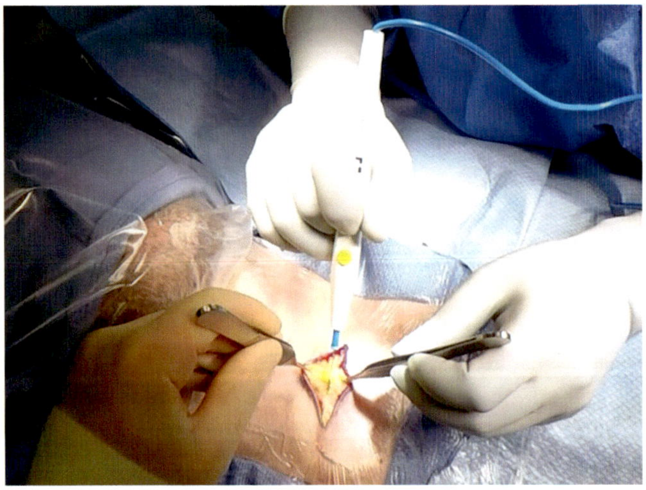

Fig. 9.2 The subcutaneous tissues and platysma were divided with electrocautery

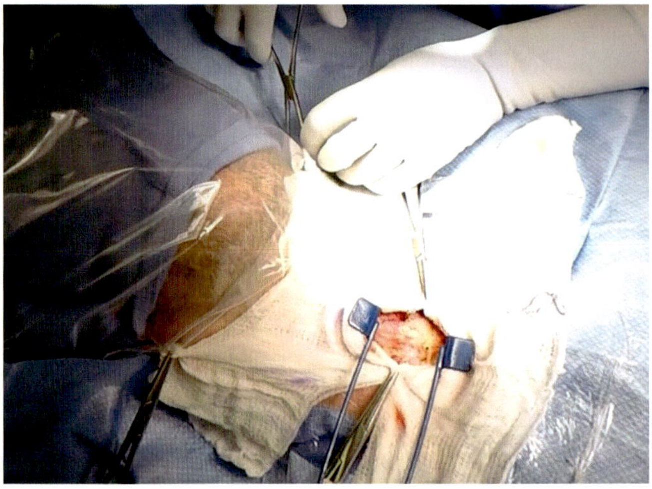

Fig. 9.4 Moist gauze was used to protect the skin edges, and an insulated spring retractor was used to provide exposure

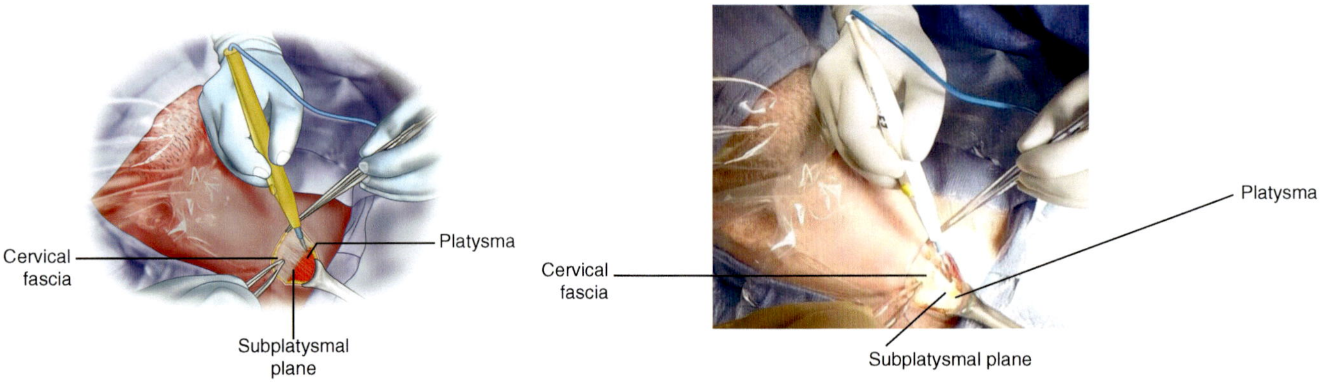

Fig. 9.3 An inferior subplatysmal flap was raised to the level of the sternal notch

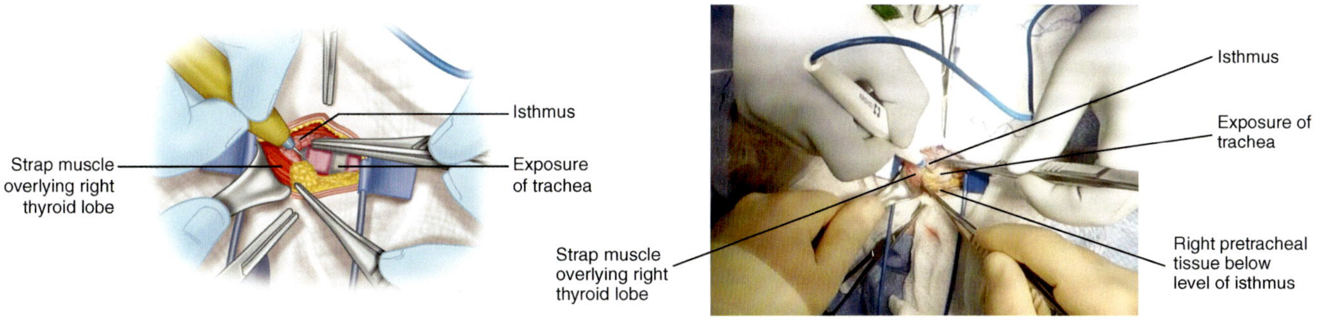

Fig. 9.5 Electrocautery was used to expose the trachea at the level of the inferior border of the isthmus

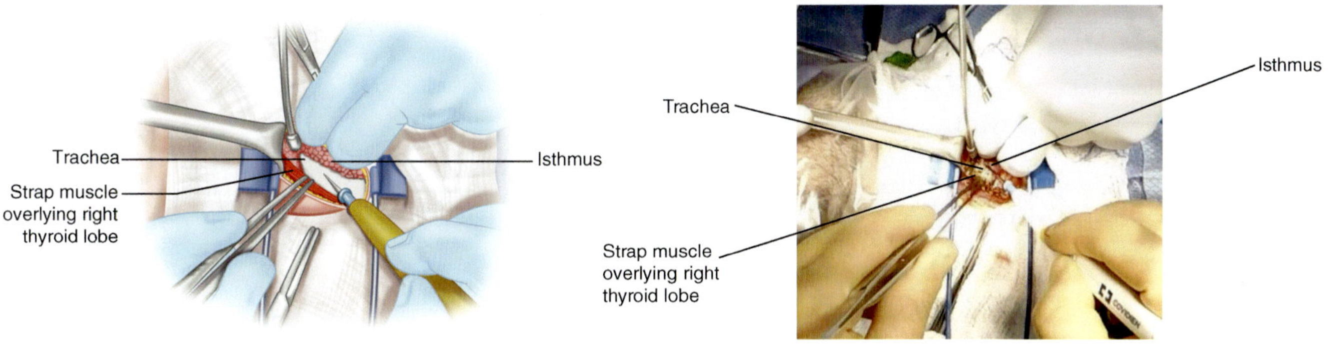

Fig. 9.6 The isthmus was divided at its junction with the right thyroid lobe using electrocautery

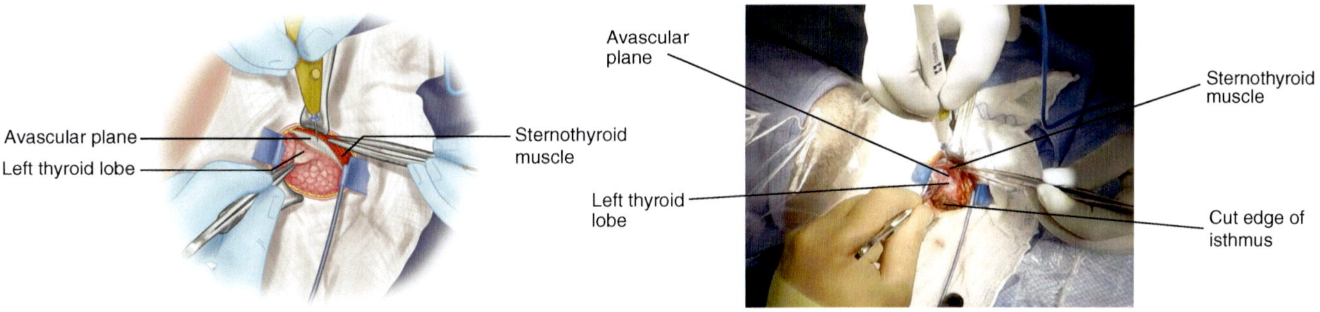

Fig. 9.7 The left strap muscles were reflected laterally, and the left thyroid lobe was mobilized medially by dividing the loose areolar tissue in this relatively avascular plane

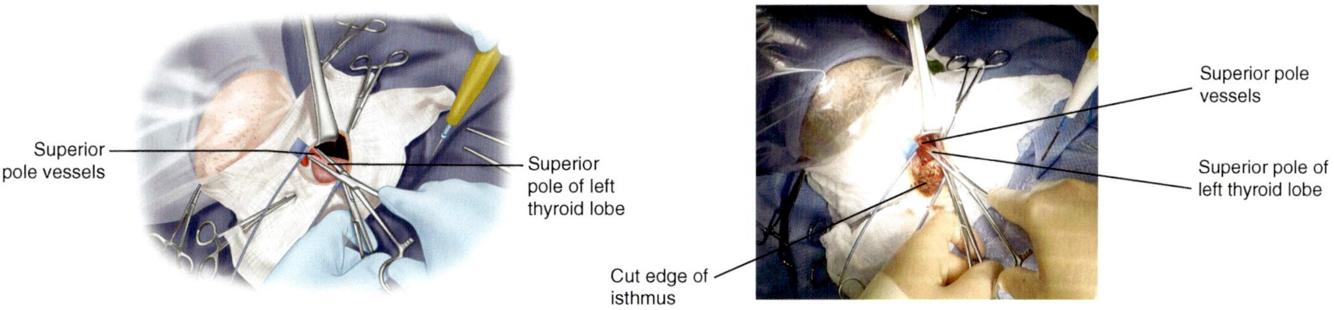

Fig. 9.8 The superior pole of the thyroid was grasped with a Kelly clamp and lifted anteriorly and laterally to facilitate exposure of the superior pole vessels

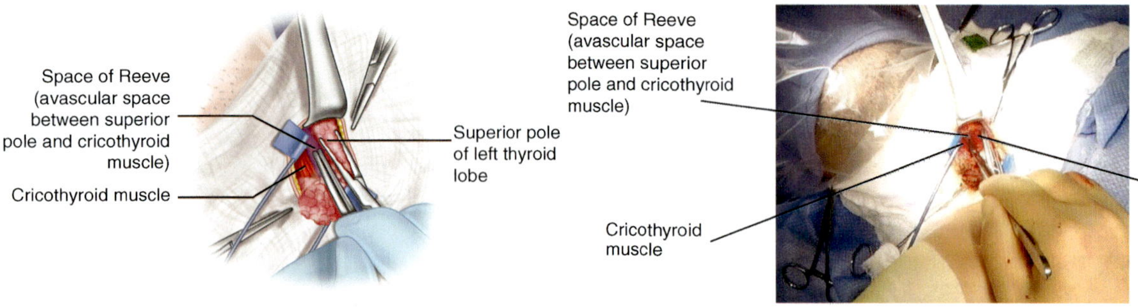

Fig. 9.9 Care was taken to avoid injury to the external branch of the superior laryngeal nerve by gingerly teasing away any muscle and tissue adhered to the thyroid capsule medially

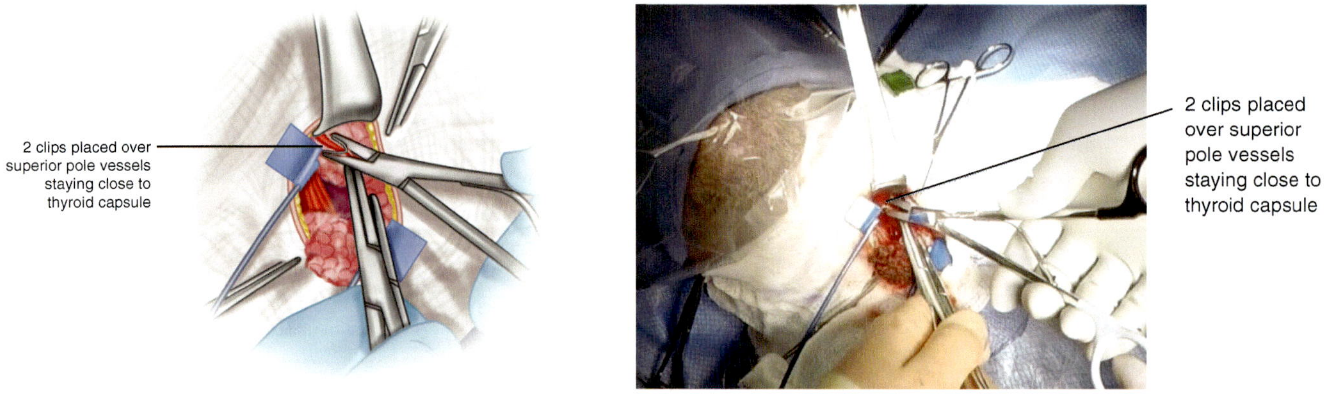

Fig. 9.10 After isolating the superior pole vessels, the vessels were doubly clipped close to the thyroid

Fig. 9.11 After the superior pole vessels were clipped, electrocautery was used to divide the tissue between the clips and the thyroid capsule. This sequence was repeated until the superior pole of the thyroid was free

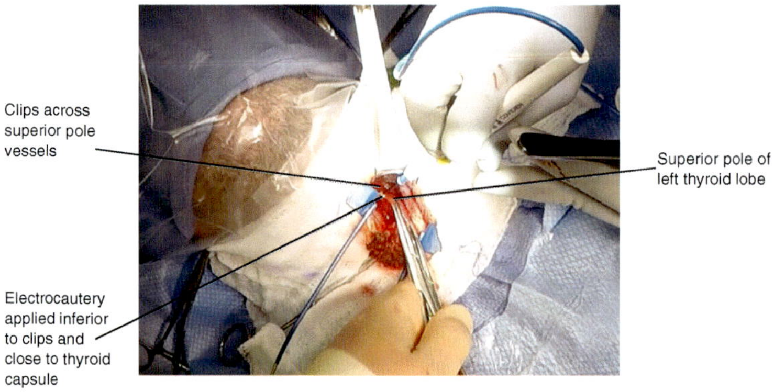

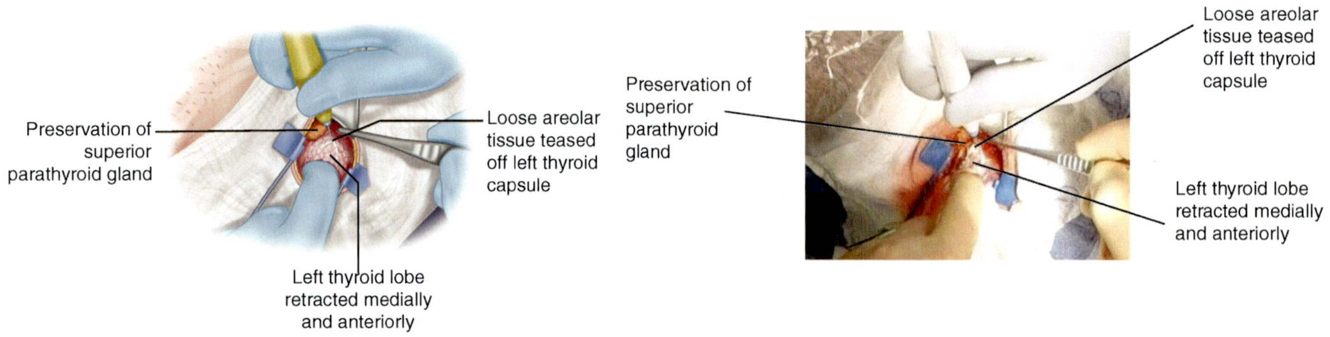

Fig. 9.12 The loose areolar tissue attached to the thyroid capsule was gently swept posteriorly. This maneuver enabled the preservation of both the superior and inferior parathyroid glands

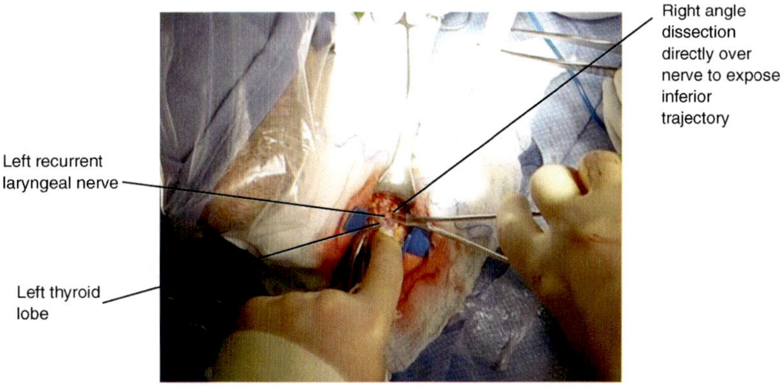

Fig. 9.13 The recurrent laryngeal nerve was identified close to its insertion in the larynx, and a right-angle dissector was used to trace the nerve inferiorly

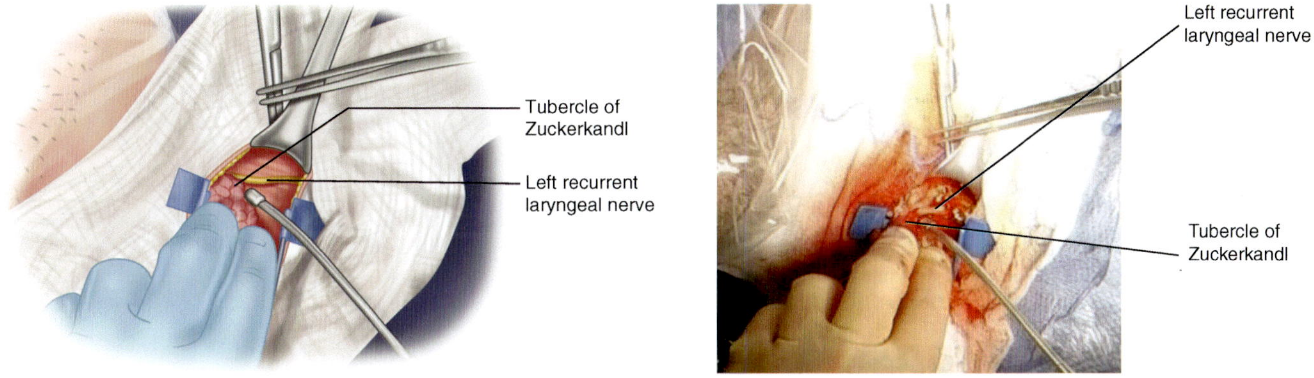

Fig. 9.14 The left recurrent laryngeal nerve was further exposed

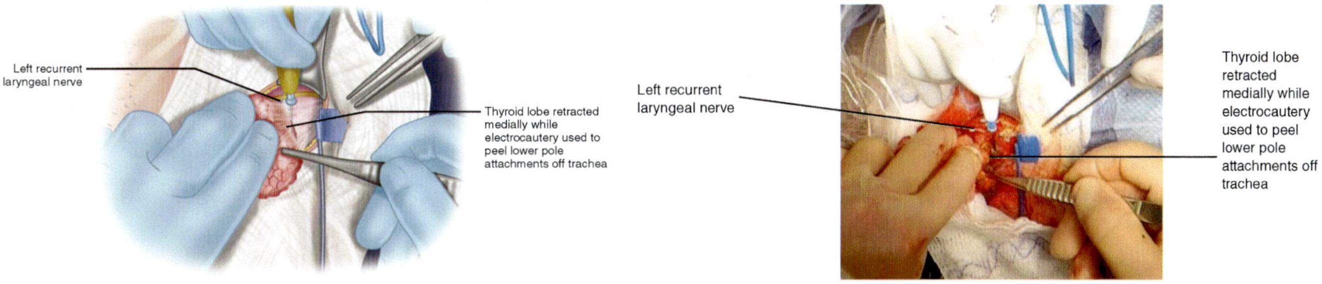

Fig. 9.15 With the recurrent laryngeal nerve in view, the lower pole attachments were clipped close to the thyroid capsule and ligated with electrocautery down to the level of the trachea

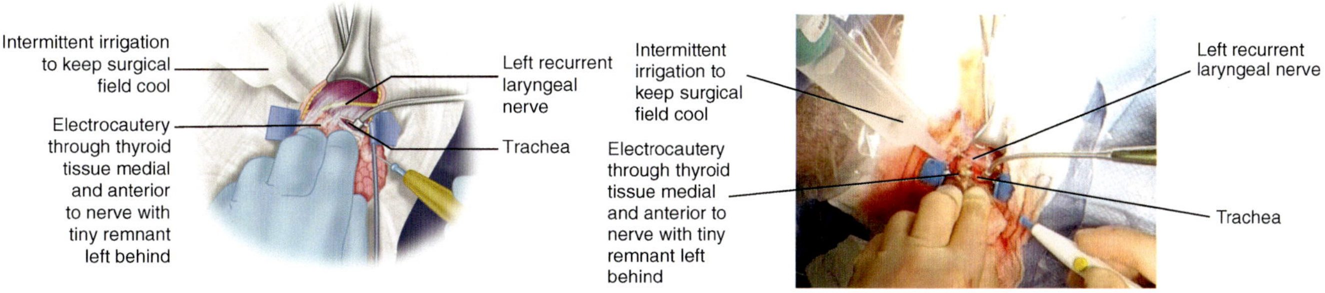

Fig. 9.16 With the entire trajectory of the nerve in view, the thyroid tissue medial and anterior to the nerve was incised with electrocautery, leaving a tiny remnant in the adherent zone for safety reasons. Intermittent irrigation was used during this maneuver to keep the surgical field cool

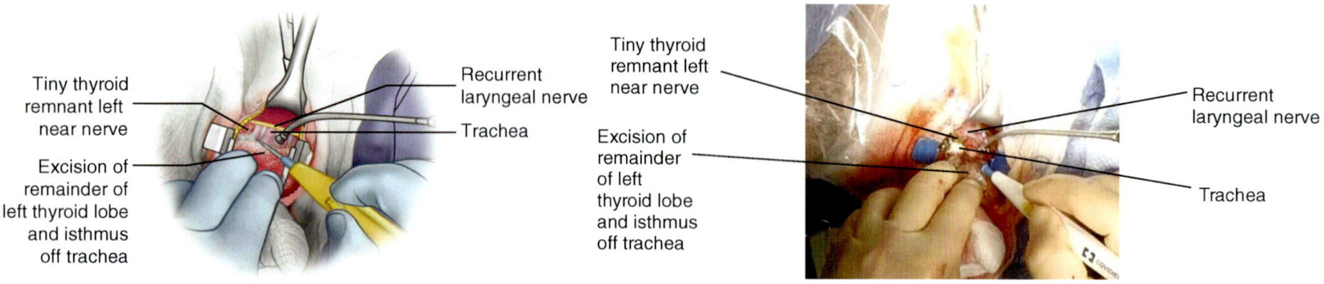

Fig. 9.17 The isthmus and pyramidal lobe were removed with the specimen

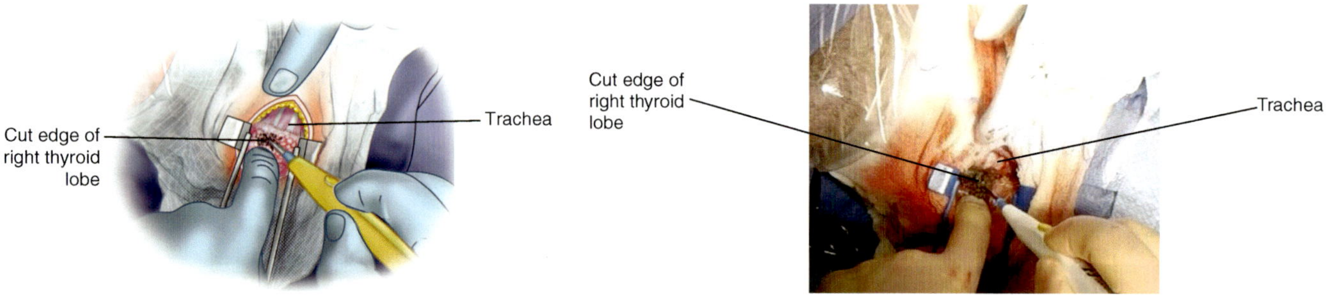

Fig. 9.18 Electrocautery was applied to the cut edge of the right lobe for hemostasis

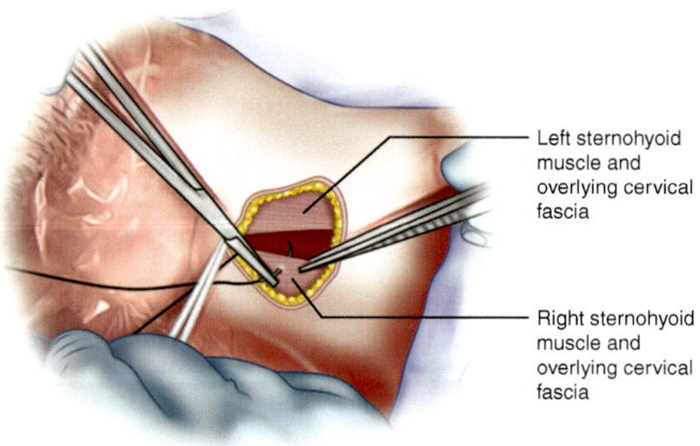

Fig. 9.19 The sternothyroid was approximated with one 4-0 silk figure-of-eight stitch, and the sternohyoid and cervical fascia were reapproximated with a running 4-0 silk stitch to provide coverage of the trachea

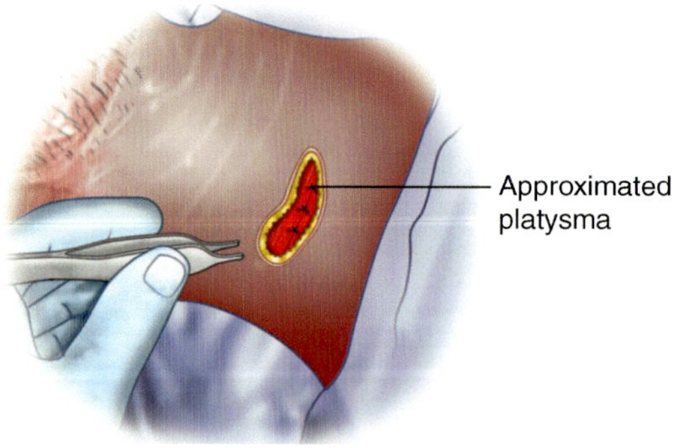

Fig. 9.20 The platysma was reapproximated with interrupted 4.0 silk stitches

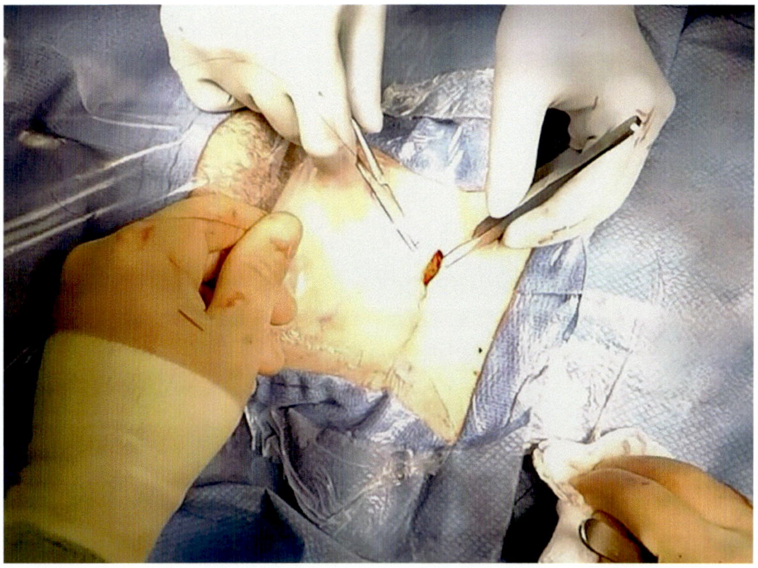

Fig. 9.21 The skin was closed with a running subcuticular 4-0 Monocryl stitch and topped with Steri-Strips

Suggested Reading

Chen H. Fine needle aspiration biopsy of the thyroid: thyroid lobectomy and total thyroidectomy. In: Fischer J, Jones D, Pomposelli F, Upchurch G, Klimberg V, Schwaitzberg S, Bland K, editors. Fischer's mastery of surgery. 6th ed. Philadelphia: Wolters Kluwer Health/Lippincott Williams & Wilkins; 2012. p. 468–78.

Haugen BR, Alexander EK, Bible KC, Doherty GM, Mandel SJ, Nikiforov YE, et al. 2015 American Thyroid Association Management Guidelines for adult patients with thyroid nodules and differentiated thyroid cancer: the American Thyroid Association Guidelines Task Force on Thyroid Nodules and Differentiated Thyroid Cancer. Thyroid. 2016;26(1):1–133.

Patel KN, Yip L, Lubitz CC, Grubbs EG, Miller BS, Shen W, et al. The American Association of Endocrine Surgeons Guidelines for the definitive surgical management of thyroid disease in adults. Ann Surg. 2020;271(3):e21–93.

10 Total Thyroidectomy and Ipsilateral Central Lymph Node Dissection for the Management of Papillary Thyroid Carcinoma

Adam Ofri and Mark Sywak

Introduction

The current American Thyroid Association (ATA) Guidelines recommend total thyroidectomy for intermediate and high-risk differentiated thyroid cancer (DTC) patients with either T3, N1, or M1 disease [1]. Patients with low-risk DTC can undergo either total thyroidectomy or lobectomy; however, the decision-making is dependent on whether radioactive iodine (RAI) therapy is likely to be recommended. Our total thyroidectomy technique employs an energy-based vessel-sealing device (LigaSure®) for vessel ligation and routine neural integrity monitoring (NIM). The safety and efficiency of the "sutureless thyroidectomy" have been well documented, and we have incorporated this approach into our practice for over 15 years [2]. Though the routine use of NIM for the preservation of the recurrent laryngeal nerve (RLN) and external branch of the superior laryngeal nerve (EBSLN) remains controversial [3], we continue to use this as an adjunct in our technique to confirm nerve function rather than as a primary means to identify the nerve. NIM is particularly useful in the setting of difficult re-operative surgery and complex thyroid cancer procedures.

Central lymph node dissection (CLND) is recommended for patients, with clinically involved central nodes and should be considered in T3 or C1Nb patients; or if it will impact further therapy. The typical pattern of nodal spread for papillary thyroid carcinomas (PTC) is central then lateral [4]; thus, the most common site of metastatic PTC is at level VI lymph nodes [5]. Cervical lymph node spread can occur early in PTC with evidence of subclinical metastases in T1a PTC [6, 7]. Studies have shown the benefit of routine CLND in PTC, with lower post-operative thyroglobulin levels and a reduction in the need for re-operation in the central compartment, with no increase in long-term morbidity [6, 8].

Pre-operative preparation requires careful consultation with the patient to obtain informed consent, with a discussion of the potential risks and benefits of the procedure. All patients must undergo an assessment of the vocal fold function with either fibre-optic laryngoscopy, vocal fold ultrasound, or voice handicap questionnaire. In the setting of known thyroid cancer, we recommend that fibre-optic laryngoscopy be performed in all cases. It is important to note that pre-existing vocal cord paralysis can occur in both benign and malignant thyroid diseases [9].

Procedure

A 40-year-old female was referred to our endocrine surgical service for the management of subclinical thyrotoxicosis and incidentally discovered papillary thyroid carcinoma. The patient was undergoing investigations prior to commencing assisted reproductive treatment with in vitro fertilisation. She was found to have a mildly suppressed thyroid-stimulating hormone (TSH) of 0.12 mU/L (0.45–4.12 mU/L). There were no overt symptoms of thyrotoxicosis, and she had a regular menstrual cycle. Her past history was unremarkable, aside from previous surgery for a paraumbilical hernia. She gave no history of prior radiation exposure. There was a family history of benign multinodular goitre in a paternal uncle. On physical examination, she had a firm 15-mm right thyroid nodule; there was no palpable lymphadenopathy, and she looked clinically euthyroid. Thyroid ultrasound identified a multinodular goitre with a suspicious 17-mm heterogeneous right thyroid nodule with microcalcifications (TIRADS 5). There was a suspicious 8-mm irregular nodule in the left thy-

A. Ofri
School of Medicine, University of New South Wales, St Leonards, NSW, Australia

Department of Surgery, Royal North Shore Hospital, St Leonards, NSW, Australia

M. Sywak (✉)
University of Sydney Endocrine Surgery Unit, Royal North Shore Hospital, St Leonards, NSW, Australia

Department of Endocrine and Oncology Surgery, Royal North Shore Hospital, St Leonards, NSW, Australia
e-mail: marksywak@nebsc.com.au

A. Shifrin (ed.), *Atlas of Thyroid Surgery*, https://doi.org/10.1007/978-3-030-93673-0_10

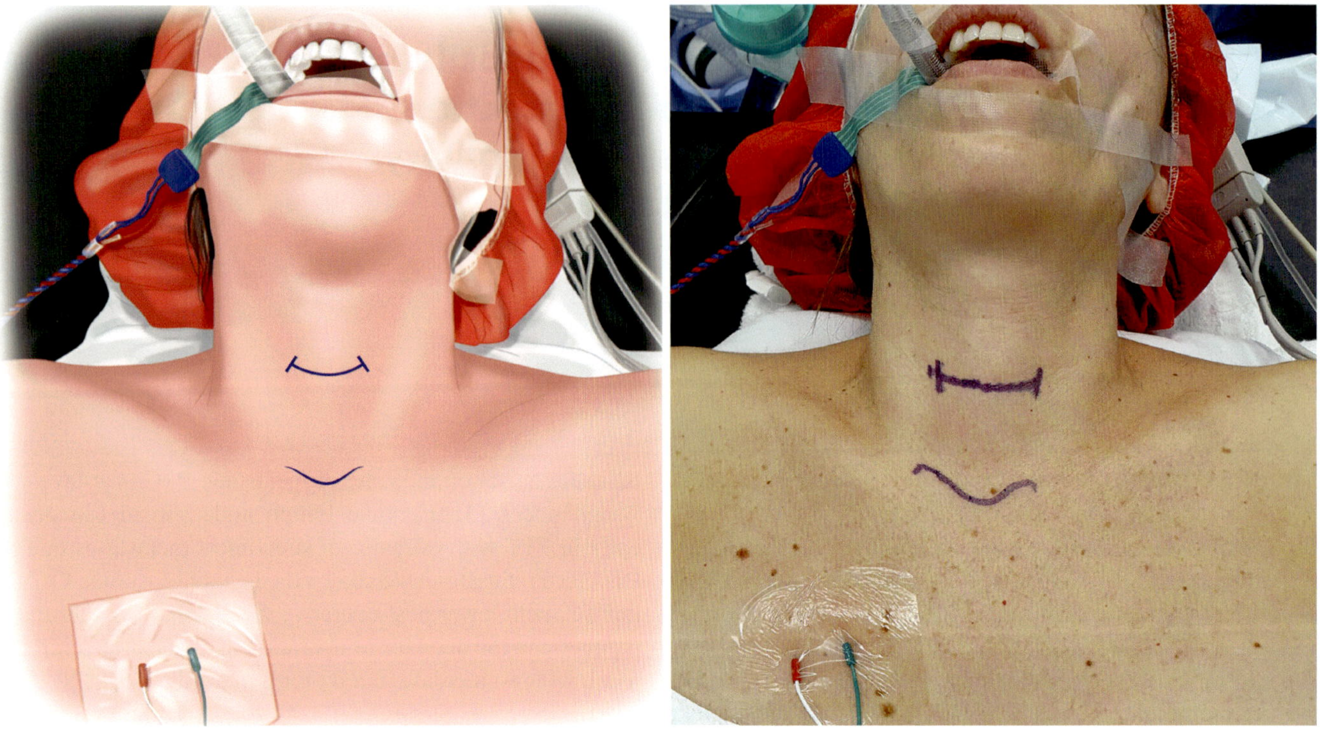

Fig. 10.1 A central 4-cm transverse marking is placed in an appropriate cervical skin crease

roid lobe (TIRADS 5). In addition, there were two hypoechoic suspicious right central compartment lymph nodes. Fine-needle biopsy of the right and left thyroid nodules confirmed papillary thyroid carcinoma (Bethesda VI). In view of the multifocal papillary thyroid cancer and suspicious central compartment lymph nodes, the patient was consented for, and underwent, total thyroidectomy and CLND.

At surgery, the patient is routinely intubated with a NIM electromyogram (EMG) tracheal tube, with right-sided chest leads placed to facilitate a working NIM system. Under general anaesthetic, the patient is placed in a supine position with both arms in complete adduction and cervical extension. A central 4-cm transverse marking is placed in an appropriate cervical skin crease (Fig. 10.1). Incision site and bilateral superficial cervical plexus blocks are performed (Fig. 10.2). The skin is prepared with 10% povidone-iodine solution. The surgery commences with a blade incision to the skin and electrocautery to divide through subcutaneous tissue and platysma. A combination of electrocautery and blunt dissection is used to create sub-platysmal flaps in a plane anterior to the anterior jugular vessels, assisted by Monehan and then Kocher retractors (Fig. 10.3). The superior flap dissection extends to the cricothyroid and the inferior flap to the sternal notch. Fascia is opened in the midline longitudinally (Fig. 10.4) and the strap muscles separated. Sternohyoid and sternothyroid are individually divided transversely with LigaSure if required to facilitate thyroid access (Fig. 10.5). Capsular dissection of the strap muscles off the thyroid is performed with diathermy and blunt dissection to facilitate superior and inferior exposure of the thyroid – assisted by Kocher and Langenbeck retractors. The remnant thyroglossal duct is dissected free using electrocautery, taking care to completely excise the thyroglossal remnant. The pyramidal lobe is mobilised at the superior aspect of the thyroid isthmus (Fig. 10.6). The anteriorly, associated Delphian lymph node is included in this dissection. Once this is dissected free superiorly, it is then retracted to facilitate in creating a plane deep into the thyroid isthmus. Right-angle forceps are used to further dissect the plane anterior to the trachea, with LigaSure used to divide the isthmus completely (Fig. 10.7). Division of the thyroid isthmus is not performed if the thyroid cancer is centrally located. The remnant duct and Delphian node are then completely excised and sent for histopathological assessment.

At this stage, the ipsilateral carotid sheath is opened, and vagal nerve stimulation (V1) is performed to confirm recurrent laryngeal nerve function (Fig. 10.8). Once confirmed, the pathological hemithyroid is mobilised, initially with lateral dissection and division of the middle thyroidal vein. The superior pole is grasped with Kelly forceps and retracted antero-infero-medially by the surgeon, with retraction by the

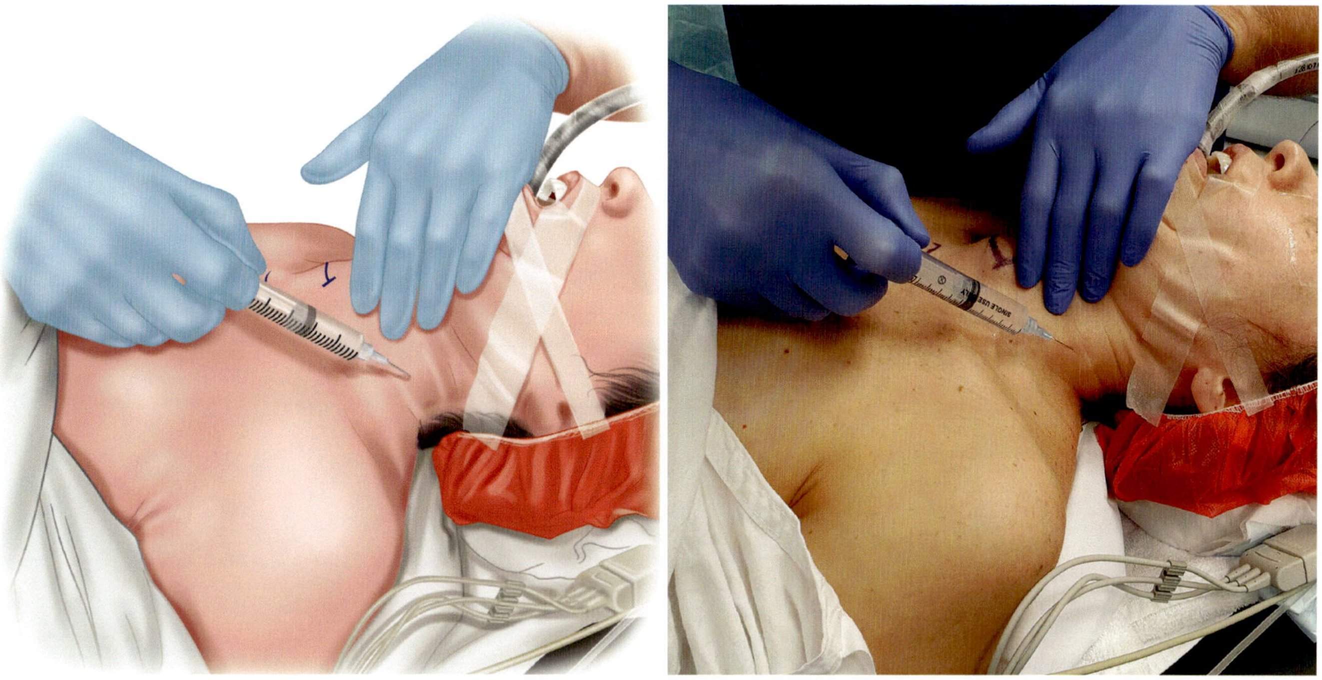

Fig. 10.2 Incision site and bilateral superficial cervical plexus blocks are performed

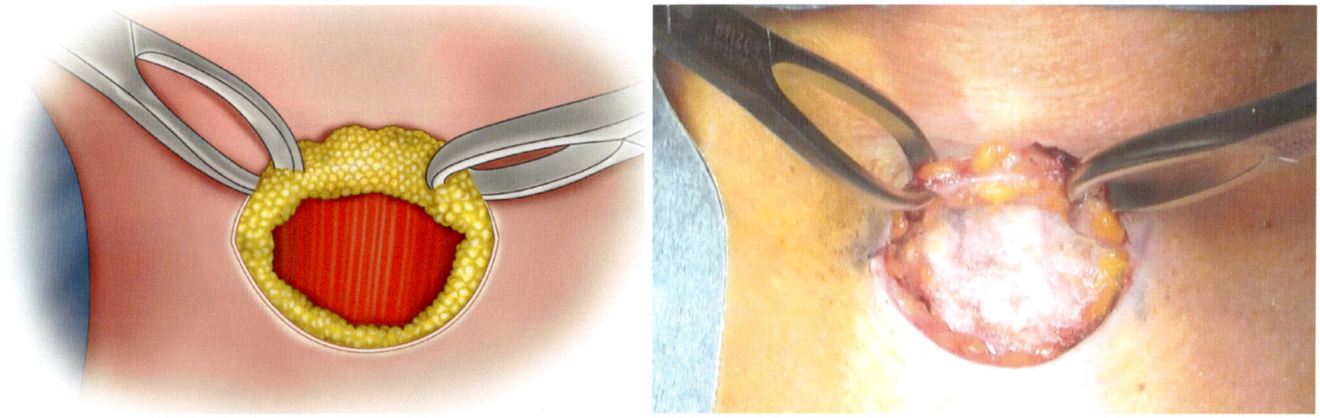

Fig. 10.3 Sub-platysmal flaps created in a plane anterior to the anterior jugular vessels

assistant using Langenbeck retractors (Fig. 10.9). Capsular dissection of the superior pole is performed with diathermy and LigaSure, focusing on identifying the ipsilateral EBSLN. Once visually identified, NIM testing confirms identification and cricothyroid muscle twitching is visualised; the nerve is then preserved (Fig. 10.10), and further dissection is performed to completely release the superior pole. The inferior pole is then retracted superomedially (Fig. 10.11). The inferior parathyroid is identified and its vascular pedicle preserved through a capsular dissection approach. Once the gland is medialised, the key focus is the identification of the ipsilateral RLN. Sharp and blunt dissection is performed behind the tubercle of Zuckerkandl; identifying the inferior thyroidal artery and the RLN. Exposure of the RLN is performed by blunt dissection on the nerve with fine mosquito forceps (Fig. 10.12). The RLN is followed distally and proximally, ensuring that the bifurcation to the anterior and posterior branches is confirmed. The NIM probe is used to confirm

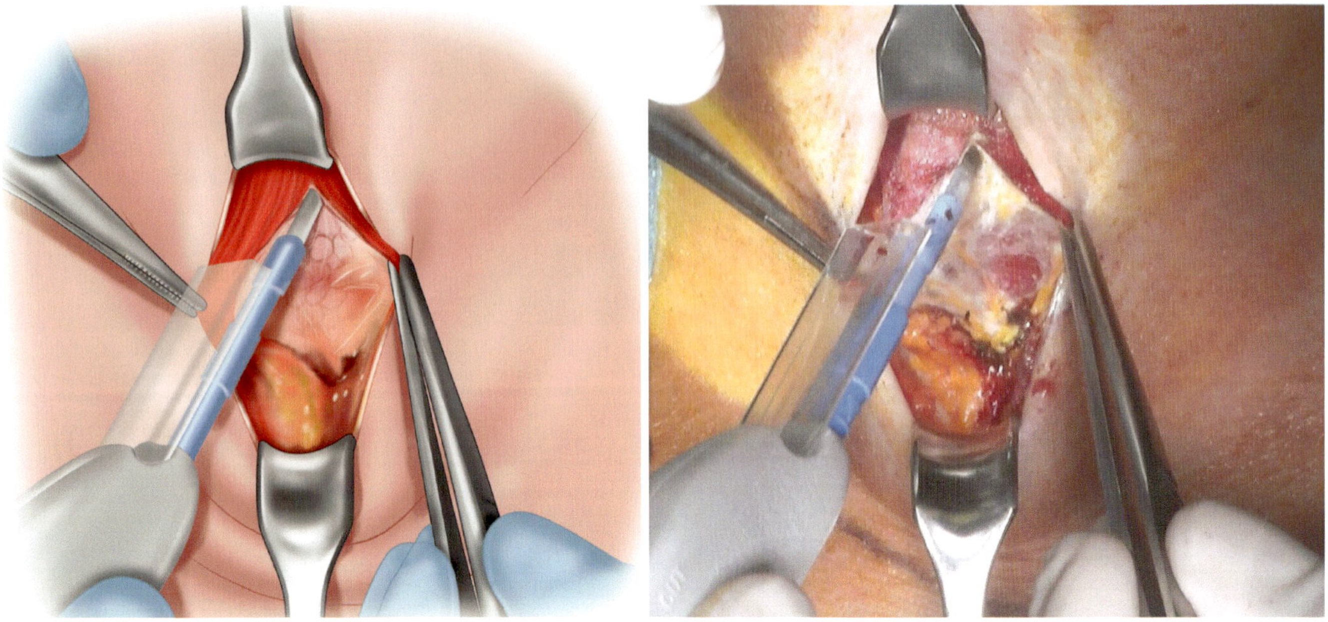

Fig. 10.4 Fascia is opened in the midline longitudinally

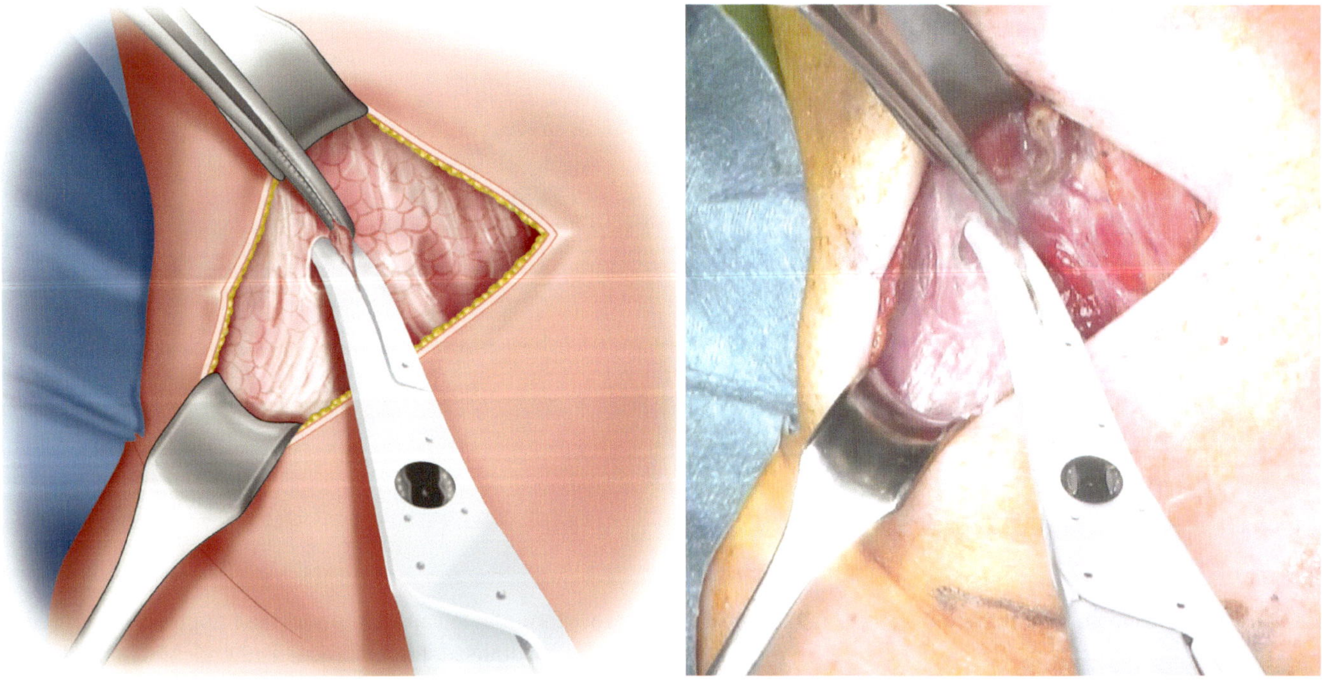

Fig. 10.5 Sternohyoid and sternothyroid are divided transversely with LigaSure to facilitate thyroid access

nerve integrity (Fig. 10.13). Tissue overlying the RLN is dissected free; a suture ligation may be required in close proximity to the RLN in the region of the ligament of Berry to avoid thermal injury to the nerve with the energy device. The superior parathyroid gland is identified and preserved in this region. Once the thyroid is dissected free from the RLN, midline tracheal adhesions are divided with electrocautery and LigaSure. Prior to the division of the Ligament of Berry, a final NIM stimulation is performed to confirm RLN function, ensuring the nerve has not been injured or inadvertently compressed in a ligature. Sharp dissection is then used to divide the tissue anterior to the ligament of Berry, and the hemithyroid specimen is reviewed prior to sending for histopathological assessment (Fig. 10.14).

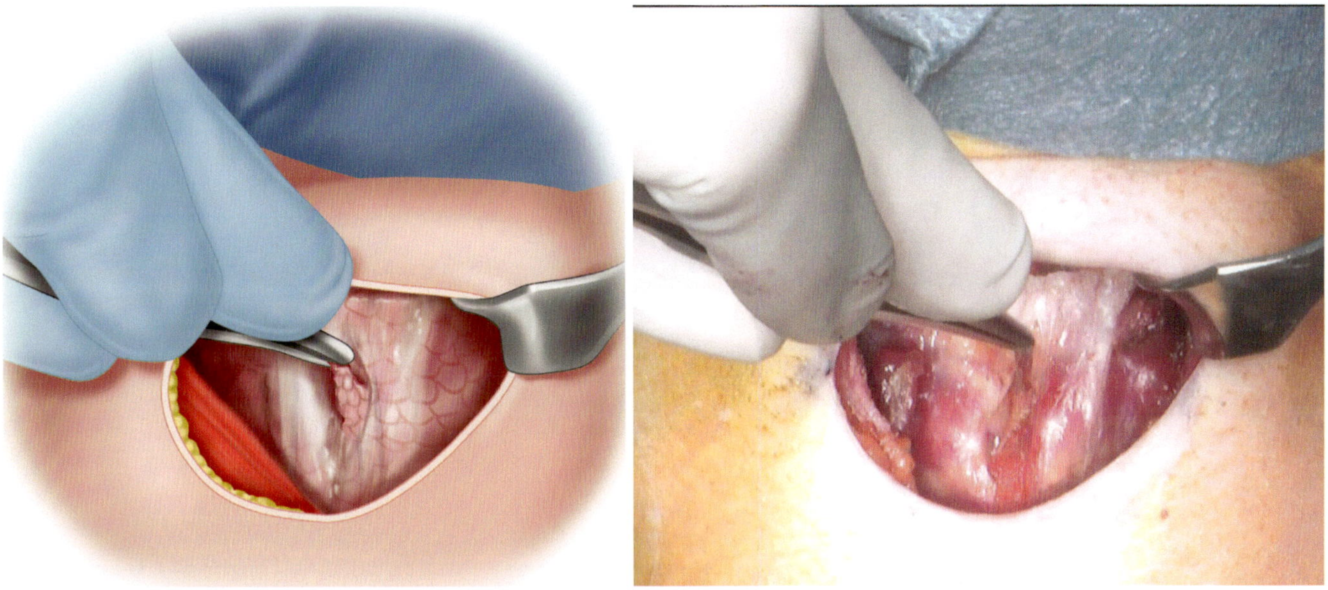

Fig. 10.6 The pyramidal lobe is mobilised at the superior aspect of the thyroid isthmus

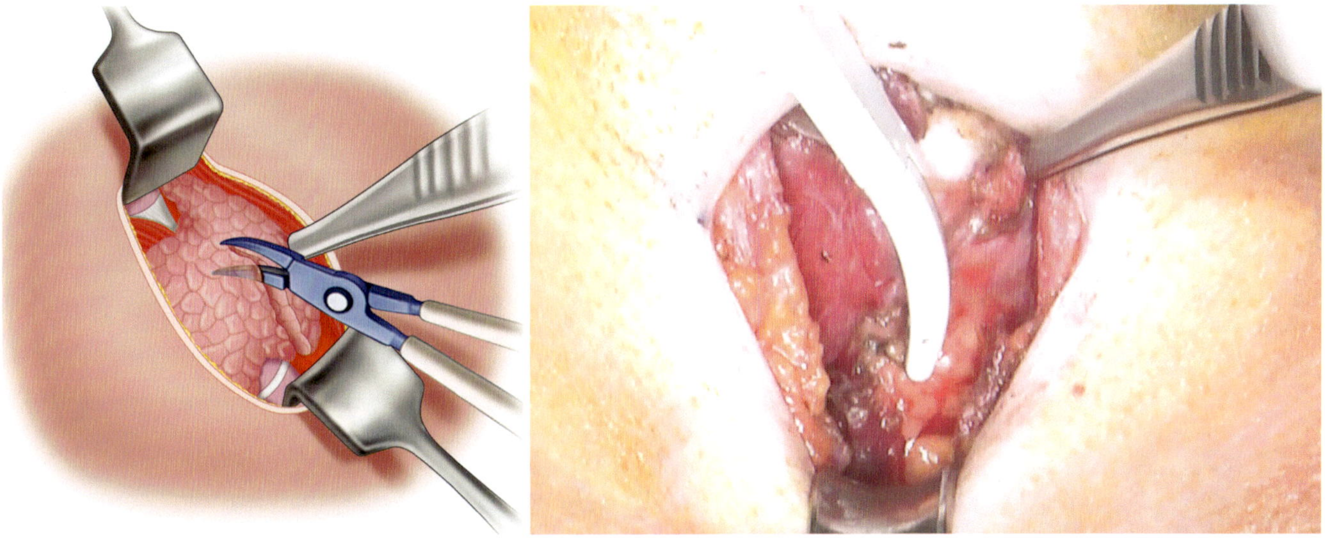

Fig. 10.7 Right-angle forceps are used to dissect the plane anterior to the trachea, with LigaSure used to divide the isthmus completely

An ipsilateral central node dissection is then commenced removing levels VI and VII lymph node compartments. The medial border of the dissection is the contra-lateral aspect of the trachea, the lateral border is the ipsilateral carotid artery, and the inferior extent is superior to the brachiocephalic vein. Dissection is performed to the depth of the prevertebral fascia and involves skeletonisation of the ipsilateral RLN and cervical Oesophagus. Visual inspection and digital palpation can identify involved nodes (Fig. 10.15). The RLN is surrounded by the nodal packet, and careful dissection should be performed, with interval confirmation of nerve integrity (Fig. 10.16). The lymph node compartment is split along the course of the RLN and is often removed in two separate components. The inferior aspect of the nodal compartment extends to involve the thyrothymic ligament, and LigaSure is used to divide the thyrothymic ligament and confirm haemostasis (Fig. 10.17). Ipsilateral central node dissection typically requires autotransplantation of the inferior parathyroid gland. Prior to commencing on the contralateral side, a second vagal stimulation is performed (V2) to confirm the integrity of the RLN throughout its course (Fig. 10.18).

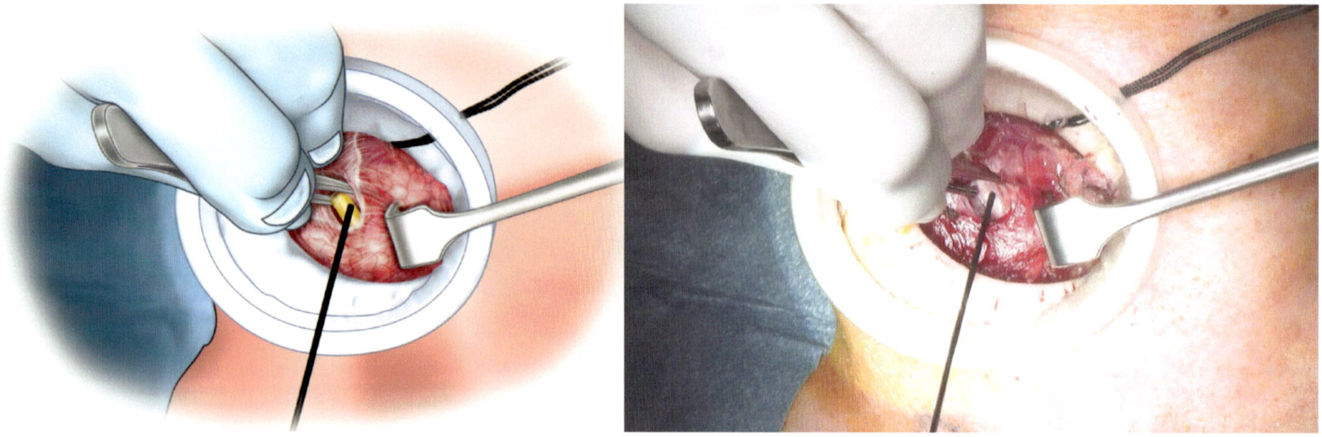

Fig. 10.8 V1 is performed to confirm recurrent laryngeal nerve function

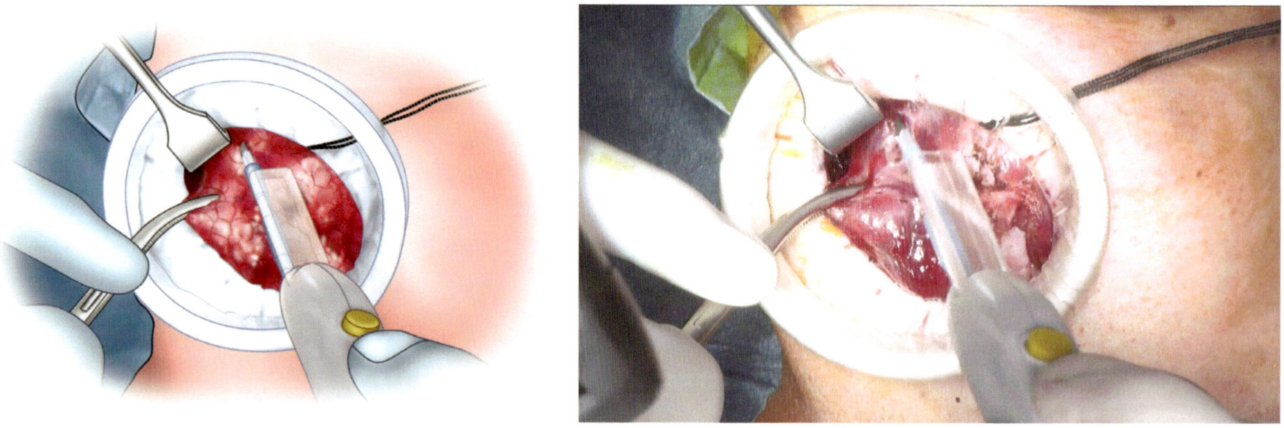

Fig. 10.9 The superior pole is grasped with Kelly forceps and retracted antero-infero-medially by the surgeon, with retraction by the assistant with Langenbeck retractors

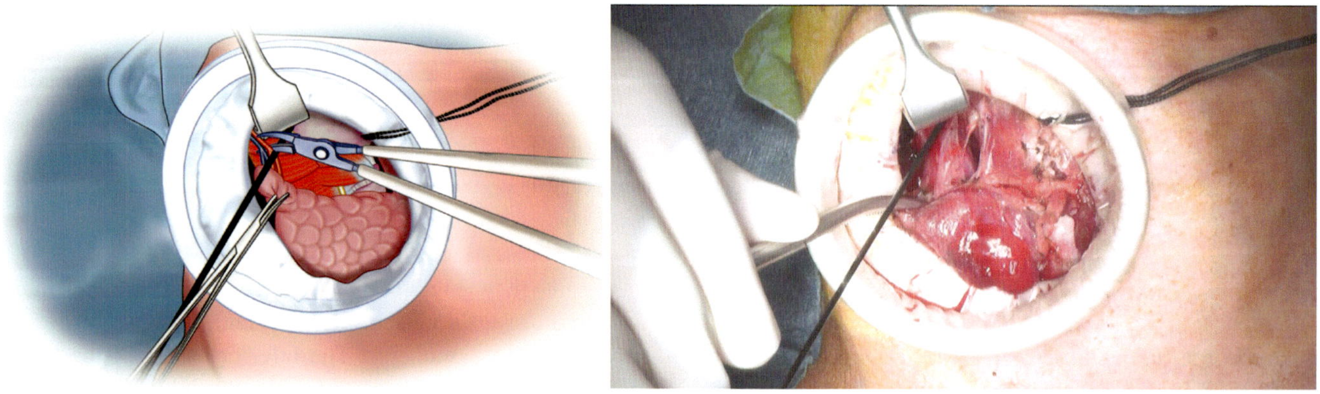

Fig. 10.10 Once visually identified, NIM testing confirms identification of the EBSLN and cricothyroid muscle twitching is visualised

Contra-lateral hemithyroidectomy is performed in the same fashion as the pathologically involved side.

At the conclusion of the procedure, normal saline irrigation is applied to the cavity to confirm haemostasis. A Valsalva manoeuvre of 30–40-cm H_2O is performed by the anaesthetist to facilitate the identification of any potential bleeding sites. Once haemostasis is confirmed, we routinely apply small pieces of oxidised regenerated cellulose for further haemostasis (Fig. 10.19). In a large cavity, we would place a 10Fr circular drain, secured on the skin with

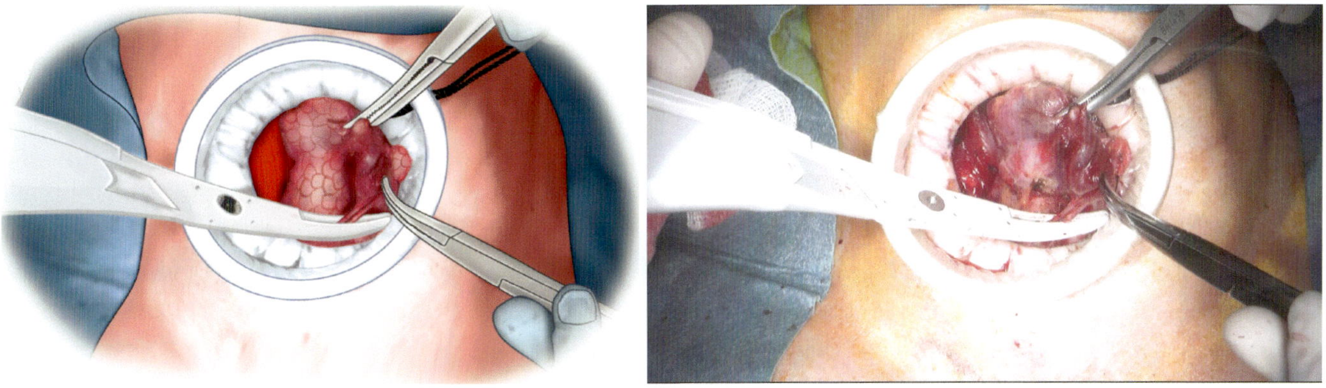

Fig. 10.11 The inferior pole is retracted superomedially prior to facilitating inferior parathyroid identification

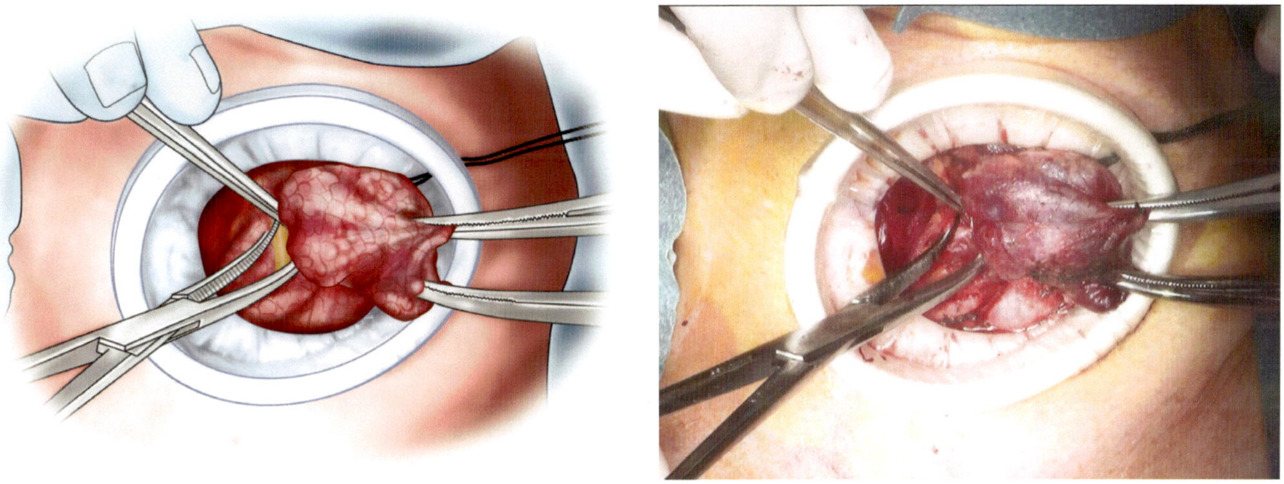

Fig. 10.12 Exposure of the RLN is performed by blunt dissection on the nerve, with fine mosquito forceps

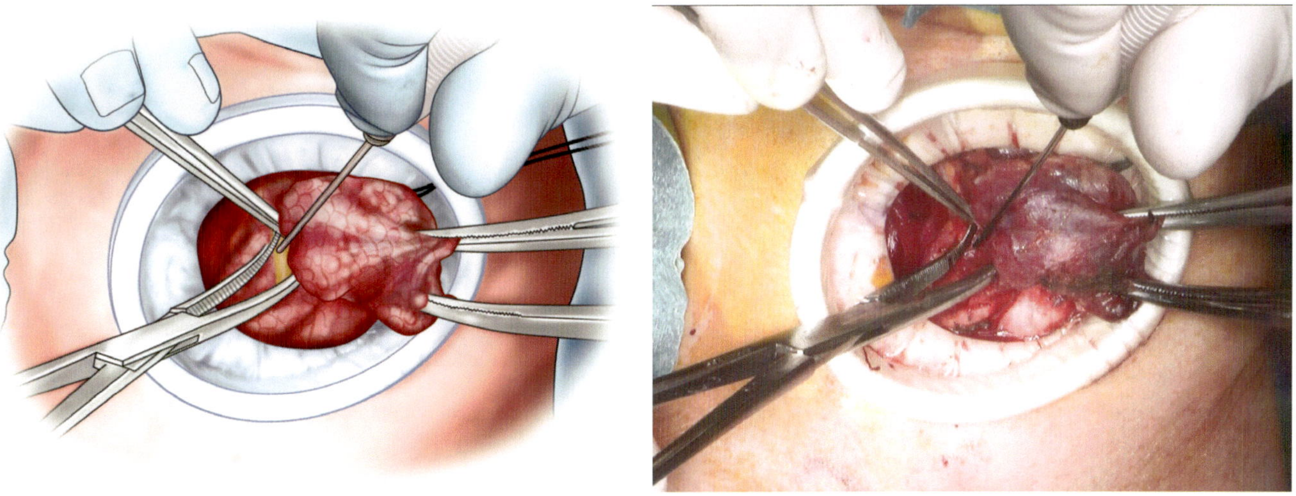

Fig. 10.13 After ensuring that the bifurcation of the RLN to its anterior and posterior branches, the NIM probe is used to confirm nerve integrity

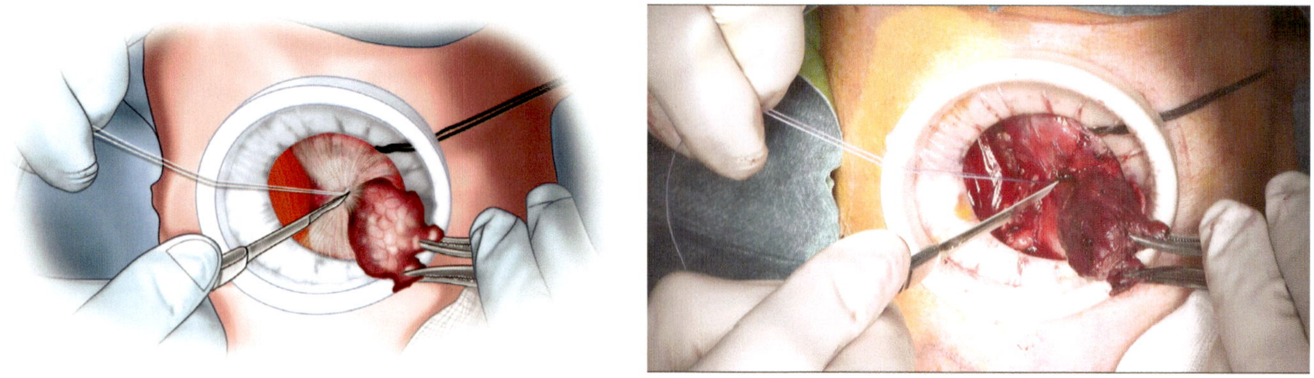

Fig. 10.14 Sharp dissection is used to divide tissue anterior to the ligament of Berry

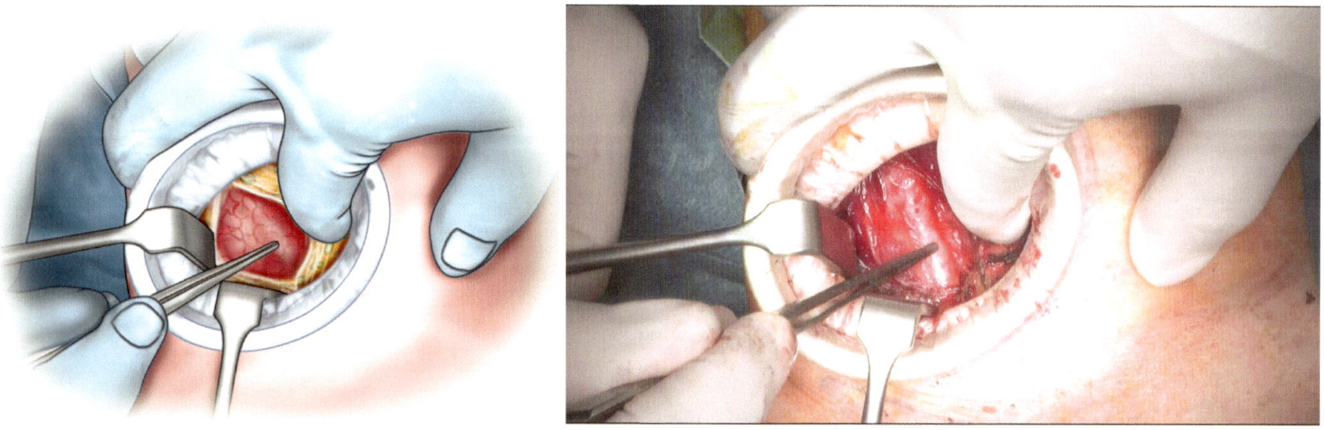

Fig. 10.15 When performing a central lymph node dissection, visual inspection and digital palpation can identify involved nodes

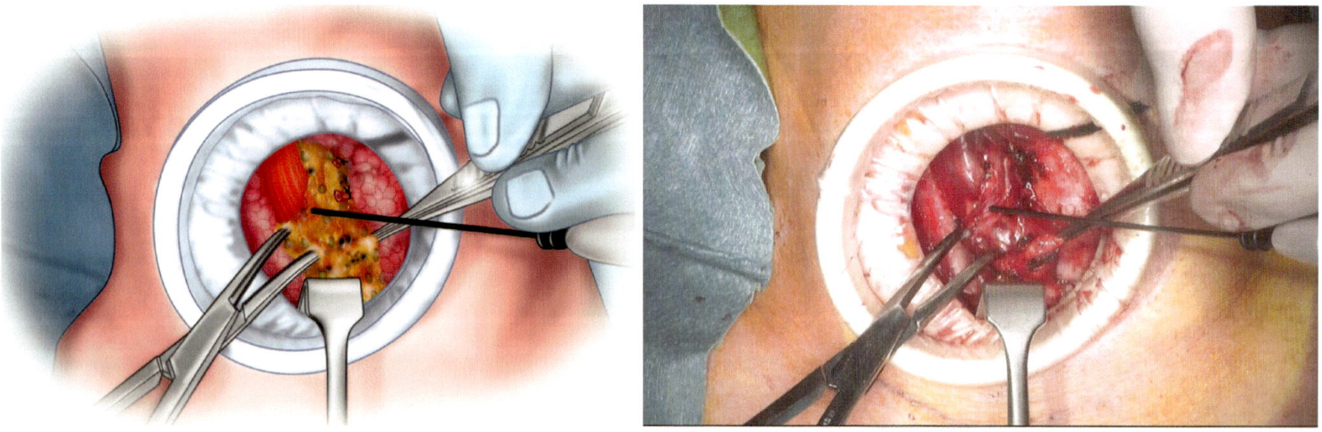

Fig. 10.16 The nodal packet surrounds the RLN, and careful dissection should be performed, with interval confirmation of nerve integrity

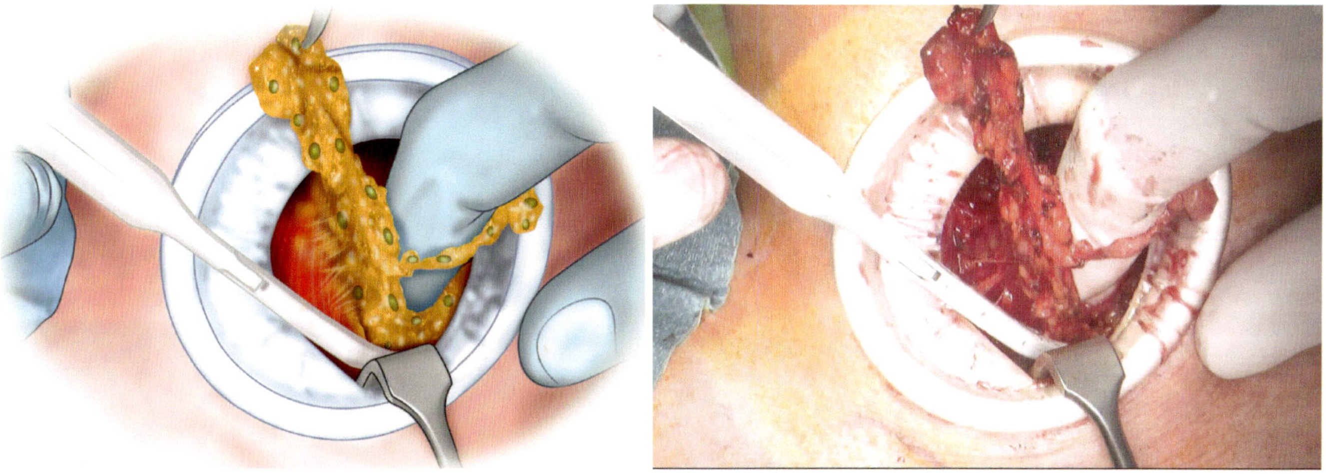

Fig. 10.17 The inferior aspect of the nodal compartment extends to involve the thyro-thymic ligament, and LigaSure is used to divide the thyro-thymic ligament and confirm haemostasis

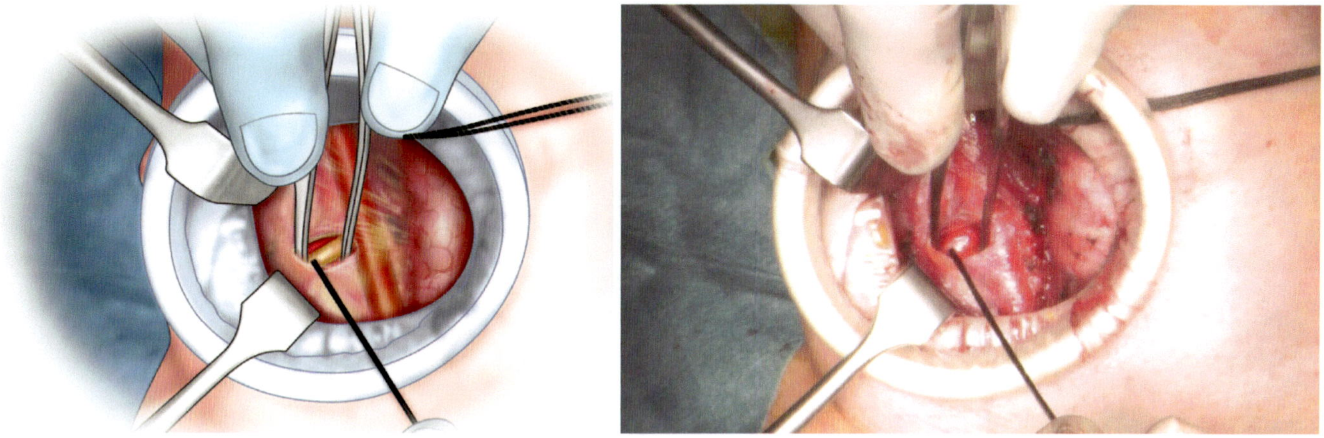

Fig. 10.18 V2 performed to confirm integrity of the RLN throughout its course prior to commencing the contra-lateral side

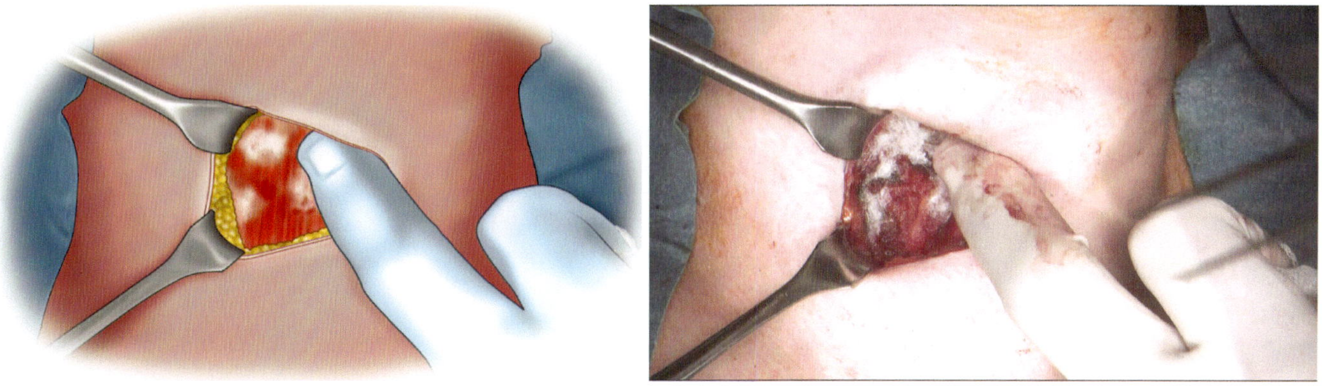

Fig. 10.19 Routine application of small pieces of oxidised regenerated cellulose for further haemostasis

a silk stitch. The midline strap muscles are re-approximated with a running 3-0 Vicryl suture, leaving a small inferior defect (Fig. 10.20). If required, autotransplantation of parathyroid is performed prior to closing the platysma. Dissection is performed onto the right sternocleidomastoid (Fig. 10.21). The parathyroid is fragmented, mixed with 1 ml of saline and injected into the sternocleidomastoid (Fig. 10.22). The platysma is then re-approximated with interrupted 3-0 Vicryl sutures (Fig. 10.23). A continuous 4-0 Monocryl suture is used to close the skin with a single Steri-Strip™ applied along the length of the wound (Fig. 10.24).

The patient is commenced on appropriate weight-adjusted dosing of thyroxine (1.6 ug/kg/day). Routine calcium replacement is commenced (calcium carbonate 1200 mg bd). Parathyroid hormone (PTH) and corrected serum calcium are

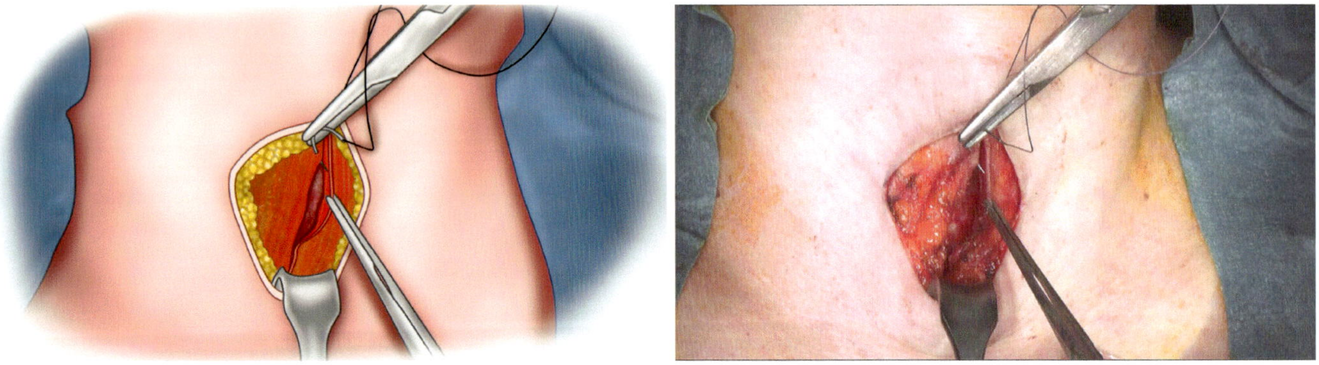

Fig. 10.20 Midline strap muscles are re-approximated with a running 3-0 Vicryl suture, leaving a small inferior defect

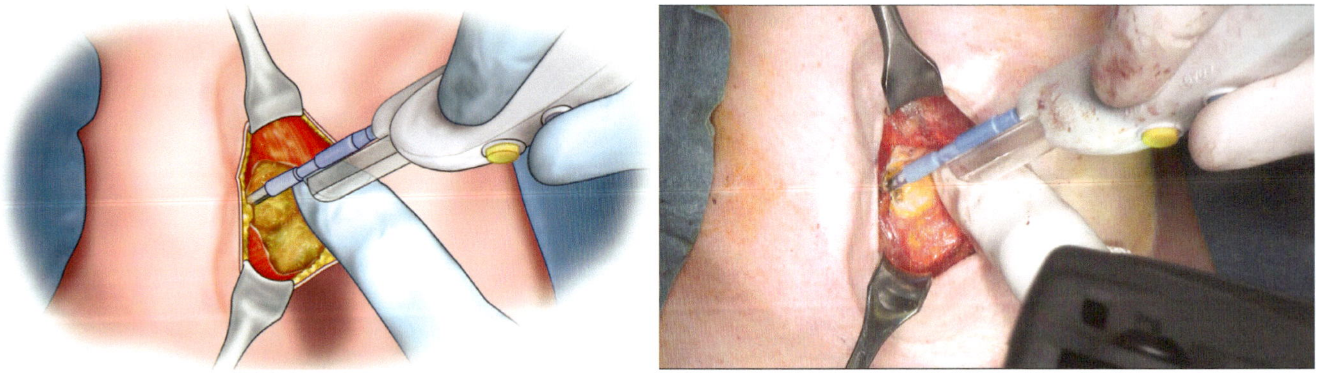

Fig. 10.21 Dissection onto the right sternocleidomastoid to create a pocket for autotransplantation

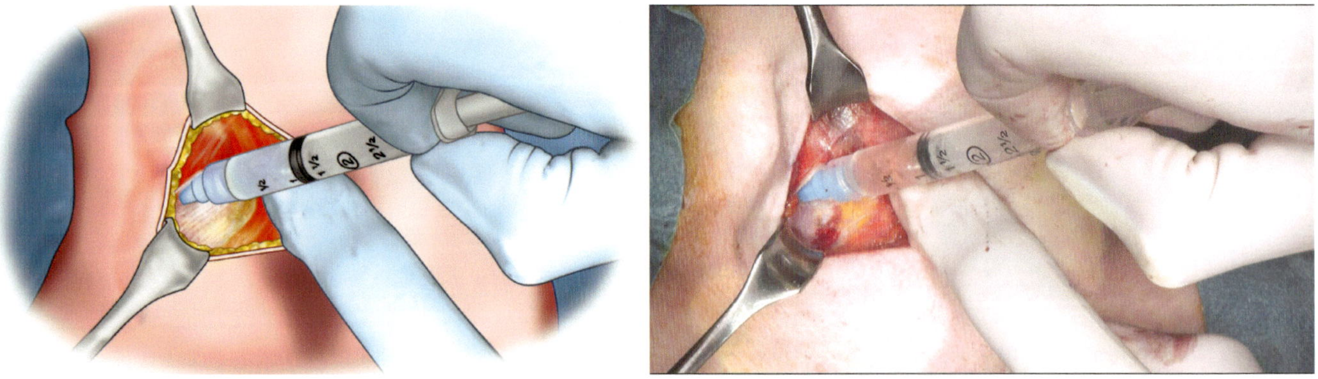

Fig. 10.22 The fragmented parathyroid is mixed with 1 ml of saline and injected into the sternocleidomastoid

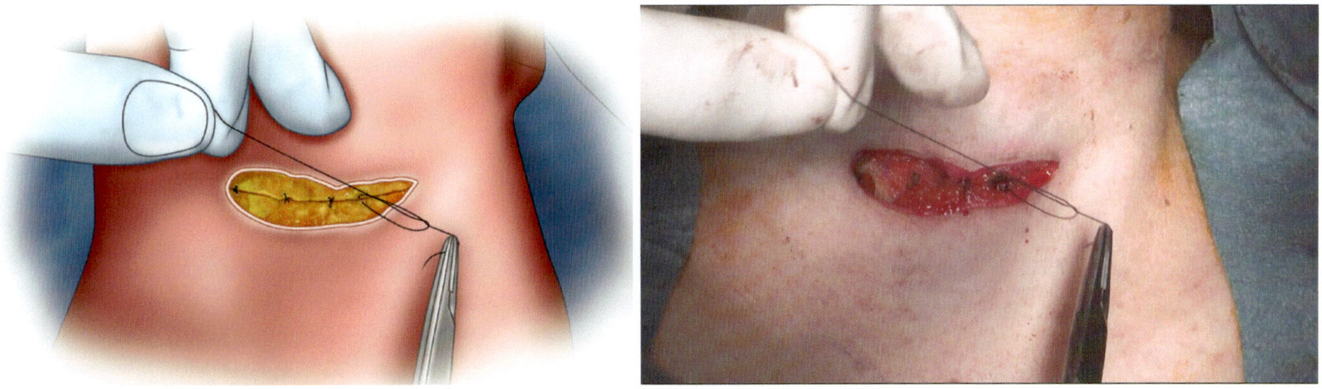

Fig. 10.23 The platysma is re-approximated with interrupted 3-0 Vicryl sutures

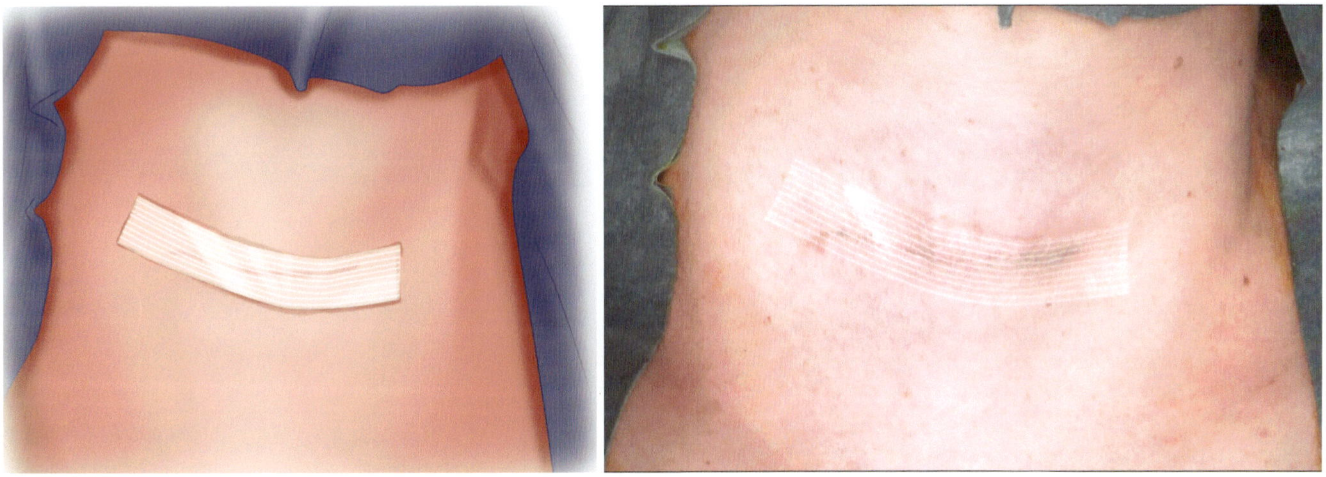

Fig. 10.24 A continuous 4-0 Monocryl suture is used to close the skin with a single Steri-Strip™ applied along the length of the wound

measured in the recovery suite and daily until discharge. Discharge typically occurs on the first post-operative day. An ice pack is applied to the wound intermittently for 48 h, and the members of the nursing staff are instructed to observe carefully for respiratory distress and evidence of neck hematoma. Patients commence neck exercises post-operatively and continue until their clinic follow-up. The final pathology in this case revealed right-sided 25-mm PTC and left-sided multifocal PTC, all clear of margins, with 4/4 involved lymph nodes. The patient was discussed at a multidisciplinary meeting and has undergone radioactive iodine treatment.

References

1. Haugen BR, et al. 2015 American Thyroid Association Management Guidelines for adult patients with thyroid nodules and differentiated thyroid cancer: the American Thyroid Association Guidelines Task Force on Thyroid Nodules and Differentiated Thyroid Cancer. Thyroid. 2016;26(1):1–133.
2. O'Neill CJ, et al. Sutureless thyroidectomy: surgical technique. ANZ J Surg. 2011;81(7–8):515–8.
3. Cirocchi R, et al. Intraoperative neuromonitoring versus visual nerve identification for prevention of recurrent laryngeal nerve injury in adults undergoing thyroid surgery. Cochrane Database Syst Rev. 2019;1:CD012483.
4. Thompson AM, et al. A preoperative nomogram for the prediction of ipsilateral central compartment lymph node metastases in papillary thyroid cancer. Thyroid. 2014;24(4):675–82.
5. Clark OH, Duh QY, Kebebew E, editors. Textbook of endocrine surgery. New Delhi, India: JP Medical Ltd; 2016.
6. Grodski S, et al. Routine level VI lymph node dissection for papillary thyroid cancer: surgical technique. ANZ J Surg. 2007;77(4):203–8.
7. So YK, et al. Subclinical lymph node metastasis in papillary thyroid microcarcinoma: a study of 551 resections. Surgery. 2010;148(3):526–31.
8. Popadich A, et al. A multicenter cohort study of total thyroidectomy and routine central lymph node dissection for cN0 papillary thyroid cancer. Surgery. 2011;150(6):1048–57.
9. Kay-Rivest E, et al. Preoperative vocal cord paralysis and its association with malignant thyroid disease and other pathological features. J Otolaryngol Head Neck Surg. New Delhi, India, 2015;44:35.

Hemithyroidectomy with *en bloc* Ipsilateral Central Node Dissection for Low-Risk Papillary and Medullary Thyroid Cancer

11

Frank Weber, Andreas Machens, and Henning Dralle

Introduction

Advances in morphologic and molecular tumor characterization, tumor epidemiology, and clinical outcome research have allowed for a more balanced view on the risk-benefit profile of thyroid cancer surgery [1]. The concept of personalized thyroid surgery, prompted by the advent of less invasive surgical techniques, rises to the challenge posed by the current epidemic of low-risk thyroid cancers, shifting the focus to risk minimization.

A large body of evidence indicates that survival for low-risk papillary thyroid cancer is comparable irrespective of whether lobectomy or total thyroidectomy has been performed [2]. Current American Thyroid Association (ATA) management guidelines recommend lobectomy for unifocal, node-negative, intrathyroid papillary thyroid cancer up to a tumor size of 4 cm [3]. However, some risk factors, including vascular invasion or aggressive tumor histology, are hard to verify before, or by frozen section analysis during, the operation.

The reduction of surgical trauma must be weighed against the oncological adequacy of the operation. Absent definitive evidence about the benefit-risk balance of prophylactic lymph node dissection, the identification of lymph node metastasis is pivotal. Patients with low-risk papillary thyroid cancers referred to the authors are notified during the informed consent discussion about the option of lobectomy with *en bloc* ipsilateral central lymph node dissection. Increasingly, more medullary thyroid cancers are also diagnosed early [4, 5]. Current evidence suggests that desmoplasia-negative medullary thyroid cancer has not spread to lymph nodes [6], opening a window of opportunity for pursuing a unilateral resection strategy. This personalized concept relies on intraoperative frozen section analysis. Based on the frozen section, a risk-based approach by hemithyroidectomy with *en bloc* ipsilateral central lymph node dissection for intrathyroid, desmoplasia-negative sporadic medullary thyroid cancer is favored. Conceptually, this surgical approach may also be useful in patients harboring low-risk papillary thyroid cancer, sparing these patients an increased risk of morbidity after total thyroidectomy with postoperative radioiodine treatment.

Procedure

A 52-year-old patient with a right-sided thyroid nodule was referred with a diagnosis of medullary thyroid cancer prompted by a calcitonin level of 515 pg/ml (<8.4 pg/mL). High-resolution neck ultrasonography showed an 11-mm large nodule within the right thyroid lobe without enlarged lymph nodes. The patient was provided with the option of hemithyroidectomy with ipsilateral central lymph node dissection, which he consented to, subject to the absence of desmoplasia and lymph node metastases on intraoperative frozen section analysis.

For a level operative field and optimal visual magnification, the patient is placed in a supine position. The neck is extended with a shoulder roll tucked underneath, moving the larynx and brachiocephalic vessels upward (Fig. 11.1).

Surgery is performed under general anesthesia and, by using magnifying glasses (x2.5), bipolar coagulation and continuous nerve monitoring. Short-acting muscle relaxants are used for intubation only but avoided for the rest of the operation to preclude interference with intraoperative nerve monitoring.

F. Weber (✉) · H. Dralle
Department of General, Visceral and Transplantation Surgery, Section of Endocrine Surgery, University of Duisburg-Essen, Essen, Germany
e-mail: Frank.Weber@uk-essen.de

A. Machens
Department of Visceral, Vascular and Endocrine Surgery, Martin Luther University Halle-Wittenberg, Halle (Saale), Germany

A. Shifrin (ed.), *Atlas of Thyroid Surgery*, https://doi.org/10.1007/978-3-030-93673-0_11

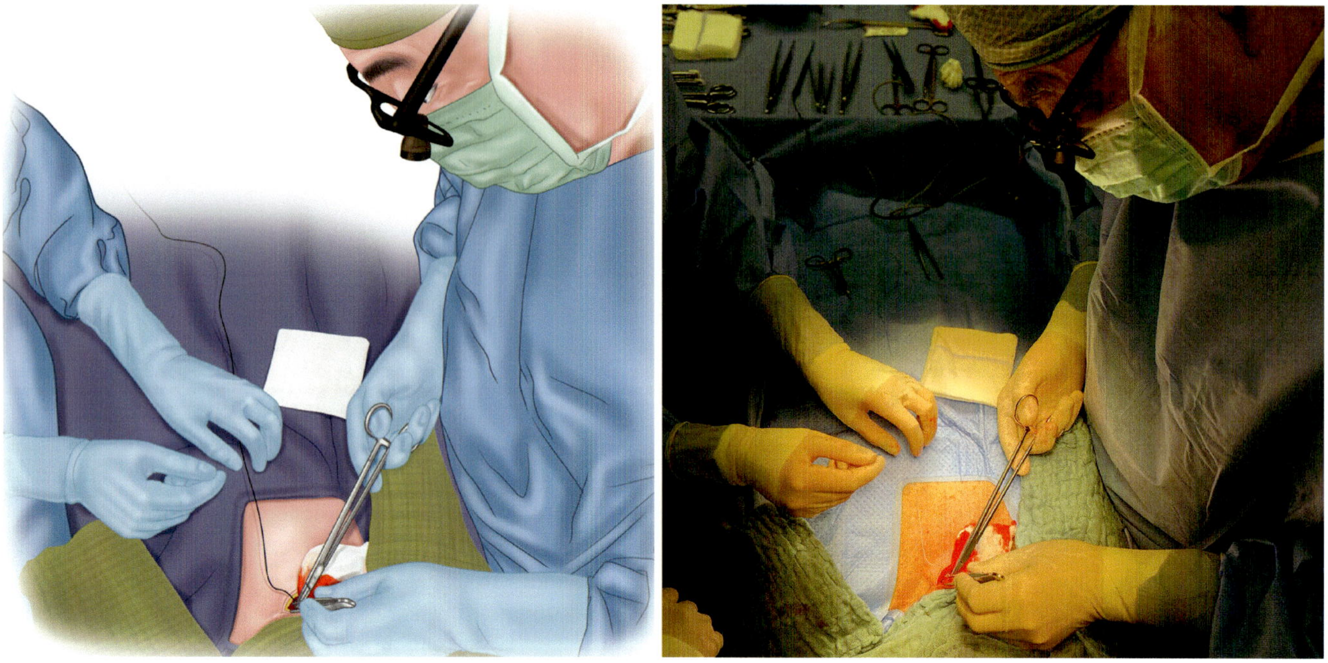

Fig. 11.1 For a level operative field and optimal visual magnification, the patient is placed in a supine position. The neck is extended with a shoulder roll tucked underneath, moving the larynx and brachiocephalic vessels upward

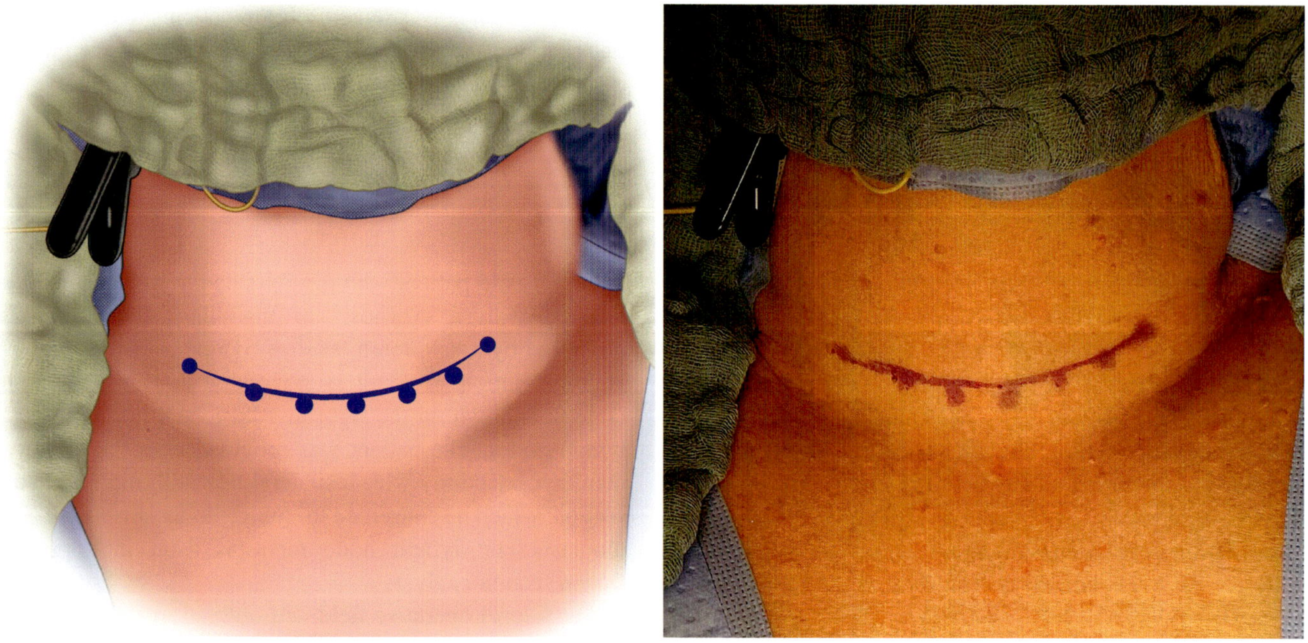

Fig. 11.2 The line of incision is outlined three-quarters of an inch above the sternal notch, in or parallel to normal skin creases

The line of incision is outlined three-quarters of an inch above the sternal notch, in or parallel to normal skin creases (Fig. 11.2). This Kocher collar incision can be extended laterally within the same horizontal line to accommodate lateral lymph node dissection, which may be required when lymph node metastases are identified on intraoperative frozen section analysis.

Superior and inferior platysma flaps are raised, preserving the anterior jugular veins if possible (Fig. 11.3). The superior platysma flap is held in place by Ethibond 2-0 support sutures extending over the anesthesia screen and tensioned in adults by two 500-cc infusion bottles. The inferior platysma flap is secured by a small vessel retractor, which is fixed with draping tape.

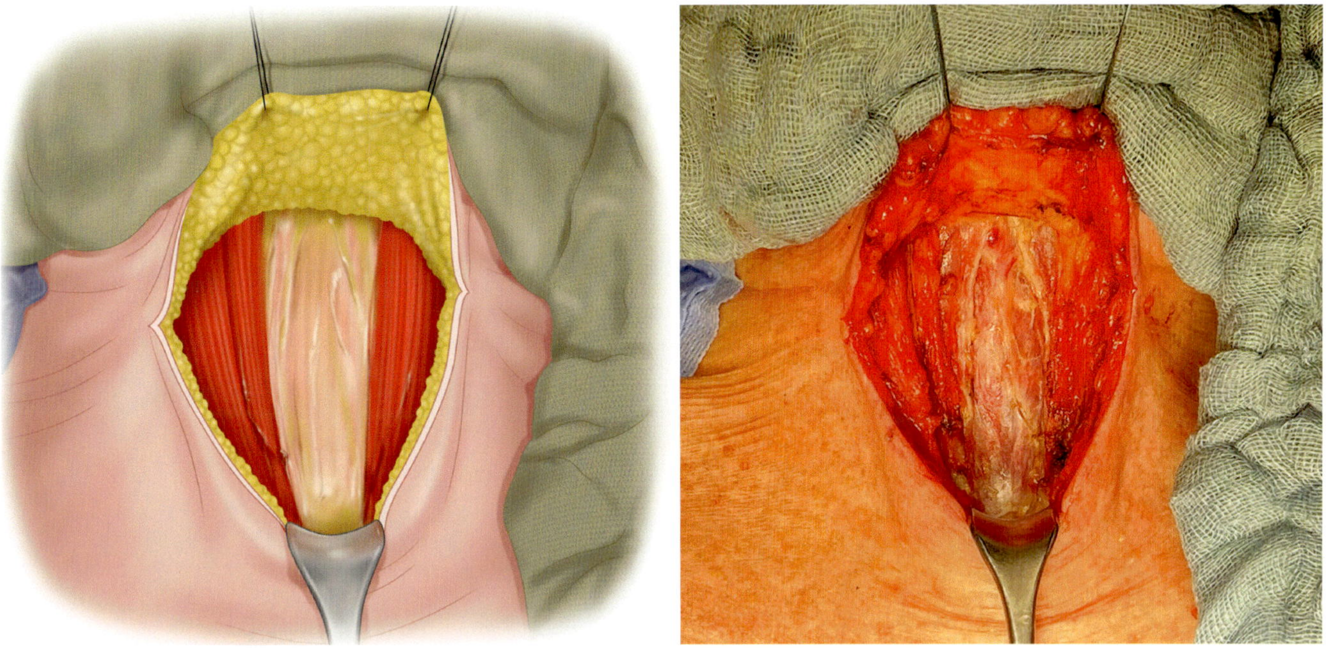

Fig. 11.3 Superior and inferior platysma flaps are raised. The superior platysma flap is held in place by tensioned Ethibond 2-0 support sutures, whereas the inferior platysma is secured with a small vessel retractor

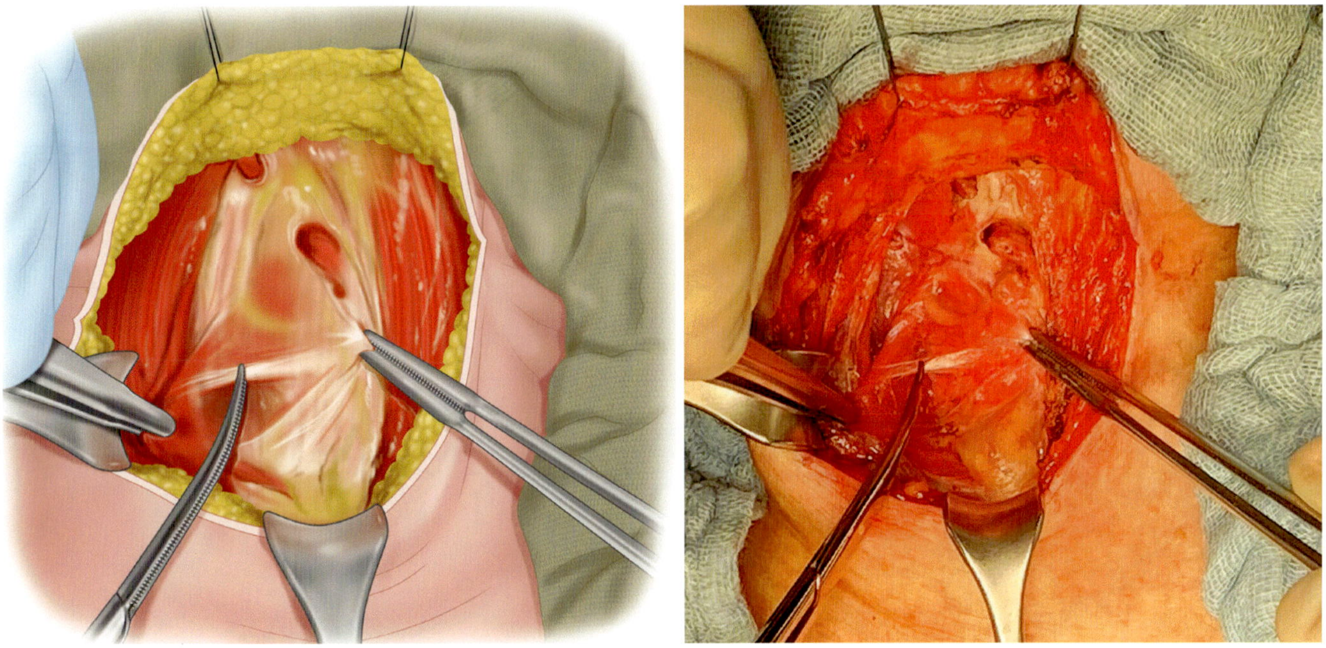

Fig. 11.4 The strap muscles are separated at the linea alba colli to access the loose connective tissue that fills the space between the undersurface of the right strap muscles and the right thyroid lobe

The strap muscles are separated at the linea alba colli to access the loose connective tissue that fills the space between the undersurface of the right strap muscle and the right thyroid lobe (Fig. 11.4).

The dissection is carried forward toward the right vascular sheath, and the middle thyroid vein, also referred to as Kocher's vein, is identified and ligated (Fig. 11.5).

The thyroid lobe is displaced medially using a large vein retractor. The path of the vagus nerve, running between the carotid artery and internal jugular vein, is identified and confirmed electrophysiologically using a handheld stimulating probe (Fig. 11.6).

Using meticulous dissection, the vagus nerve is dissected circumferentially over a distance of 1 cm. A 2-mm

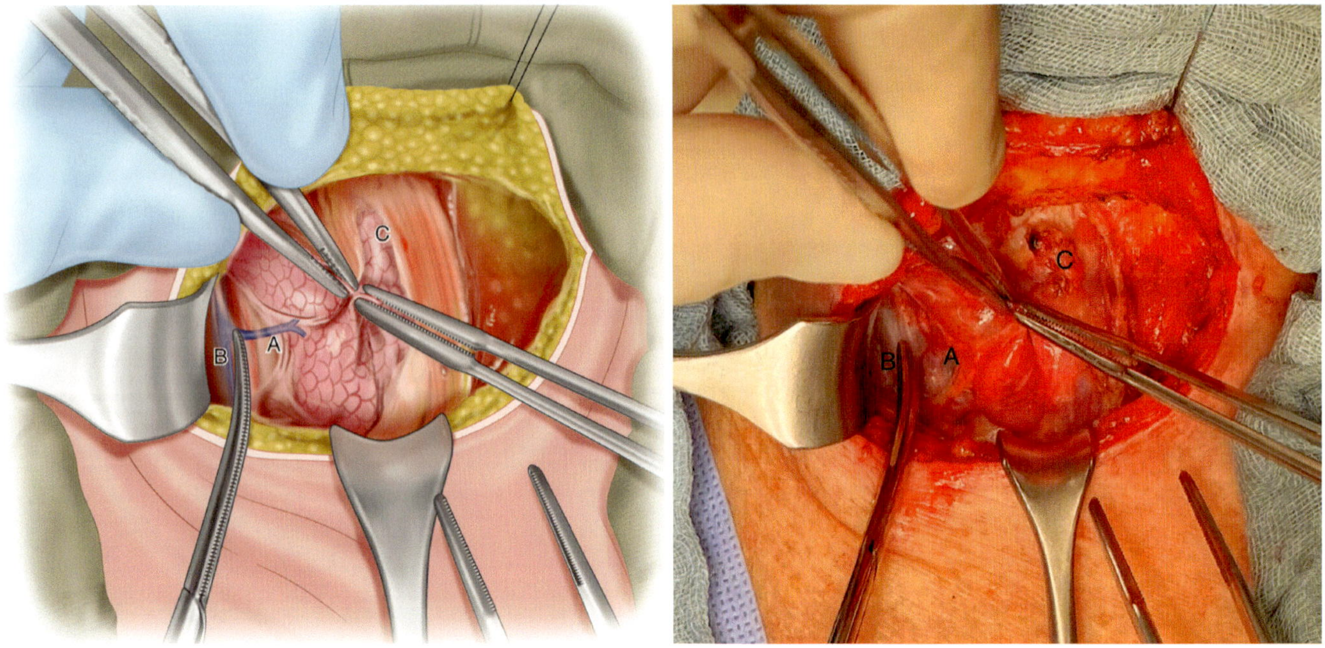

Fig. 11.5 The dissection is carried forward toward the right vascular sheath. Kocher's vein is identified and ligated. (**a**) Kocher's vein. (**b**) Internal jugular vein. (**c**) Pyramidal lobe

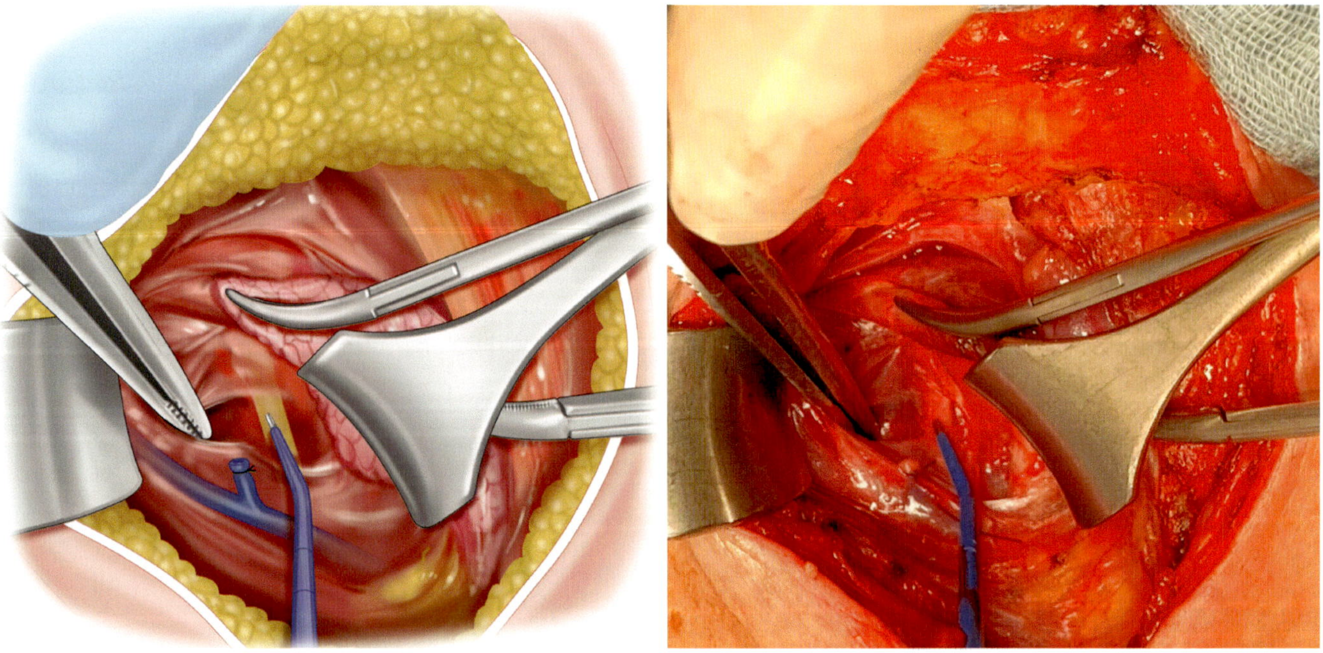

Fig. 11.6 With the right thyroid lobe displaced medially with a vein retractor, the route of the vagus nerve between the carotid artery and internal jugular vein is identified and mapped electrophysiologically using a handheld stimulating probe (blue)

clip electrode is fastened on the dissected vagus nerve segment for continuous nerve stimulation (Fig. 11.7a). For male patients, a 3-mm clip electrode may be better suited. Placement of the clip electrode is easier when nerve retractors or small Overholt clamps are used to expose the dissected nerve segment (Fig. 11.7b and Fig. 11.7c). Feeding microvasculature and the thin sheath of the vagus nerve are carefully preserved during dissection and electrode placement.

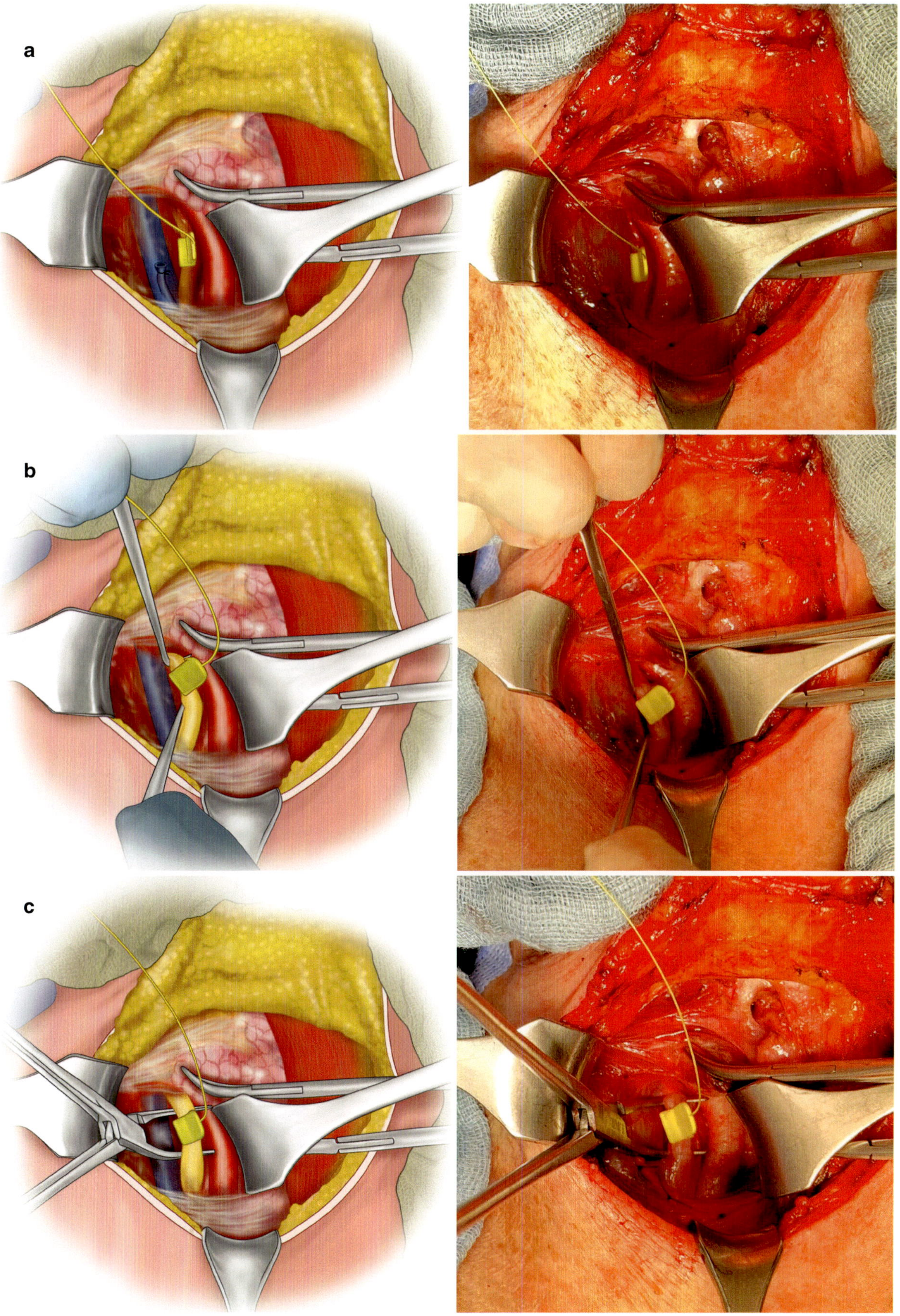

Fig. 11.7 (**a**) After circumferential meticulous circumferential dissection over a distance of 1 cm, preserving vagus sheath and feeding microvasculature, a clip electrode is fastened on the vagus nerve for continuous intraoperative nerve stimulation. Placement of the clip electrode is accomplished by nerve retractors (**b**) or a small Overholt clamp (**c**)

The right thyroid lobe is displaced medially. The recurrent laryngeal nerve is traced electrophysiologically along its course using a handheld stimulatory probe (Fig. 11.8).

Hemithyroidectomy with *en bloc* dissection of the ipsilateral central neck compartment (level 6, dotted area) starts with the lower central lymph nodes, progressing in a caudal-to-cranial direction (Fig. 11.9).

The lower parathyroid gland is identified, and the line of dissection is adapted to maintain adequate perfusion (Fig. 11.10). If preservation *in situ* is unfeasible, the completely

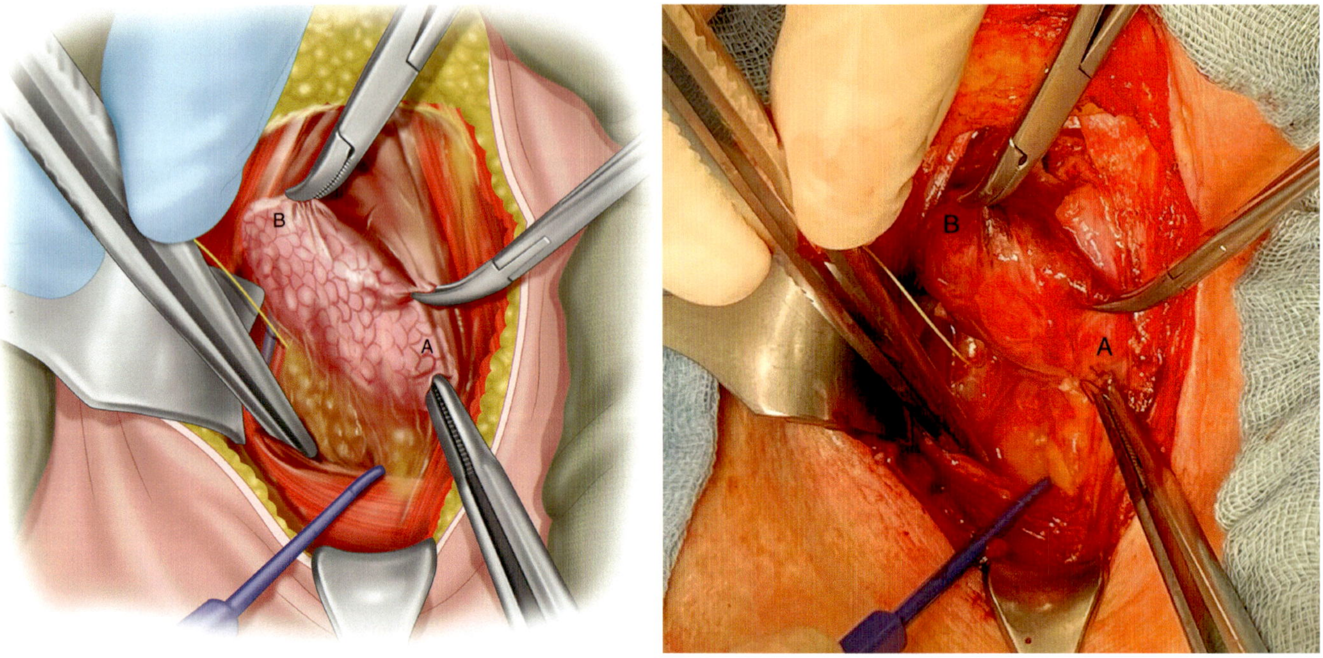

Fig. 11.8 After medial displacement of the right thyroid lobe, the right recurrent laryngeal nerve is electrophysiologically traced along its course using a handheld stimulatory probe (blue). (**a**) Lower thyroid pole. (**b**) Upper thyroid pole

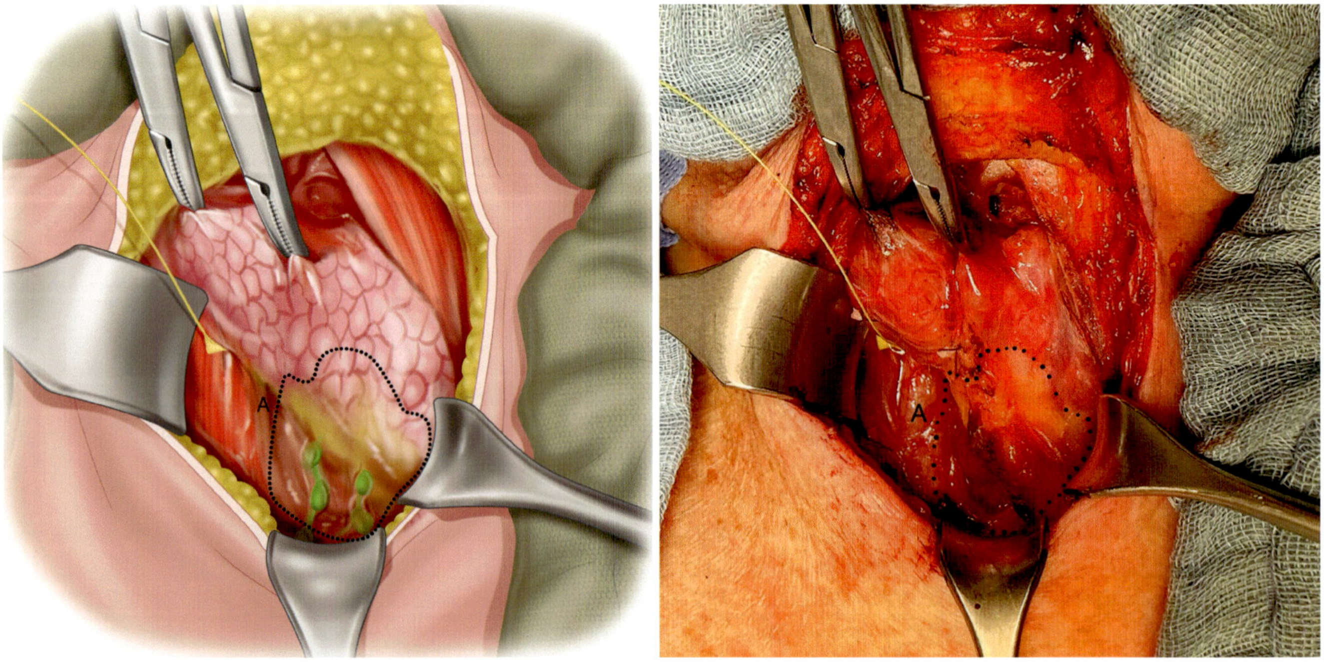

Fig. 11.9 Hemithyroidectomy with *en bloc* dissection of the ipsilateral central neck compartment (level 6, dotted area) starts with the lower central lymph nodes, progressing in a caudal-to-cranial direction. (**a**) Carotid artery

devascularized parathyroid gland is minced and autografted in small slivers into the right sternocleidomastoid muscle.

The central lymph node dissection proceeds from the level of the brachiocephalic vessels cephalad along the trachea (Fig. 11.11). Resection of the thyrothymic ligament generally is unnecessary.

The right thyroid lobe, taking the isthmus, pyramidal lobe, and Delphian lymph node with it, is eventually severed from the left thyroid lobe (Fig. 11.12).

The window presented by the right sternothyroid-laryngeal triangle is delineated to expose the upper pol vessels and the external branch of the superior laryngeal

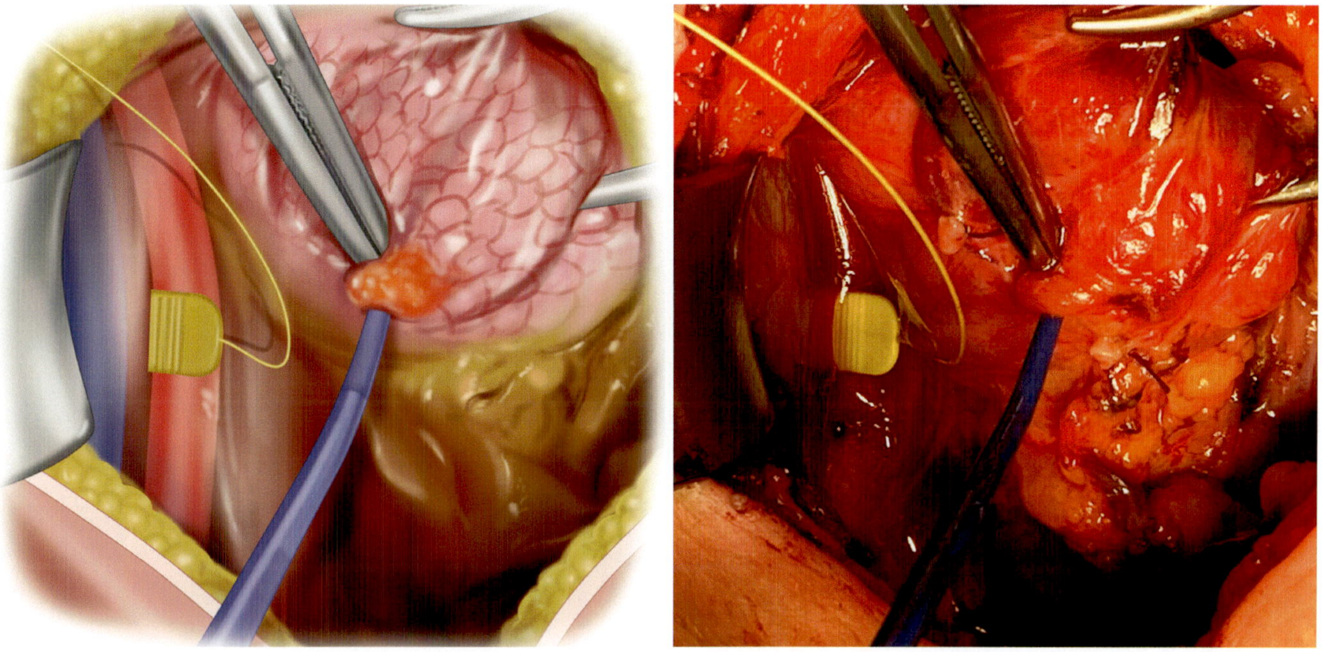

Fig. 11.10 Identification of the right lower parathyroid gland, the perfusion of which is checked for adequacy

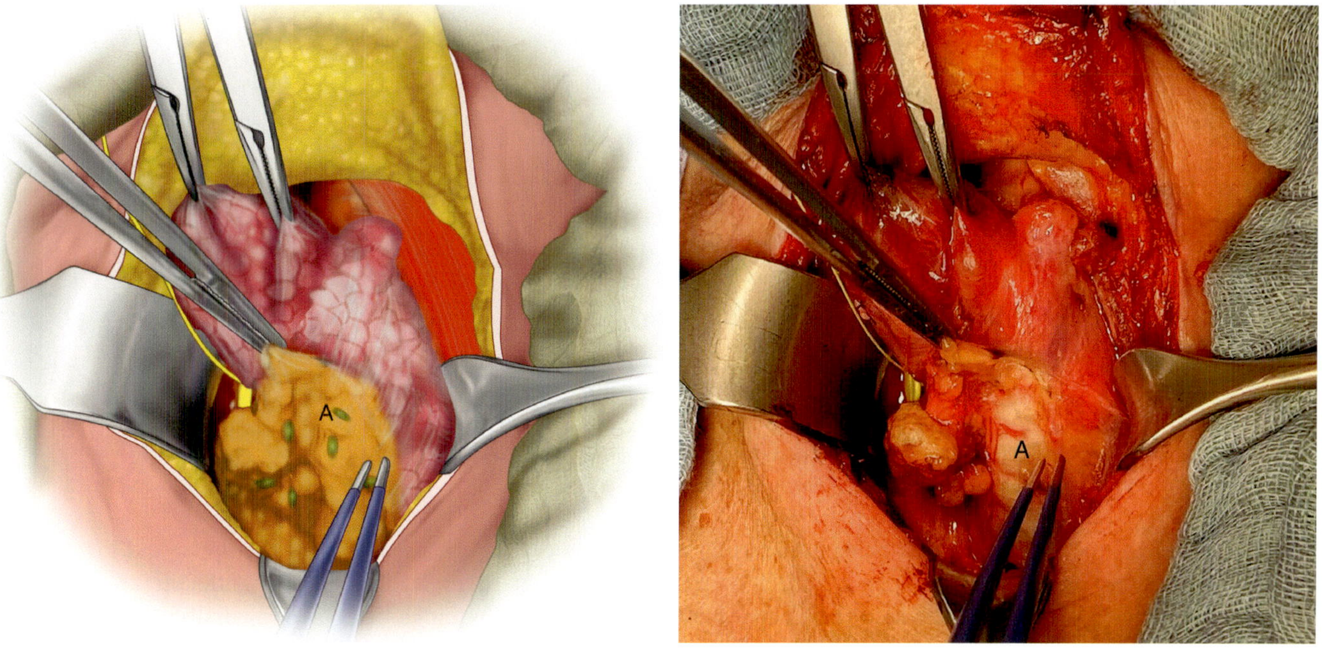

Fig. 11.11 The right central lymph node dissection proceeds from the level of the brachiocephalic vessels cephalad along the trachea (A)

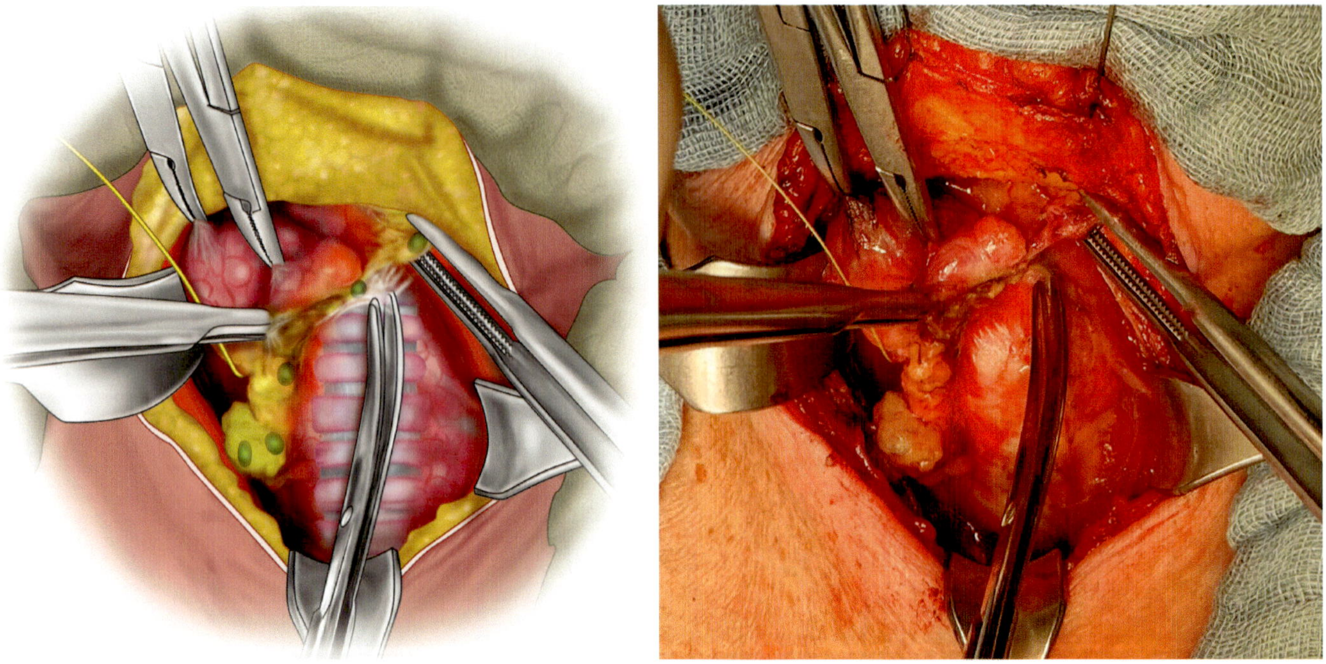

Fig. 11.12 The right thyroid lobe, taking the isthmus, pyramidal lobe, and Delphian lymph node with it, is severed from the undissected left thyroid lobe

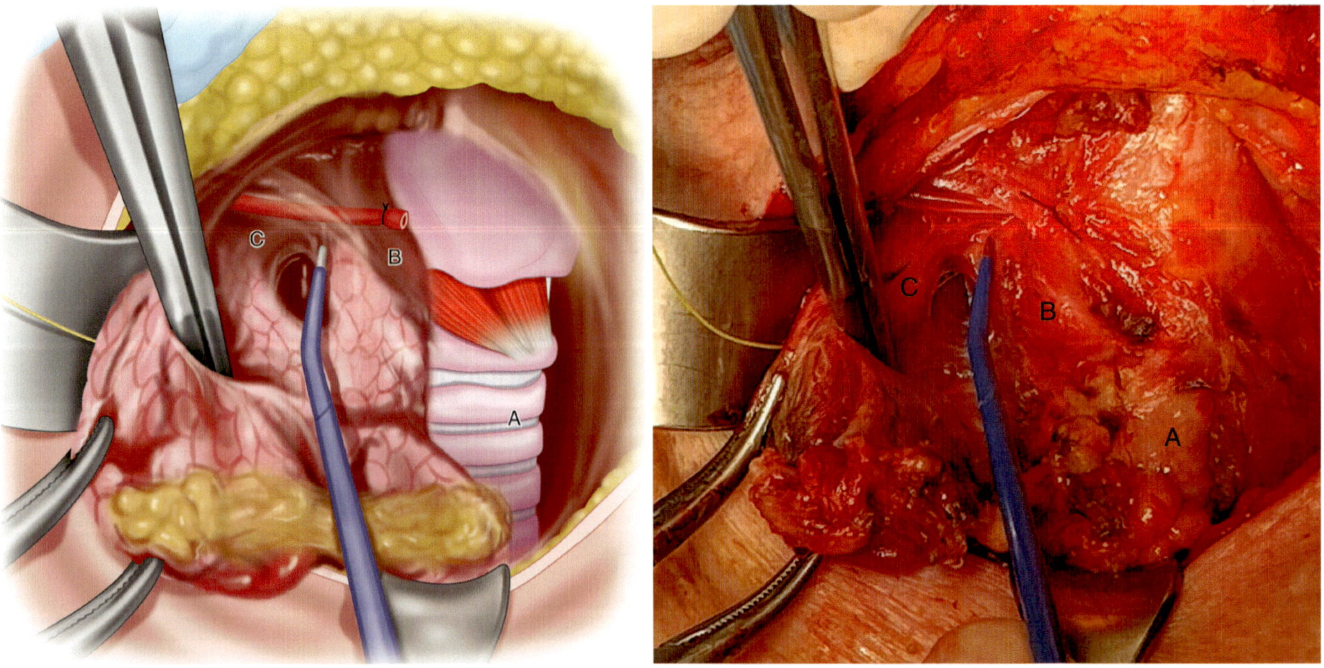

Fig. 11.13 The window of the right sternothyroid-laryngeal triangle is delineated to expose the upper pole vessels and the external branch of the superior laryngeal nerve, the course of which is mapped with a handheld stimulating probe (blue). (**a**) Trachea. (**b**) Cricothyroid muscle (**c**) Upper thyroid pole

nerve. The route of the external branch is identified using a handheld stimulating probe (Fig. 11.13).

The upper pole vessels are divided between small Overholt clamps and ligated near the thyroid capsule one after the other (Fig. 11.14).

Pean clamps are used to grasp the upper and lower parts of the right thyroid lobe. Using gentle, nerve-monitored traction, the thyroid lobe rotates medially. Particular care should be exercised to ensure that the tension exerted by the

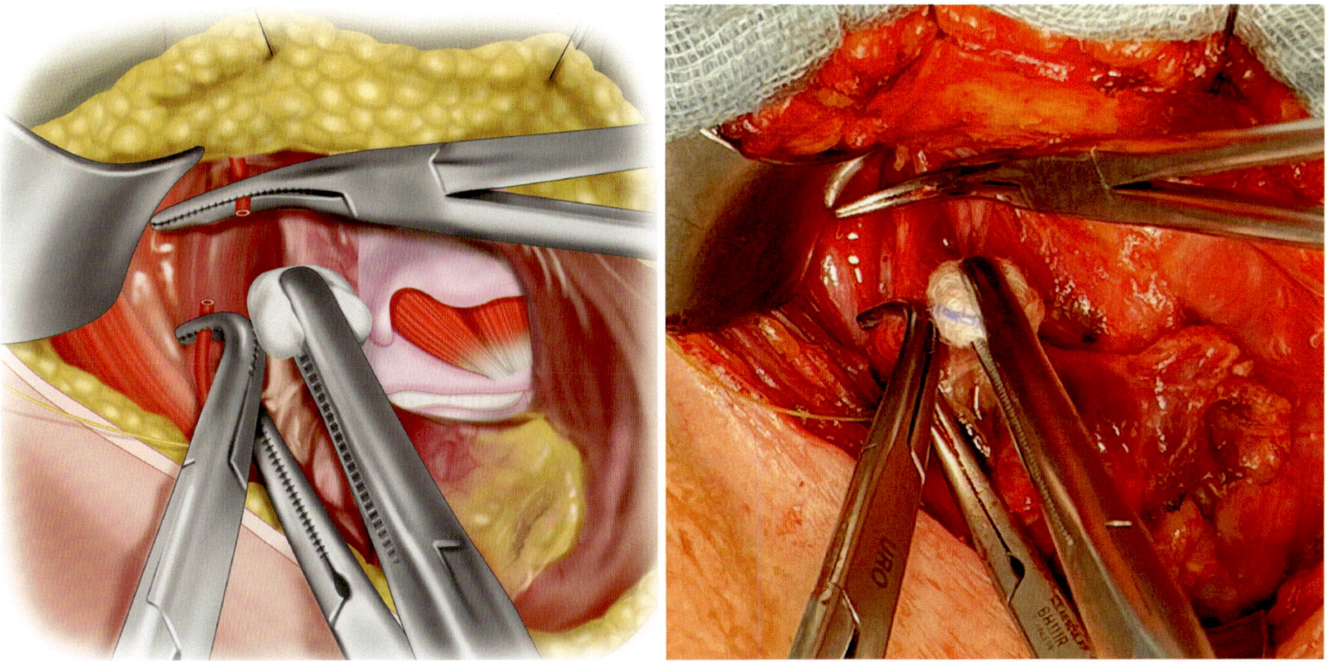

Fig. 11.14 The upper pole vessels are divided between small Overholt clamps and ligated near the thyroid capsule one after the other

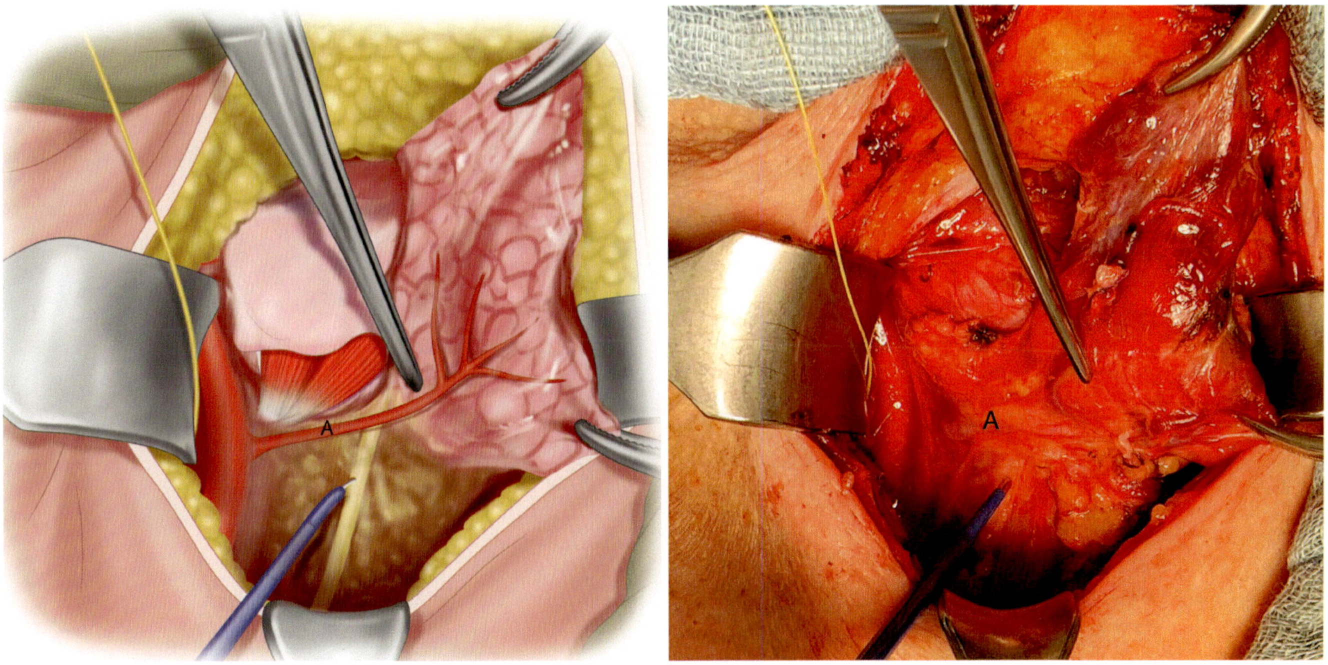

Fig. 11.15 Surgeon's view of the operative field with the thyroid gland displaced medially. The right lower parathyroid gland (forceps) is identified. The right recurrent laryngeal nerve, coursing underneath the inferior thyroid artery (A), has been electrophysiologically traced using a handheld stimulating probe (blue)

Pean clamps is strictly vertical, just enough to expose the operative field (Fig. 11.15).

The anatomic path of the recurrent laryngeal nerve, including extralaryngeal branching, is identified (Fig. 11.16). This is even more imperative when the thyroid gland is mobilized closer at the ligament of Berry (Fig. 11.17). The terminal branches of the lower thyroid artery are cut and ligated close to the thyroid capsule. Retronerval lymph node dissection should be undertaken only when the tumor has spread to level 6 lymph nodes.

Advancing cephalad, the right upper parathyroid gland and its feeding vessels are identified (Fig. 11.18). The line of

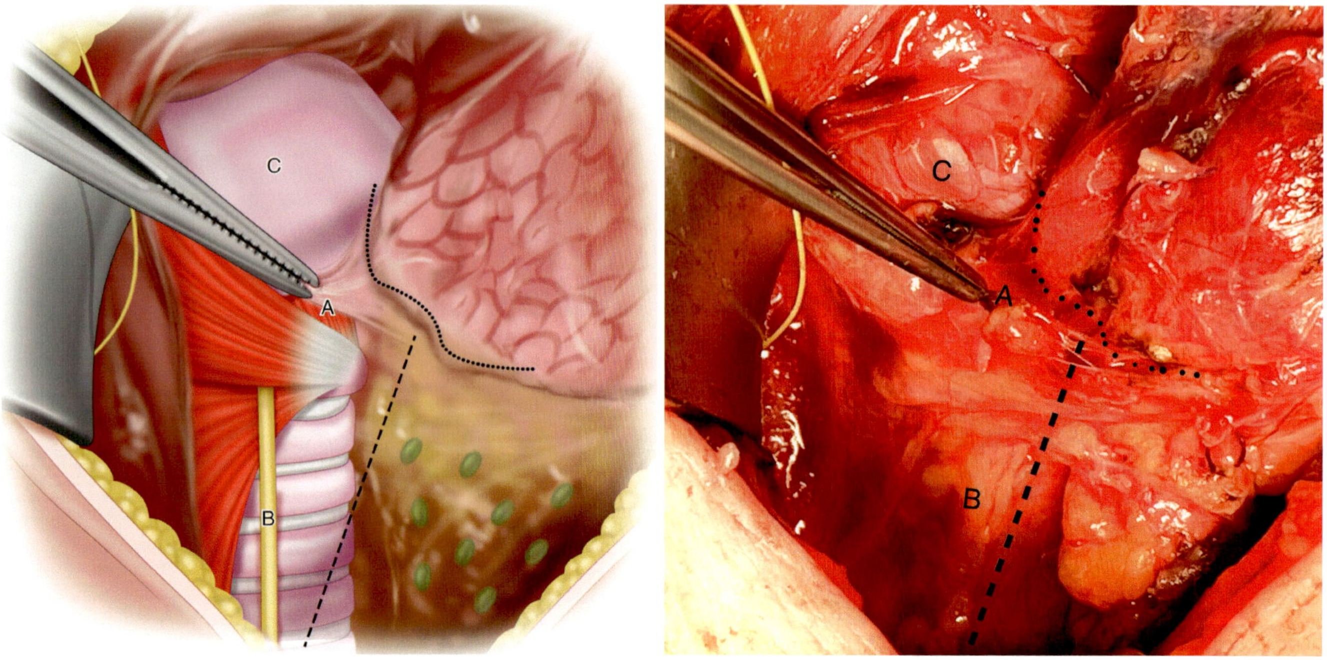

Fig. 11.16 Upward retraction of the right thyroid lobe and ipsilateral central lymph nodes, exposing the ligament of Berry (dotted line). The line of dissection is kept anterior to the plane of the recurrent laryngeal nerve and parathyroid glands (broken line). (**a**) Lower parathyroid gland. (**b**) The recurrent laryngeal nerve. (**c**) Cricothyroid muscle

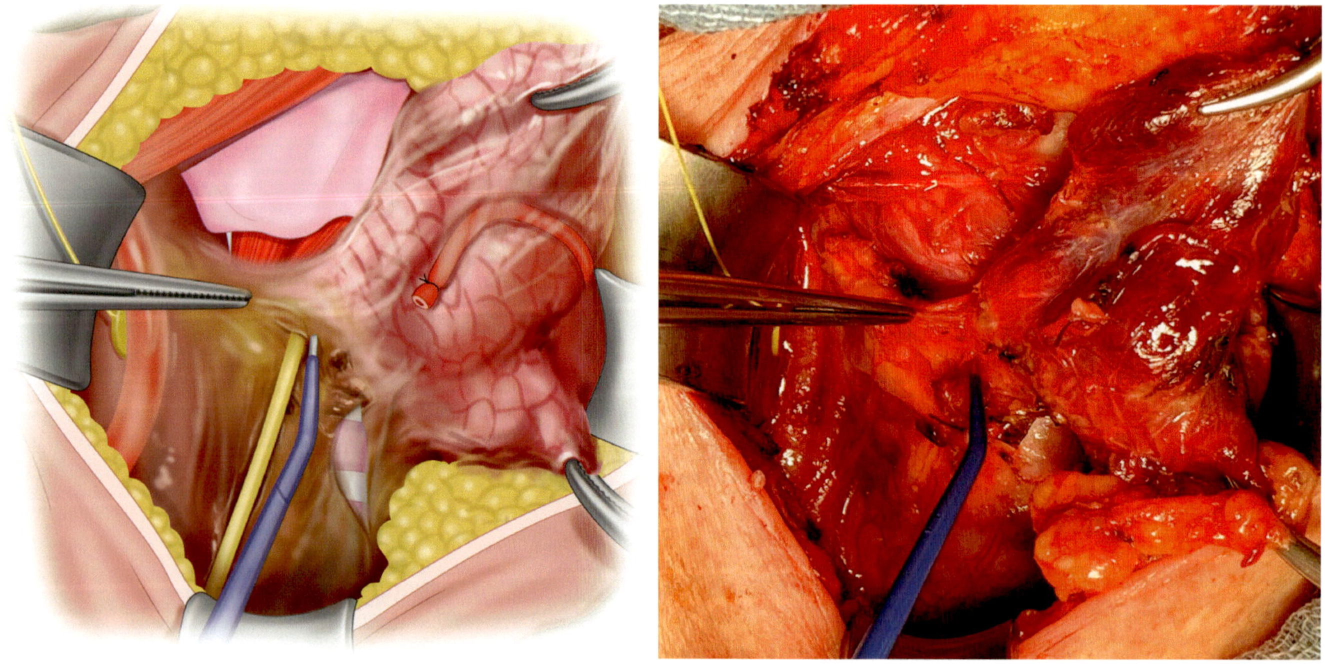

Fig. 11.17 Dissection of the right thyroid lobe off the ligament of Berry. The line of dissection must be kept near the thyroid capsule to preserve perfusion of the upper parathyroid gland and spare the superior laryngeal nerve

dissection is kept close to the thyroid capsule to preserve the blood supply of the upper thyroid pole and to spare the superior laryngeal nerve (Fig 11.19).

Upon completion, one contiguous surgical specimen is sent for frozen section analysis, which comprises the right thyroid lobe (marked with a 4-0 suture at its upper pole for orientation) and ipsilateral central lymph nodes (Fig. 11.20). When the tumor is confined to the thyroid and desmoplasia-negative, as in this patient, the contralateral lobe can be spared, so that the operation is ended.

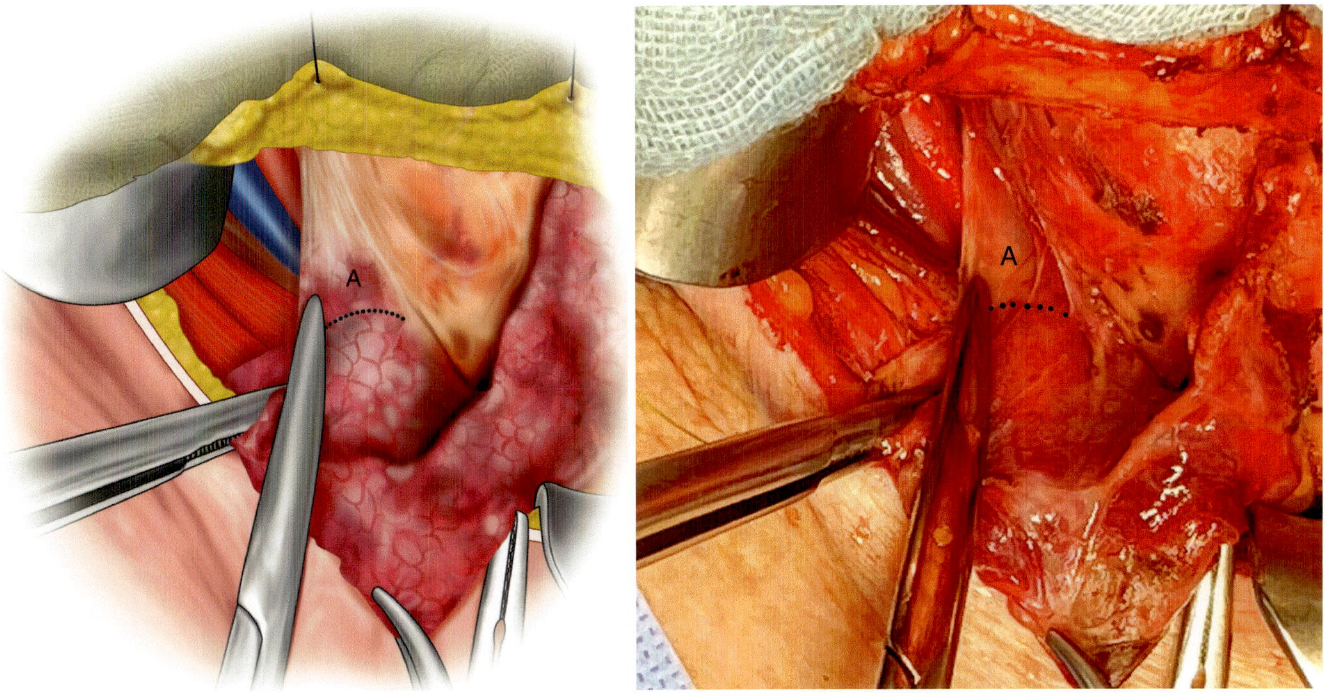

Fig. 11.18 Medial view of the upper parathyroid gland with intended line of dissection (dotted line). (**a**) Parathyroid gland

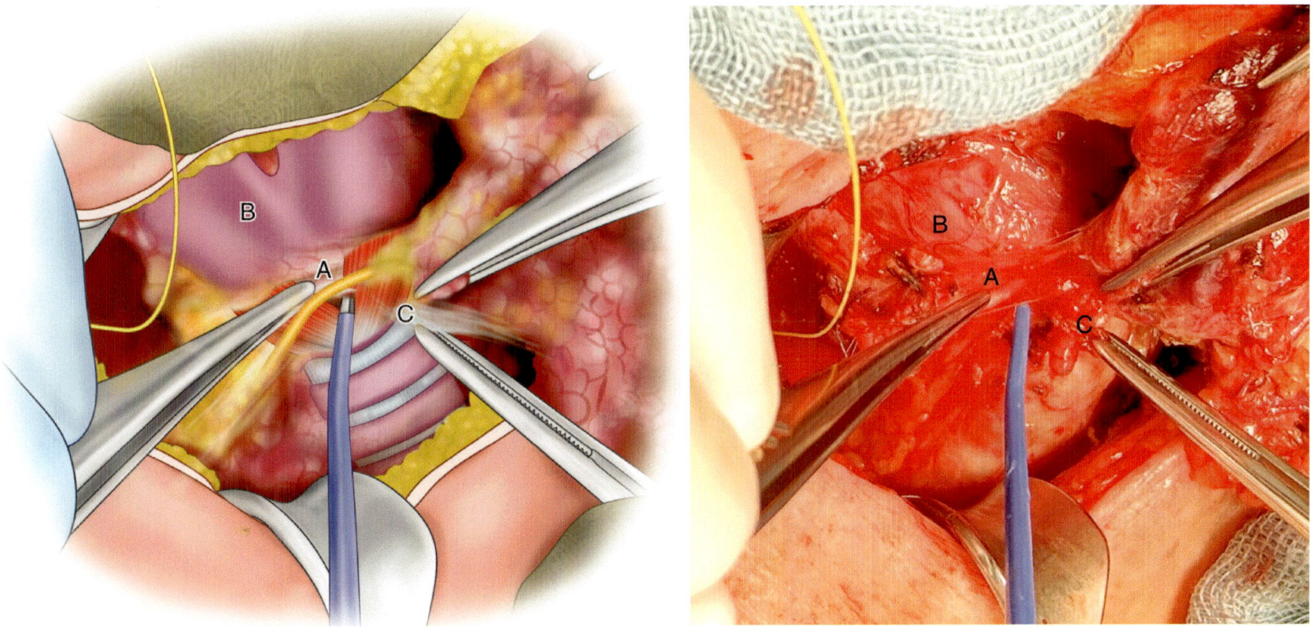

Fig. 11.19 High laryngeal entry of the right recurrent laryngeal nerve, necessitating meticulous dissection of nearby thyroid and lymphatic tissue. (**a**) The recurrent laryngeal nerve. (**b**) Cricothyroid muscle. (**c**) Lymphatic tissue

Before closing the skin, a wound drain may be placed, which typically is removed on the second postoperative day (Fig. 11.21). The sternohyoid and sternothyroid (strap) muscles (Fig. 11.22) and subcutaneous tissues (Fig. 11.23) are approximated using absorbable 4-0 braided interrupted sutures. Finally, the skin is closed using titan clips, which are also removed on the second postoperative day.

Definitive histopathology confirmed the intraoperative frozen section analysis, revealing a 10-mm large, desmoplasia-negative, and node-negative (0/6) medullary thyroid cancer confined to the right thyroid lobe. The patient made an uneventful recovery, and reached a biochemical cure on the second postoperative day, when his serum calcitonin had fallen to 5.1 pg/ml (<8.4 pg/mL).

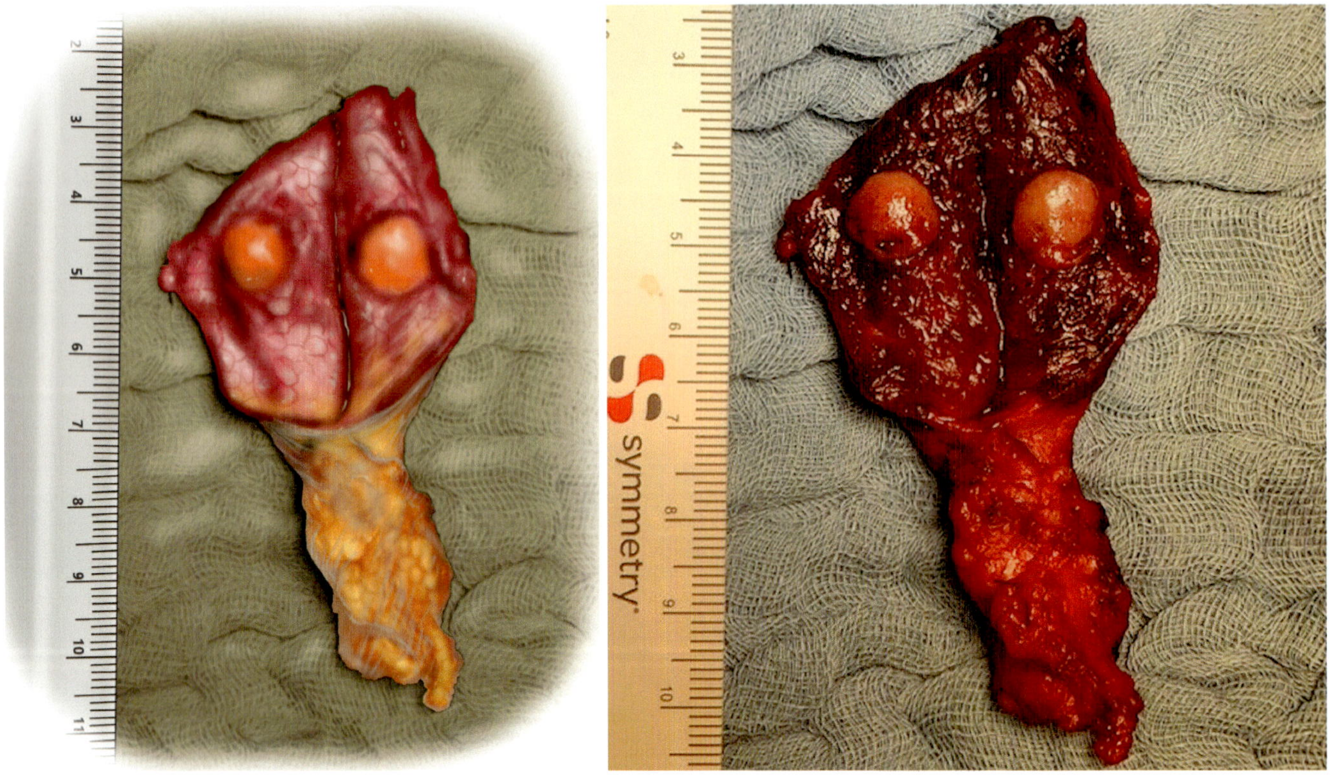

Fig. 11.20 The removed surgical specimen, encompassing the right thyroid lobe and right central lymph nodes, before being sent for frozen section analysis

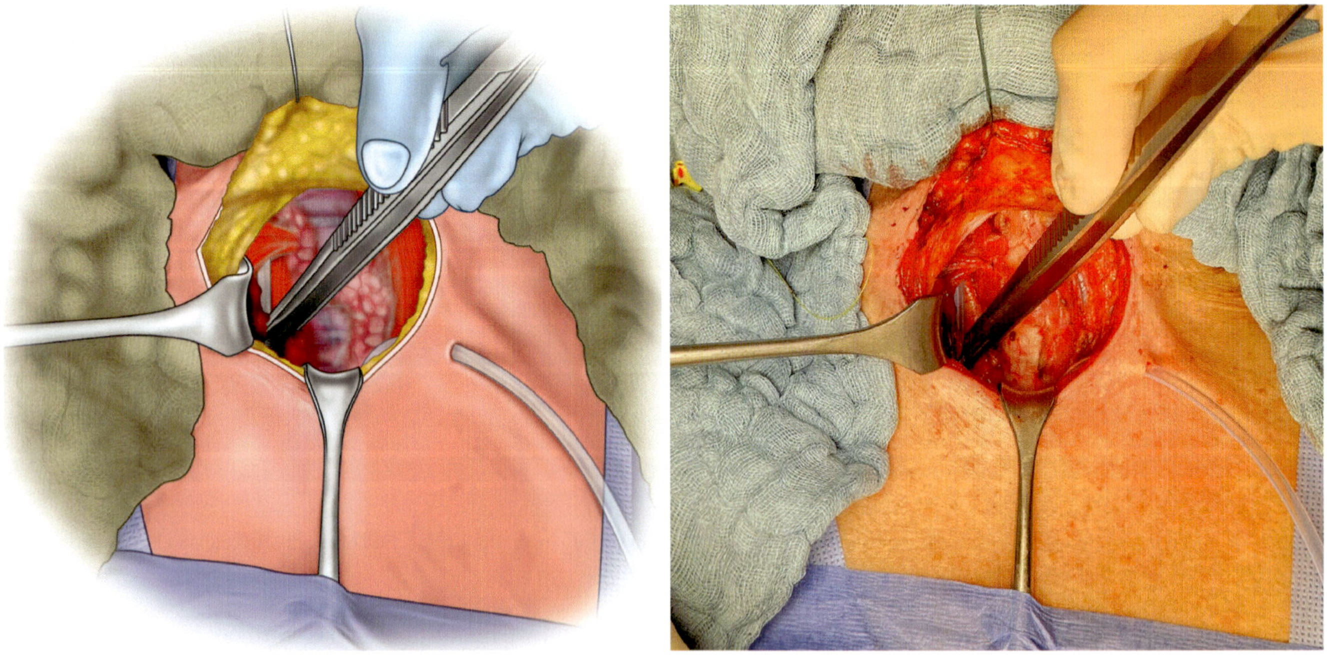

Fig. 11.21 Placement of a Blake drain before wound closure

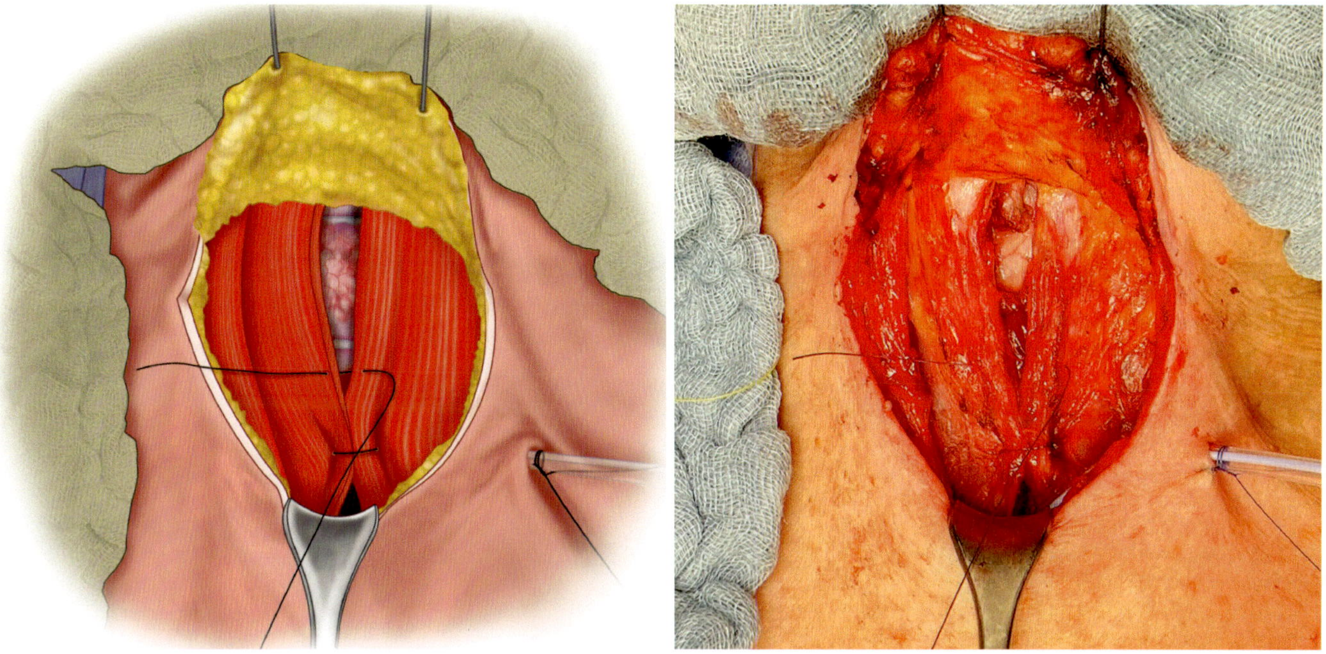

Fig. 11.22 Approximation of the strap muscles using absorbable 4-0 braided interrupted sutures

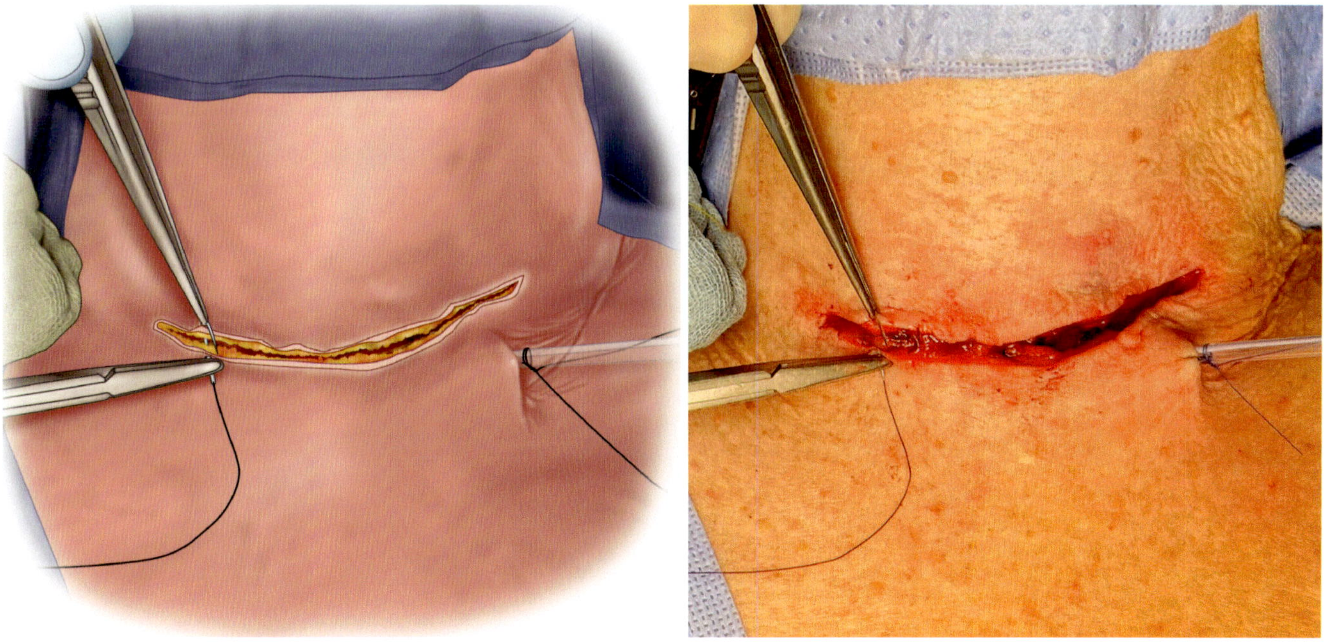

Fig. 11.23 Subcutaneous wound closure using absorbable 4-0 braided interrupted sutures

References

1. Welch HG, Doherty GM. Saving thyroids – overtreatment of small papillary cancers. N Engl J Med. 2018;379:310–2.
2. Hartl DM, Hadoux J, Guerlain J, Breuskin I, Haroun F, et al. Risk-oriented concept of treatment for intrathyroid papillary thyroid cancer. Best Pract Res Clin Endocrinol Metab. 2019;33(4):101281.
3. Haugen BR, Alexander EK, Bible KC, Doherty GM, Mandel SJ, Nikiforov YE, et al. American Thyroid Association management guidelines for adult patients with thyroid nodules and differentiated thyroid cancer. Thyroid. 2016;26(1):1–133.
4. Lorenz K, Machens A, Dralle H. Extent of resection in intrathyroidal medullary thyroid cancer. Chirurg. 2020;91:1017–24.
5. Machens A, Lorenz K, Dralle H. Prediction of biochemical cure in patients with medullary thyroid cancer. Br J Surg. 2020;107:695–704.
6. Koperek O, Scheuba C, Cherenko M, Neuhold N, De Micco C, Schmid KW, et al. Desmoplasia in medullary thyroid carcinoma: a reliable indicator of metastatic potential. Histopathology. 2008;52:623–30.

Video-Assisted Thyroidectomy

12

Marco Raffaelli, Carmela De Crea, Francesco Pennestrì, Celestino Pio Lombardi, and Rocco Bellantone

Introduction

Historically, surgical access for neck endocrine diseases has been performed using a traditional Kocher access, implying a wide skin incision, which results in a visible large scar in the neck [1]. During the last two decades, the introduction of minimally invasive surgery interested all the fields of general surgery, and endocrine surgery was not an exception [2]. Indeed, after the description of the first successful case of endoscopic parathyroidectomy by Gagner [3] in 1996, several minimally invasive approaches for thyroidectomy and parathyroidectomy were developed [1, 4–11]. The different approaches described for thyroidectomy include the endoscopic technique [1, 5, 6, 9, 10], video-assisted procedure and mini-access, nonendoscopic operations [11], the last implying a smaller incision without the use of an endoscope and thus without the advantages of endoscopic magnification for adequate visualization of neck structures. The approach with the endoscope can be classified respectively in purely endoscopic [3, 5, 9, 12] and video-assisted procedures [6, 7, 13], depending on the need or not of CO_2 insufflation. The totally endoscopic techniques include procedures with cervical access [1, 9] and procedures with extracervical access [5, 12], which require the use of external devices (retractors) in order to create and maintain the working space for dissection and trocar positioning [9].

Video-assisted thyroidectomy (VAT) is a central, completely gasless approach that reproduces all the steps of conventional surgery, with the endoscope becoming a tool that allows the surgeon to perform the same operation through a smaller skin incision [6]. The approach is similar to the procedure that Miccoli and coworkers initially described for parathyroidectomy and successfully adopted for thyroidectomy [7, 14].

Twenty years after its first description, VAT is now one of the most broadly diffused minimally invasive approaches to thyroidectomy [15–17].

The explanation of the success of VAT resides in its safety and reproducibility in different clinical settings. Moreover, the similarity of VAT to conventional thyroidectomy allows one to exploit the typical advantages of minimally invasive procedures in terms of cosmetic results and postoperative course, without relevant changes in surgical technique [18–21]. After its initial descriptions, VAT has been evolving [22]. Indeed, the procedure initially limited to selected benign thyroid pathologies has now become a notable procedure in the surgical armamentarium for the treatment of thyroid surgical diseases, within the boundaries of its selection criteria [17, 20].

Being video assisted, VAT is performed under both direct and endoscopic vision [6], gaining the advantages of magnified vision for most critical steps of the surgical procedure. Indeed, thanks to endoscope magnification, the recurrent laryngeal nerve (RLN) and parathyroid glands can be adequately identified and preserved [23, 24]. Moreover, the endoscope allows for easy visualization of the external branch of the superior laryngeal nerve (EBSLN) in most of the cases of VAT [25].

Early after the first experiences with minimally invasive thyroidectomy, several small single institution reports

M. Raffaelli (✉) · C. De Crea
Division of Endocrine and Metabolic Surgery, Fondazione Policlinico Universitario Agostino Gemelli IRCCS, Università Cattolica del Sacro Cuore, Rome, Italy
e-mail: Marco.Raffaelli@unicatt.it

F. Pennestrì
Division of Endocrine and Metabolic Surgery, Fondazione Policlinico Universitario Agostino Gemelli IRCCS, Rome, Italy

C. P. Lombardi
Division of Endocrine Surgery, Fondazione Policlinico Universitario Agostino Gemelli IRCCS, Università Cattolica del Sacro Cuore, Rome, Italy

R. Bellantone
Center of Endocrine and Obesity Surgery, Fondazione Policlinico Universitario Agostino Gemelli IRCCS, Università Cattolica del Sacro Cuore, Rome, Italy

A. Shifrin (ed.), *Atlas of Thyroid Surgery*, https://doi.org/10.1007/978-3-030-93673-0_12

[1, 4–6, 12, 13, 26], two multicenter studies [19, 27], and several large retrospective studies [16, 28–31] have been published confirming the reproducibility and safety of VAT. Specifically addressed advantages of VAT over conventional thyroidectomy are better cosmetic results and lower postoperative pain [32, 33]. These results have been further validated in two well-designed randomized controlled trials by Gal et al. [34] and El Labban [35], showing the superiority of VAT over conventional surgery in terms of cosmetic results and reduced postoperative distress.

Noteworthy to mention is that the additional advantage of VAT is the reduced incidence and severity of early voice and swallowing postthyroidectomy symptoms compared to conventional surgery [36].

Furthermore, a recent retrospective cost analysis shows that the cost of VAT appears to be equal to that of conventional thyroidectomy [37].

Finally, a recent meta-analysis demonstrated that VAT reduced immunosuppression, which can be considered proof of its minimally invasive nature [38].

Low invasiveness and similarity with the conventional procedure of VAT render this approach feasible and particularly suitable, in experienced hands, under locoregional anesthesia (cervical block) [39], showing the best results in patients with relative contraindications for general anesthesia.

In this chapter, we describe the surgical technique of minimally invasive video-assisted thyroidectomy, which has been routinely performed at our department since 1998 [6], addressing the specific indication of the technique.

Indications

An accurate patient selection plays a key role in successful VAT accomplishment. In the early experience of the technique, indications were quite limited (single nodule <3 cm in largest diameter, thyroid estimate volume ≤20 mL, small nodules with suspicious or indeterminate cytology, small pretoxic or toxic adenoma); contraindications at the beginning of the experience included thyroiditis and prior neck surgery [20]. With increasing experience, the selection criteria for VAT have been widened. Extended indications included thyroiditis patients who have undergone video-assisted thyroid lobectomy needing completion thyroidectomy and selected cases of Graves' disease, where VAT can be performed safely with results comparable with conventional surgery [40].

The extensive use of fine-needle aspiration biopsy in clinical practice has increased the diagnosis of small thyroid nodules with indeterminate or suspicious cytology. This group of patients probably represents the ideal candidates for VAT. Indeed, the initial concerns regarding the adequacy of the resection of VAT in the treatment of papillary thyroid carcinoma (PTC) were overcome by several studies demonstrating its safety in selected cases of PTC [41–43]. In 2005, we demonstrated that thyroid gland manipulation is not significantly different between VAT and conventional thyroidectomy, without additional risks of thyroid capsule rupture and thyroid cell seeding related to the surgical technique [21].

Moreover, the completeness of the resection achieved with VAT resulted in a similar way to that of conventional surgery in selected cases of PTC with a comparable rate of recurrence in the short-to-medium term follow-up [43, 44]. These results have been further confirmed in a recent series of patients who underwent VAT for PTC followed up for a time period longer than 10 years [17], in which a very low recurrence rate was observed, comparable to that of conventional surgery.

After acquiring adequate experience with the technique and supported by the previous optimal results in terms of safety and completeness of the surgical resection, we standardized a video-assisted lymph-node dissection of the central compartment [43, 45].

From a purely technical point of view, it should be considered that the endoscope shows specific advantages. Indeed, it allows a meticulous exploration of the central compartment and enables the identification of even slightly enlarged lymph nodes that might be overlooked at open surgery.

Video-assisted approach with central access allows to performing a formal central neck compartment dissection when needed, providing optimal results in terms of the completeness of the oncological resection and the number of removed nodes, with an overall outcome comparable to that of the open counterpart [43, 46, 47]. However, the preoperative evidence of central neck lymph node metastases still represents a contraindication for the video-assisted method [46, 47].

Patients carrying RET oncogene mutation for familial forms of medullary thyroid carcinoma but not even expressing the disease (absence of detectable nodules and basal/stimulated calcitonin in the normal range) are excellent candidates for VAT [48].

In summary, today, in our experience, the eligibility criteria for VAT include thyroid nodules ≤35 mm in diameter, estimated thyroid volume ≤30 ml, selected cases of PTC, RET gene mutation carriers, concomitant thyroiditis, and selected cases of Graves' disease [20].

Operative Technique

Patient and Surgical Team Positions

The patient is positioned supine on the operating table with the neck in slight extension and the arms tucked on each side. The less neck extension may contribute to the decreased postoperative pain observed in VAT with respect to conventional surgery. The skin is prepped from the lower lip to the nipples in a fashion similar to conventional thyroidectomy. However, the area of the surgical incision may also be covered by a transparent dressing (Tegaderm, for example) to protect the skin edges.

The surgical team is composed of the surgeon and two assistants, of which one handles the endoscope (Fig. 12.1). The monitor is placed in front of the surgeon, who is positioned on the right side of the patient. A second additional monitor is usually placed in front of the assistants, who are on the left side of the patient. The absence of any external support allows modulating the position of the endoscope in relation to the different steps of the dissection. This represents an important advantage of the video-assisted procedure over purely endoscopic techniques. The tip of the endoscope is usually oriented toward the patient's head, but it can be changed to explore the upper mediastinum when a concomitant central compartment lymphadenectomy is required.

Anesthesia

Thyroid surgery and VAT are usually performed under general anesthesia with endotracheal intubation. However, with the increasing experience, the feasibility of VAT under local anesthesia (LA-VAT) with a superficial cervical block (Fig. 12.2) has been demonstrated [39]. In our experience, besides the patients showing specific contraindications for general anesthesia, the indications to LA-VAT are mainly based on the patient's and surgeon's preference.

Surgical Instruments

Most of the surgical instruments necessary for VAT are usually available in operating theaters, and it is not a source of additional costs. The only instruments not used in conventional thyroidectomy are small, special spatulas and spatula-shaped aspirators (2–3 mm in diameter), which are useful in dissection. They come from ear, nose and throat and plastic surgery and are reusable (Fig. 12.3). Sealing systems (LigaSure Precise™, Harmonic Focus Plus®, Thunderbeat Open Fine Jaw (OFJ)®, Caiman®) have been proved to be

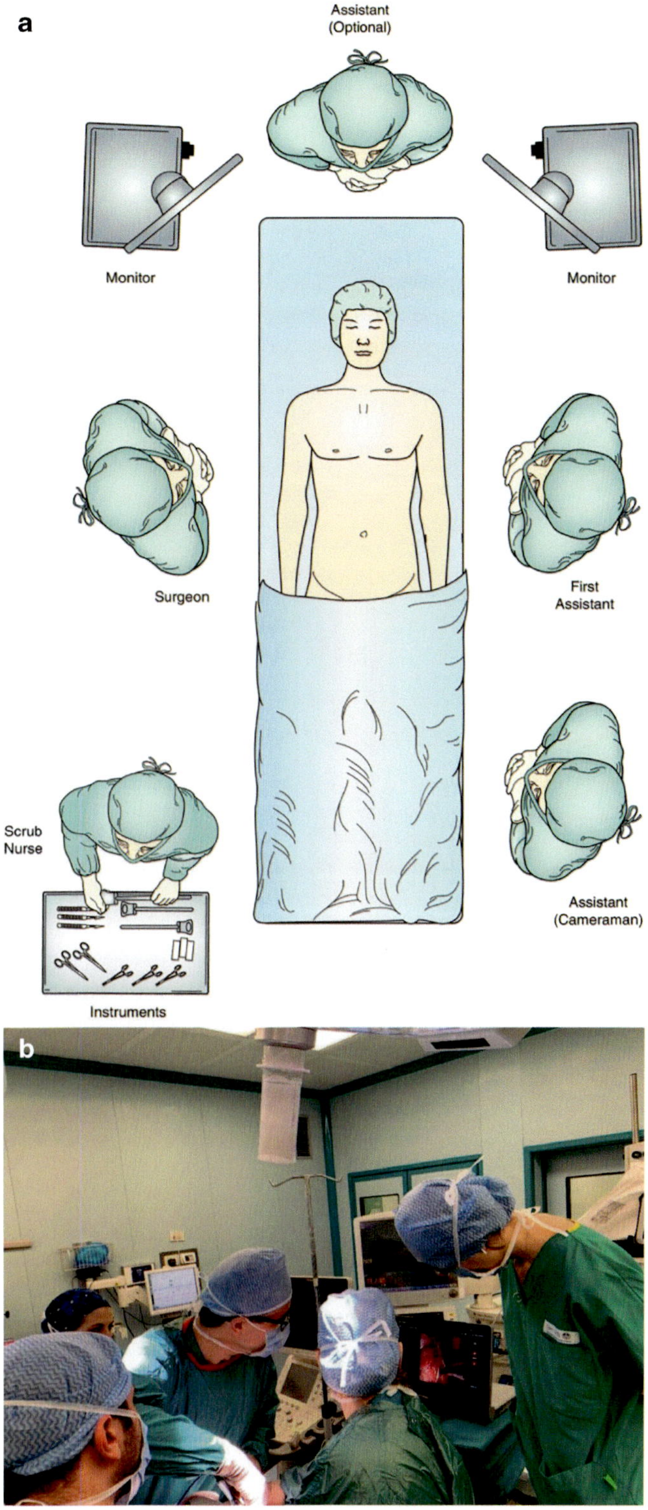

Fig. 12.1 (**a**) Operating room setting and position of the surgical team. (From Raffaelli et al. [50]; with permission). (**b**) Position of the surgical team in VAT using the Nanoscope™ System Arthrex, a small (1.9 mm) single-use camera system that combines imaging sensors, LED lights, and image and operative room integration and control. (Unpublished personal experience)

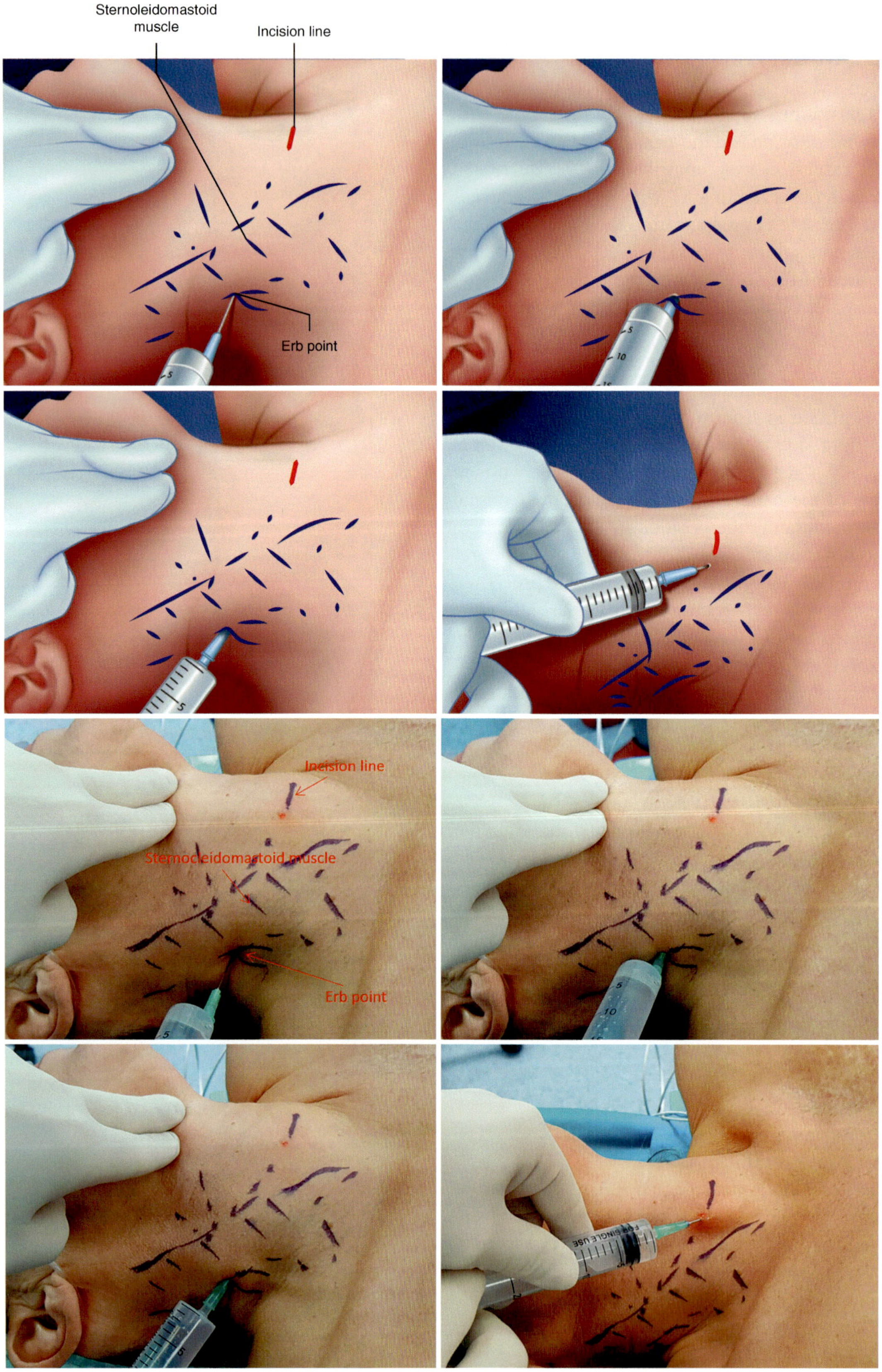

Fig. 12.2 Superficial cervical block. The cervical block is performed with the patient in the operating room. A mixture of bupivacaine 0.25% and carbocaine 0.5% is used as locoregional anesthetic. A 4-cm, 23-gauge needle is inserted at the midpoint along the posterior border of the sternocleidomastoid muscle on the affected side, and the tip is directed anteriorly. After having aspirated first, a 10-mL bolus of the bupivacaine-carbocaine mixture is injected. The needle is then directed toward the midline, and an additional 5 mL bolus of the anesthetic mixture is injected while the needle is withdrawn. Then a bolus of 5-mL of the anesthetic is administered along the incision line at an intermediate level between the sternal notch and the cricoid cartilage in the midline

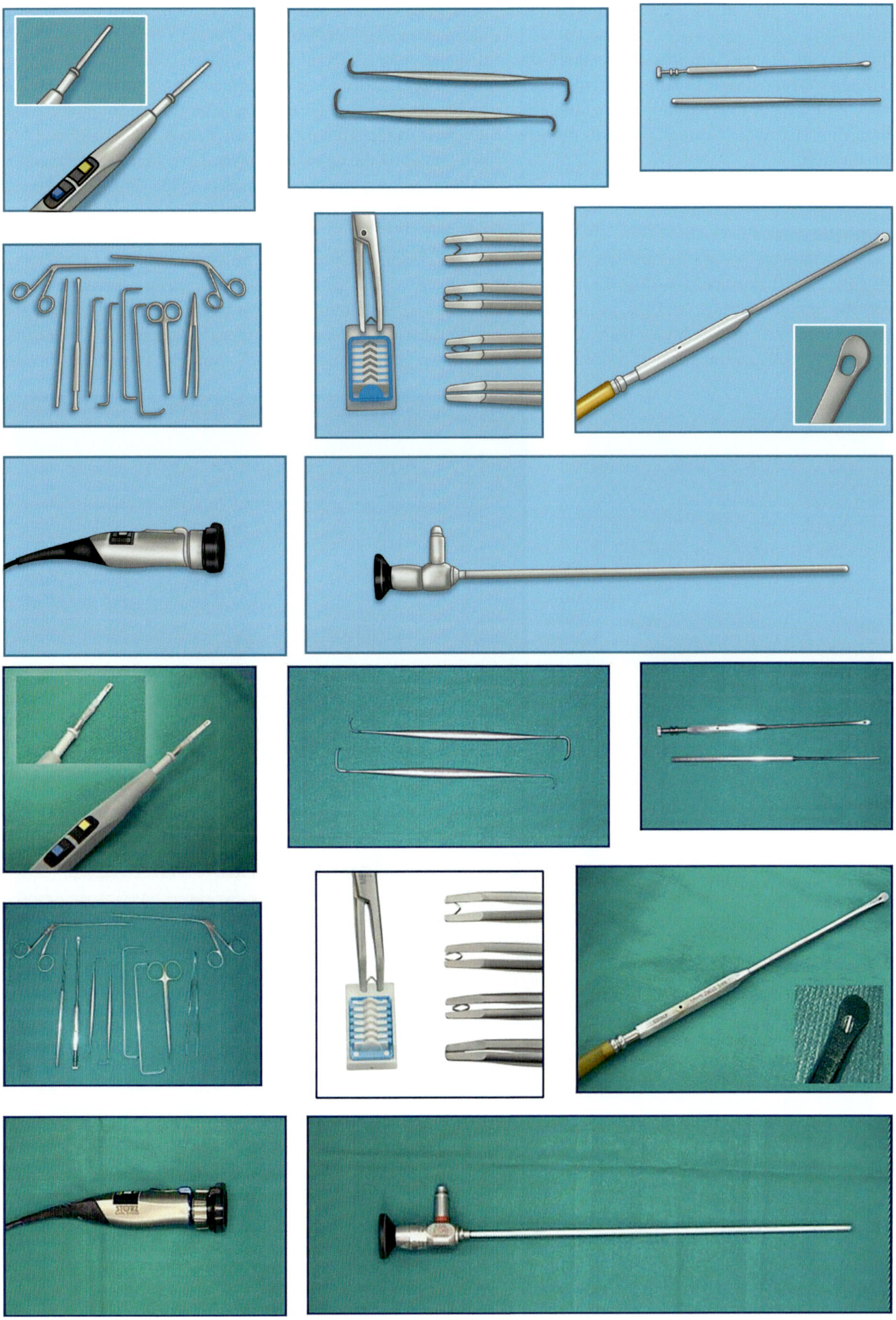

Fig. 12.3 Surgical instruments for VAT

effective during VAT since they allow the surgeon to reduce the operative time [49].

From a technical point of view, considering the small size of the skin incision, probably the ideal sealing systems would be those endowed with a long, freely rolling stem, similar to the CS-14 Ultracision Harmonic Scalpel® model, unfortunately out of production.

Surgical Technique

A small (1.5–2 cm), central skin incision (Fig. 12.4) is performed between the cricoid cartilage and the sternal notch (Fig. 12.5). The skin incision is usually higher than in conventional cervicotomy and can also be modulated according to the neck conformation and thyroid position. However, the skin incision is usually performed just below (1 cm) the cricoid cartilage in order to obtain an optimal exposure and safe control of the upper thyroid vascular pedicle. The skin incision would be ideally placed in an existing skin wrinkle to optimize the aesthetic result. After incising the platysma muscle (Fig. 12.6) and preparing the upper and lower flaps (Fig. 12.7), the cervical *linea alba* is opened as far as possible (Fig. 12.8), taking care to avoid any minimal bleeding. The thyroid lobe (on the affected side) is then separated from the strap muscles by means of small conventional retractors (Farabeuf retractors), which are also used to maintain open operative space (Fig. 12.9). The thyroid lobe is medially retracted, while the strap muscles are laterally retracted using the two Farabeufs. At this point, the endoscope (5 mm – 30°) and the dedicated

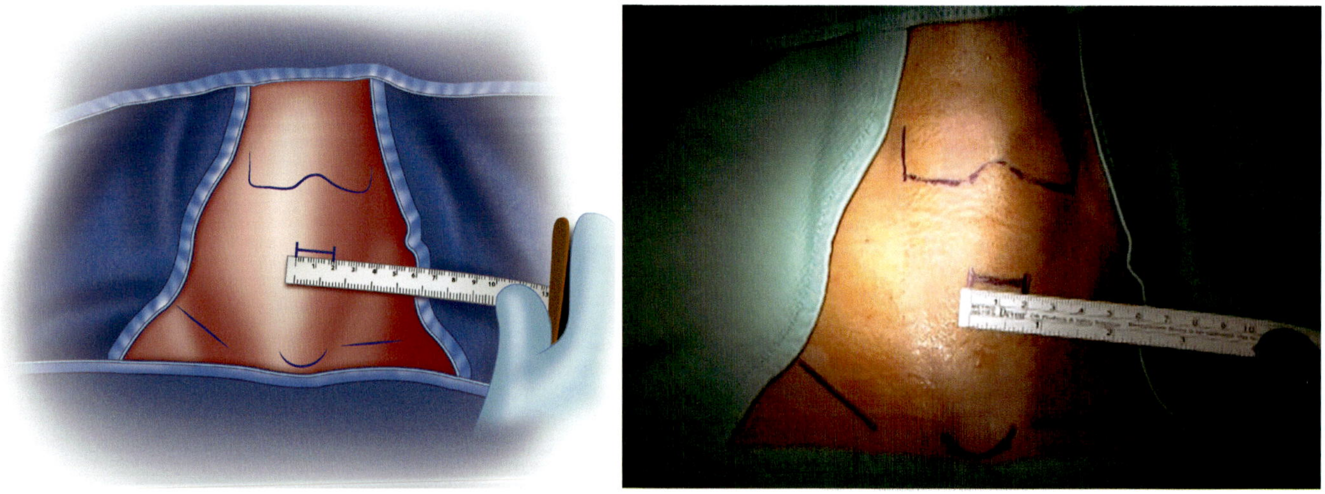

Fig. 12.4 A small skin incision (1-5-2 cm) is performed

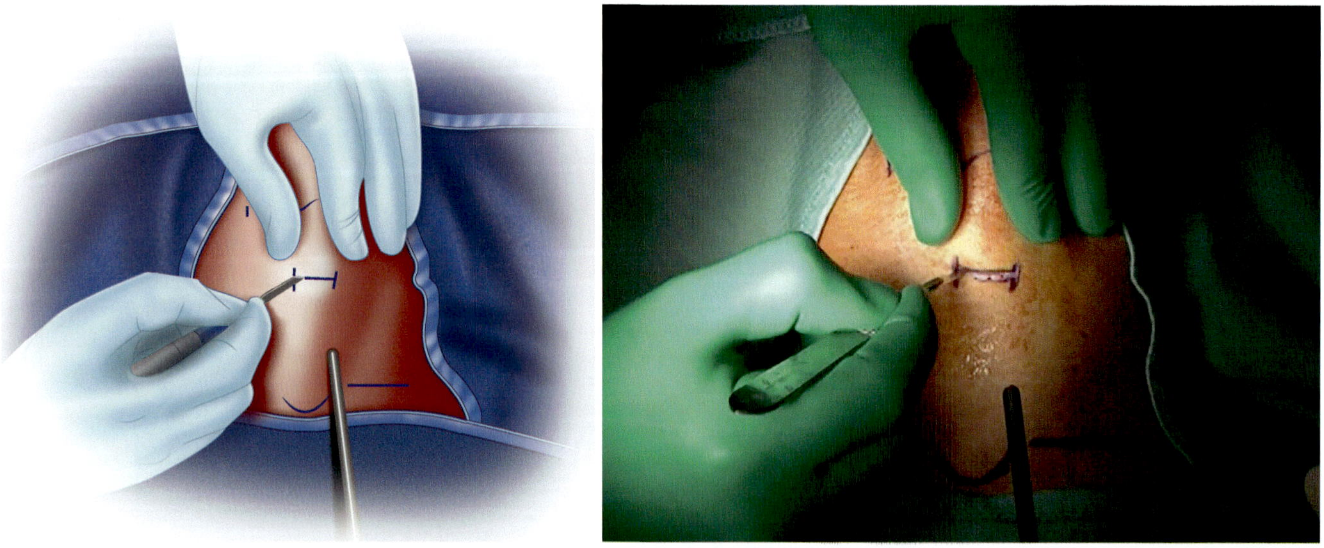

Fig. 12.5 The incision was carried out with the scalpel blade through the skin and subcuticular fat tissue

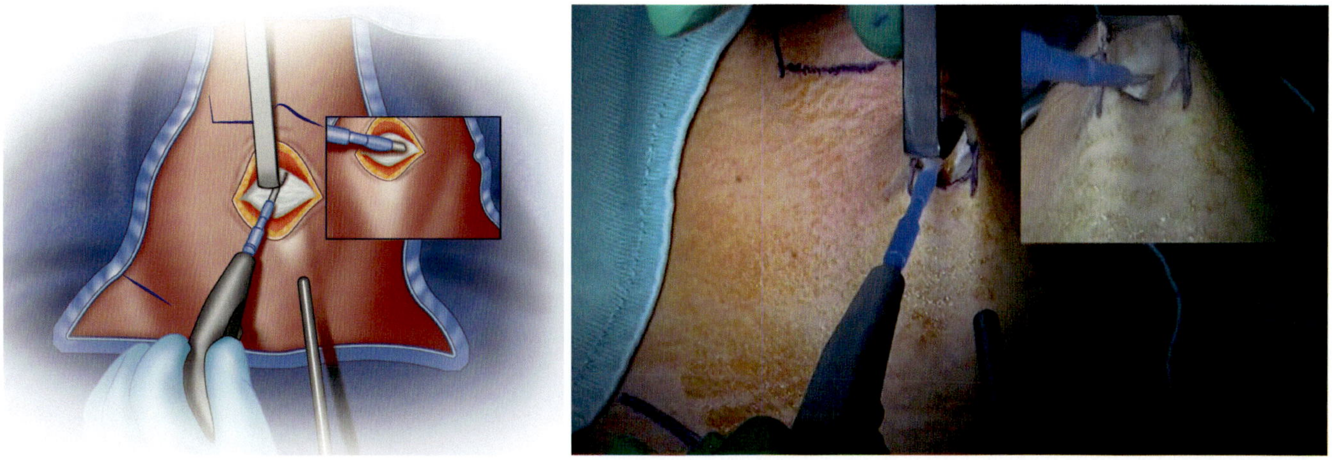

Fig. 12.6 Incision of the platysma muscle in order to prepare the upper and lower flaps

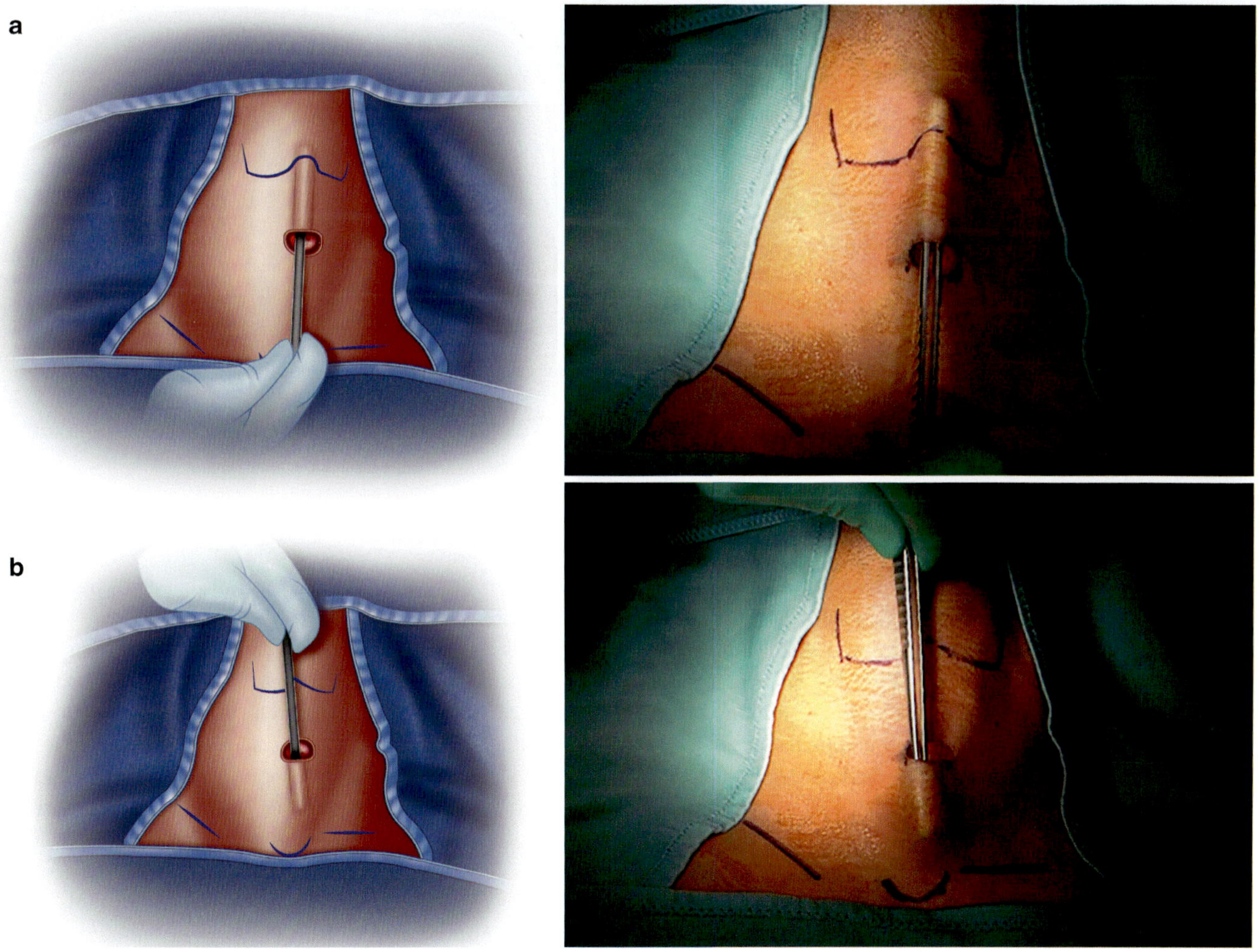

Fig. 12.7 Upper (a) and lower (b) flaps

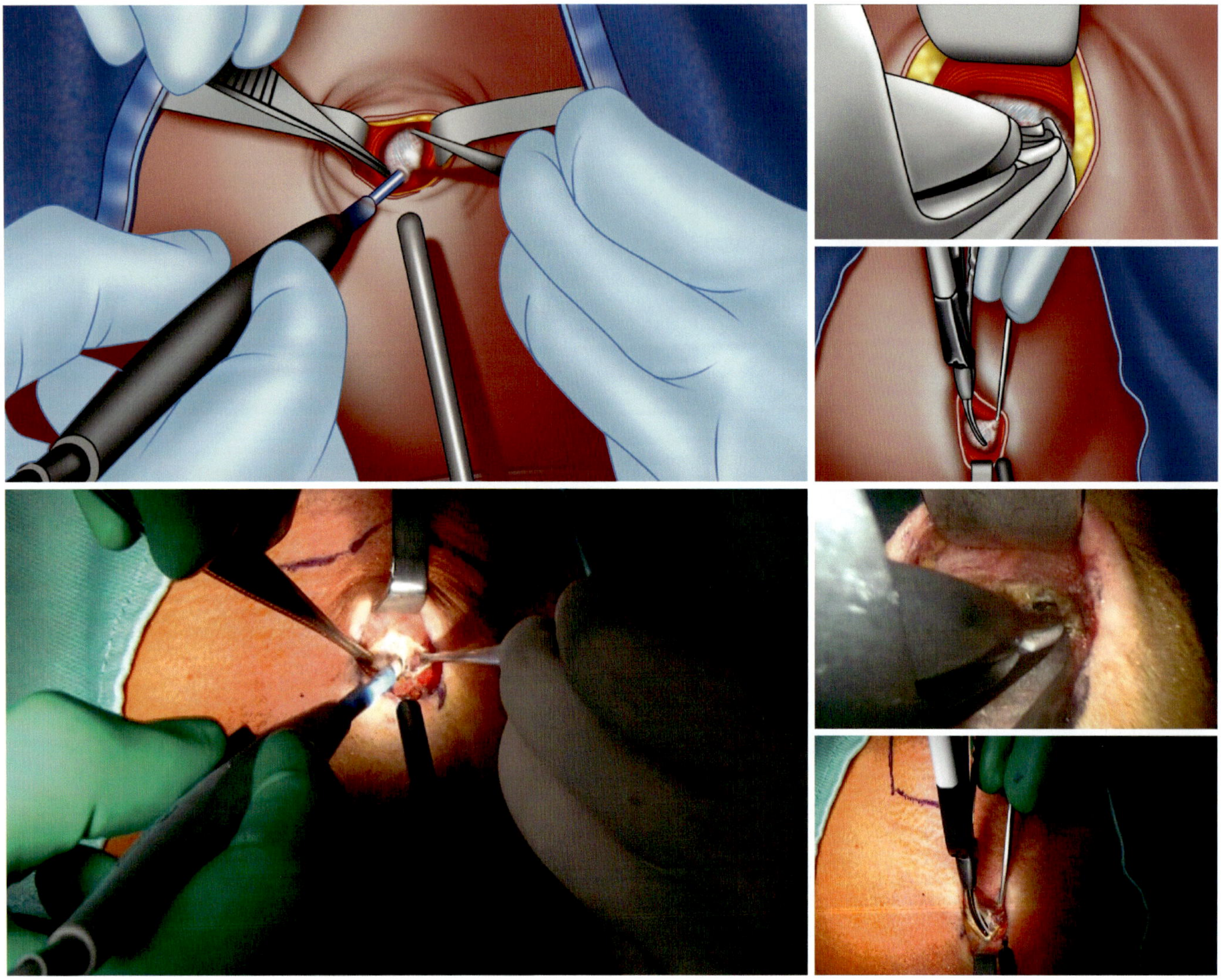

Fig. 12.8 The cervical *linea alba* is opened as far as possible

small surgical instruments (2 mm in diameter) are introduced through the single skin incision. The first step of the procedure consists in completely freeing the thyroid gland in order to have good exposure of the prevertebral fascia, which represents the posterior aspect of the dissection. The middle thyroid vein, if present, is sectioned to gain complete access to the prevertebral fascia. The medial and lateral edges of the dissection are, respectively, the tracheoesophageal groove and the medial aspect of the common carotid artery. If intraoperative neuromonitoring is used, the identification and stimulation of the vagus nerve are then performed as the first step of the surgical procedure (Fig. 12.10a). If continuous intraoperative nerve monitoring is used, the automated periodic stimulation (APS) electrode is placed at the level of the vagus nerve, prepared for about 1 cm (Fig. 12.10b).

The dissection is carried out by a blunt technique using two dedicated instruments (spatulas); one of the instruments is connected to an aspiration system. After its complete separation from the muscles, the thyroid lobe is retracted downward, in order to expose the upper pole vessels; these are dissected using the spatula and the spatula-shaped aspirator (Fig. 12.11). During this phase, it is usually possible to identify the EBSLN, thanks to the magnification of the endoscope (Fig. 12.12). The upper pole vessels are then either selectively clipped and cut or directly cut using a sealing system (Fig. 12.13). During this step, special attention

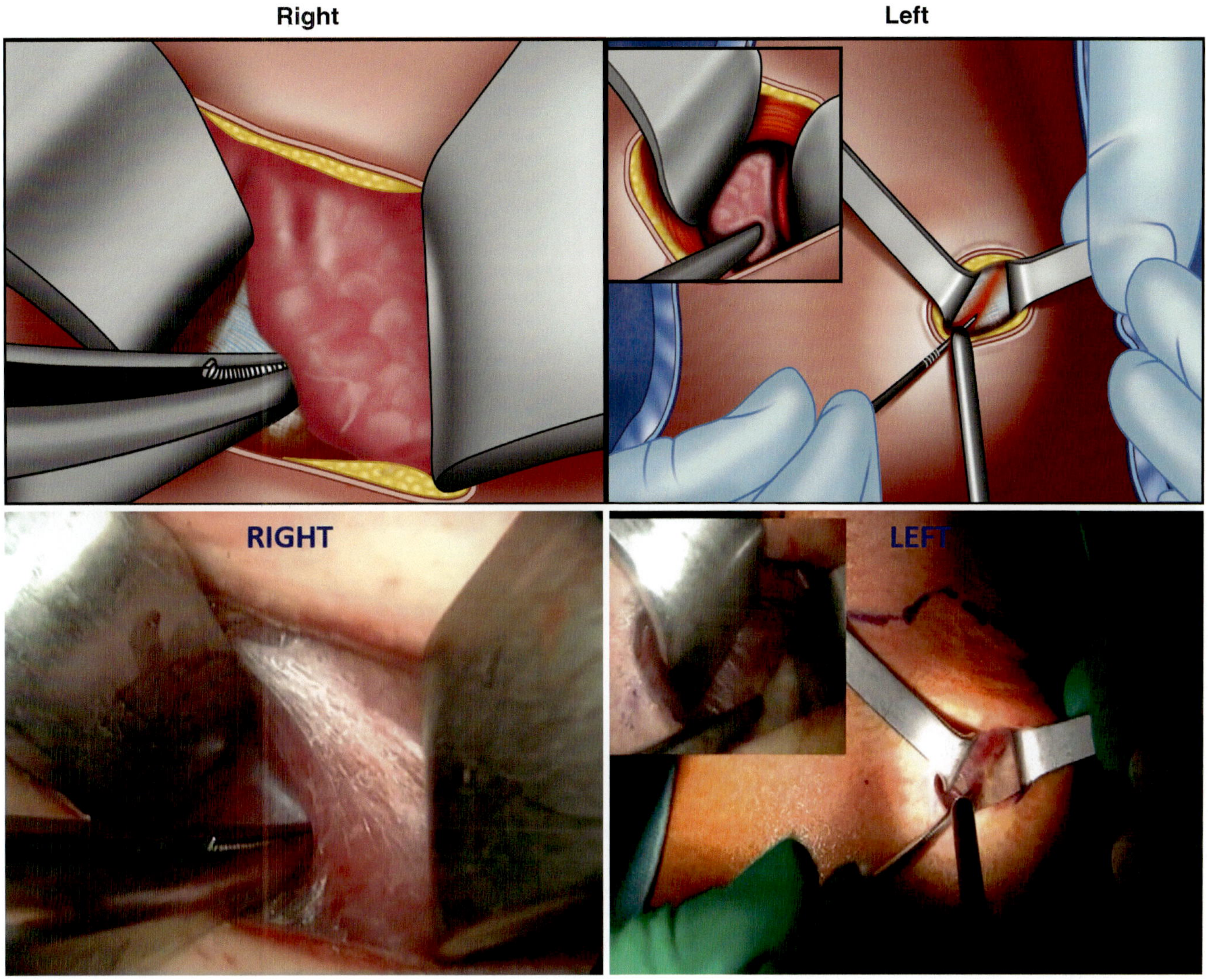

Fig. 12.9 Blunt dissection frees the thyroid lobe from the strap muscle. Then the operative space is created by two conventional Farabeuf divaricators that retract the thyroid lobe medially and the strap muscles laterally, maintaining an adequate working space. To note, the lateral limit of the operative space is the common carotid artery, easily exposed by means of the lateral Farabeuf. After creating the operative space, the 5-mm-30° endoscope and the 2-mm dedicated instruments are introduced through the same central access. In cases in which intraoperative neuromonitoring is used, predissection vagus nerve stimulation can easily be accomplished as the very first step of the surgical procedure

should be paid to controlling the tip of the energy device in order to avoid pharynx or larynx thermal injury. After complete dissection of the upper pole, the thyroid lobe is retracted medially by means of the *Farabeuf* retractor to identify the RLN under endoscopic vision (Fig. 12.14). The magnification (two- to three fold) of the endoscope allows a straightforward identification of the RLN. Gentle medial traction on the thyroid lobe, in order to avoid any inadvertent stretch injury to the RLN, and lateral traction on the strap muscles allow to improve the exposition of the inferior thyroid artery, thus facilitating the identification of the RLN, typically found where it crosses the inferior thyroid artery. The Zuckerkandl tubercle can be another useful landmark for the identification of the RLN, as in conventional procedure. If intraoperative neuromonitoring is used, once the RLN is identified, it is stimulated in order to check the predissection function (Figs. 12.15 and 12.16). Thus, the RLN is prepared and bluntly dissected (Fig. 12.17), under endoscopic vision,

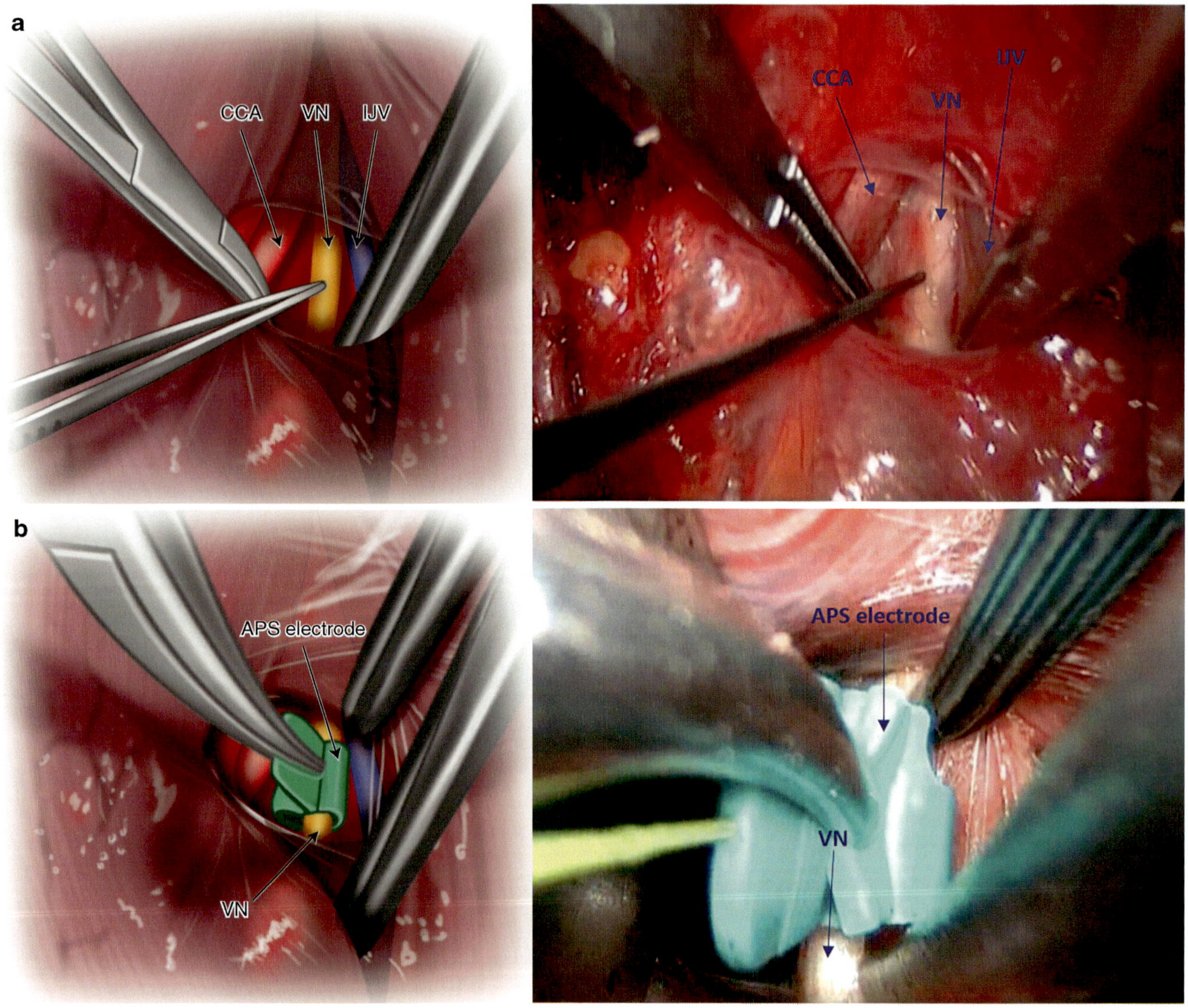

Fig. 12.10 (**a**) Stimulation of the vagus nerve (VN) using intermittent neuromonitoring. CCA-common carotid artery; IJV-internal jugular vein. (**b**) In case continuous monitoring is used, it is necessary to position the automated periodic stimulation (APS) electrode at the level of the VN prepared for about 1 cm

with an upward direction from the mediastinum toward its entry point in the larynx. At this point, the superior parathyroid gland is identified at the level of the posterior aspect of the thyroid lobe (Fig. 12.18).

The parathyroid glands are identified and preserved with adequate vascularization supply, facilitated by the assistance of the endoscopic magnification.

The thyroid lobe is then extracted (Fig. 12.19) from the skin incision, and the procedure is accomplished under endoscopic and direct vision (Fig. 12.20). During the maneuver of thyroid lobe extraction, it is of utmost importance to avoid excessive traction, which can result in inadvertent stretch injury to the nerve.

After identifying and preserving the inferior parathyroid gland (Fig. 12.21), the lower vascular pole is selectively dissected by means of a conventional tie, clip, or energy device. It is important to carry out a completely bloodless dissection facilitated by using a spatula-shaped aspirator. At this step of the procedure, it is of the utmost importance to check again the RLN and the parathyroid glands. Although the separation of the thyroid from the trachea is usually carried out using a sealing system (Fig. 12.22), dissection close to the nerve can be accomplished by means of a titanium clip or conventional ligature in order to avoid the risk of a thermal injury to the RLN. At the end of the thyroid lobe resection, the RLN and the ipsilateral vagus nerve are stimulated (postdissection stimulation).

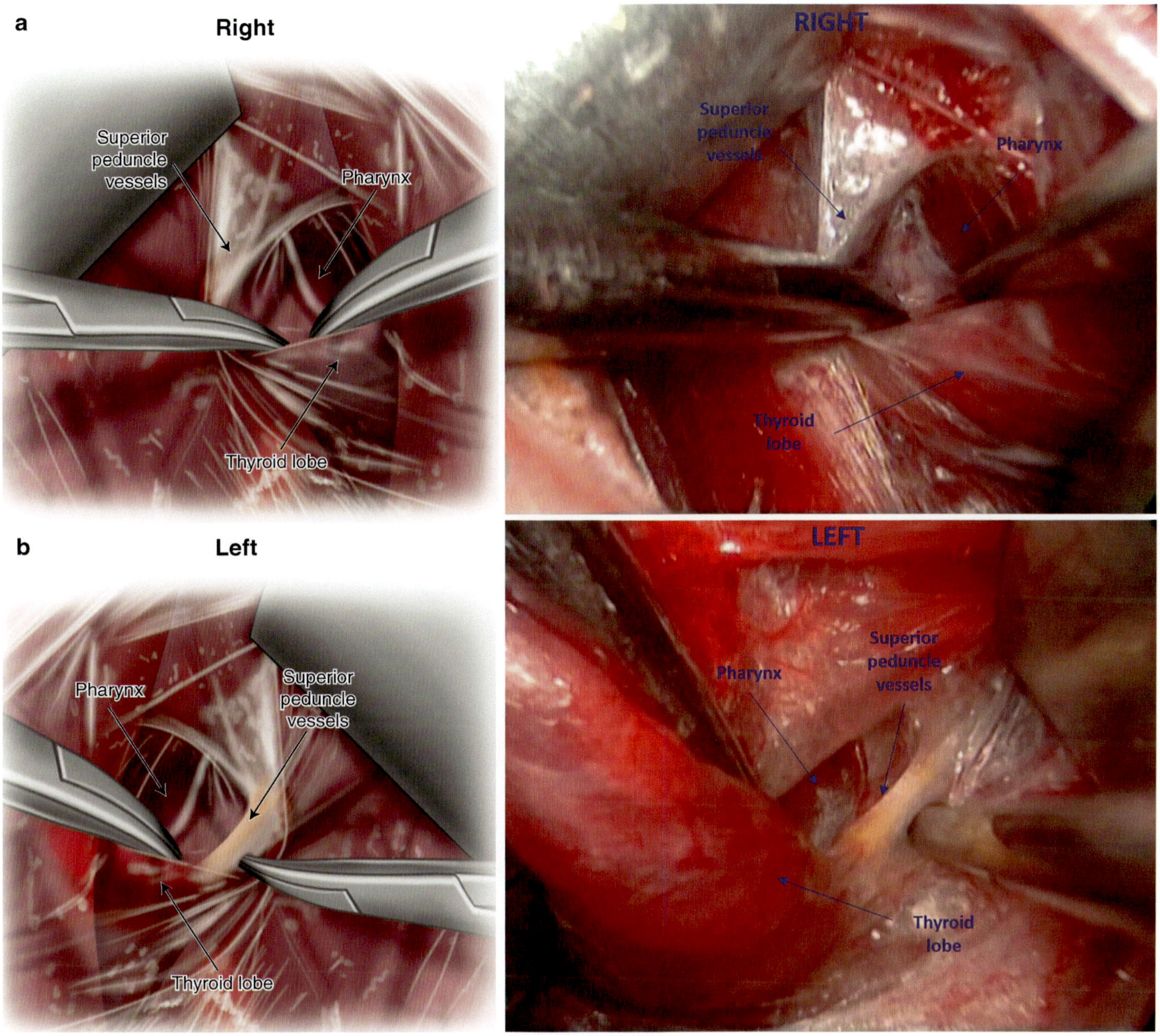

Fig. 12.11 The thyroid lobe is retracted downward and laterally to expose the upper pole vessels that are prepared with blunt dissection by means of a dedicated spatula and spatula-shaped aspirator. (**a**) Right side. (**b**) Left side

The isthmus is sectioned using a sealing device in case of thyroid lobectomy. If total thyroidectomy is planned, the same steps are performed on the contralateral side. In the case of total thyroidectomy, before proceeding to the contralateral lobe dissection, the dissected lobe is repositioned in its original cervical space in order to optimize the surgical working space. After checking the hemostasis, the strap muscles are sutured along the midline, and the same is done for the platysma. The skin is closed by means of a nonresorbable subcuticular running suture (Fig. 12.23) or by a skin sealant. Generally, no position of drain required. Hemostatic agents can be used and placed in the operating field, such as the Tabotamp Fibrillar® (Ethicon).

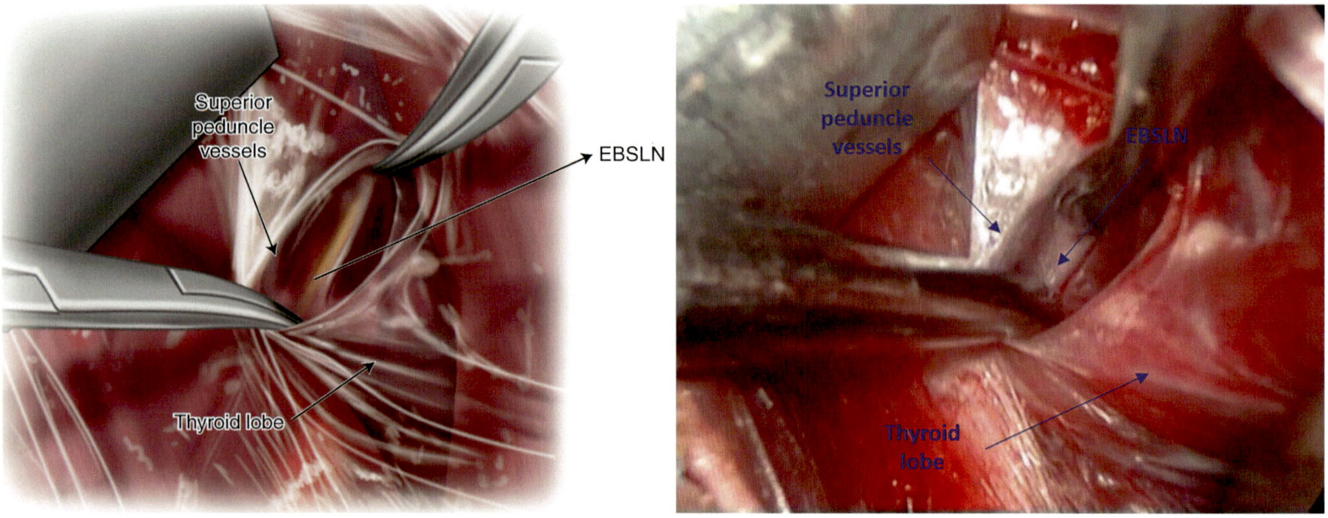

Fig. 12.12 Identification of the external branch of the superior laryngeal nerve (EBSLN)

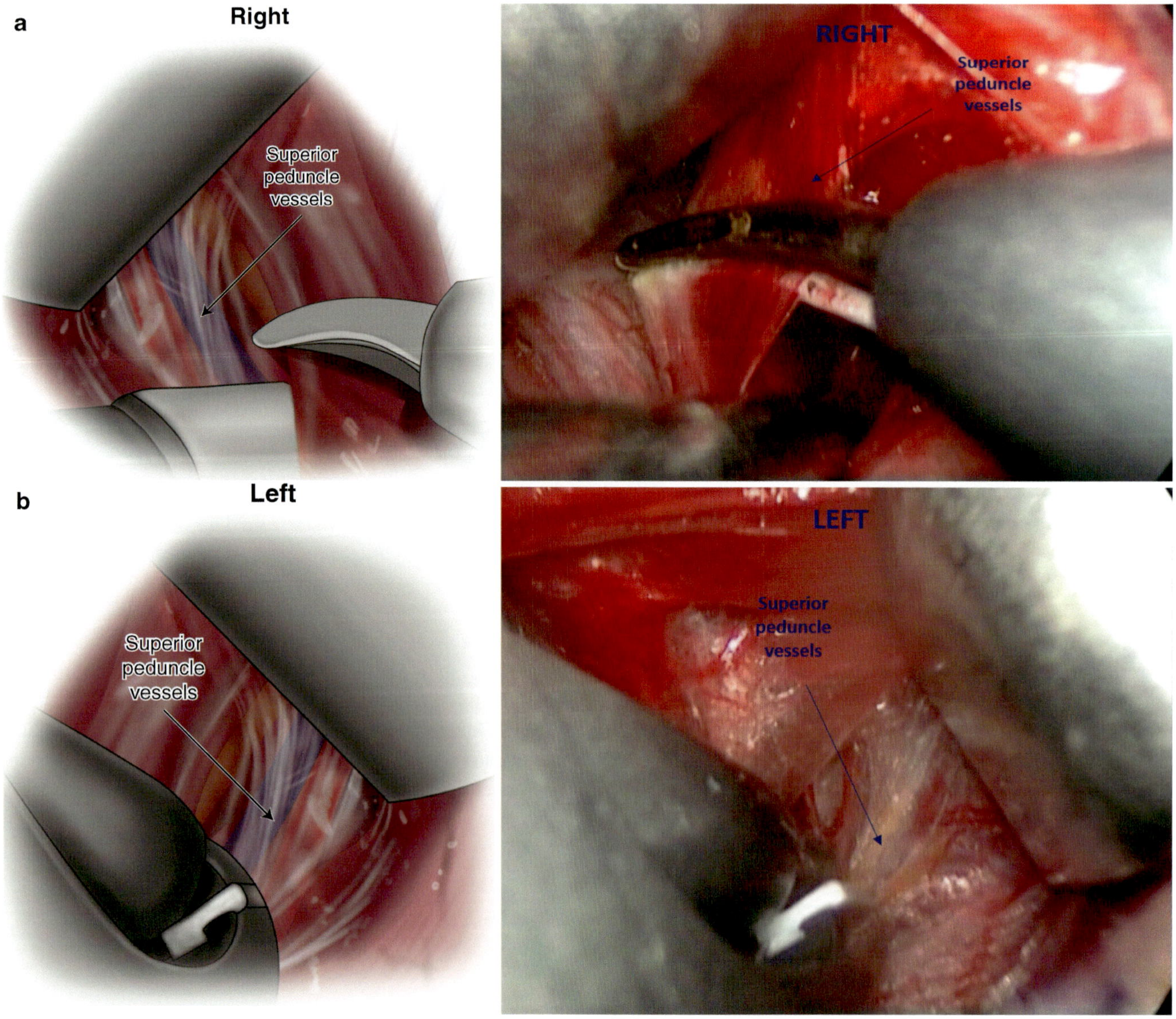

Fig. 12.13 The upper pedicle vessels are then selectively dissected using a sealing system (in this case, Harmonic Focus Plus®), with special attention to preserving the EBSLN. (**a**) Right side. (**b**) Left side

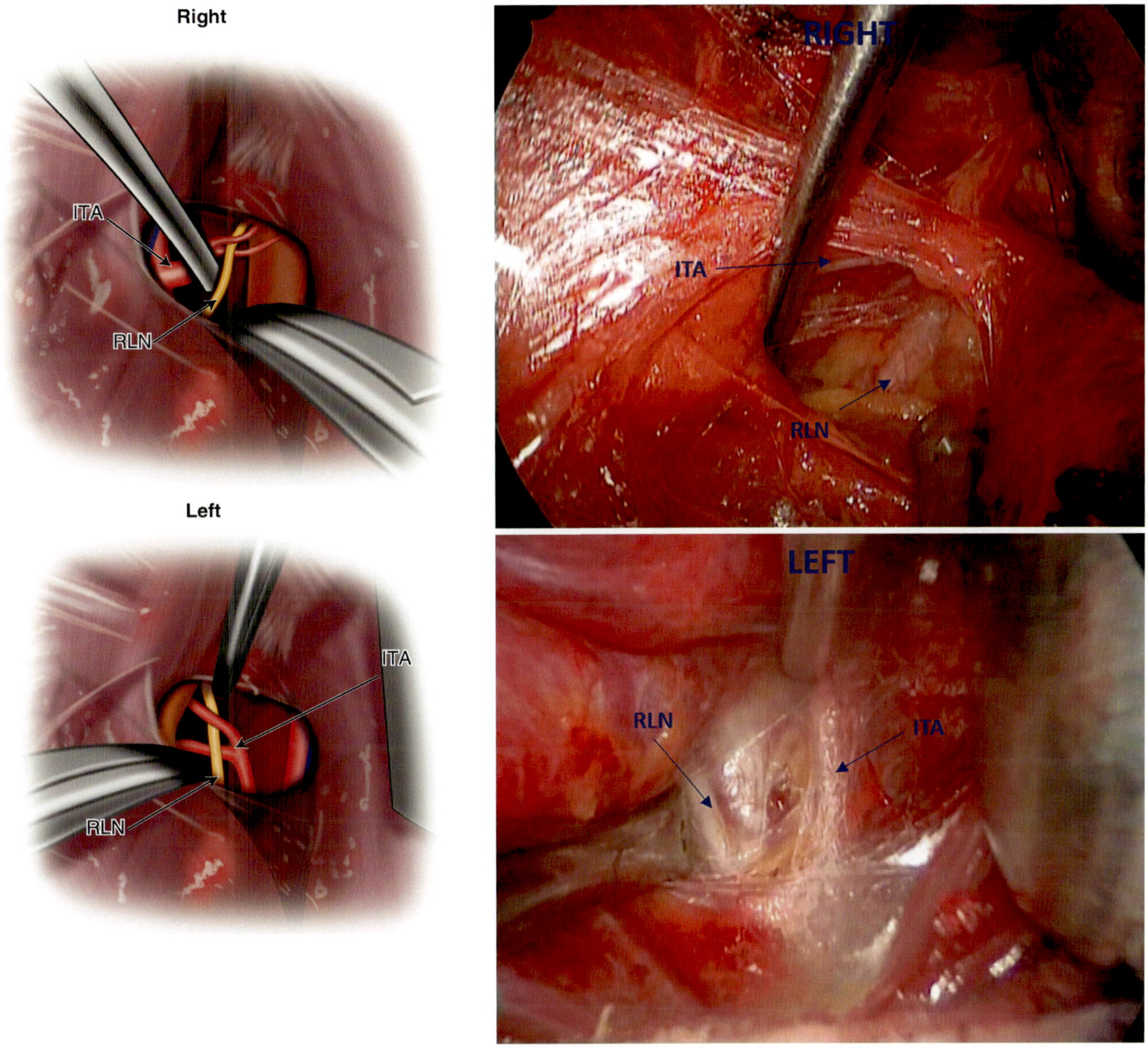

Fig. 12.14 Endoscopic identification of the recurrent laryngeal nerve (RLN). ITA-inferior thyroid artery

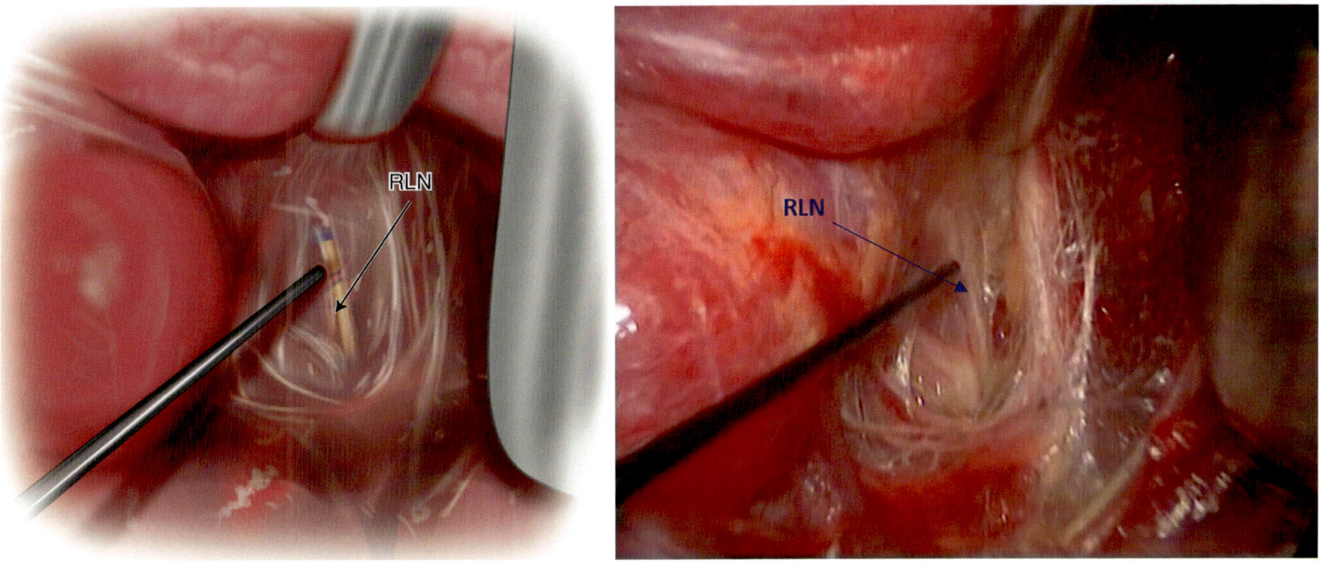

Fig. 12.15 Stimulation of the recurrent laryngeal nerve (RLN) using intermittent neuromonitoring

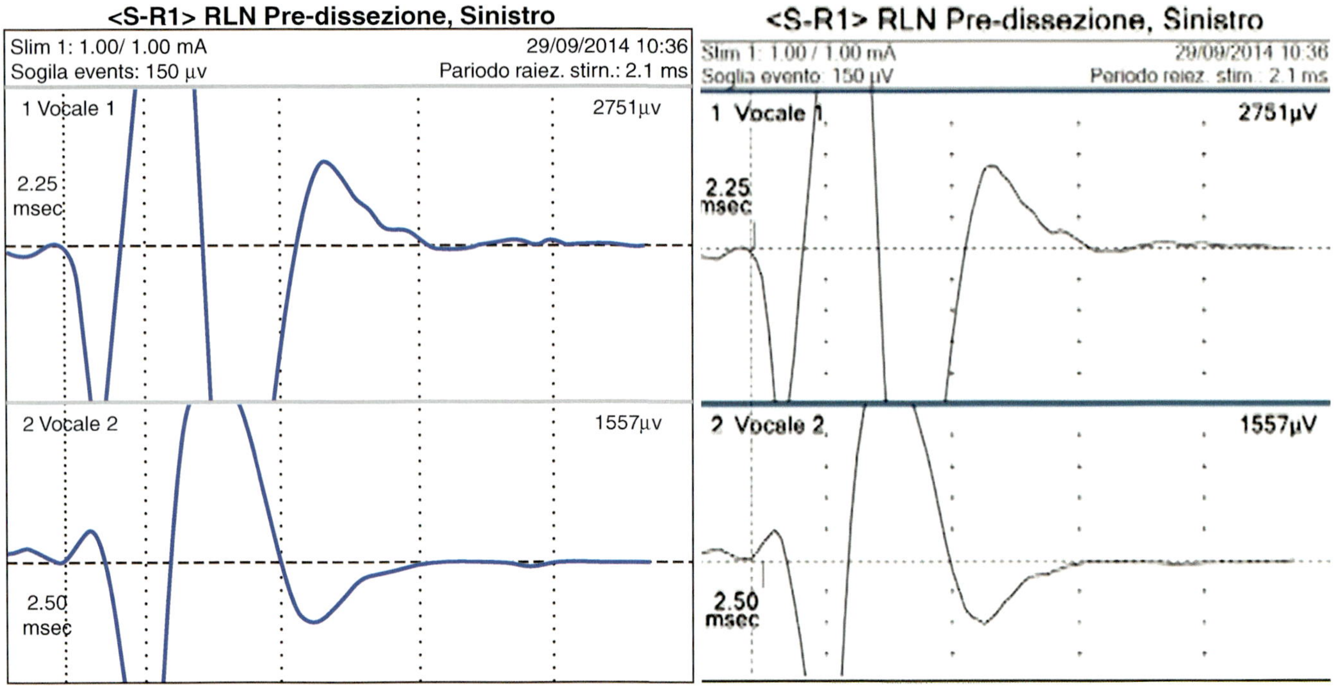

Fig. 12.16 Biphasic curve of the electromyographic potential following recurrent laryngeal nerve (RLN) stimulation

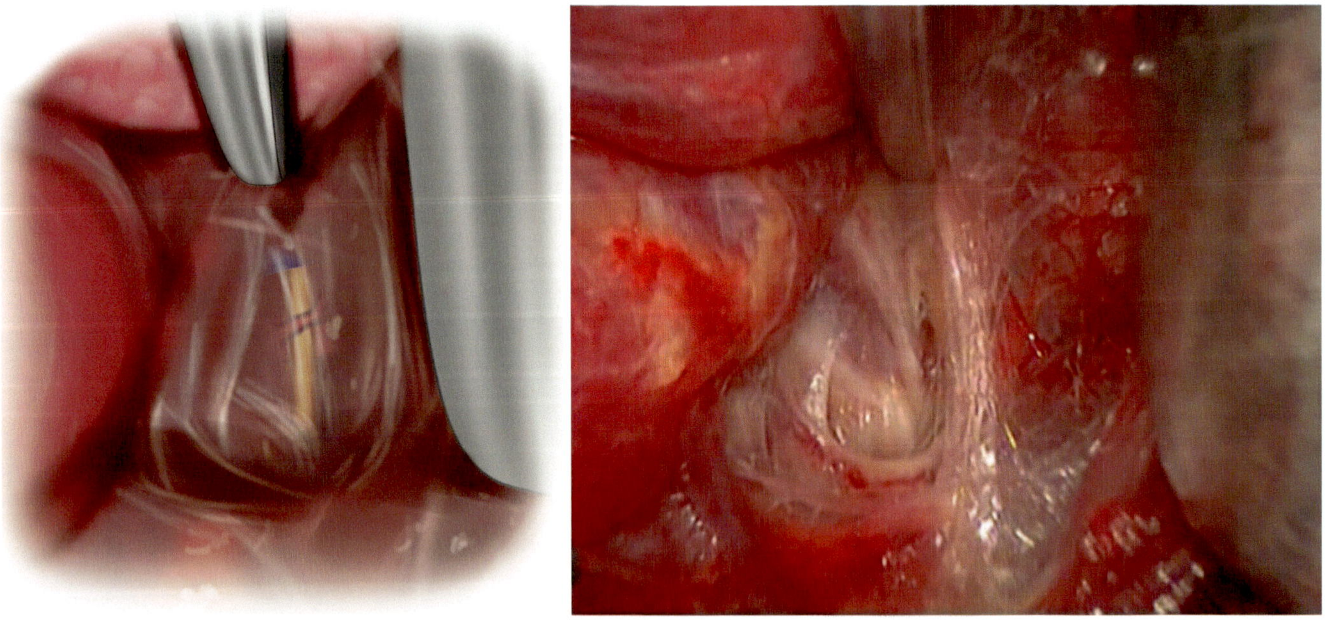

Fig. 12.17 Once identified, the recurrent laryngeal nerve (RLN) is prepared and bluntly dissected, under endoscopic vision, with an upward direction from the mediastinum toward its entry point in the larynx. ITA-inferior thyroid artery

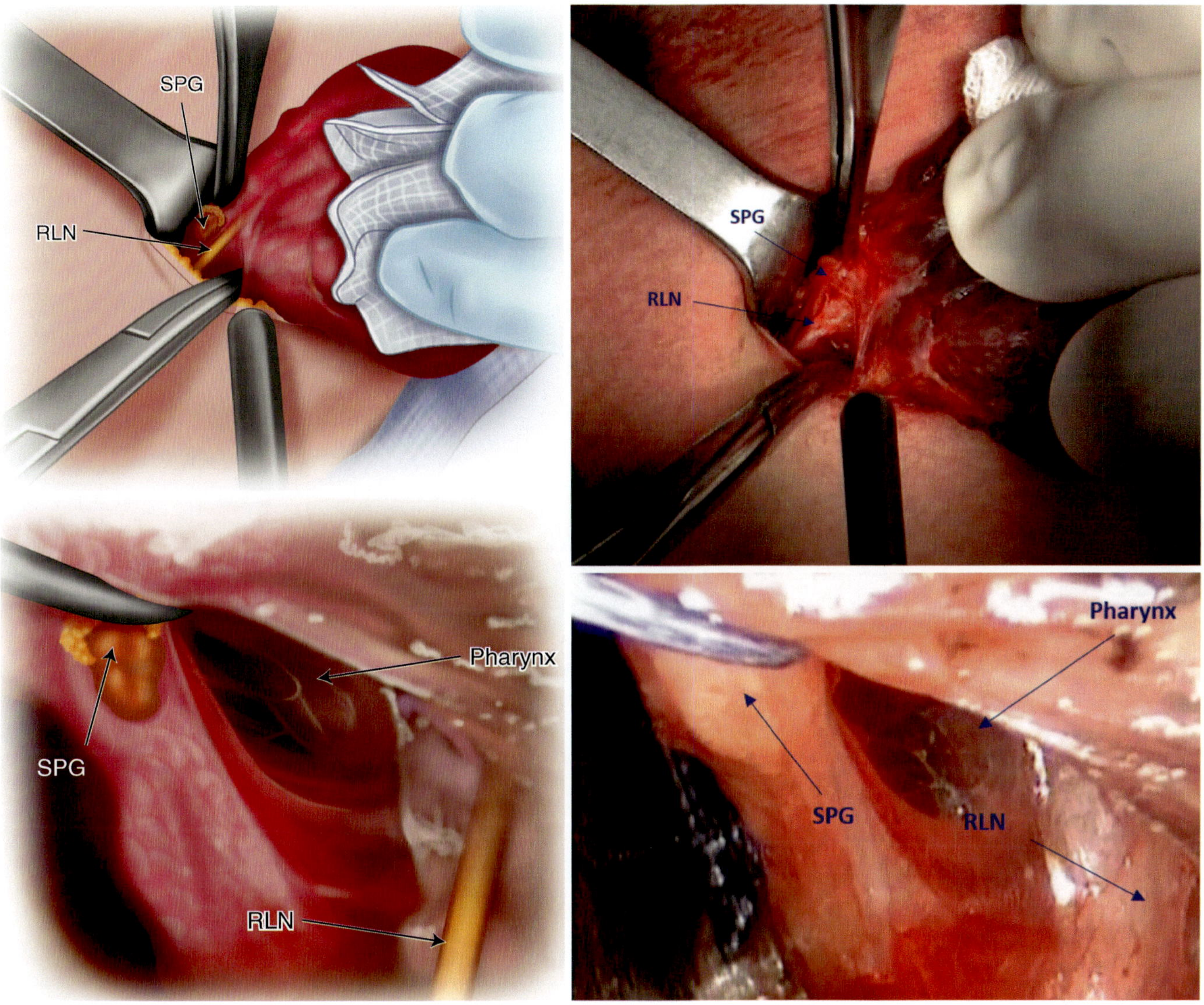

Fig. 12.18 The superior parathyroid gland (SPG) is identified at the level of the posterior aspect of the thyroid lobe. RLN-recurrent laryngeal nerve

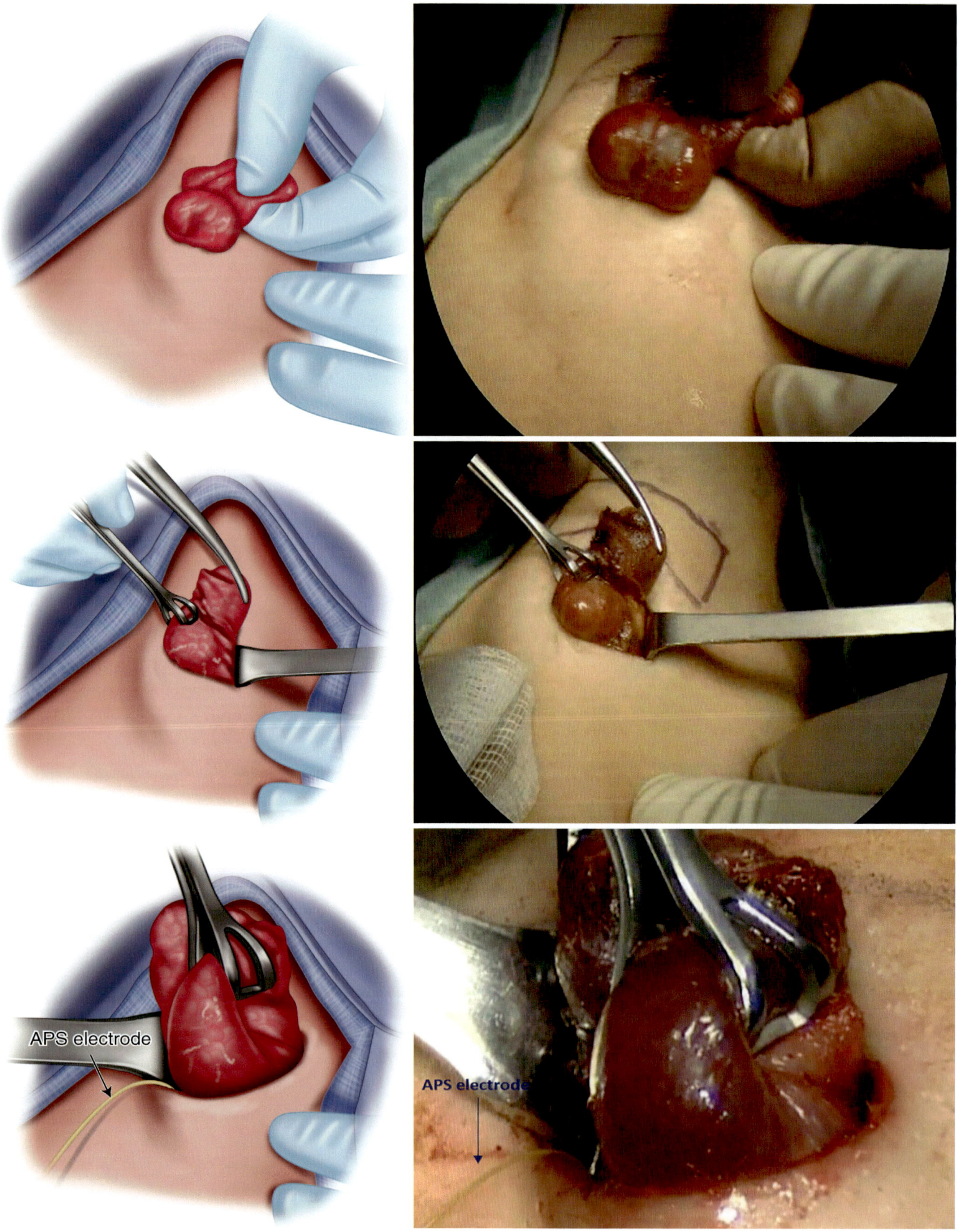

Fig. 12.19 Extraction of the thyroid lobe

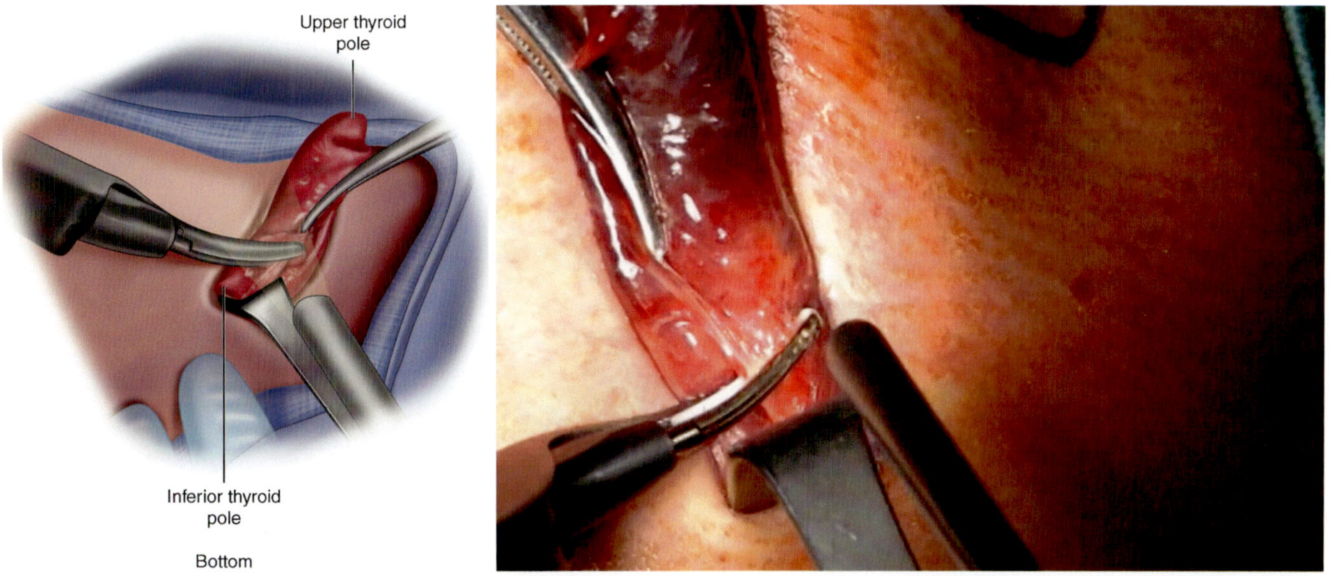

Fig. 12.20 At this point, the procedure is completed under endoscopic and direct vision

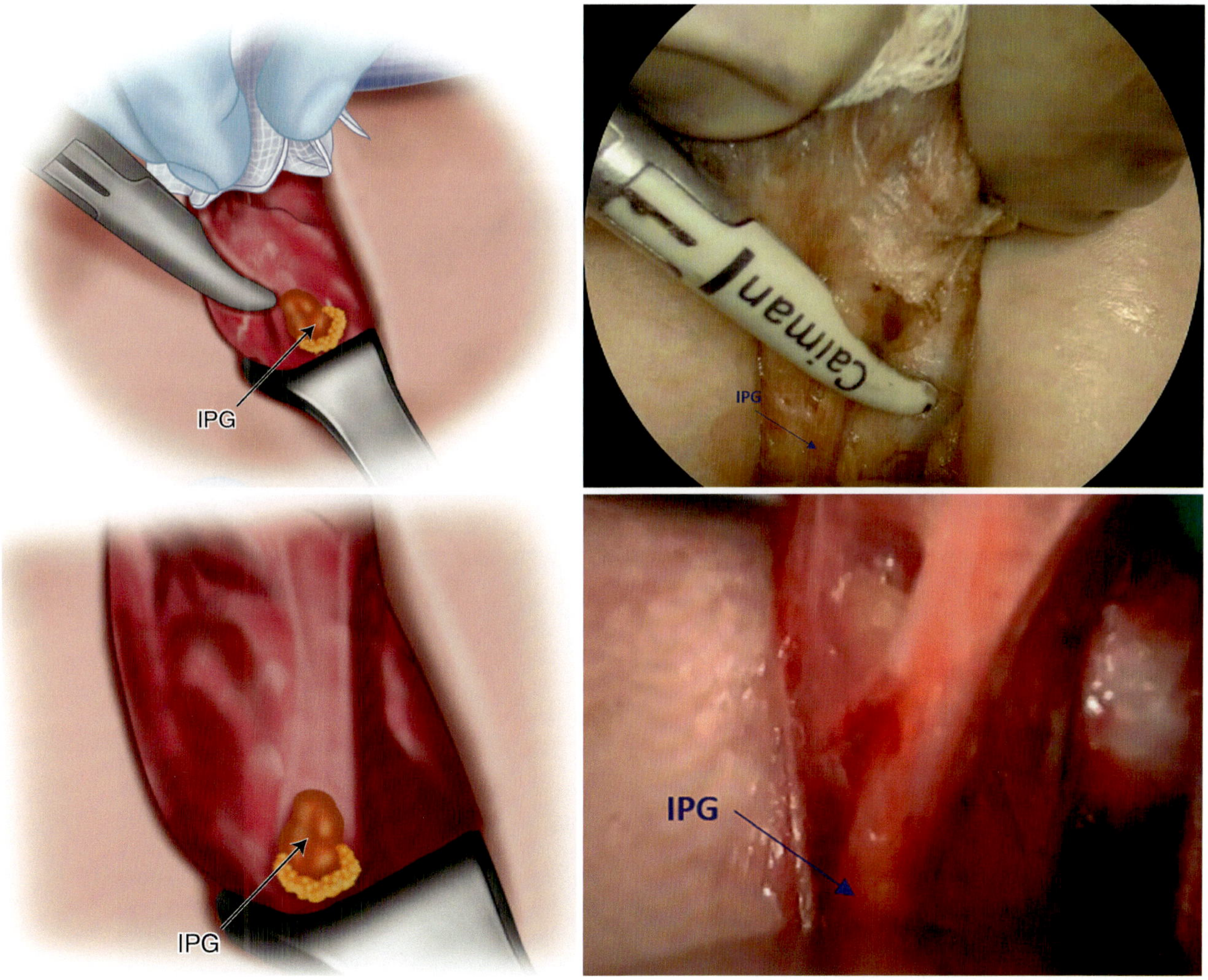

Fig. 12.21 The inferior parathyroid gland (IPG) is identified at the level of the anterior and inferior aspects of the thyroid lobe. The inferior thyroid vessels are selectively clipped and cut, or directly cut using a sealing system

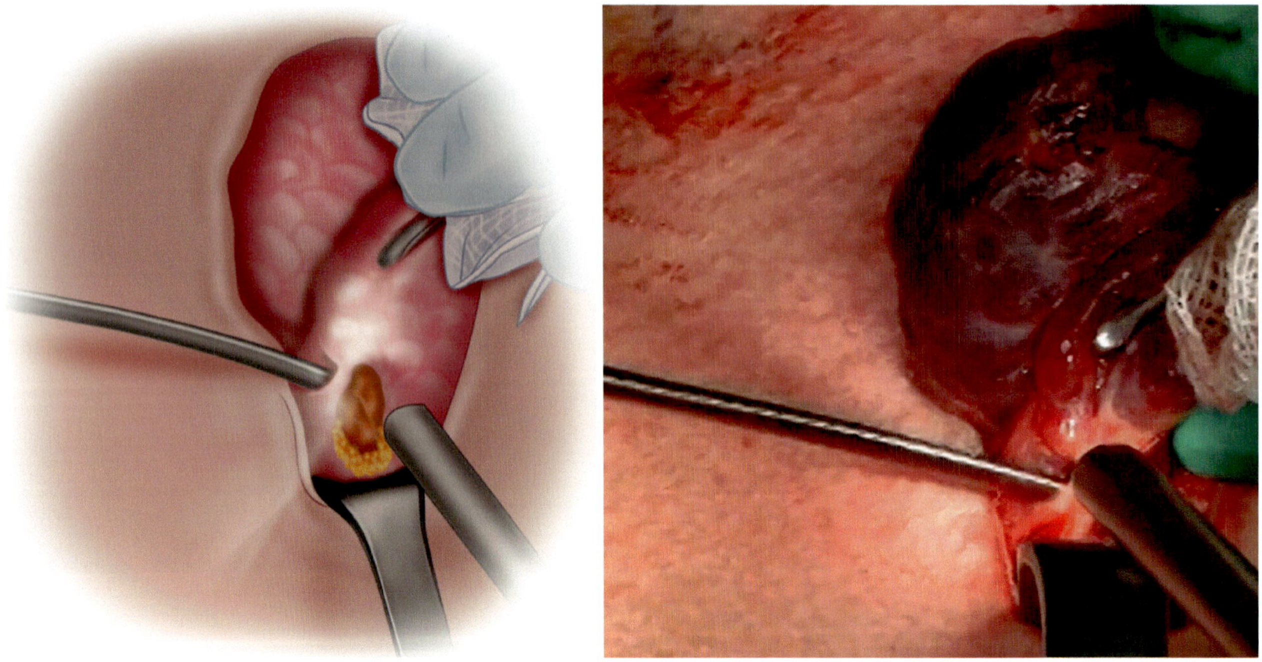

Fig. 12.21 (continued)

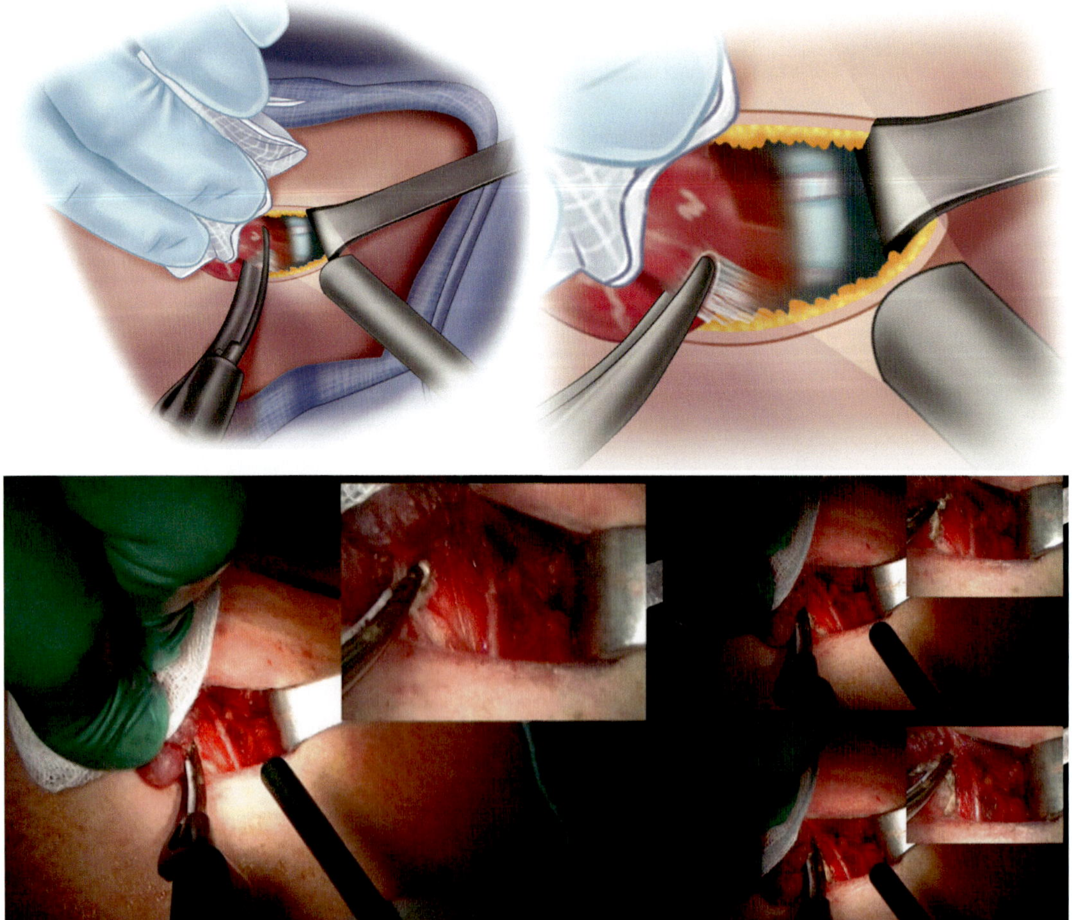

Fig. 12.22 The dissection of the thyroid lobe from the trachea is usually carried out using a sealing system

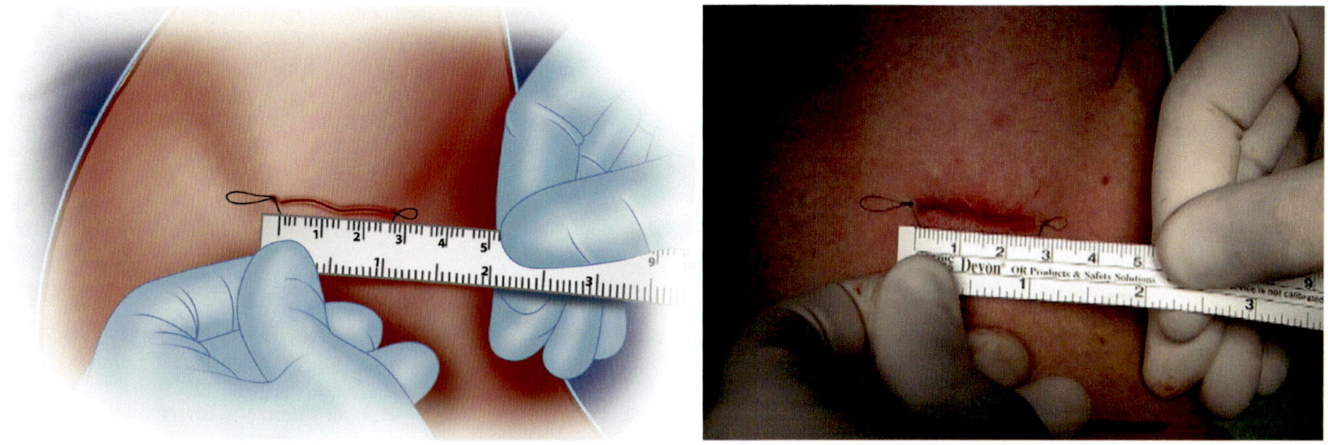

Fig. 12.23 The skin is closed by means of a nonabsorbable subcuticular running suture

Conclusions

From our experience of more than 20 years, we can reaffirm the concept that VAT is a safe procedure that is not burdened by an increase of complication rate or additional costs. Furthermore, this technique offers advantages in terms of cosmetic results and postoperative pain. VAT represents a valid option also in cases of "low-risk" papillary thyroid carcinomas with excellent oncologic outcomes.

References

1. Yeung GH. Endoscopic surgery of the neck: a new frontier. Surg Laparosc Endosc. 1998;8(3):227–32. http://www.ncbi.nlm.nih.gov/pubmed/9649050. Accessed 11 Dec 2018.
2. Duh Q-Y. Presidential address: minimally invasive endocrine surgery--standard of treatment or hype? Surgery. 2003;134(6):849–57. https://doi.org/10.1016/S0039.
3. Gagner M. Endoscopic subtotal parathyroidectomy in patients with primary hyperparathyroidism. Br J Surg. 1996;83(6):875. http://www.ncbi.nlm.nih.gov/pubmed/8696772. Accessed 11 Dec 2018.
4. Inabnet WB III, Jacob BP, Gagner M. Minimally invasive endoscopic thyroidectomy by a cervical approach. Surg Endosc. 2003;17(11):1808–11. https://doi.org/10.1007/s00464-002-8760-7.
5. Ikeda Y, Takami H, Tajima G, et al. Total endoscopic thyroidectomy: axillary or anterior chest approach. Biomed Pharmacother. 2002;56 Suppl 1:72s–8s. http://www.ncbi.nlm.nih.gov/pubmed/12487257. Accessed 11 Dec 2018.
6. Bellantone R, Lombardi CP, Raffaelli M, Rubino F, Boscherini M, Perilli W. Minimally invasive, totally gasless video-assisted thyroid lobectomy. Am J Surg. 1999;177(4):342–3. http://www.ncbi.nlm.nih.gov/pubmed/10326857. Accessed 11 Dec 2018.
7. Miccoli P, Berti P, Conte M, Bendinelli C, Marcocci C. Minimally invasive surgery for thyroid small nodules: preliminary report. J Endocrinol Investig. 1999;22(11):849–51. https://doi.org/10.1007/BF03343657.
8. Mourad M, Ngongang C, Saab N, et al. Video-assisted neck exploration for primary and secondary hyperparathyroidism. Surg Endosc. 2001;15(10):1112–5. https://doi.org/10.1007/s004640090017.
9. Gagner M, Inabnet WB. Endoscopic thyroidectomy for solitary thyroid nodules. Thyroid. 2001;11(2):161–3. https://doi.org/10.1089/105072501300042848.
10. Miccoli P, Pinchera A, Cecchini G, et al. Minimally invasive, video-assisted parathyroid surgery for primary hyperparathyroidism. J Endocrinol Investig. 1997;20(7):429–30. https://doi.org/10.1007/BF03347996.
11. Ferzli GS, Sayad P, Abdo Z, Cacchione RN. Minimally invasive, nonendoscopic thyroid surgery. J Am Coll Surg. 2001;192(5):665–8. http://www.ncbi.nlm.nih.gov/pubmed/11333106. Accessed 11 Dec 2018.
12. Ohgami M, Ishii S, Arisawa Y, et al. Scarless endoscopic thyroidectomy: breast approach for better cosmesis. Surg Laparosc Endosc Percutan Tech. 2000;10(1):1–4. http://www.ncbi.nlm.nih.gov/pubmed/10872517. Accessed 19 Dec 2018.
13. Mourad M, Saab N, Malaise J, et al. Minimally invasive video-assisted approach for partial and total thyroidectomy. Surg Endosc. 2001;15(10):1108–11. https://doi.org/10.1007/s004640090018.
14. Miccoli P, Bendinelli C, Conte M, Pinchera A, Marcocci C. Endoscopic parathyroidectomy by a gasless approach. J Laparoendosc Adv Surg Tech – Part A. 1998;8(4):189–94. https://doi.org/10.1089/lap.1998.8.189.
15. Miccoli P, Biricotti M, Matteucci V, Ambrosini CE, Wu J, Materazzi G. Minimally invasive video-assisted thyroidectomy: reflections after more than 2400 cases performed. Surg Endosc. 2016;30(6):2489–95. https://doi.org/10.1007/s00464-015-4503-4.
16. Lombardi CP, Raffaelli M, De Crea C, D'Amore A, Bellantone R. Video-assisted thyroidectomy: lessons learned after more than

one decade. Acta Otorhinolaryngol Ital. 2009;29(6):317–20. http://www.ncbi.nlm.nih.gov/pubmed/20463836. Accessed 15 Dec 2018.
17. Bellantone R, Raffaelli M, De Crea C, et al. Video-assisted thyroidectomy for papillary thyroid carcinoma: oncologic outcome in patients with follow-up ≥ 10 years. World J Surg. 2018;42(2):402–8. https://doi.org/10.1007/s00268-017-4392-x.
18. Bellantone R, Lombardi CP, Bossola M, et al. Video-assisted vs conventional thyroid lobectomy: a randomized trial. Arch Surg. 2002;137(3):301–4; discussion 305. http://www.ncbi.nlm.nih.gov/pubmed/11888453. Accessed 13 Dec 2018.
19. Miccoli P, Bellantone R, Mourad M, Walz M, Raffaelli M, Berti P. Minimally invasive video-assisted thyroidectomy: multiinstitutional experience. World J Surg. 2002;26(8):972–5. https://doi.org/10.1007/s00268-002-6627-7.
20. Sessa L, Lombardi CP, De Crea C, Raffaelli M, Bellantone R. Video-assisted endocrine neck surgery: state of the art. Updat Surg. 2017;69(2):199–204. https://doi.org/10.1007/s13304-017-0467-3.
21. Lombardi CP, Raffaelli M, Princi P, et al. Safety of video-assisted thyroidectomy versus conventional surgery. Head Neck. 2005;27(1):58–64. https://doi.org/10.1002/hed.20118.
22. Bakkar S, Materazzi G, Biricotti M, et al. Minimally invasive video-assisted thyroidectomy (MIVAT) from A to Z. Surg Today. 2016;46(2):255–9. https://doi.org/10.1007/s00595-015-1241-0.
23. Bellantone R, Lombardi CP, Raffaelli M, Boscherini M, De Crea C, Traini E. Video-assisted thyroidectomy. J Am Coll Surg. 2002;194(5):610–4. http://www.ncbi.nlm.nih.gov/pubmed/12022601. Accessed 11 Dec 2018.
24. Miccoli P, Fregoli L, Rossi L, et al. Minimally invasive video-assisted thyroidectomy (MIVAT). Gland Surg. 2020;9(Suppl 1):S1–5. https://doi.org/10.21037/gs.2019.12.05.
25. Berti P, Materazzi G, Conte M, Galleri D, Miccoli P. Visualization of the external branch of the superior laryngeal nerve during video-assisted thyroidectomy. J Am Coll Surg. 2002;195(4):573–4. https://doi.org/10.1016/S1072-7515(02)01338-8.
26. Wilhelm T, Metzig A. Endoscopic minimally invasive thyroidectomy: first clinical experience. Surg Endosc. 2010;24(7):1757–8. https://doi.org/10.1007/s00464-009-0820-9.
27. Terris DJ, Angelos P, Steward DL, Simental AA. Minimally invasive video-assisted thyroidectomy: a multi-institutional North American experience. Arch Otolaryngol Head Neck Surg. 2008;134(1):81–4. https://doi.org/10.1001/archoto.2007.22.
28. Miccoli P, Berti P, Frustaci GL, Ambrosini CE, Materazzi G. Video-assisted thyroidectomy: indications and results. Langenbeck's Arch Surg. 2006;391(2):68–71. https://doi.org/10.1007/s00423-006-0027-7.
29. Lombardi CP, Raffaelli M, Princi P, De Crea C, Bellantone R. Video-assisted thyroidectomy: report of a 7-year experience in Rome. Langenbeck's Arch Surg. 2006;391(3):174–7. https://doi.org/10.1007/s00423-006-0023-y.
30. Lombardi CP, Raffaelli M, Princi P, De Crea C, Bellantone R. Video-assisted thyroidectomy: report on the experience of a single center in more than four hundred cases. World J Surg. 2006;30(5):794–800; discussion 801. https://doi.org/10.1007/s00268-005-0390-5.
31. Minuto MN, Berti P, Miccoli M, et al. Minimally invasive video-assisted thyroidectomy: an analysis of results and a revision of indications. Surg Endosc. 2012;26(3):818–22. https://doi.org/10.1007/s00464-011-1958-9.
32. Miccoli P, Berti P, Raffaelli M, Materazzi G, Baldacci S, Rossi G. Comparison between minimally invasive video-assisted thyroidectomy and conventional thyroidectomy: a prospective randomized study. Surgery. 2001;130(6):1039–43. https://doi.org/10.1067/msy.2001.118264.
33. Miccoli P, Rago R, Massi M, et al. Standard versus video-assisted thyroidectomy: objective postoperative pain evaluation. Surg Endosc. 2010;24(10):2415–7. https://doi.org/10.1007/s00464-010-0964-7.
34. Gal I, Solymosi T, Szabo Z, Balint A, Bolgar G. Minimally invasive video-assisted thyroidectomy and conventional thyroidectomy: a prospective randomized study. Surg Endosc. 2008;22(11):2445–9. https://doi.org/10.1007/s00464-008-9806-2.
35. El-Labban GM. Minimally invasive video-assisted thyroidectomy versus conventional thyroidectomy: a single-blinded, randomized controlled clinical trial. J Minim Access Surg. 2009;5(4):97–102. https://doi.org/10.4103/0972-9941.59307.
36. Lombardi CP, Raffaelli M, De Crea C, et al. Long-term outcome of functional post-thyroidectomy voice and swallowing symptoms. Surgery. 2009;146(6):1174–81. https://doi.org/10.1016/j.surg.2009.09.010.
37. Byrd JK, Nguyen SA, Ketcham A, Hornig J, Gillespie MB, Lentsch E. Minimally invasive video-assisted thyroidectomy versus conventional thyroidectomy: a cost-effective analysis. Otolaryngol Head Neck Surg. 2010;143(6):789–94. https://doi.org/10.1016/j.otohns.2010.08.002.
38. Zheng C, Liu S, Geng P, et al. Minimally invasive video-assisted versus conventional open thyroidectomy on immune response: a meta analysis. Int J Clin Exp Med. 2015;8(2):2593–9.
39. Lombardi CP, Raffaelli M, Modesti C, Boscherini M, Bellantone R. Video-assisted thyroidectomy under local anesthesia. Am J Surg. 2004;187(4):515–8. https://doi.org/10.1016/j.amjsurg.2003.12.030.
40. Berti P, Materazzi G, Galleri D, Donatini G, Minuto M, Miccoli P. Video-assisted thyroidectomy for Graves? Disease: report of a preliminary experience. Surg Endosc. 2004;18(8):1208–10. https://doi.org/10.1007/s00464-003-9225-3.
41. Miccoli P, Elisei R, Materazzi G, et al. Minimally invasive video-assisted thyroidectomy for papillary carcinoma: a prospective study of its completeness. Surgery. 2002;132(6):1070–4. https://doi.org/10.1067/msy.2002.128694.
42. Bellantone R, Lombardi CP, Raffaelli M, et al. Video-assisted thyroidectomy for papillary thyroid carcinoma. Surg Endosc. 2003;17(10):1604–8. https://doi.org/10.1007/s00464-002-9220-0.
43. Lombardi CP, Raffaelli M, de Crea C, et al. Report on 8 years of experience with video-assisted thyroidectomy for papillary thyroid carcinoma. Surgery. 2007;142(6):944–51. https://doi.org/10.1016/j.surg.2007.09.022.
44. Miccoli P, Pinchera A, Materazzi G, et al. Surgical treatment of low- and intermediate-risk papillary thyroid cancer with minimally invasive video-assisted thyroidectomy. J Clin Endocrinol Metab. 2009;94(5):1618–22. https://doi.org/10.1210/jc.2008-1418.
45. Lombardi CP, Raffaelli M, De Crea C, Sessa L, Rampulla V, Bellantone R. Video-assisted versus conventional total thyroidectomy and central compartment neck dissection for papillary thyroid carcinoma. World J Surg. 2012;36(6):1225–30. https://doi.org/10.1007/s00268-012-1439-x.
46. Bellantone R, Lombardi CP, Raffaelli M, Boscherini M, Alesina PF, Princi P. Central neck lymph node removal during minimally invasive video-assisted thyroidectomy for thyroid carcinoma: a feasible and safe procedure. J Laparoendosc Adv Surg Tech – Part A. 2002;12(3):181–5. https://doi.org/10.1089/10926420260188074.
47. Miccoli P, Elisei R, Donatini G, Materazzi G, Berti P. Video-assisted central compartment lymphadenectomy in a patient with a positive RET oncogene: initial experience. Surg Endosc Other Interv Tech. 2007;21(1):120–3. https://doi.org/10.1007/s00464-005-0642-3.
48. Miccoli P, Elisei R, Berti P, et al. Video assisted prophylactic thyroidectomy and central compartment nodes clearance in two RET gene mutation adult carriers. J Endocrinol Investig. 2004;27(6):557–61. https://doi.org/10.1007/BF03347478.
49. Miccoli P, Berti P, Raffaelli M, Materazzi G, Conte M, Galleri D. Impact of Harmonic Scalpel on operative time during video-assisted thyroidectomy. Surg Endosc. 2002;16(4):663–6. https://doi.org/10.1007/s00464-001-9117-3.
50. Raffaelli M, Traini E, Lombardi CP, Bellantone R. Minimally invasive video-assisted parathyroidectomy: how to correctly approach of the adenoma. In: Shifrin A, editor. Atlas of parathyroid surgery. New York: Springer; 2020.

Robotic Total Thyroidectomy via Bilateral Axillo-Breast Approach (BABA)

13

Hyunsuk Suh

Introduction

The bilateral axillo-breast approach (BABA) robotic thyroidectomy is one of the most comprehensive remote-access or "scarless" thyroid surgery techniques. The combination of a robotic platform and four widely spaced and symmetrical incisions across the chest provides the most ideal triangulation as well as refined maneuverability of the instruments. Furthermore, it provides the most familiar orientation and midline view of the thyroid. The readily extensible subplatysmal flap ensures adequate working space for larger goiters and advanced thyroid cancer, including lateral neck lymph node metastasis, leading to an improved overall quality of life in eliminating relatively large visible cervical scars, especially in those with a history of hypertrophic or keloid scar formation [1, 2].

The BABA technique was initially described by Dr. Youn in 2004 at the Seoul National University in South Korea. The technique was initially performed endoscopically, but the robotic platform was adopted just a few years later for its advantages, such as enhanced 3D visualization with 10x magnification, superior dexterity with endo-wrist function, and surgeon autonomy [3]. Its safety and efficacy have been well established over the years, driven by excellent surgical and oncologic outcomes as well as patient satisfaction [4, 5].

The BABA robotic technique can have a relatively steeper learning curve (35–40 cases) [6], but the overall efficacy and safety have been well established in Asia and the first series of 200 cases performed in the United States (recently submitted for publication). These outcome-based studies show that the robotic BABA technique is a very comprehensive treatment option for benign and malignant diseases of the thyroid and applicable to the US patient population with comparable excellent results and low rates of both standard and technique-specific complications.

H. Suh (✉)
Suh Scarless Thyroid Surgery Center, Norman/Clayman Endocrine Institute, Hospital for Endocrine Surgery, Tampa, FL, USA

Procedure

A 32-year-old woman presented to the endocrine surgery service with left isthmic 3.5-cm and 1.6-cm multifocal papillary thyroid cancer. During her workup, the patient was found to have contralateral lateral neck level 3 lymph node metastasis. Given the findings, the patient had opted for the BABA robotic total thyroidectomy with bilateral central neck and right modified radical neck dissection.

For the BABA technique, patient positioning is very similar to the open thyroidectomy with neck extension and arms relaxed on the side, exposing the axillary skin creases (Fig. 13.1). Neuromonitoring for the recurrent laryngeal nerve is routinely utilized to assist with early nerve localization and the evaluation of its function throughout the surgery. Depending on the device, the nerve stimulator cord can be attached to the robotic instrument, such as a hook cautery. After the hydrodissection using diluted (1:200,000) epinephrine solution along the subcutaneous flap space, four 8-mm skin incisions are made along the anterior axillary skin creases and peri-areolar margins. Then a blunt dissection is performed using a vascular tunneller. Trocars are inserted, and the flap space is completed under direct visualization. The robotic arms are docked, maintaining a wide-angle separation (Fig. 13.2) with the camera in arm 2 and the energy device (i.e., Hook, Harmonic scalpel, etc.) in arm 3. Graspers (i.e., ProGrasp, Cardiere, etc.) and dissectors/forceps (i.e., Maryland bipolar) are inserted in arms 1 and 4 to provide two opposing instruments for ideal traction and countertraction. A familiar view of the anterior neck is achieved with exposed strap muscles and bilateral sternocleidomastoid muscles (Fig. 13.3).

The remaining steps of the surgery are similar to open thyroidectomy. The medial raphe is divided, and the exposed isthmus is divided using the energy device (Fig. 13.4). Then lateral dissection is performed to separate the strap muscles down to the carotid sheath while providing medial retraction of the thyroid gland using the contralateral grasper. The inferior parathyroid gland should be

A. Shifrin (ed.), *Atlas of Thyroid Surgery*, https://doi.org/10.1007/978-3-030-93673-0_13

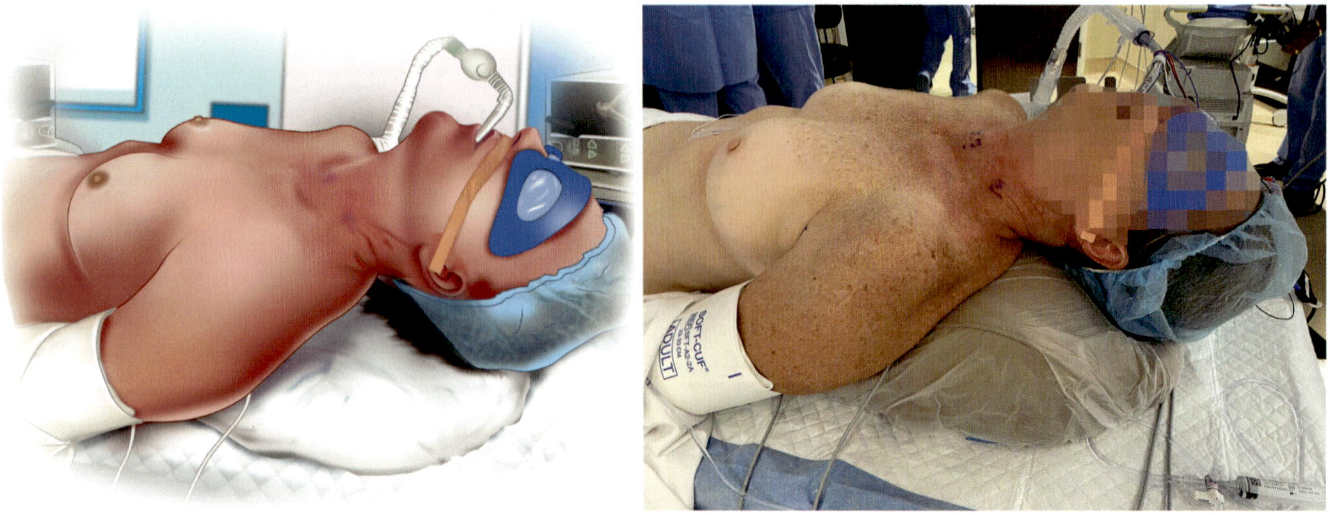

Fig. 13.1 Patient positioning is very similar to open thyroid surgery. Neck is extended, and arms are down to the side, exposing the anterior axillary skin folds

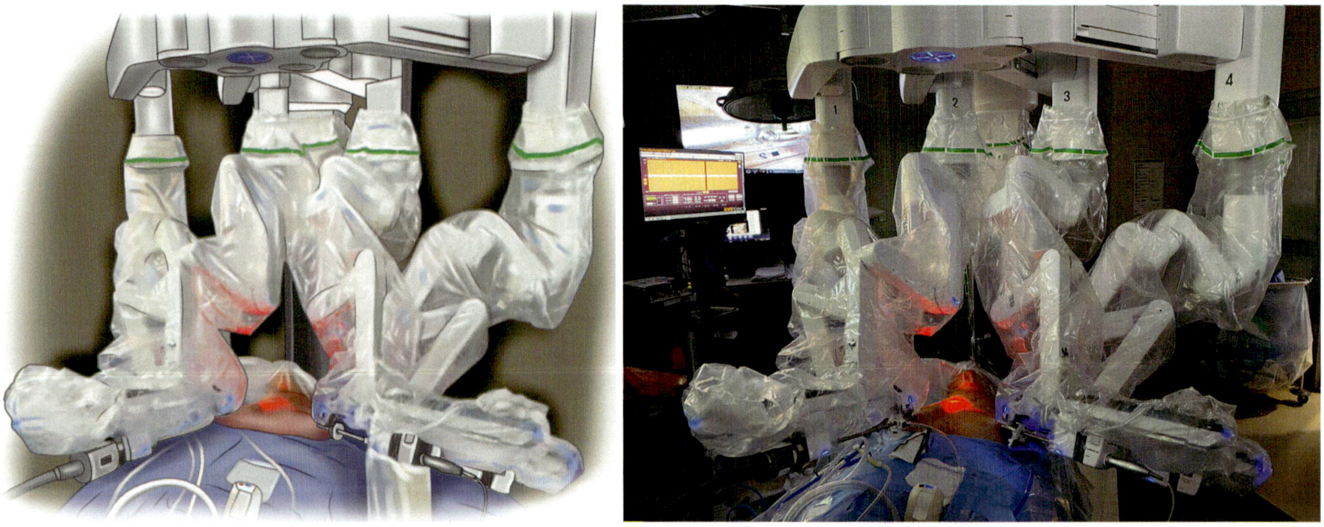

Fig. 13.2 Robot arms are widely spaced, providing an ideal triangulation, depth perception, and working space. Robot arm collision is minimized

localized, along with its pedicle (Fig. 13.5a). The carotid artery is exposed, and the vagus nerve is tested using the robotic hook cautery. Subsequently, the recurrent laryngeal nerve is localized and dissected distally toward the insertion site (Fig. 13.5b).

Once the nerve has been localized, the inferior parathyroid gland is dissected off the thyroid. The recurrent laryngeal nerve is dissected caudal to cranial, and the ligament of Berry is sharply divided. The inferior thyroid artery is dissected and divided while preserving any branches to the inferior and superior parathyroid glands. The superior parathyroid glands are dissected off with anteromedial retraction of the thyroid gland (Fig. 13.5c). The superior pole is isolated circumferentially with exploration of the cricothyroid space. The superior-pole vessel is clearly isolated and explGred for the external branch of the superior laryngeal nerve prior to dividing the vessels. The contralateral lobe is removed in a similar fashion. The bilateral axillary instruments are swapped (grasper and dissectors), given the reversed role in thyroid retraction and dissection (Fig. 13.6). The superior-pole vessels can be clipped and divided using the robotic clip applier (Fig. 13.7). The two breast trocar instruments (robotic

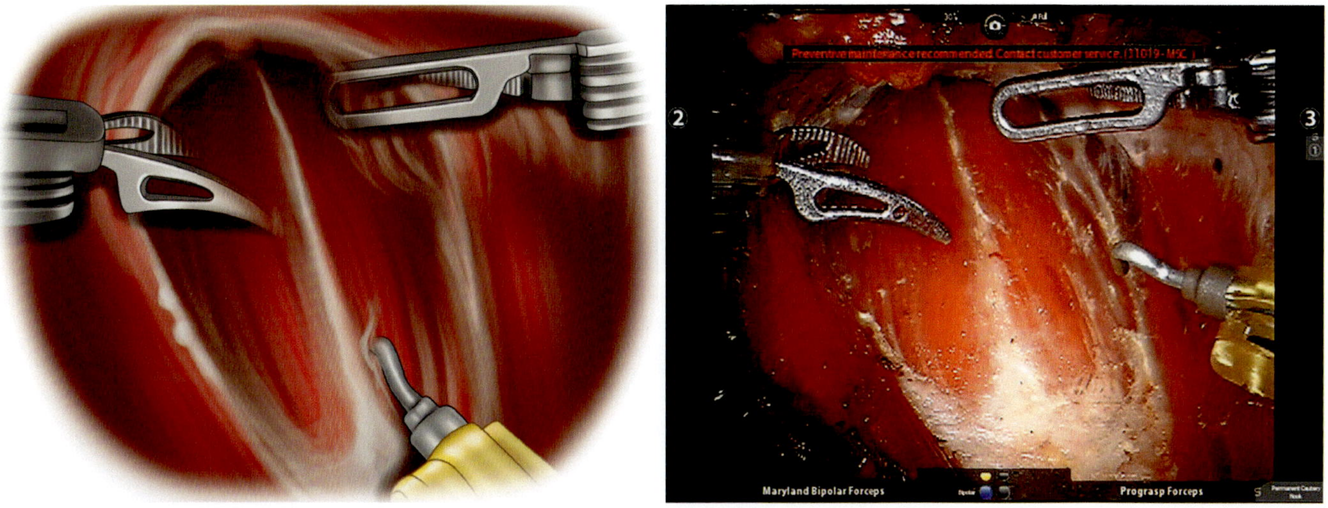

Fig. 13.3 Completion of subplatysmal flap with midline visualization of strap muscles and bilateral sternocleidomastoid muscles. Triangulation with two opposing instruments (left Maryland dissector and right ProGrasp grasper) and an energy device (hook cautery monopolar)

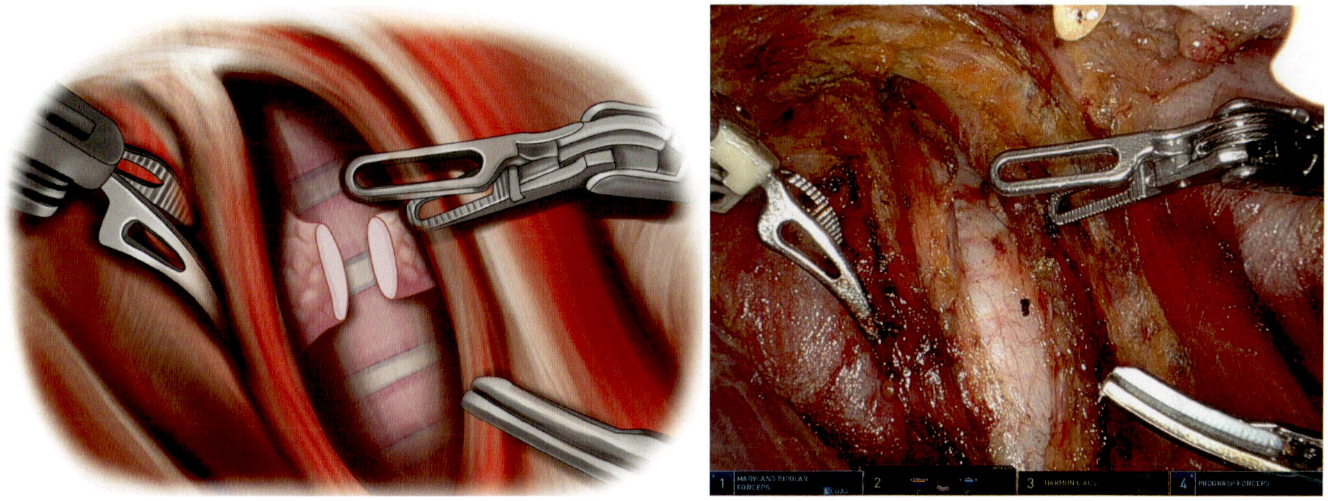

Fig. 13.4 Strap muscle is divided along the median raphe, and isthmus is divided, exposing the trachea

camera and energy devices) can be swapped depending on your preference.

Once the thyroidectomy has been completed, therapeutic central neck dissection is performed. For right central neck dissection, anteromedial lymph nodes were dissected first (Fig. 13.8a). Then the posterolateral lymph nodes were dissected (Fig. 13.8b). Subsequently, the right modified radical neck dissection is performed by extending the subcutaneous flap to expose the sternocleidomastoid (SCM) muscle (Fig. 13.9). The SCM muscle is retracled laterally using a percutaneous suture held by an external fixed retractor (Fig. 13.10). The carotid artery and internal jugular vein are dissected using a Cardiere grasper, while the vagus nerve is preserved (Fig. 13.11a). Jugular and prevertebral lymph nodes are dissected (Fig. 13.11b). The spinal accessory nerve is localized and preserved for lateral neck level 2 and 3 dissection (Fig. 13.12a, b).

Once the dissection is completed and hemostasis has been achieved, the strap muscle is closed (Fig. 13.13). For specimen extraction, an endoscopic specimen retrieval bag is used and typically removed through the left axillary trocar site. In general, axillary skin is very elastic and accommodating, but for large specimens, the trocar track can be dilated and the skin incision can be extended.

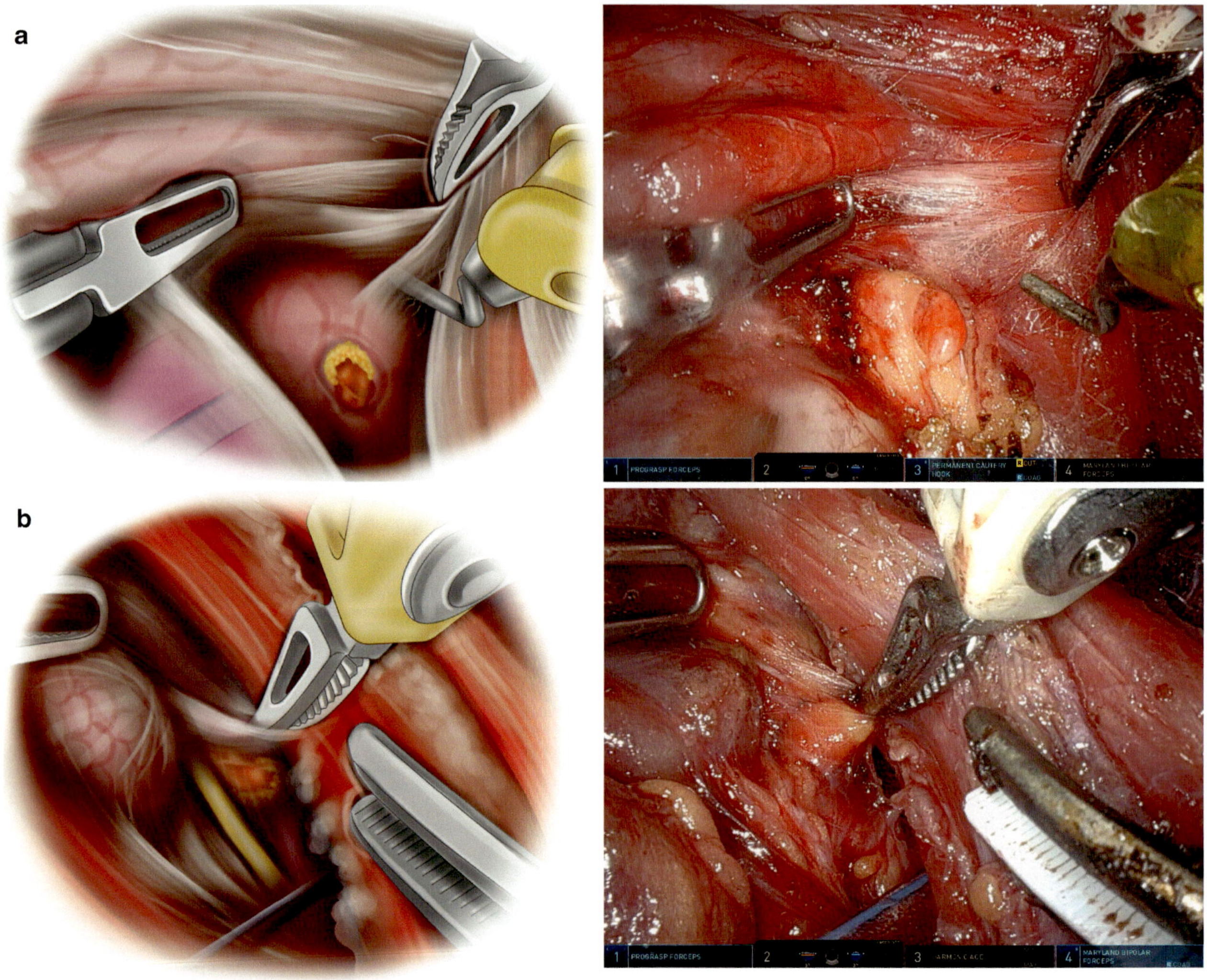

Fig. 13.5 (**a**) Strap muscle is dissected laterally to expose the inferior parathyroid gland. (**b**) The recurrent laryngeal nerve is localized and dissected distally toward the insertion site while the superior parathyroid gland is dissected off with anteromedial retraction of the thyroid gland

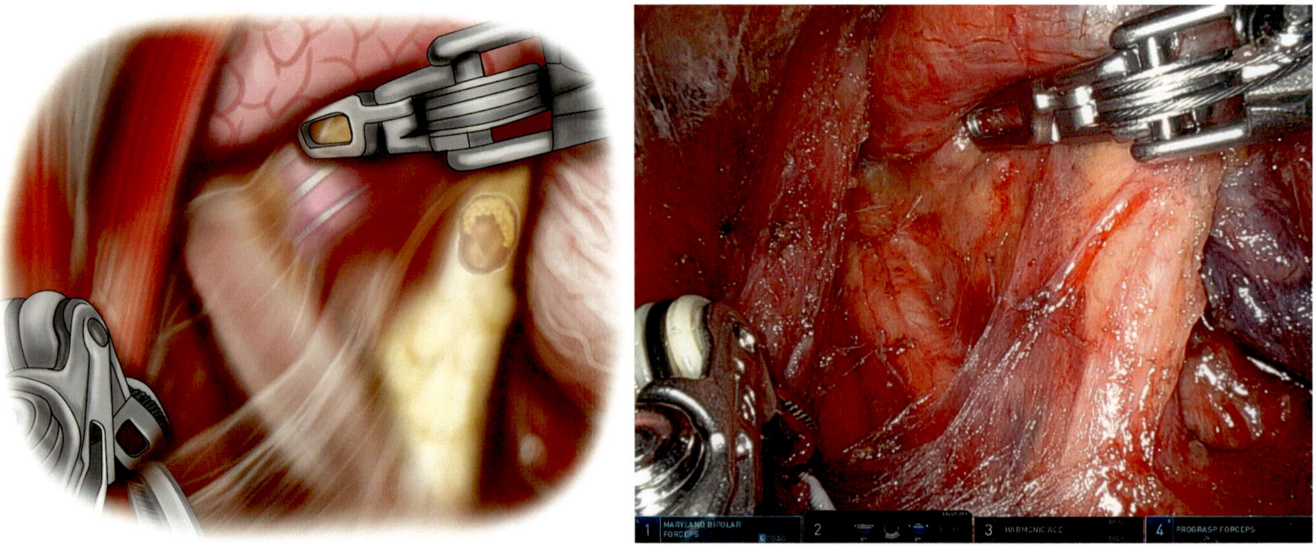

Fig. 13.6 The contralateral lobe is removed in a similar fashion. The bilateral axillary instruments are swapped (grasper and dissectors), given the reversed role in thyroid retraction and dissection

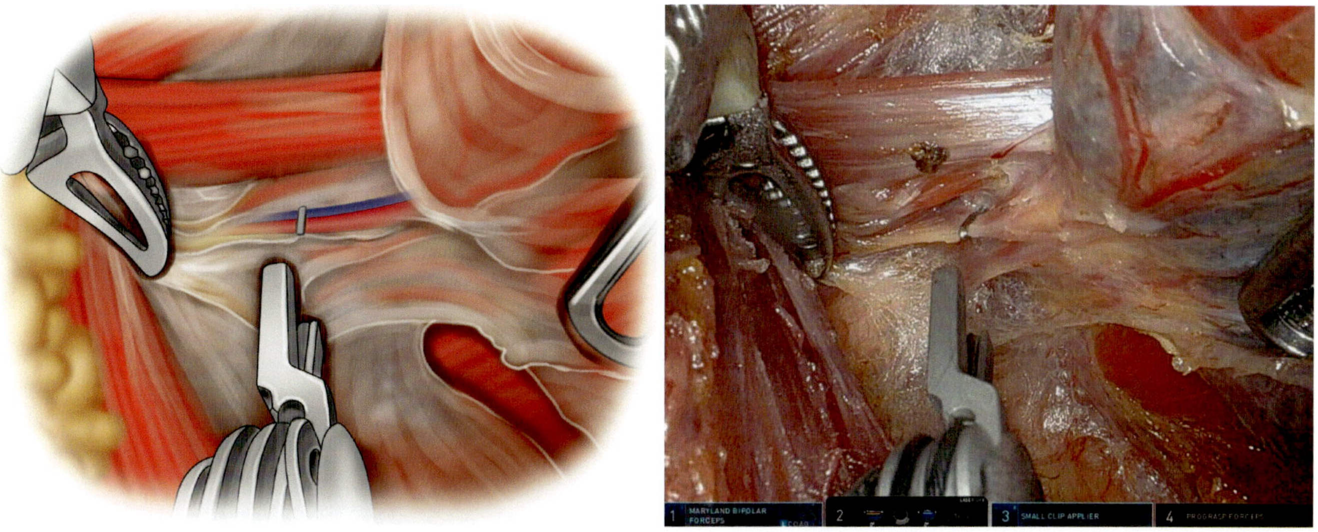

Fig. 13.7 The superior-pole vessels can be clipped and divided using the robotic clip applier

a

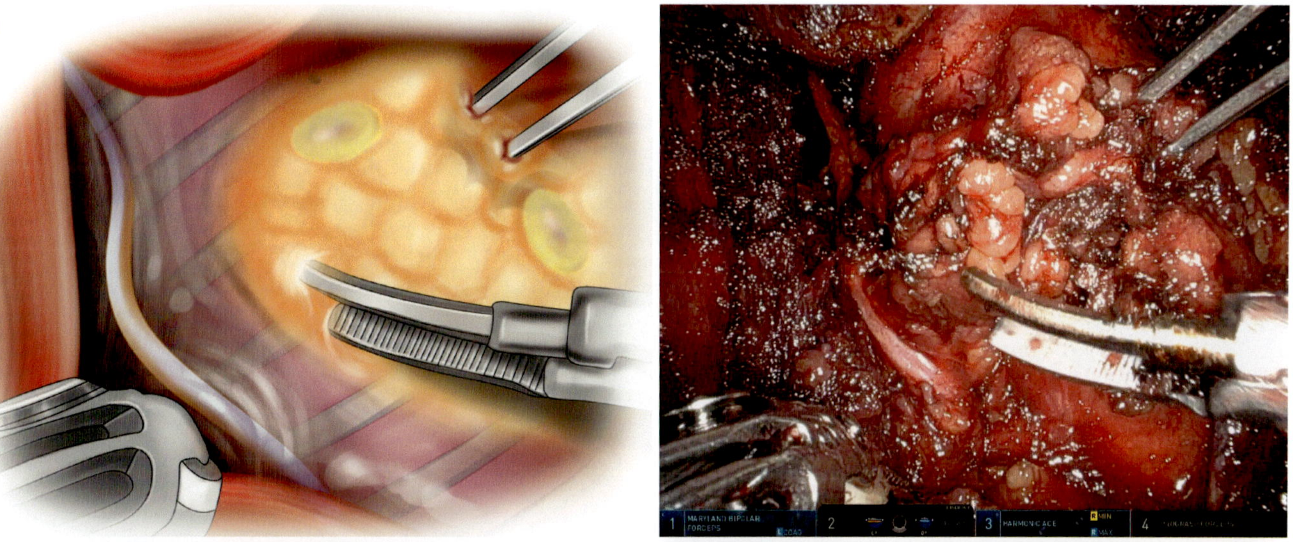

b

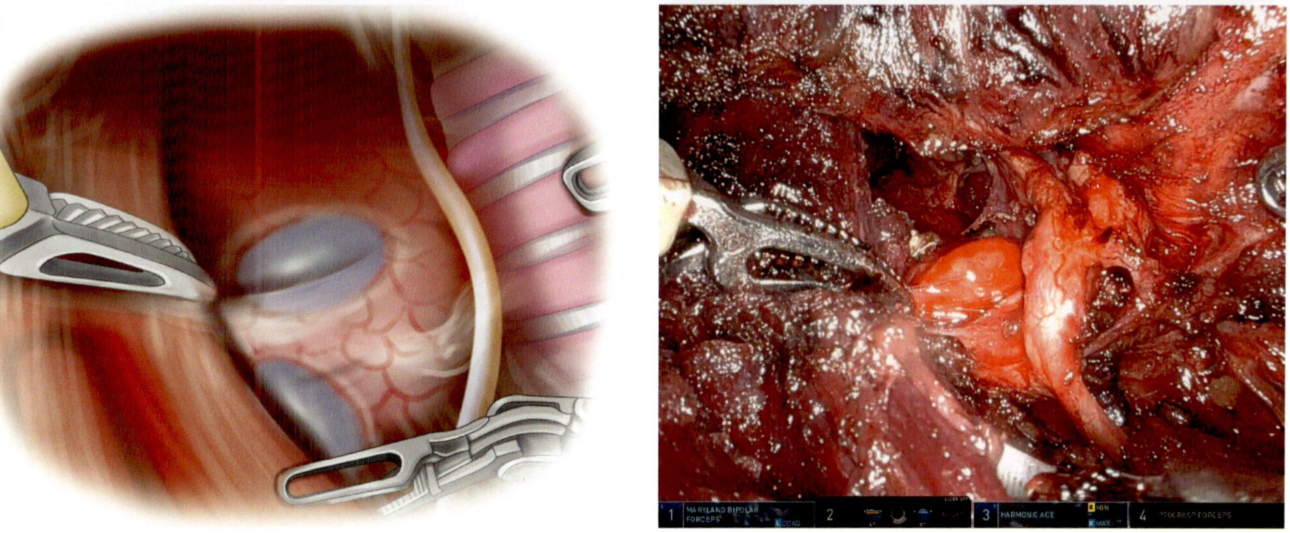

Fig. 13.8 (**a**) Anteromedial lymph nodes are dissected. (**b**) Posterolateral lymph nodes are dissected

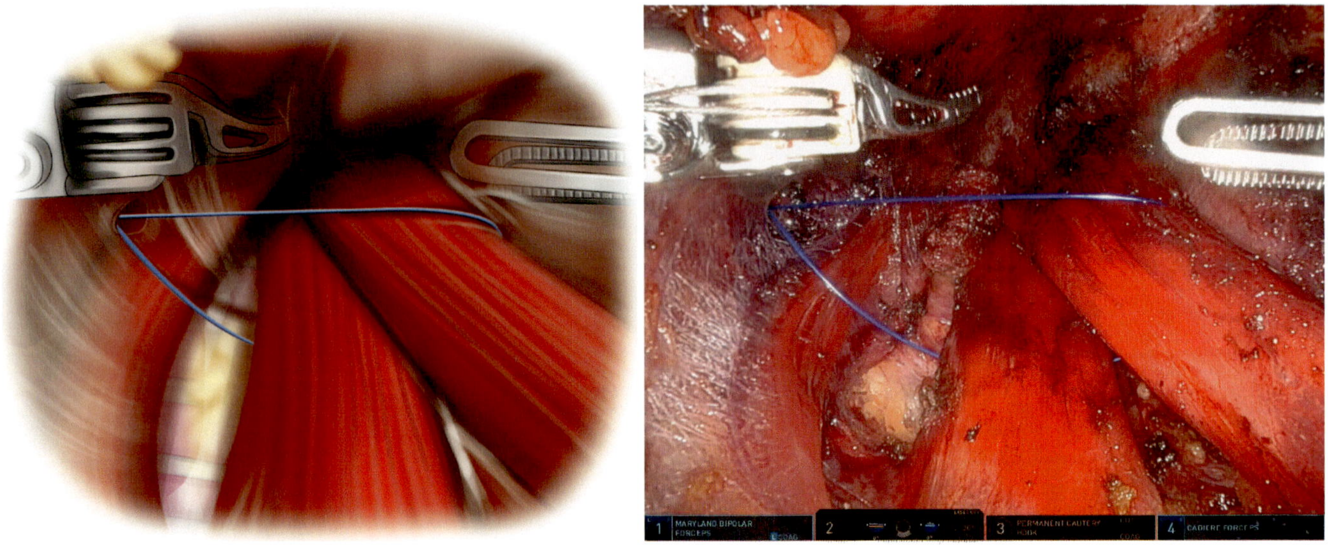

Fig. 13.9 Right modified radical neck dissection is performed by extending the subcutaneous flap to expose the SCM muscle

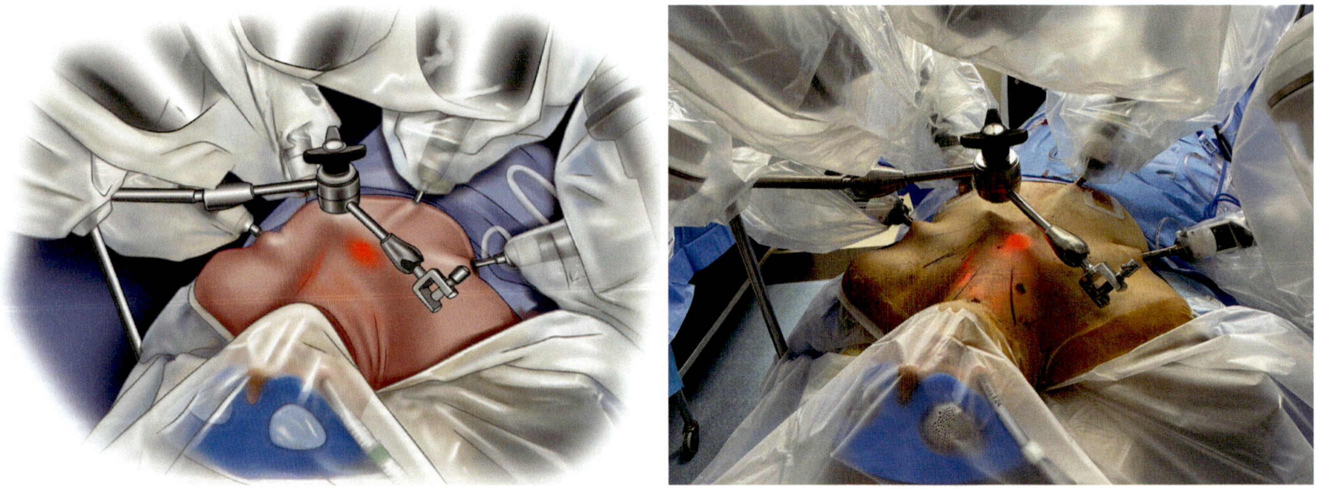

Fig. 13.10 The SCM muscle is retracted laterally using a percutaneous suture held by an external fixed retractor

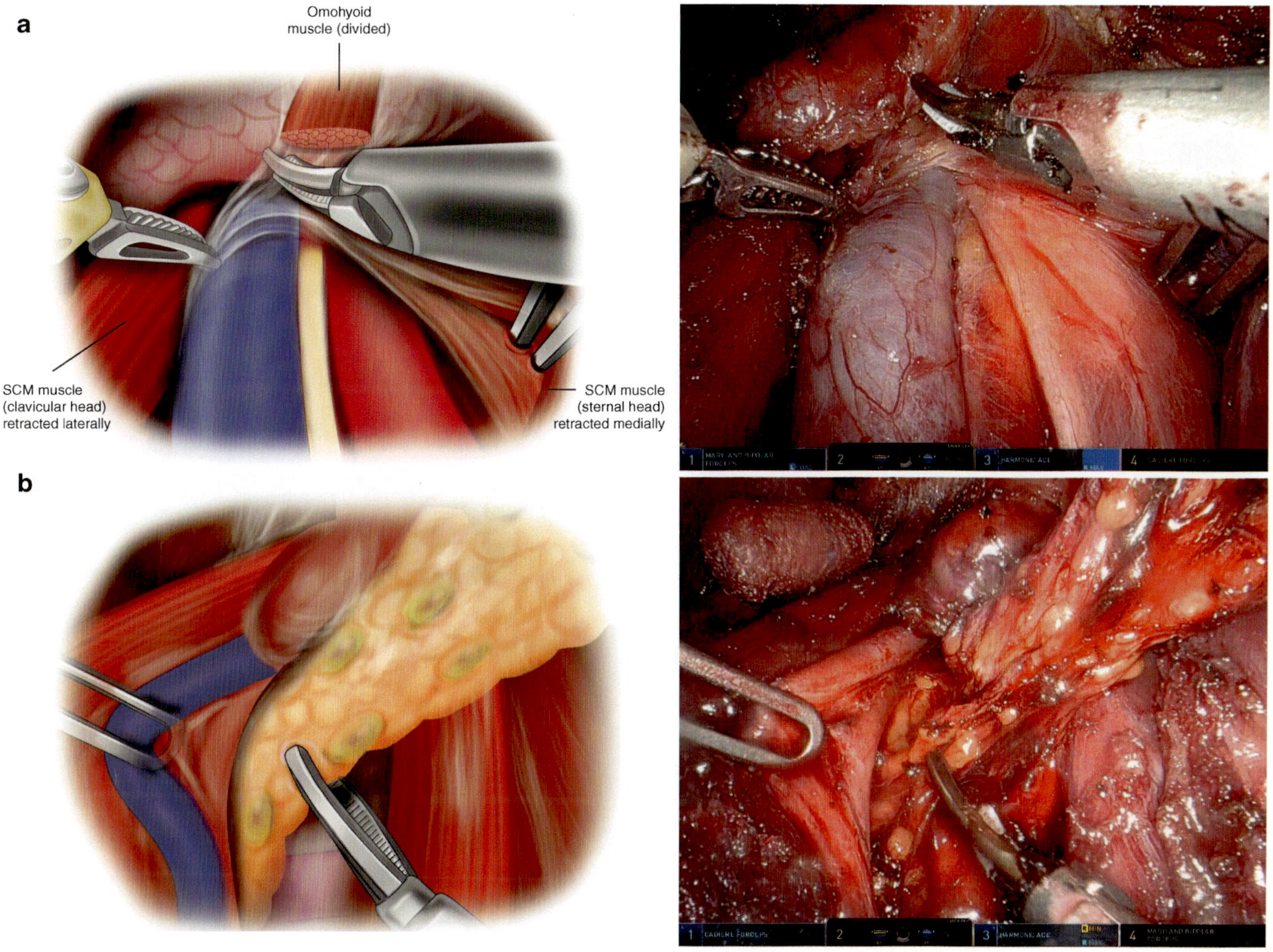

Fig. 13.11 (**a**) The carotid artery and internal jugular vein are dissected using a Cardiere grasper, while the vagus nerve is preserved. (**b**) Jugular and prevertebral lymph nodes are dissected

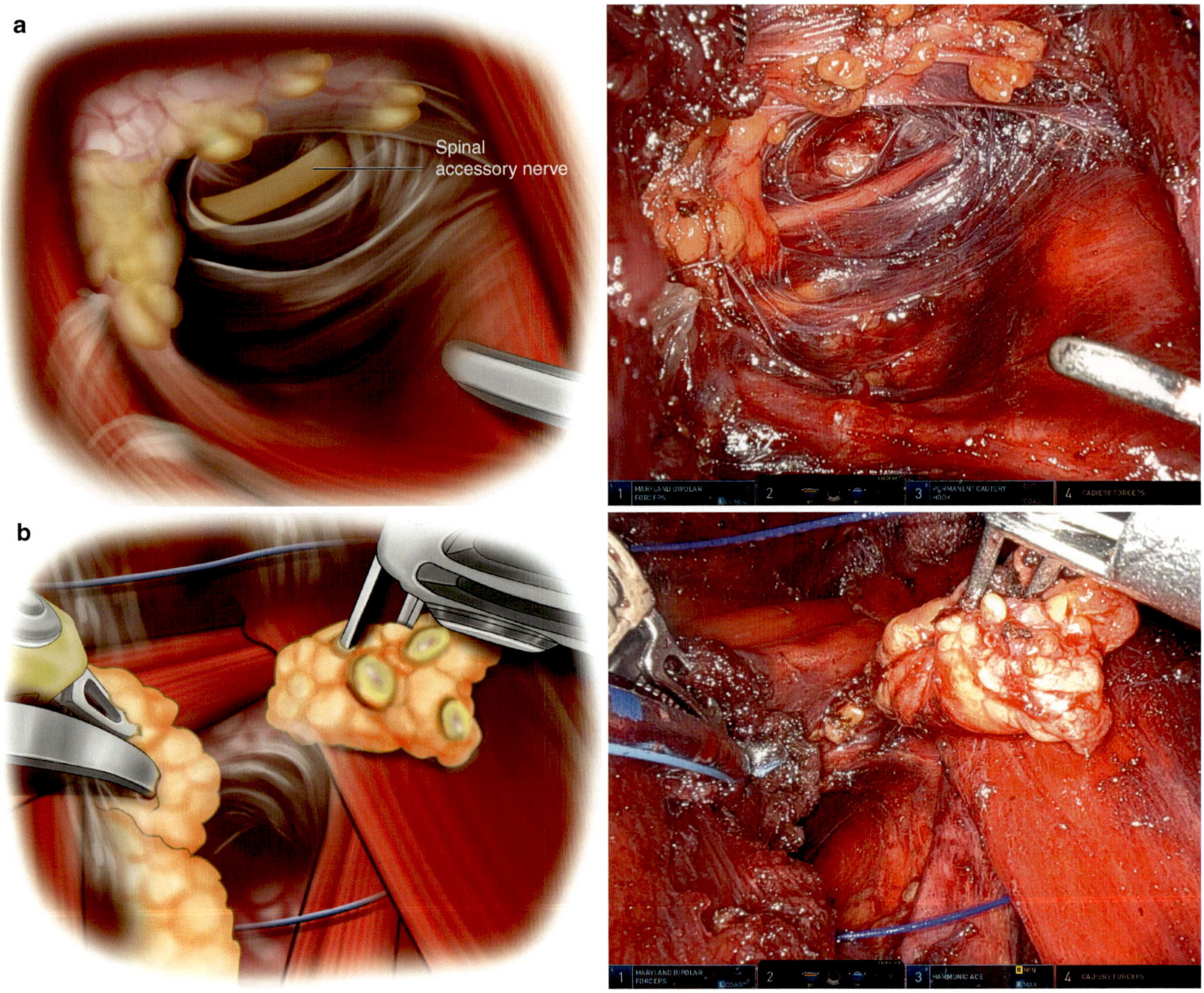

Fig. 13.12 (**a**, **b**) The spinal accessory nerve is well localized and preserved for lateral neck level 2 and 3 dissection

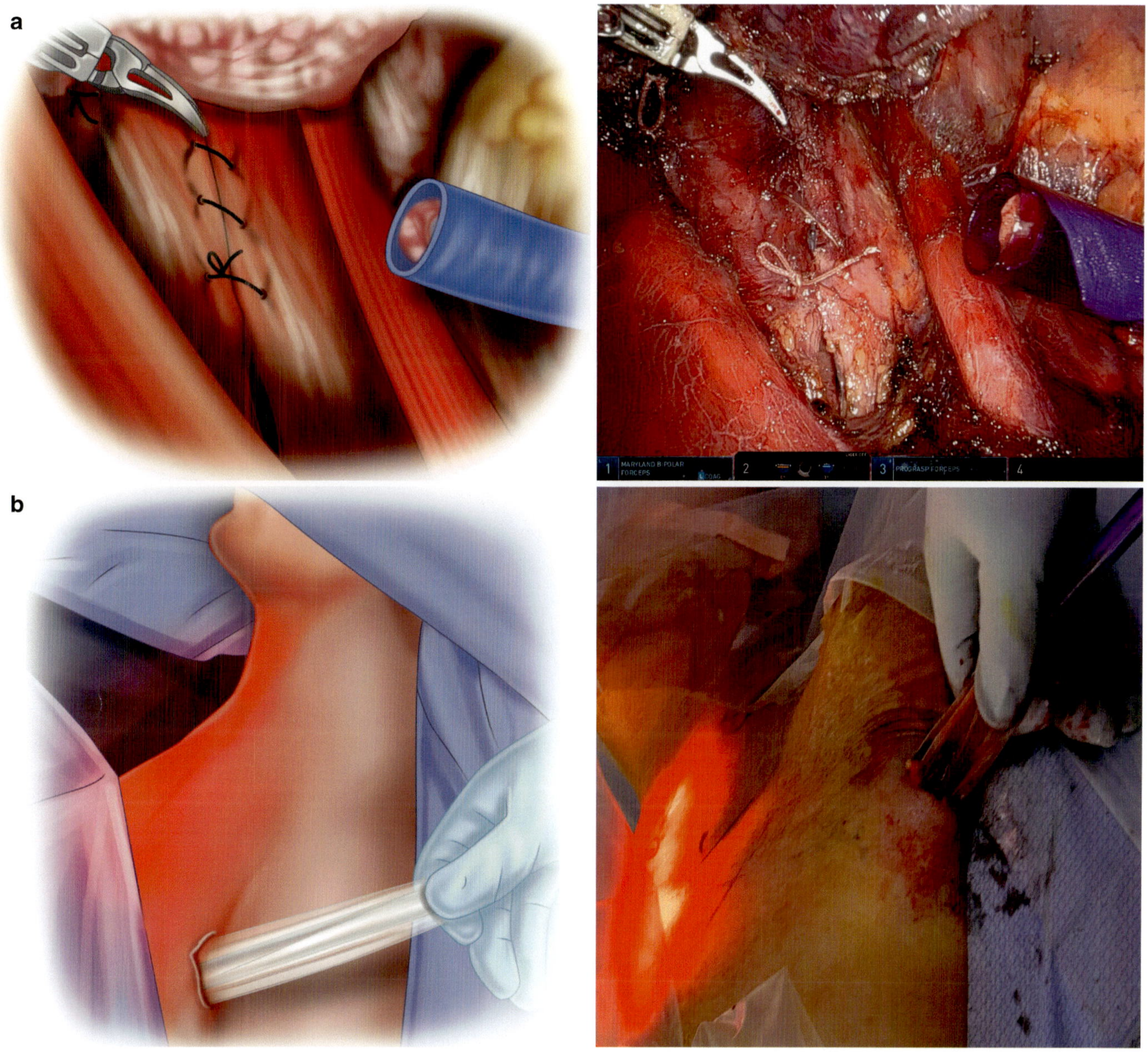

Fig. 13.13 (**a**, **b**) Once the dissection is completed and hemostasis has been achieved, strap muscle is closed

References

1. Choi Y, Lee JH, Kim YH, et al. Impact of post thyroidectomy scar on the quality of life of thyroid cancer patients. Ann Dermatol. 2014;26:693–9.
2. Arora A, Swords C, Garas G, et al. The perception of scar cosmesis following thyroid and parathyroid surgery: a prospective cohort study. Int J Surg. 2016;25:38–43.
3. Choe JH, Kim SW, Chung KW, et al. Endoscopic thyroidectomy using a new bilateral axillo-breast approach. World J Surg. 2007;31:601–6.
4. Lee KE, Kim E, Koo DH, et al. Robotic thyroidectomy by bilateral axillo-breast approach: review of 1026 cases and surgical completeness. Surg Endosc. 2013;27:2955–62.
5. Chai YJ, Suh H, Woo JW, et al. Surgical safety and oncological completeness of robotic thyroidectomy for thyroid carcinoma larger than 2 cm. Surg Endosc. 2017;31:1235–40.
6. Liu SYW, Kim JS. Bilateral axillo-breast approach robotic thyroidectomy: review of evidence. Gland Surg. 2017;6:250–7.

14 Transoral Endoscopic Total Thyroidectomy via Vestibular Approach (TOETVA)

Joon-Hyop Lee, Sihoon Lee, and Young Jun Chai

Introduction

Transoral thyroidectomy is the first true "scarless" minimally invasive approach, unlike its predecessors such as transaxillary, bilateral axillo-breast, and retroauricular approaches, because it does not involve any incision on the skin. The concept was first proposed by Witzel in 2008, when he demonstrated the first proof-of-concept hybrid transoral thyroidectomy with human cadavers and animals [1]. In the early stages of its development, the approach was sublingual (Fig. 14.1), meaning that the access was made through the oral cavity inside the mandible [1–3]. But as several cases of recurrent laryngeal and mental nerve injuries were reported in the early stages of its clinical application, the sublingual route lost its position as the primary oral access [4]. The alternative method was the vestibular approach (Fig. 14.1), first demonstrated in 2011, in which the access point was repositioned exterior to the mandible and beneath the platysma muscle layer [5]. This approach gained increasing popularity among endocrine surgeons, and in 2016, Anuwong published the first large-scale human transoral endoscopic thyroidectomy vestibular approach (TOETVA) study, including 60 cases [6]. In this landmark study, the postoperative complication rates of the novel approach were reported to be comparable to the conventional open and minimally invasive thyroidectomies. The same group subsequently published a comparison study of 432 TOETVA and open thyroidectomy cases, which were matched by propensity scores [7]. The postoperative results of this study were comparable as well. At the moment, TOETVA is being conducted in more than 80 institutions across over 30 countries [8]. The advantages of TOETVA, apart from its scarless nature, include median symmetric view, which allows total thyroidectomy to be done without additional incisions, minimal transoral specific complications such as mental nerve injury and/or oral infection, and easy access to the central lymph nodes due to its cephalocaudal orientation [8].

J.-H. Lee (✉)
Department of Surgery, Gachon University College of Medicine, Gil Medical Center, Incheon, Republic of Korea
e-mail: deftnovice@gachon.ac.kr

S. Lee
Gachon Medical Research Institute, Gachon University College of Medicine, Gil Medical Center, Incheon, Republic of Korea

Y. J. Chai
Department of Surgery, Seoul Metropolitan Government-Seoul National University, Boramae Medical Center, Seoul, Republic of Korea

Indication and Contraindication of TOETVA

TOETVA has just passed its juvenile stage in its development as a feasible surgical approach and is starting to be spread across the world. The procedure, however, remains relatively reserved to a select group of experts compared to open or other minimally invasive thyroidectomies. There are no absolute inclusion and exclusion criteria, which may differ according to the surgeons' experience level of TOETVA. In general, the criteria are similar to those of other minimally invasive thyroidectomies [8]. (1) Benign tumors or follicular neoplasms that are 3 cm or smaller in its largest diameter and (2) differentiated thyroid carcinomas that are 2 cm or smaller in its largest diameter without evidence of lymph node metastasis may be feasible indications. For experienced surgeons, however, the indication may be extended to include controlled Graves' disease and differentiated thyroid carcinomas larger than 2 cm in diameter with evidence of suspicious central lymph node metastasis. On the other hand, total thyroidectomy should be limited to lesions that do not require central neck node dissection for those with less experience to prevent complications such as bilateral recurrent laryngeal nerve palsies or hypoparathyroidism. Exclusion criteria consist of patients with (1) a history of radiation in the head, neck, or upper mediastinum or of previous neck surgery; (2) evidence of suspicious lateral lymph node, distant metastases, or tracheal/esophageal/posterior infiltration; and (3) medullary and poorly/undifferentiated histology.

A. Shifrin (ed.), *Atlas of Thyroid Surgery*, https://doi.org/10.1007/978-3-030-93673-0_14

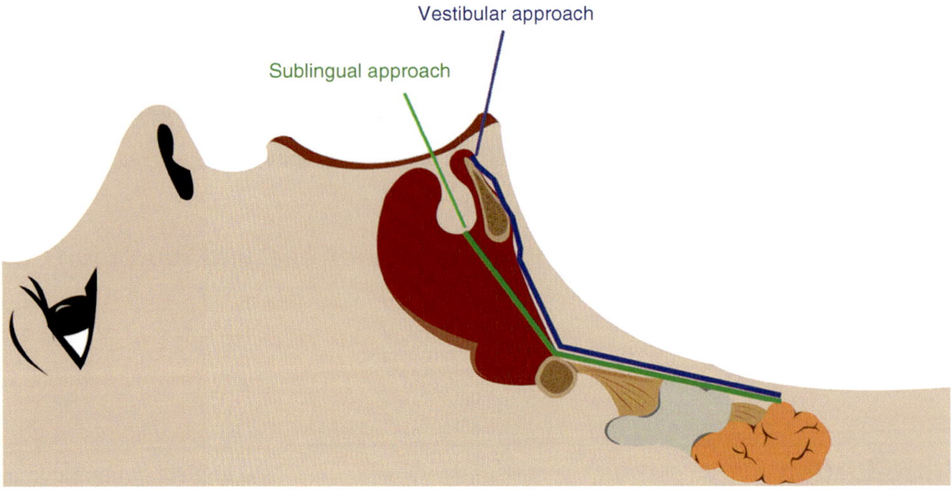

Fig. 14.1 Schematics of sublingual and vestibular access of transoral thyroidectomy

Procedure

Position and Preparation

The patient is placed in a lithotomy position with the neck extended under general anesthesia (Fig. 14.2). Either nasotracheal or oral intubation is possible. The monitor is positioned between the legs of the patient. The surgeon faces the monitor on the head side of the patient, and the assistant and nurse are positioned on the left side and right side of the surgeon, respectively, for right-handed surgeons (vice versa for left-handed surgeons). The type and dosage of preoperative prophylactic antibiotics do not differ from those of open thyroidectomy.

Skin marking should be done on the skin of the neck area to indicate the thyroid notch, cricothyroid cartilage, medial borders of the sternocleidomastoid muscles (SCM), sternal notch, and midline for orientation purposes (Fig. 14.3). The oral cavity is disinfected with chlorhexidine-soaked gauzes. The disinfectant solution should not be poured freely into the oral cavity as it may flow into the nasal cavity and cause adverse effects on the olfactory nerves.

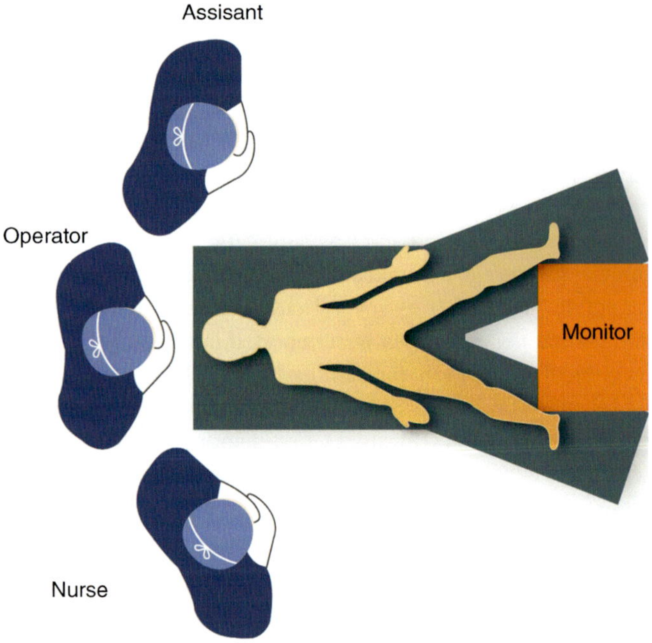

Fig. 14.2 Operating room setting; the patient is in lithotomy position, and the monitor is placed between the legs. The surgeon faces the monitor on the head side of the patient, and the assistant and nurse are positioned on the left and right side of the surgeon, respectively

Incision

The incisions are situated at the lower buccal mucosa. The main 11-mm incision is made at the center of the oral vestibule, and the auxiliary 5-mm incisions are made at both sides (Fig. 14.4a). Attention should be paid to position the main incision nearer the lip rather than the inferior buccal gingiva and leave at least 1 cm of spare buccal mucosa in order to facilitate the angulation of the camera during operation and mucosal suture at the end of surgery. Furthermore, the 5-mm trocar incisions should be situated lateral to the canine in order to avoid mental nerve injury.

In patients without any cardiovascular history, a mixture of 0.5 ml 1:1000 epinephrine solution and 4.5 ml saline can be injected into the incision site prior to the incision in order to reduce profuse mucosal bleeding (Fig. 14.4b).

Flap Formation

Through the middle incision, the periosteum of the mental protuberance should be visualized after resecting the mentalis muscles. After identifying the periosteal layer, a vascular graft tunneler is used to create the initial part of the flap

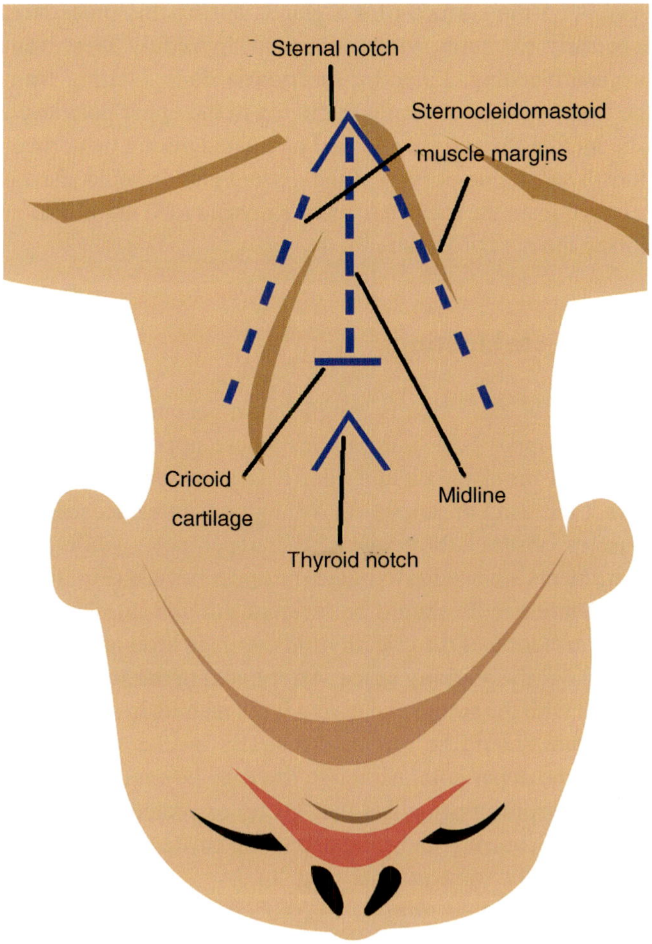

Fig. 14.3 Skin marking to demarcate the important structures for orientation purposes

over the mandible down to the level of the larynx. When gliding the tunneler over the mandible, it should feel as if the surgeon is attempting to scratch the bone with the instrument to ensure access to the subplatysmal layer. A blunt-tipped 10-mm trocar is then inserted through this path, and CO_2 is connected to insufflate the working space to pressure at no higher than 6 mmHg to prevent subcutaneous emphysema. The two 5-mm trocars are inserted through the lateral incisions straight down before crossing over the chin and redirected medially after crossing the mandible (Fig. 14.5). While gliding over the chin, special attention must be paid to prevent the trocars from perforating the skin. At this stage, a 10-mm 30-degree rigid endoscope is inserted through the main trocar to visually check if both 5-mm trocars have access to the subplatysmal working space.

The extent of the flap should consist of the upper border as the top of the larynx, the lower border as the sternal notch, and the lateral borders as the medial borders of both SCM. In patients with a protruding chin, it is difficult to obtain a lower area view due to acute angulation. In such cases, the view may be more easily acquired by rotating the 30-degree rigid endoscope 180 degrees (Fig 14.6a, b).

Midline Dissection and Isthmectomy

After creating the working space, the midline of the strap muscles should be resected starting from above the thyroid notch all the way down to the sternal notch. In order to easily visualize the upper pole of the thyroid gland later on, it is important to dissect the midline as high up as possible.

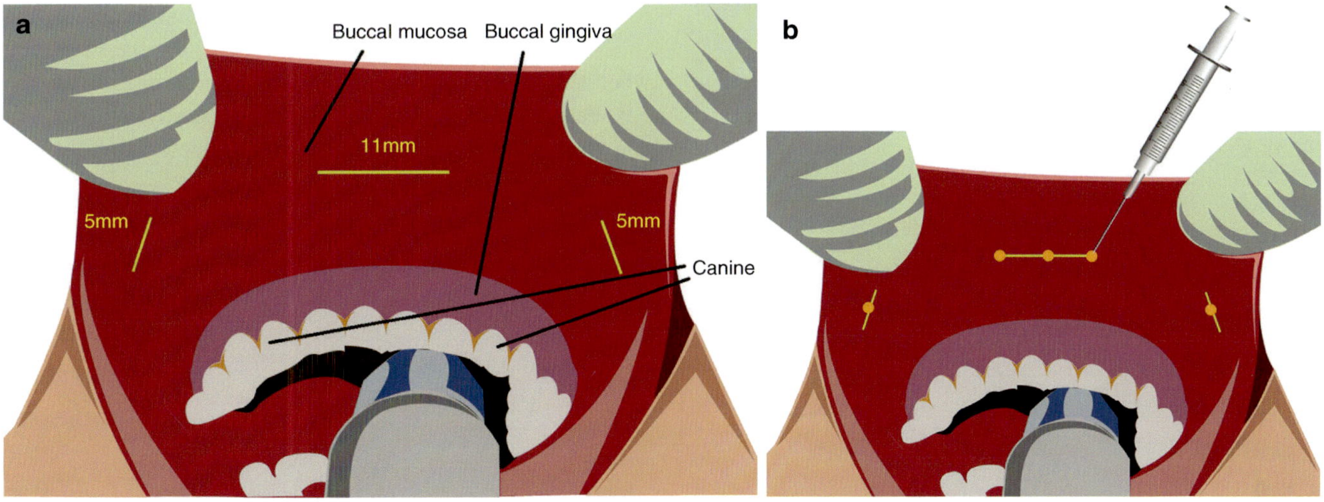

Fig. 14.4 Intraoral incision of TOETVA. (**a**) The main 11-mm incision is made in the middle of the oral mucosa. It should be situated nearer the lip than the inferior buccal gingiva, leaving at least 1 cm of buccal mucosa to facilitate camera angulation and mucosal suture. The 5-mm trocar incisions should be situated lateral to the canine in order to avoid mental nerve injury (**b**). Injection site of the saline/epinephrine mixture prior to incision. Inject 5 mm of the mixture at the red dotted area equally to reduce mucosal bleeding

The isthmus of the thyroid gland will be revealed after dissecting the midline of the strap muscles. In total thyroidectomy cases, it is advisable to dissect the isthmus evenly across the middle in order to leave some tissue for both lobes to grasp during medial traction, if there are no lesions in the isthmus. Depending on which direction it is skewed, the pyramidal lobe should be resected from the larynx and resected later *enbloc* with the closer lobe.

Lateral Dissection

By medially retracting the isthmic stump, it becomes easy to separate the strap muscles from the thyroid gland along the avascular plane. Attention should be paid to preserving the vessels on the surface of the glands during this procedure, especially for cases with concurrent thyroiditis, to prevent profuse bleeding. Lateral dissection is done, starting from the lower pole level then working up to the upper pole level. The middle thyroid vein should be ligated during this procedure. The isthmic portion of the thyroid gland should also be resected from the trachea to ensure thyroid lobe mobilization during the next procedures.

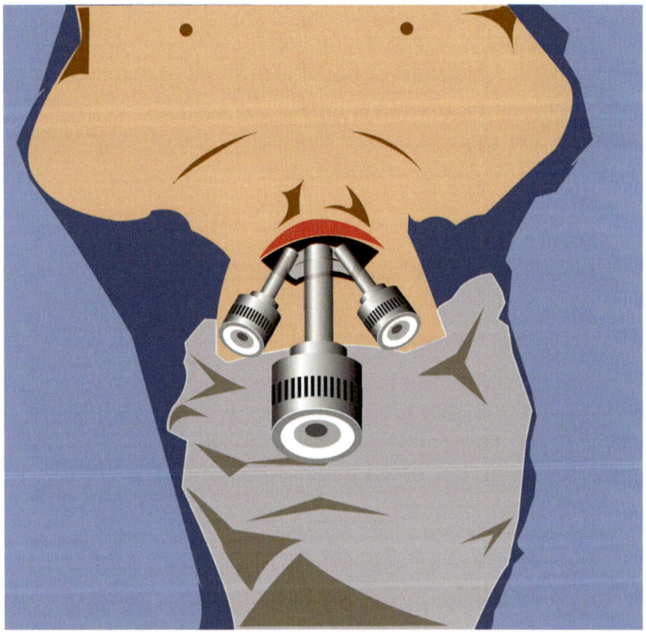

Fig. 14.5 Trocar placement

Upper Pole Ligation

After lateral dissection is completed, it becomes possible to view the upper pole. For patients whose upper pole is situated high up at the caudal end, it is necessary to laterally retract the strap muscles with 4-0 nylon sutures because the muscles obstruct the view of the upper pole, while both instruments are needed to ligate the upper vessels (Fig. 14.7). The suture needle should be inserted through the skin near the intersection of the cricothyroid cartilage level and the lateral end of the working space. After hooking the sternohyoid muscle with the suture and taking it out near its insertion site, the suture should be retracted laterally by the assistant to expose the upper pole. Although this may be enough in most cases, thyroid upper poles that go up extremely high need additional suturing and lateral traction of the sternothyroid muscles in the same manner (Fig. 14.7).

The upper pole should be grabbed with a grasper and retracted laterally and ventrally while a dissector meticulously exposes the avascular plane between the upper pole and cricothyroid muscles attached to the thyroid cartilage, also known as Joll's space (Fig. 14.8a, b). The superior thyroid vessels and certain types of the external branch of the superior laryngeal nerves (Cernea type 2) can be identified when this space is exposed [9]. It is important to ligate the connective tissue close up to the thyroid gland (Fig. 14.8c, d) and work your way up bit by bit to the superior thyroid ves-

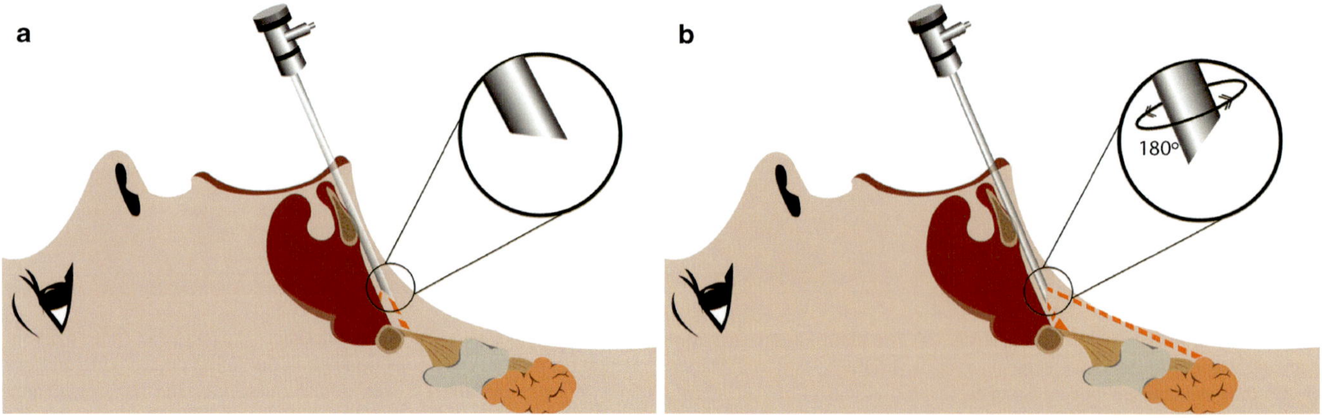

Fig. 14.6 Camera manipulation during flam formation. (**a**) During the initial phase of flap formation, visualizing the deeper sternal side may be difficult. (**b**) By rotating the 30-degree rigid endoscope 180 degrees, the visual of the lower area may be more easily acquired

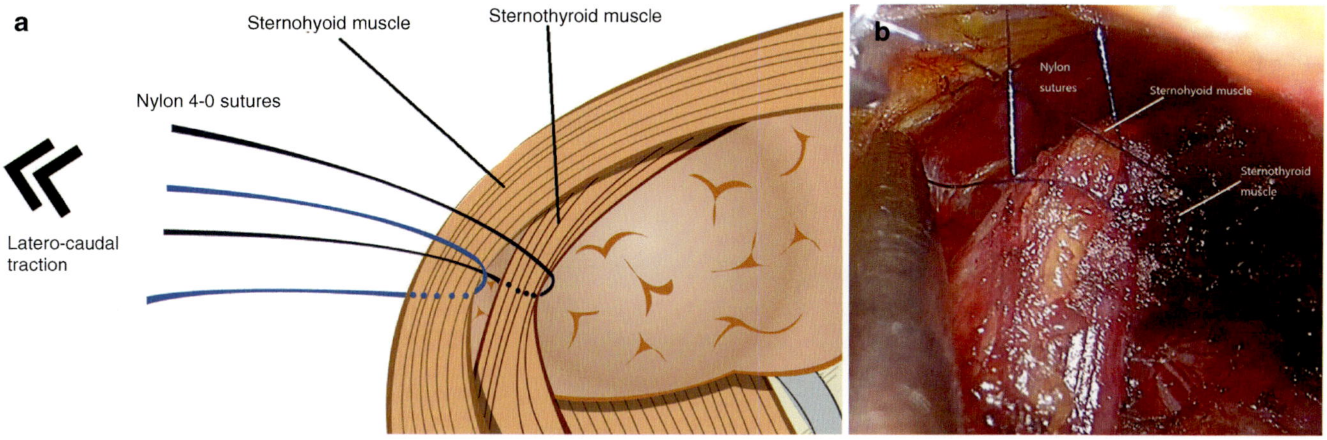

Fig. 14.7 Use of 4-0 nylon sutures to laterally retract the strap muscles

sels in order to preserve the cricothyroid muscle and superior parathyroid gland function (Fig. 14.8e, f). Each main superior vessel should be ligated separately. The posterior side of the upper pole should be dissected caudally to a level no lower than the cricothyroid cartilage to prevent recurrent laryngeal nerve (RLN) injury.

Recurrent Laryngeal Nerve Identification and Preservation

The ligated upper pole should be retracted in a medial, caudal, and ventral direction with contralateral forceps to expose Berry's ligament (Fig 14.9a, b). The most important aspect of identifying the RLN in TOETVA is safely exposing the structure at the laryngeal entry point near Berry's ligament and protecting it from thermal damage during gland resection. Meticulous use of the ipsilateral dissecting forceps, such as an endoscopic right angle, will expose the RLN without rupturing adjacent vessels (Fig 14.9c, d). Even more judicious use of energy-based surgical devices is of paramount importance in preventing inadvertent thermal damage to the nerves. One tip is to cover the exposed RLN with packed gauze and retract it laterally while using an energy device near the nerve entry point (Fig 14.9e, f). This will help prevent high-temperature fluids from directly contacting the nerves.

Lower Pole Ligation and Resection of the Gland

After safely preserving the RLN near Berry's ligament, the RLN should be exposed along its course all the way down to the lower pole level. During this procedure, each lower thyroid vessel should be ligated separately as close as possible to the thyroid gland in order to preserve the lower parathyroid gland and its function. At this point, it is possible to completely resect the thyroid lobe from the attached trachea.

Specimen Retrieval

Once the thyroid lobe is resected, the endoscope is removed and an endobag is blindly inserted through the 10-mm port with the wires removed. After reinserting the endoscope, the bag should be properly opened up for the specimen and other foreign materials, such as gauzes, to be placed in (Fig. 14.10). Because the bag cannot be extracted through the trocar, it should be pulled out along with the trocar. The trocar should be reinserted after the bag and specimen are retrieved.

Contralateral Resection

Contralateral lobectomy should be carried out in the same manner. However, consideration should be made in choosing which side to start from. In some cases, the main lesion may be too large, and additional dissection may be needed to extract the specimen. This will lead to air leakage during the subsequent lobectomy. The surgeon, therefore, may choose to start with the contralateral thyroid lobe.

Suture and Stitch-Out

After extracting both thyroid glands and making sure there is no bleeding, the midline of the strap muscles should be sutured. After removing the trocars, the resected mentalis muscle through the midline incision should be sutured with three 4-0 Vicryl stitches. The oral mucosa should be lightly stitched with five 4-0 Vicryl sutures. The lateral incisions require one 4-0 Vicryl stitch each only on the mucosal layer. The suture stump should be 0.5 cm long so it may be easily

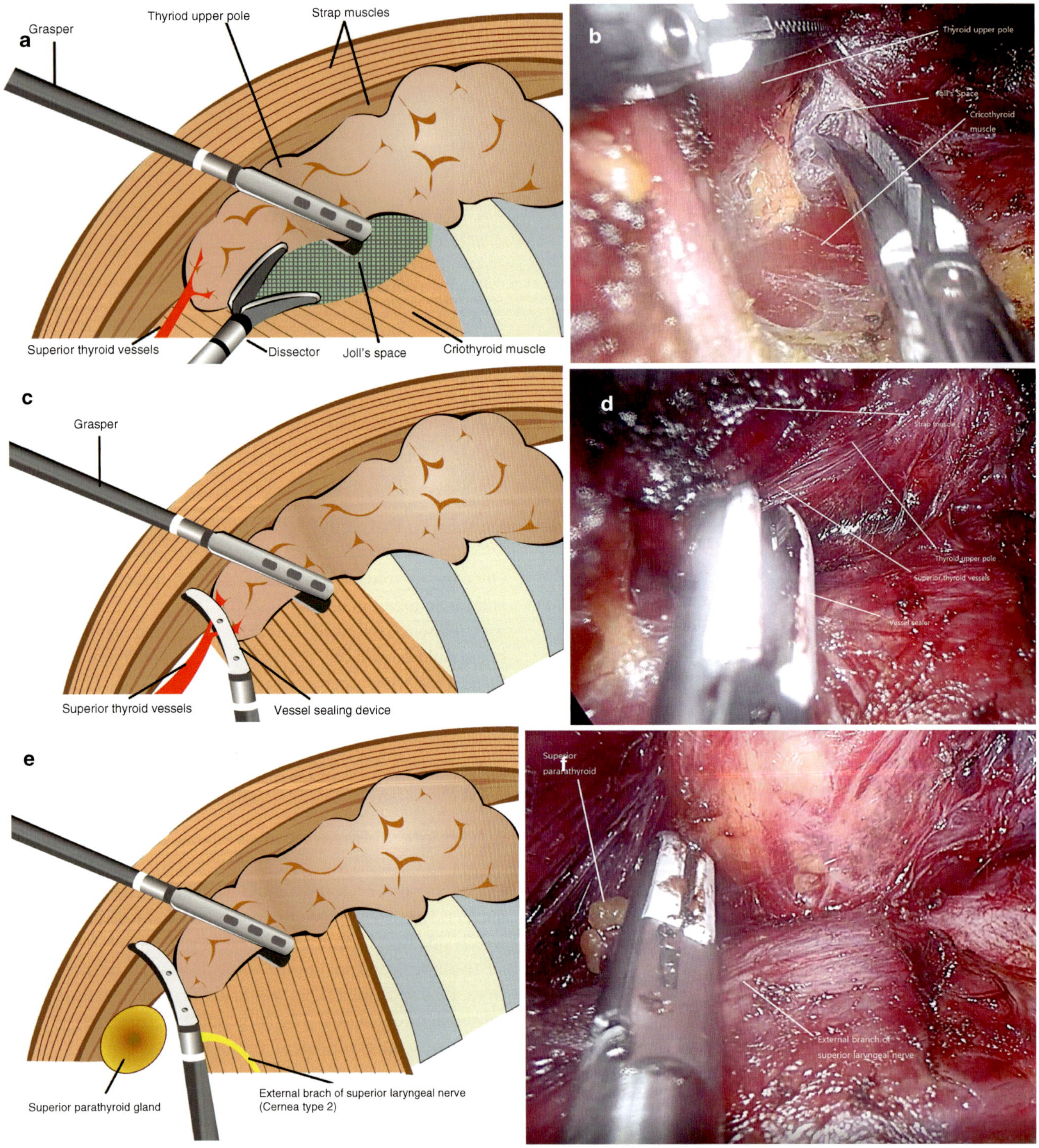

Fig. 14.8 Illustrations and images of upper pole resection. The most important point is to work bit by bit until the superior thyroid vessels are exposed. (**a**, **b**) Grab the upper pole and pull it to the ventral and lateral side away from the cricoid cartilage. Use the dissectors to expose Joll's space (in green). (**c**, **d**) Ligate the superior thyroid vessel as close as possible to the thyroid gland. By ligating the vessels and connective tissue as close to the thyroid gland as possible, the superior parathyroid and external branch of superior laryngeal nerve can be preserved (**e**, **f**)

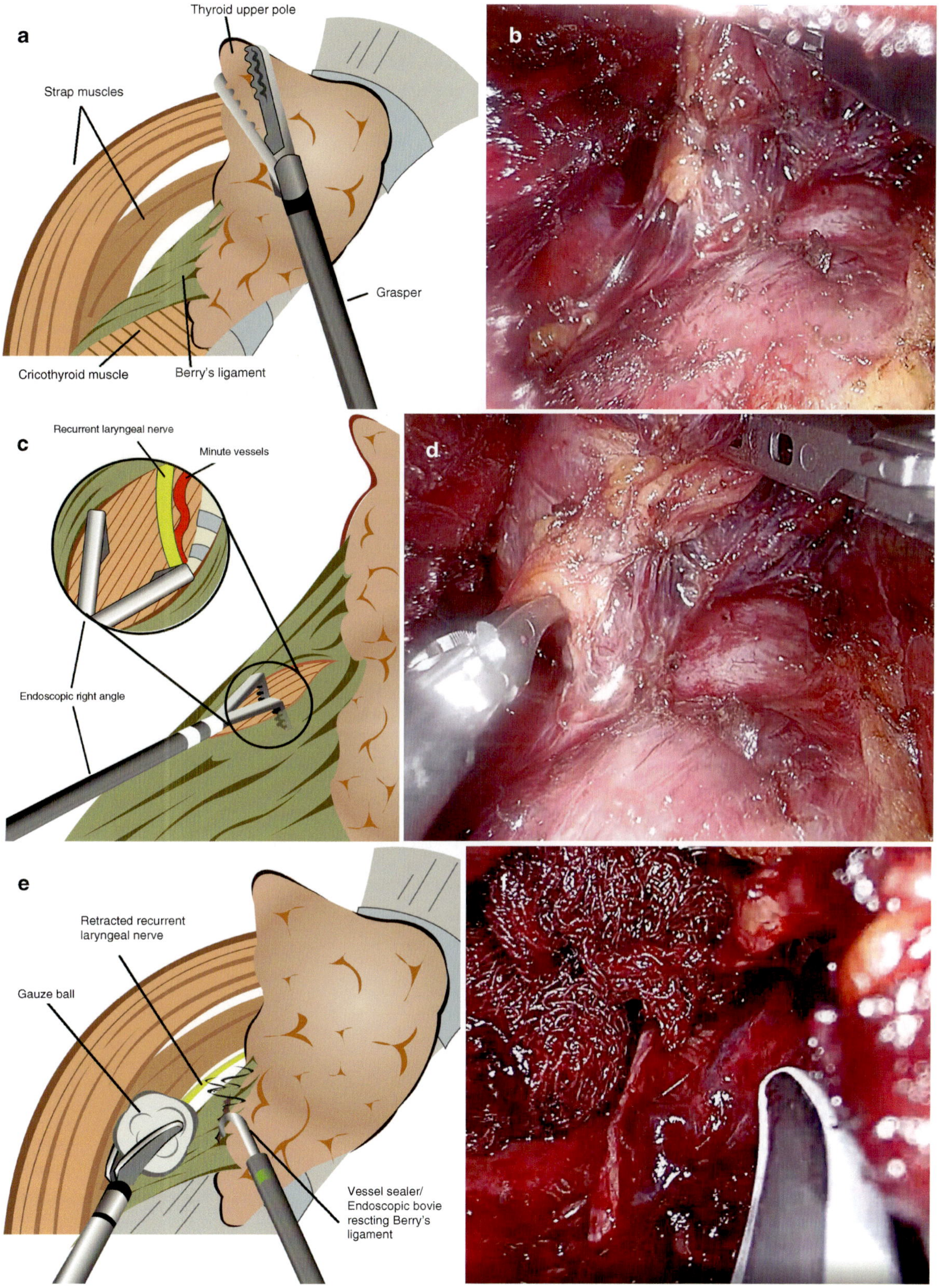

Fig. 14.9 Illustrations and images of identification of the recurrent laryngeal nerve after upper pole resection. (**a**, **b**) The mobilized upper pole should be retracted medially and caudally in order to expose Berry's ligament. (**c**, **d**) Soft tissue Berry's ligament should be meticulously dissected with an endoscopic right angle until the recurrent laryngeal nerve is revealed. (**e**, **f**) A gauze ball should be used to laterally retract the RLN while resecting the thyroid at the ligament of Berry to reduce thermal damage to the energy device

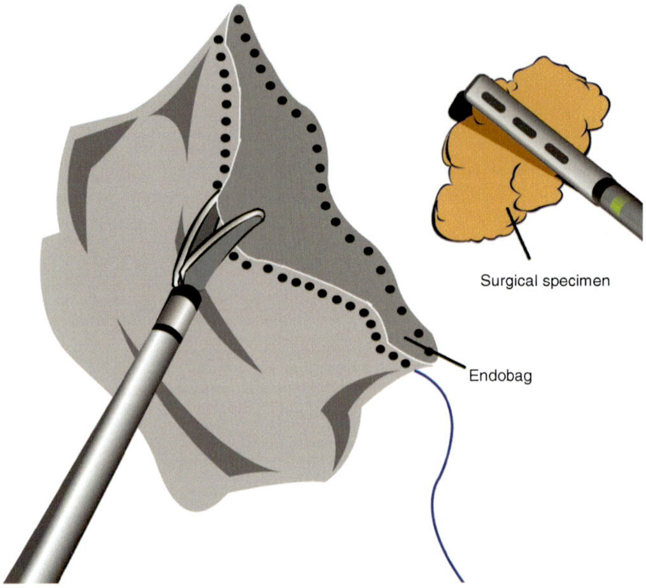

Fig. 14.10 Specimen retrieval. The endobag is blindly inserted through the 10-mm port, and the wires should be removed. After reinserting the endoscope, the bag should be properly opened up with a trocar, and a specimen should be inserted

identified 5–7 days later during the stitch-out. Routine oral hygiene care is enough after the patient is discharged 1 or 2 days after the operation.

Conclusion

TOETVA is the next step in minimally invasive thyroidectomy, whose feasibility among selected patients has been demonstrated through many clinical studies. Although TOETVA may be more technically demanding than open surgery, it possesses the potential to establish itself as a favorable approach in selected cases. Further efforts to accumulate collective experience and evidence and to pioneer new frontiers with this approach are necessary for the potential to blossom.

References

1. Witzel K, von Rahden BH, Kaminski C, Stein HJ. Transoral access for endoscopic thyroid resection. Surg Endosc. 2008;22:1871–5.
2. Benhidjeb T, Wilhelm T, Harlaar J, Kleinrensink GJ, Schneider TA, Stark M. Natural orifice surgery on thyroid gland: totally transoral video-assisted thyroidectomy (TOVAT): report of first experimental results of a new surgical method. Surg Endosc. 2009;23:1119–20.
3. Karakas E, Steinfeldt T, Gockel A, Westermann R, Kiefer A, Bartsch DK. Transoral thyroid and parathyroid surgery. Surg Endosc. 2010;24:1261–7.
4. Wilhelm T, Metzig A. Endoscopic minimally invasive thyroidectomy (eMIT): a prospective proof-of-concept study in humans. World J Surg. 2011;35:543–51.
5. Richmon JD, Pattani KM, Benhidjeb T, Tufano RP. Transoral robotic-assisted thyroidectomy: a preclinical feasibility study in 2 cadavers. Head Neck. 2011;33:330–3.
6. Anuwong A. Transoral endoscopic thyroidectomy vestibular approach: a series of the first 60 human cases. World J Surg. 2016;40:491–7.
7. Anuwong A, Ketwong K, Jitpratoom P, Sasanakietkul T, Duh QY. Safety and outcomes of the transoral endoscopic thyroidectomy vestibular approach. JAMA Surg. 2018;153:21–7.
8. Lee J-H, Chai YJ. Up-to-date evidence of transoral thyroidectomy on how to overcome the obstacles?—A review. Ann Thyroid. 2020;5:13.
9. Cernea CR, Ferraz AR, Nishio S, Dutra A Jr, Hojaij FC, dos Santos LR. Surgical anatomy of the external branch of the superior laryngeal nerve. Head Neck. 1992;14:380–3.

Transoral Endoscopic Thyroidectomy via Vestibular Approach (TOETVA)

15

Gustavo Fernández-Ranvier, Ghayth Al Awwa, and Daniela Guevara

Introduction

Traditional transcervical thyroidectomy has been a standard surgical procedure since its introduction in 1906. Advancements in surgical technique, general anesthesia, hemostasis, and neuromonitoring have made it a safe and successful procedure with low morbidity and mortality [1]. Transcervical thyroidectomy leaves the patient with a neck scar, which could be distressing, especially in patients with darker complexions and history of keloid formation [2]. Minimally invasive techniques have been developed using endoscopic and robotic approaches with the goal of avoiding disfiguring scars to the neck. These include endoscopic and robotic transaxillary thyroidectomy, both of which require a wide flap dissection and leave incisions away from the neck. None of these approaches have gained significant widespread acceptance [3]. Transoral endoscopic thyroidectomy via vestibular approach (TOETVA) has been developed since 2008 and has gained popularity and acceptance as a true scarless procedure. It can be performed with standard laparoscopic instruments, provides a clear view of vital structures, and allows access to both lobes. This approach was also shown to have postoperative outcomes comparable with the traditional open thyroidectomy [4]. Surgeons should have expertise of the open thyroidectomy technique along with laparoscopic skills to be able to adopt this procedure [5].

G. Fernández-Ranvier (✉)
Garlock Division of Surgery, Mount Sinai Hospital, New York, NY, USA
e-mail: gustavo.fernandez-ranvier@mountsinai.org

G. Al Awwa
Department of Surgery/Division of Metabolic, Endocrine, and Minimally Invasive Surgery, Icahn School of Medicine at Mount Sinai, New York, NY, USA

D. Guevara
The Garlock Division of General Surgery, Icahn School of Medicine at Mount Sinai Hospital, New York, NY, USA

Procedure

The patient is brought to the operating room and placed in a supine position with the neck mildly hyperextended (Fig. 15.1). General anesthesia is administered after nasotracheal intubation is established (orotracheal intubation is an alternative). After induction, the oral cavity and upper neck are prepped and draped in a sterile fashion (Fig. 15.2). The operating surgeon stands at the head of the bed, and the monitor is positioned at the feet (Fig. 15.3). Three incisions are made through the alveolar mucosa of the lower lip vestibule, opposite to the incisors, a 5-mm transverse medial incision along with two vertical 5 mm incisions. The two lateral incisions are just medial to the canines and just in the inner aspect of the inferior lip to avoid injury to the mental nerve (Fig. 15.4). Before port placement, a working space is created by tissue dissection through the mentalis muscle with the use of electrocautery and/or blunt dissection with special care to avoid injury to the overlying skin (Fig. 15.5). Subsequently, hydrodissection is performed with a Veress needle, where about 60 cc of a mixture of NaCl containing epinephrine (1 mg in 500-cc NaCl) is injected to create a space beneath the platysma, which is then dilated with a blunt dissector (Anuwong dilator, Kelly Wick tunneler, or Hegar dilators) (Fig. 15.6). Given the advances in laparoscopic image quality and increased maneuverability with the smaller port, we find that using three 5-mm ports is sufficient for most cases. The central port can easily be upsized, either initially or later in the case, if required. A 5-mm port is placed first through the central incision and then over the mandible, advancing the port about 2 cm distally to the chin, taking care to avoid penetration of the mentum skin. Next, the two lateral 5-mm ports are placed (Fig. 15.7). The surgical space is then maintained with insufflation of CO_2 at a pressure of 6-mm Hg. A 30-degree 5-mm camera is then placed through the central port. A Maryland dis-

A. Shifrin (ed.), *Atlas of Thyroid Surgery*, https://doi.org/10.1007/978-3-030-93673-0_15

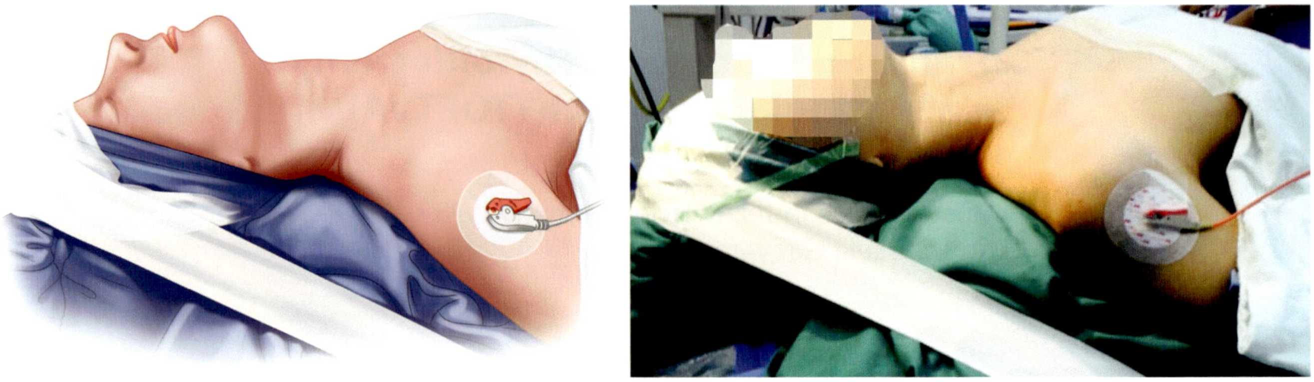

Fig. 15.1 A side view of the patient's neck in mild hyperextension. A shoulder roll is used, as well as cushioning under the neck and head for support. Tape is used for stability

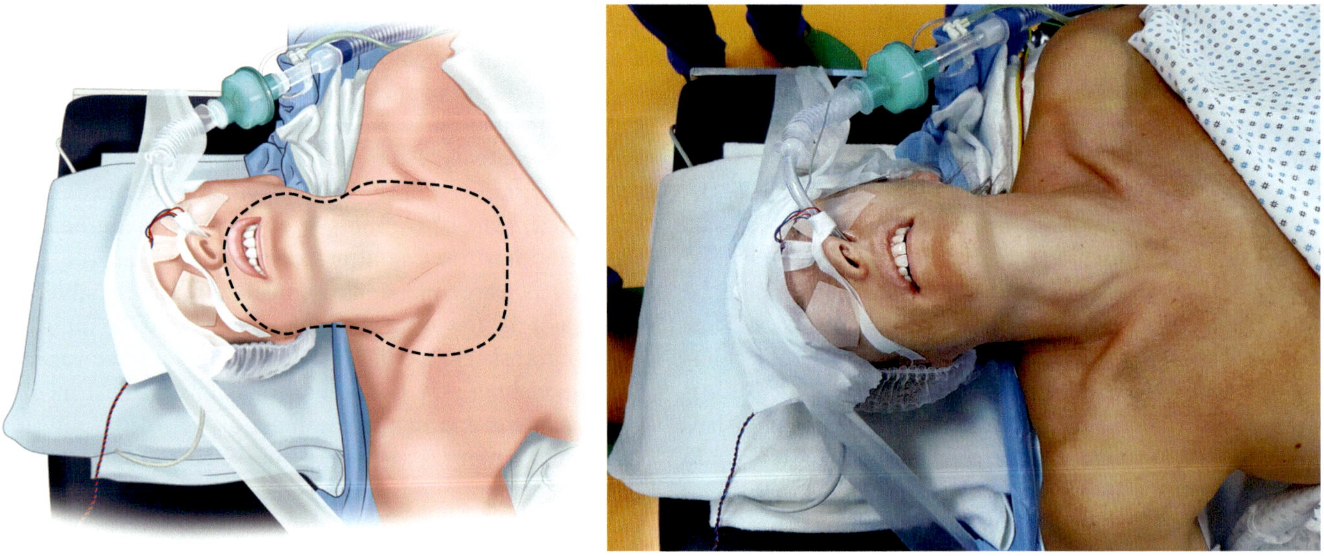

Fig. 15.2 Above view of the neck in hyperextension. Nasotracheal tube is in place with the nerve monitoring system

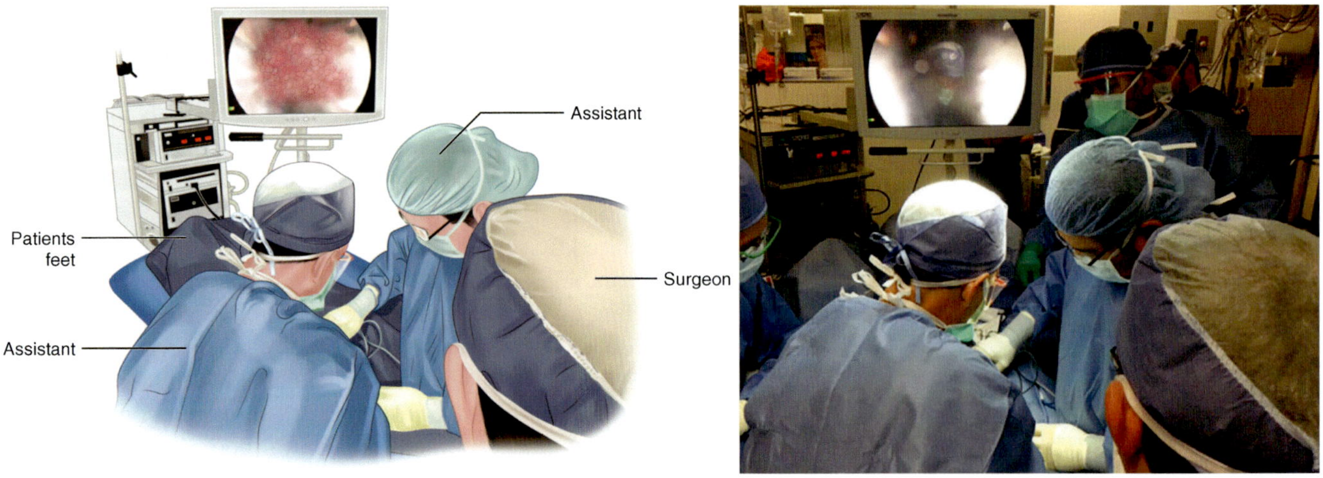

Fig. 15.3 The surgeon is situated at the head of the patient with two assistants, one to either side. The endoscopic tower is at the foot of the patient

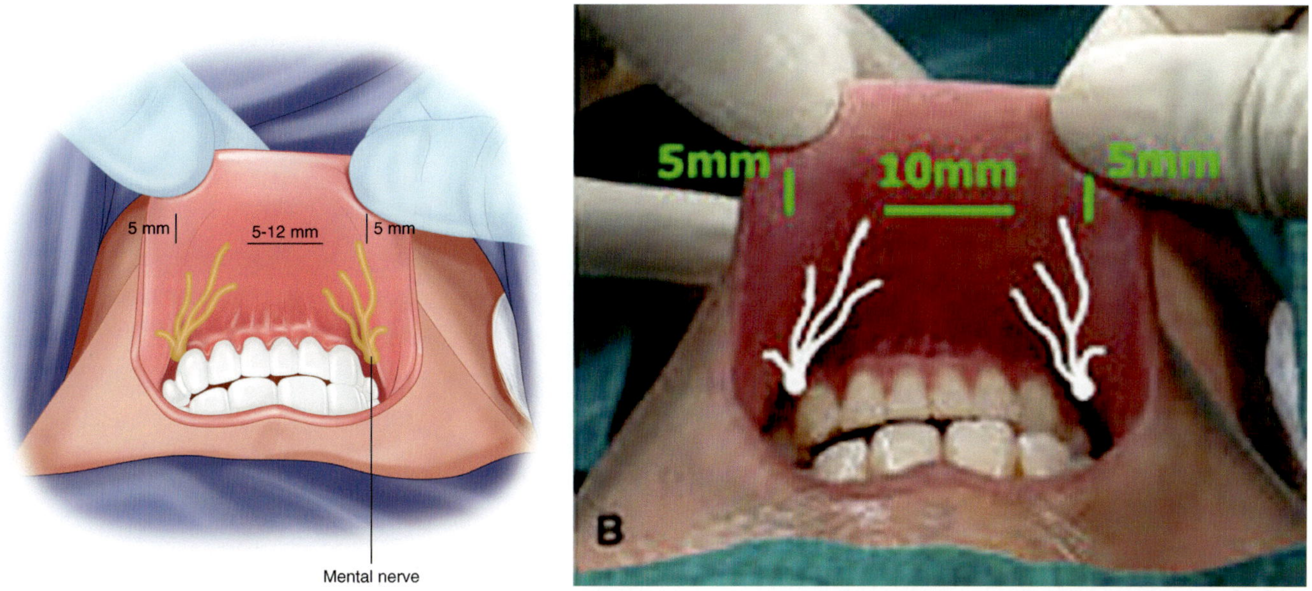

Fig. 15.4 Three incisions are made along the inner surface of the lower lip. Lateral incisions medial to the canines will help avoid the mental nerve

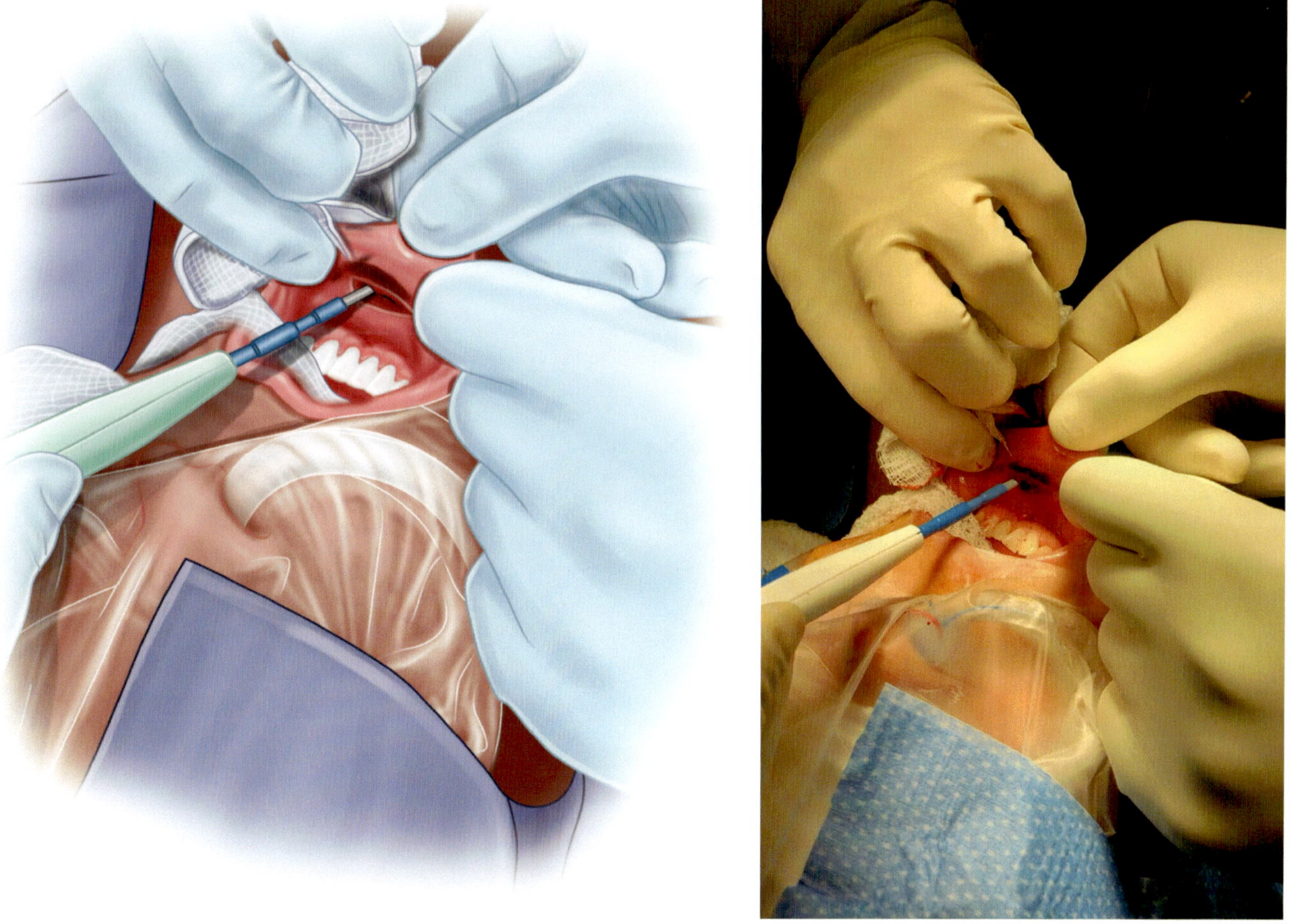

Fig. 15.5 Electrocautery and blunt dissection with a hemostat are used to pass through the mentalis muscle

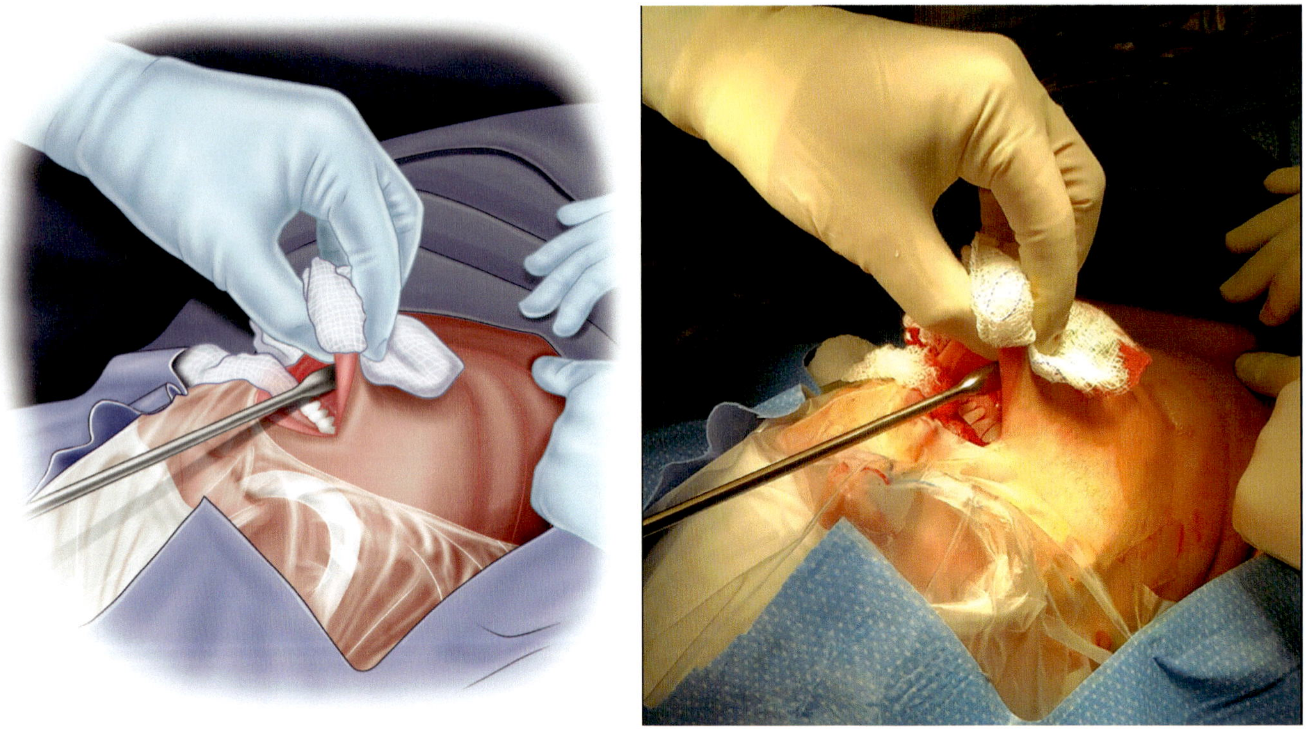

Fig. 15.6 A Veress needle with approximately 60 cc of NaCl mixed with dilute epinephrine is passed through the central incision and injected into the subplatysmal surgical space. A dilator, pictured here, is then passed through the incisions to allow for easier placement of the laparoscopic trocars

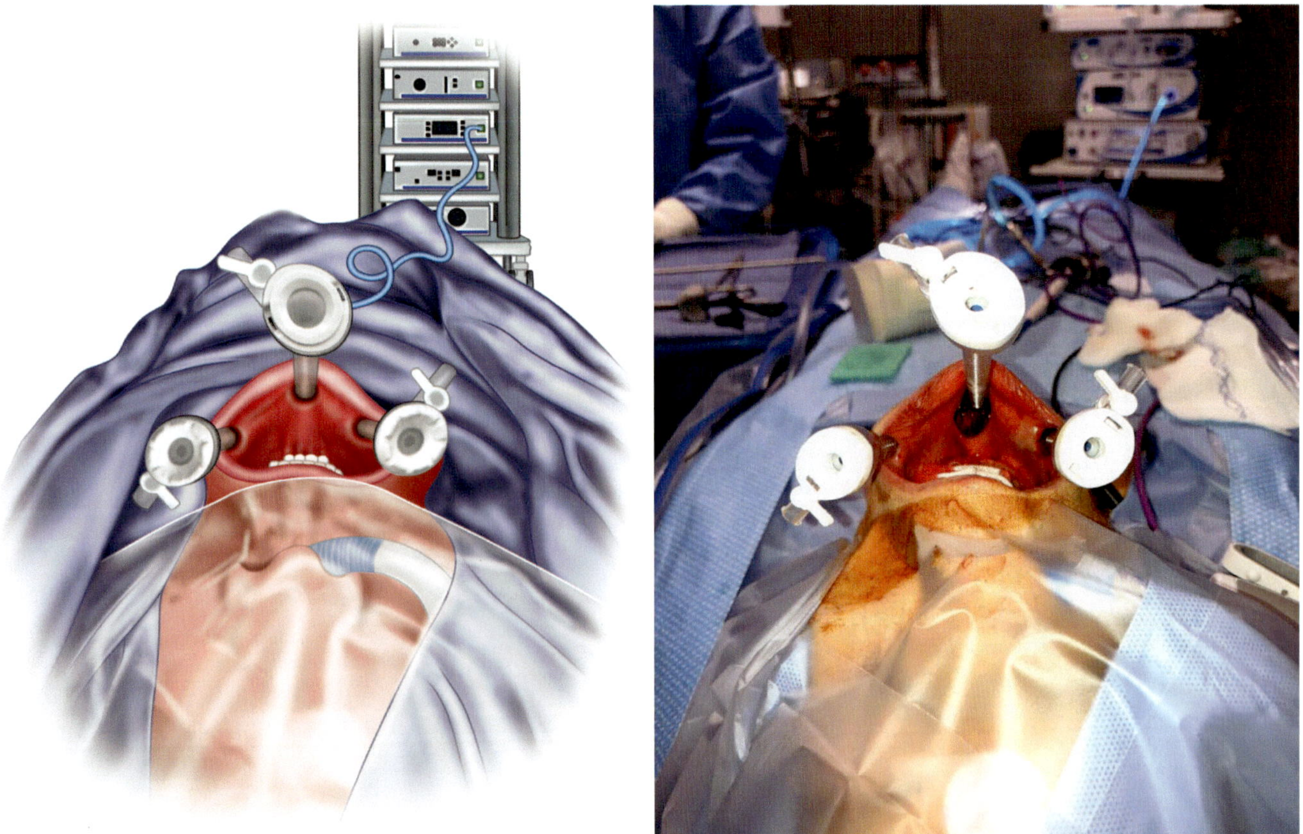

Fig. 15.7 The surgeon's view showing the final setup of three 5-mm ports. The central port can be upsized as needed for a larger camera or to remove a larger specimen if needed. This can be done initially or later in the case as required

sector and bipolar or ultrasonic energy device is used on either side of the camera for further development of the surgical space. Dissection is carried out in the caudal direction toward the sternal notch, always staying beneath the platysma muscle (Fig. 15.8). Laterally, dissecting to bilateral sternocleidomastoid muscles further enhances exposure. Once the strap muscles are visualized, they are divided in the midline to expose the thyroid gland (Fig. 15.9). The posterior surface of the strap muscles is mobilized from the underlying thyroid capsule to allow the medialization of the thyroid lobe and lateralization of the strap muscles. If optimal exposure is not accomplished by this dissection, then an exterior suture may be placed through the strap muscles for lateral retraction (Fig. 15.10). The thyroid vessels are cauterized and divided in sequence, starting with the middle thyroid veins to allow medialization of the thyroid lobe and then with the superior thyroid vessels, taking care to avoid injuring the external branch

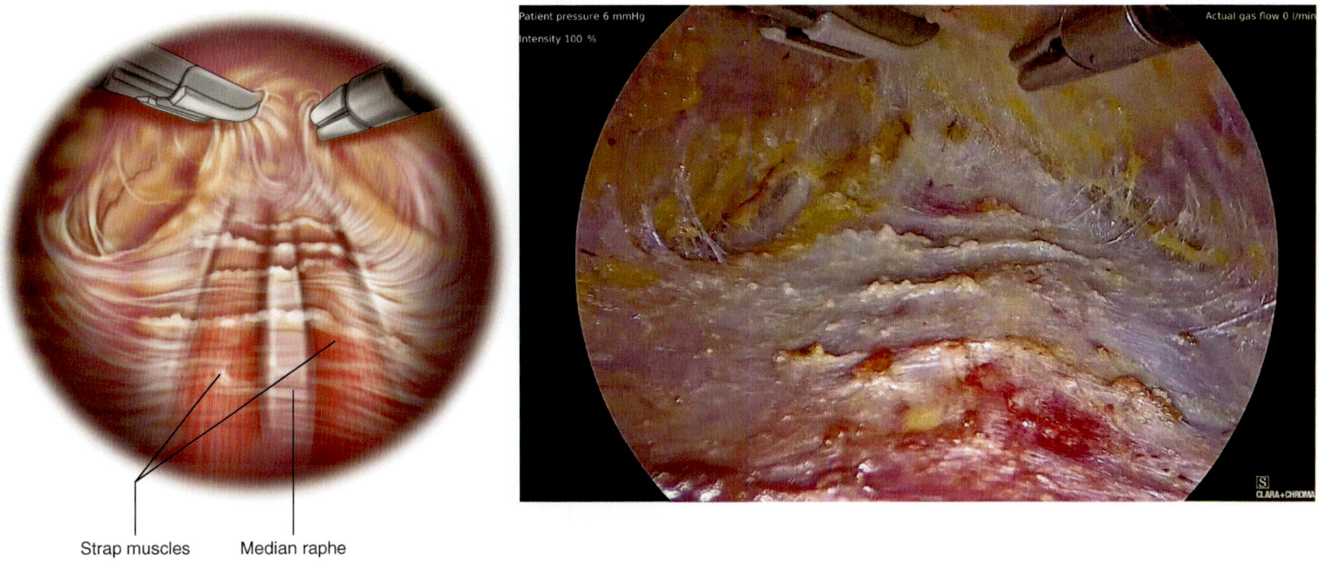

Fig. 15.8 Initial subplatysmal dissection is carried out with a Maryland dissector and a bipolar or ultrasonic energy device. Dissection is carried down to the sternal notch inferiorly and as lateral as the identification of the medial aspect of the sternocleidomastoid muscle. The strap muscles can be appreciated deep to the space

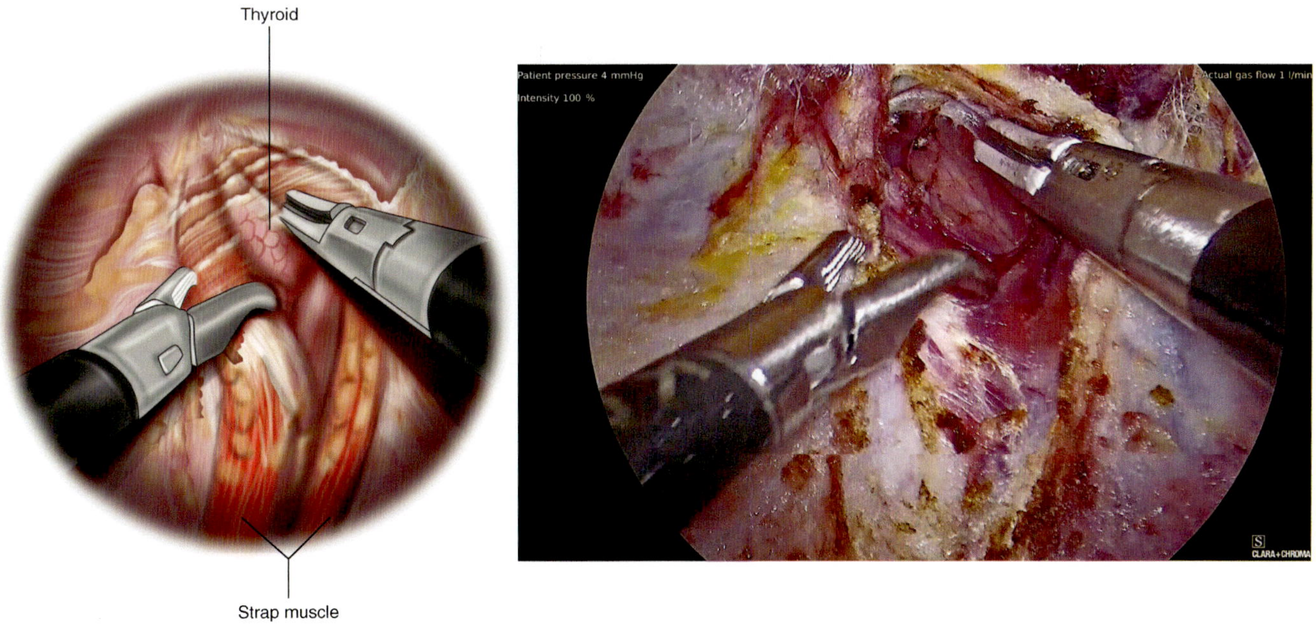

Fig. 15.9 The strap muscles are divided down the midline to expose the thyroid gland. This is easily achieved with hook electrocautery and either a bipolar or ultrasonic energy device

of the superior laryngeal nerve (Fig. 15.11). The superior lobe is then mobilized; the superior parathyroid can usually be identified and preserved in situ. The recurrent laryngeal nerve can be identified posterior and medial to the superior parathyroid gland (Fig. 15.12). The use of a nerve monitoring system is an encouraged but not mandatory tool to perform this procedure. Following the caudal dissection of the thyroid capsule will allow the identification of the inferior parathyroid gland, which should be preserved in situ. The mobilization of the inferior parathyroid gland will allow the identification of inferior thyroid vessels, which can be divided (Fig. 15.13). The same approach and technique are then applied to the contralateral lobe. The gland is then placed in an endocatch bag

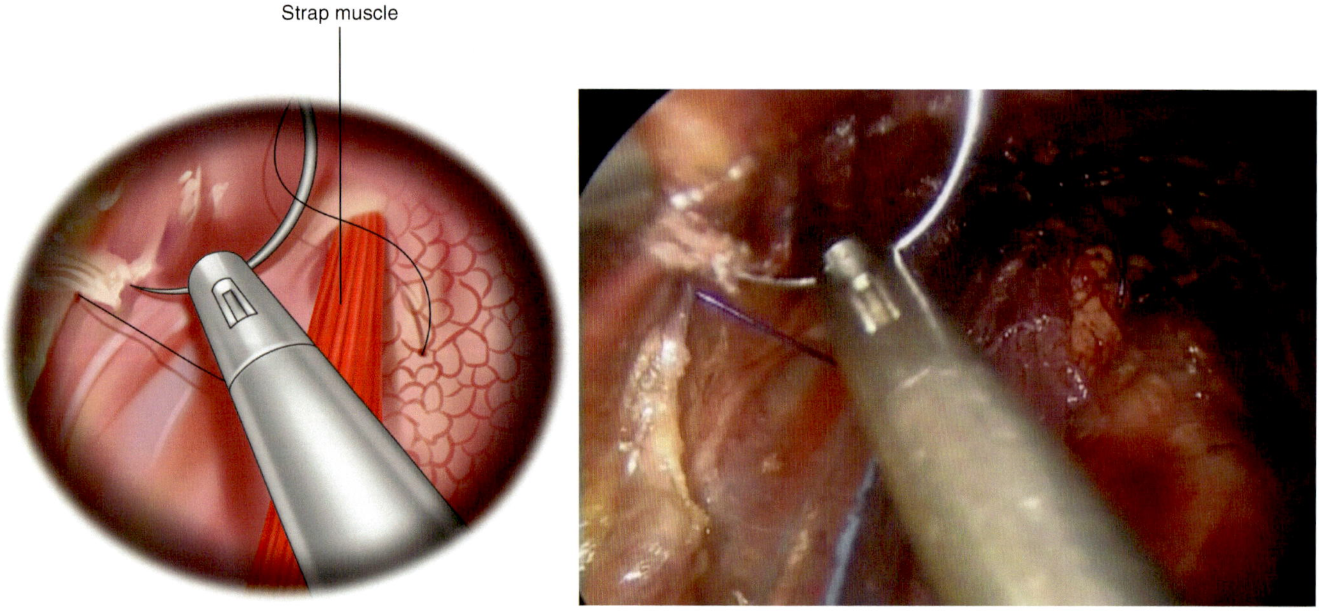

Fig. 15.10 The posterior surface of the strap muscles are mobilized from the underlying thyroid capsule to allow medialization of the thyroid lobe and lateralization of the strap muscles. If optimal exposure is not accomplished by this dissection, then an exterior suture may be placed through the strap muscles for lateral retraction

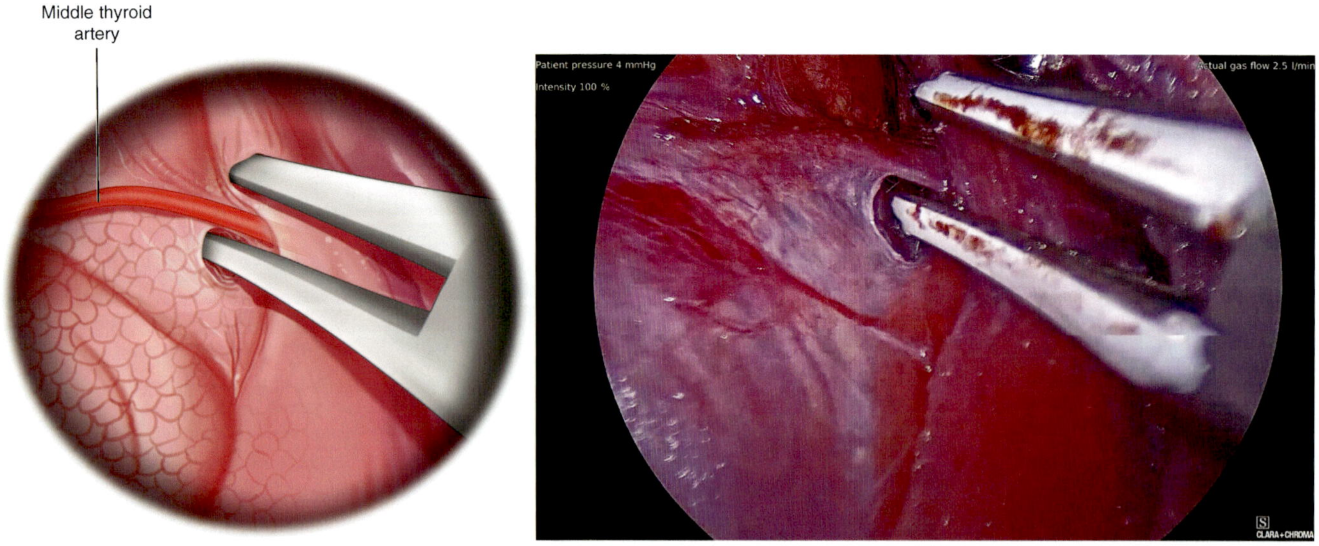

Fig. 15.11 Dissection of the thyroid gland and serial ligation of its vessels can now begin. The right middle thyroid artery pictured here is to be sealed and ligated using a bipolar or ultrasonic energy device

and brought out through the central port (Figs. 15.14, 15.15, and 15.16). The strap muscles are approximated with absorbable 3-0 self-locking sutures and the mucosa closed with 5-0 absorbable sutures (Fig. 15.17). The patient recovered well and was discharged from the hospital the same day. She was seen postoperatively with excellent results (Fig. 15.18).

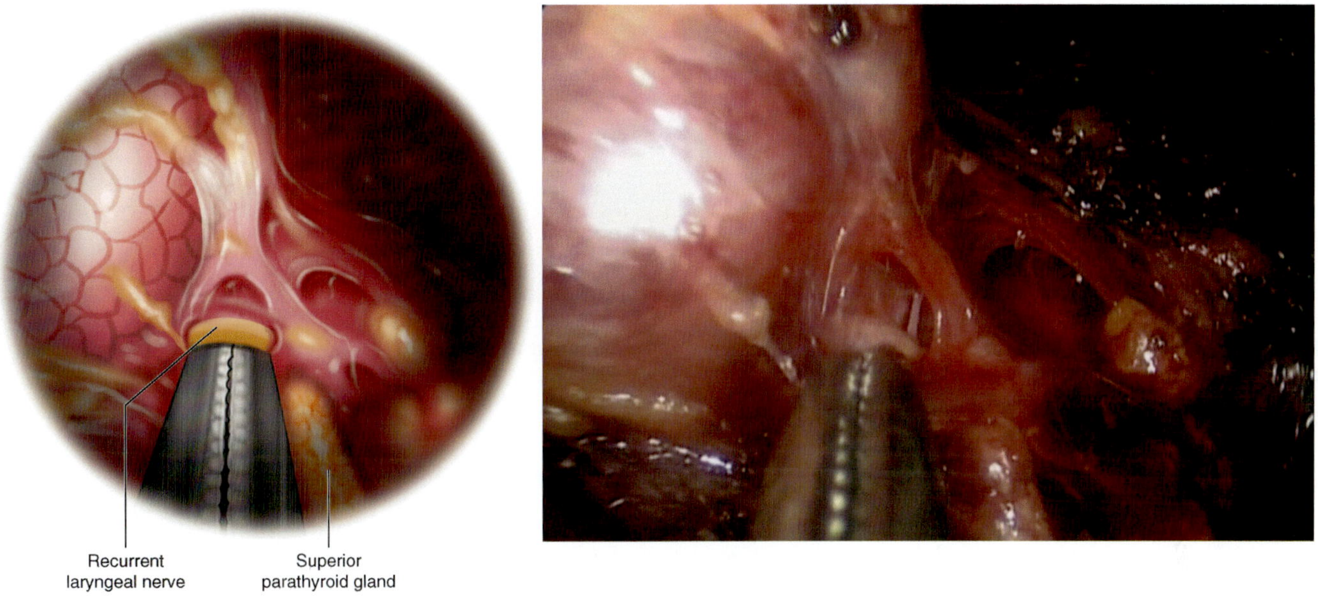

Fig. 15.12 As the superior lobe of the thyroid is mobilized, the recurrent laryngeal nerve is identified with the use of a nerve monitor attached to a Maryland dissector. The use of a nerve monitoring system is an encouraged but not mandatory tool to perform this procedure

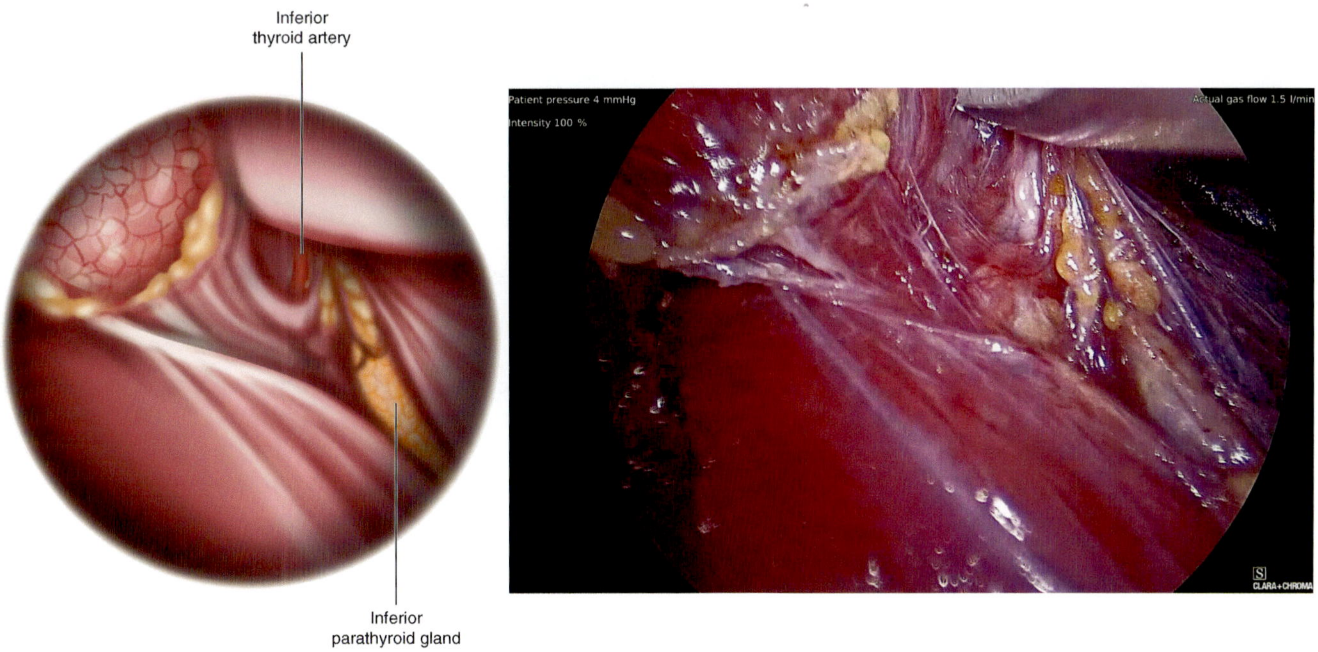

Fig. 15.13 Dissection is carried down to the inferior thyroid artery, pictured here. The inferior parathyroid gland can be appreciated and preserved in situ

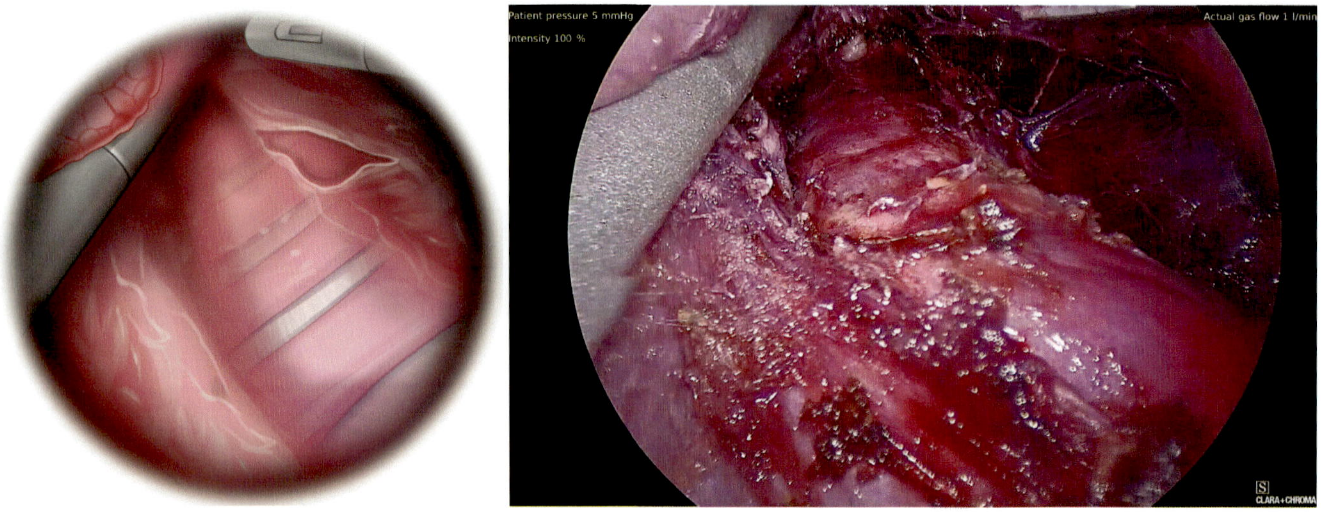

Fig. 15.14 After the same steps are repeated for the contralateral side, the dissection is complete. The thyroid is retracted to the top left of the figure, and the extent of dissection can be appreciated

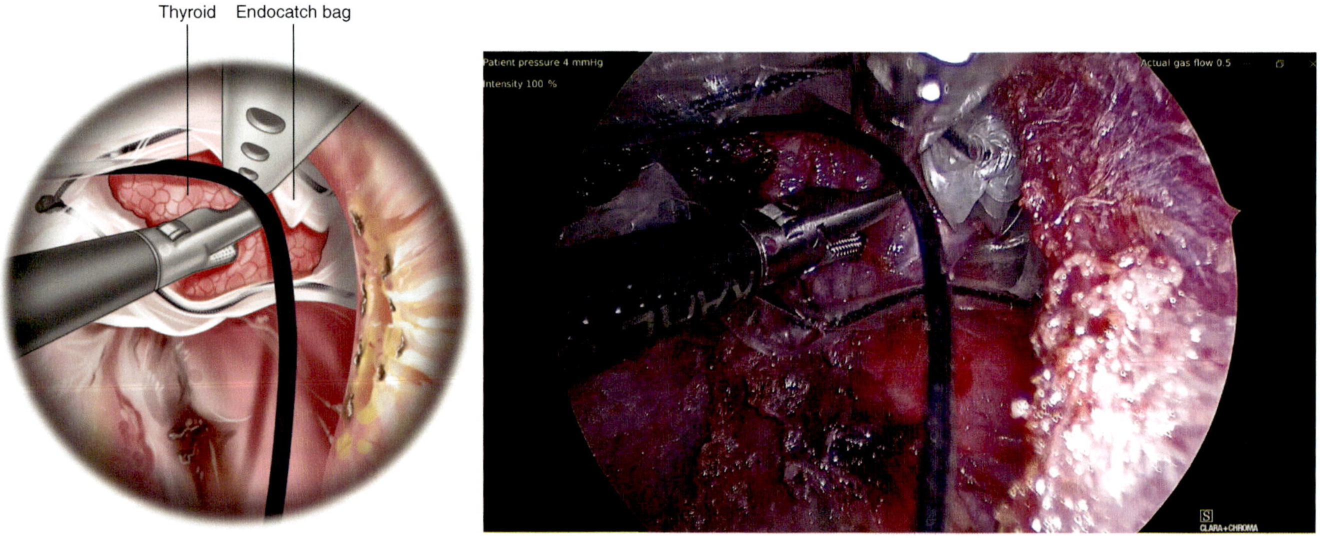

Fig. 15.15 An endocatch bag is inserted for the removal of the thyroid. The central port can be upsized if needed for the removal of the specimen

Tips and Pitfalls

- Use of clear drape on the upper face to allow visualization of the nasotracheal tube during the procedure.
- Dilute chlorhexidine mouthwash both preoperatively and prior to the start of procedure.
- The oral cavity is packed with strip gauze to avoid the accumulation of fluid.
- Use of combination of short and long acting local anesthetic for both pain and hydro-dissection during port placement.

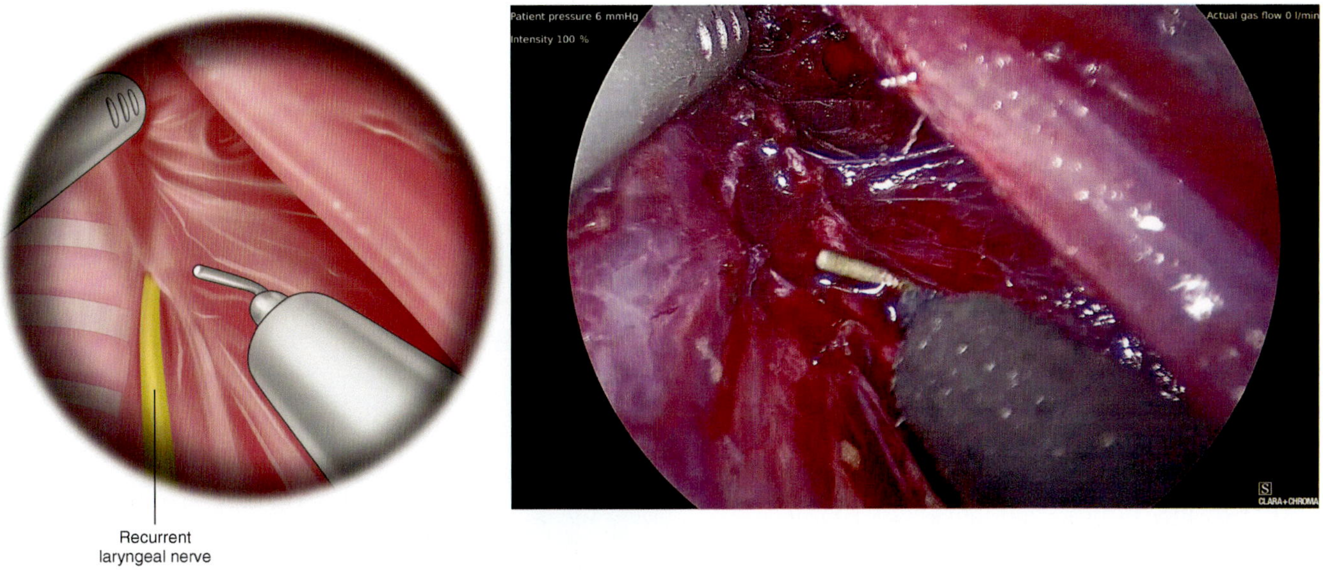

Fig. 15.16 The hook electrocautery is being used with the monitoring system, allowing detection of an intact recurrent laryngeal nerve within the tracheoesophageal groove

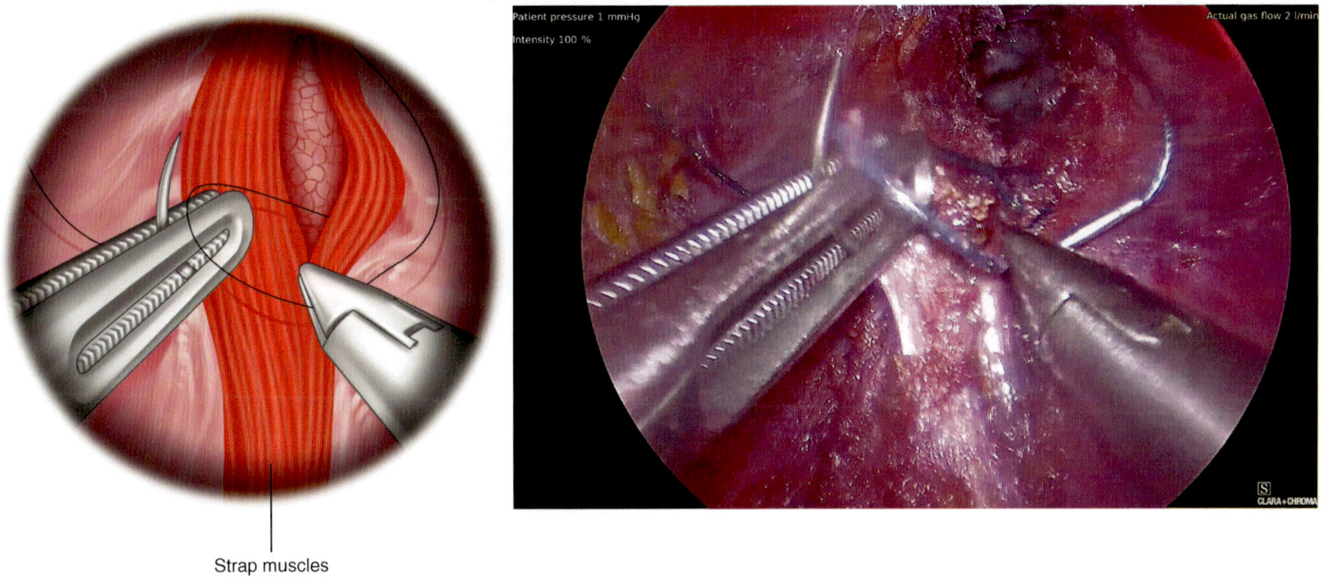

Fig. 15.17 The strap muscles are approximated with absorbable suture. The intraoral incisions are closed with 5-0 absorbable suture, usually chromic gut

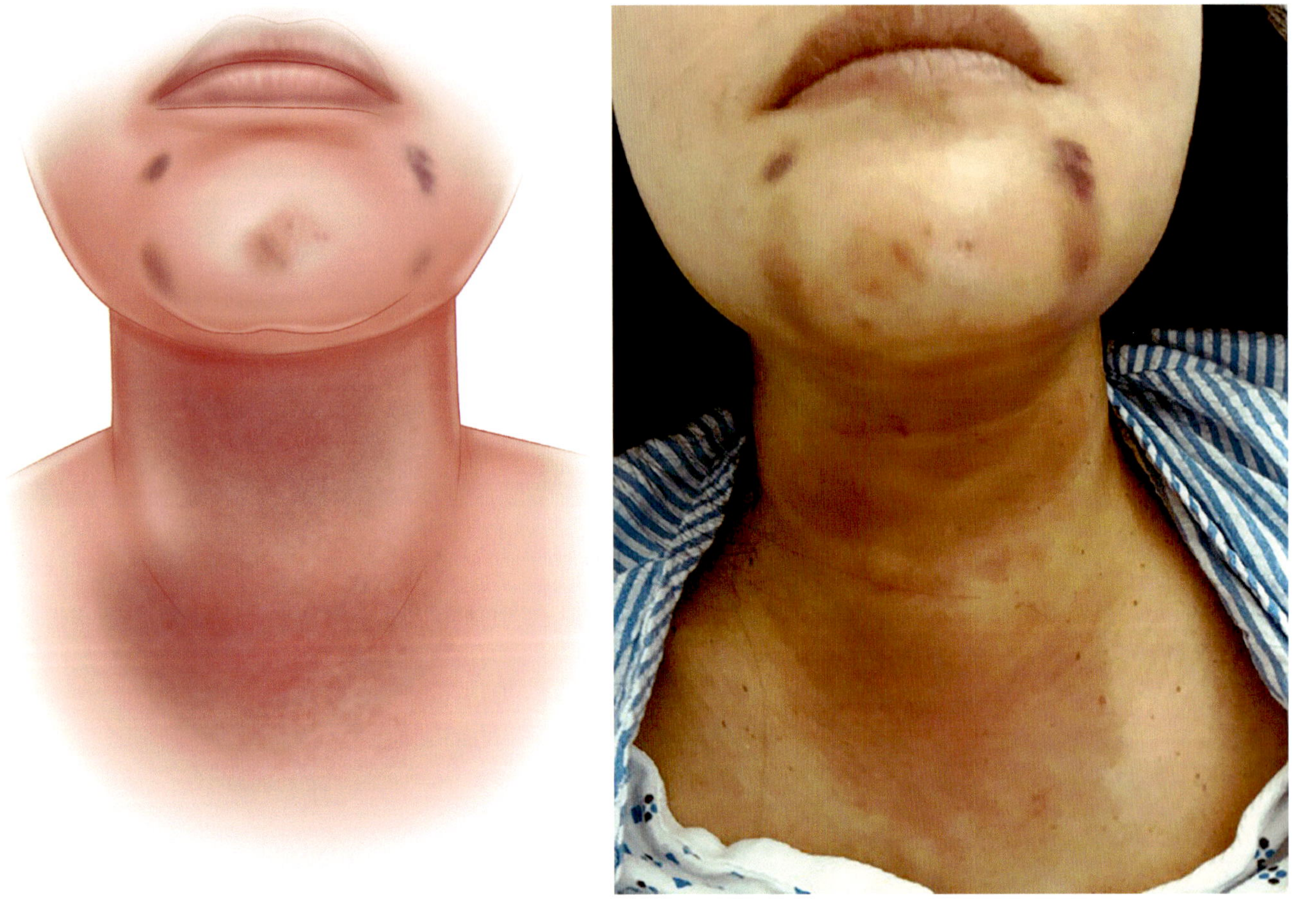

Fig. 15.18 Forty-eight hour postoperative follow-up shows normal bruising

References

1. Russell JO, et al. Minimally invasive and remote-access thyroid surgery in the era of the 2015 American Thyroid Association guidelines. Laryngoscope Investig Otolaryngol. 2016;1(6):175–9.
2. Richmon JD, Kim HY. Transoral robotic thyroidectomy (TORT): procedures and outcomes. Gland Surg. 2017;6(3):285–9.
3. Anuwong A, et al. Safety and outcomes of the transoral endoscopic thyroidectomy vestibular approach. JAMA Surg. 2018;153(1):21–7.
4. Zhang D, et al. Indications, benefits and risks of transoral thyroidectomy. Best Pract Res Clin Endocrinol Metab. 2019;33(4):101280.
5. Fernandez-Ranvier G, et al. Transoral Endoscopic Thyroidectomy Vestibular Approach. JSLS: Journal of the Society of Laparoendoscopic Surgeons. 2019;23(4):e2019.00036. https://doi.org/10.4293/JSLS.2019.00036.

Safe Thyroidectomy in Low- and Middle-Income Countries

16

Schelto Kruijff, Marianne Roberta Frederiek Bosscher, and Pim Johan Bongers

Summary

- Essentials for the treatment of thyroid pathology in low- and middle-income countries (LMICs) include sufficient knowledge of local epidemiology, cultural sensitivity, patient history and cervical ultrasonography.
- Short-term surgical missions in LMICs should only be performed when qualitative aftercare is available, treatment outcomes are reported and there is an objective to extend surgical facilities for local healthcare systems.
- The treatment of thyroid pathology should follow international thyroid management guidelines, although local circumstances, including the scarcity of equipment or medication, may require adoption of strategies towards no or less extensive surgery.
- In contrast to total thyroidectomy in high-income countries, hemithyroidectomy or extended hemithyroidectomy for large thyroid goitres and resectable malignancies are the preferred procedures in areas with limited access to thyroid hormone replacement.
- Patients should be referred when better outcomes for the patient can be expected elsewhere.

Case: A Young Patient with Advanced Thyroid Carcinoma

A 28-year-old lady in Kenia came by foot to the local hospital. She lived in a small village 300 km away from the hospital and had been suffering for years from large deformities in the left side of the neck. She experienced local pressure and had increasing difficulty swallowing, and the swelling caused her to be socially isolated in her village (Fig. 16.1). She came to the hospital with a request for treatment.

On inspection, we saw a healthy young woman with no (known) medical history. On physical examination, we saw and felt impressive lymphadenopathy on the left side of the neck in levels II, III, IV and V and a mobile nodule in the central neck at the level of the upper pole of the thyroid gland. A mobile ultrasound confirmed extensive left lymphadenopathy and minimal right lymphadenopathy and a lesion in the upper pole of the left thyroid, which was highly suspected for thyroid cancer based on the radiologic features (TIRADS 6).

Given the absence of radioactive iodine in the near and distant area, it was decided to perform a left hemithyroidectomy and level II–Vb lateral neck dissection. In this way, we aimed to achieve disease control of the left neck and primary tumor and reduce complaints of pressure and swallowing.

The decision not to perform a total thyroidectomy with central lymph node dissection and a right lateral neck dissection was taken to prevent hypoparathyroidism in the absence of calcium, hypothyroidism in the absence of thyroid hormone replacement therapy and bilateral recurrent laryngeal nerve paresis in the absence of an intensive care unit (ICU). She recovered quickly without any post-operative complications. She was discharged after 4 days, and it was agreed that she would return for additional surgical treatment in our clinic in the future if the lymphadenopathy in the right neck would increase.

Low- and Middle-Income Countries

There is general agreement that both the terms 'third world' and 'developing country' have become outdated. In general, both terms used to refer to countries with relatively poor economic and social status.

S. Kruijff · M. R. F. Bosscher
Department of Surgical Oncology, University Medical Center Groningen, Groningen, The Netherlands

P. J. Bongers (✉)
Department of Surgical Oncology, University Medical Center Groningen, Groningen, The Netherlands

A. Shifrin (ed.), *Atlas of Thyroid Surgery*, https://doi.org/10.1007/978-3-030-93673-0_16

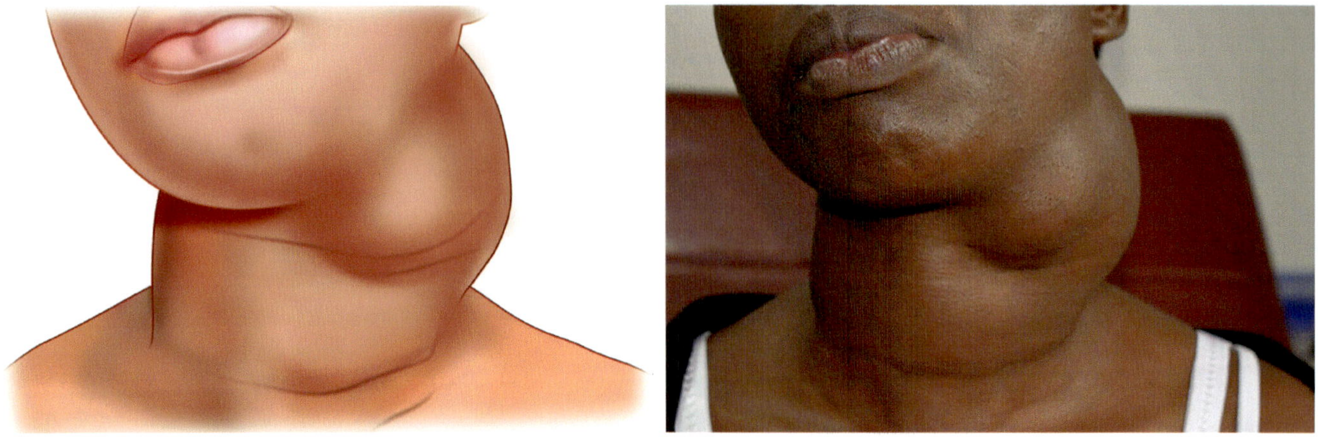

Fig. 16.1 Advanced carcinoma

Currently, the World Bank divides countries, also referred to as economies, into four income groupings: low, lower middle, upper middle, and high [1]. Annually, the gross national income (GNI) per capita is calculated, and income groupings are determined to facilitate this division. Different economic grouping systems are used by the International Monetary Fund (IMF) and the United Nations. The United Nations Development Programme (UNDP) created the Human Development Index (HDI) to assess the development of a country, not based on economic growth alone [2]. Based on a multidimensional measure of well-being, including income, education and health, countries are grouped into 'very high', 'high', 'medium' and 'low' levels of human development. In the year 2020, it classifies 151 countries as developing.

In this chapter, we will use the term 'low and middle income countries' (LMICs), adhering to the division used by the World Bank.

Healthcare system restraints vary widely and may be based on the poor accessibility of healthcare, shortage of appropriately qualified and motivated staff, lack of diagnostic and therapeutic equipment, lack of infrastructure, inadequate drug and medical supplies, bureaucracy, and poor leadership or governance. Traditionally, healthcare systems in LMICs have focused on acute care rather than chronic conditions. Therefore, medicines for chronic conditions such as iatrogenic hypothyroidism or hypoparathyroidism are less accessible than those for acute conditions.

Poverty remains correlated closely with malnourishment, less access to education, electricity, sanitation and healthcare. Citizens lacking income or health coverage are often denied access to healthcare due to obligatory individual payments.

When working in LMICs as a physician, or more specifically as a thyroid surgeon, it is important to note that differences among and within countries may be substantial in terms of economy as well as healthcare standards. Furthermore, local epidemiology differs regarding thyroid pathology. Therefore, modest expectations and an open attitude to cultural differences are vital characteristics for a successful physician or surgeon in LMICs.

For many countries in Africa and Asia, changes such as technological advances, the introduction of primary healthcare, increased literacy, access to safe water, sanitation and housing, have resulted in substantial improvements in health and life expectancy [3]. Despite this, political instability, environmental disasters, declining economic performance, unresponsive governance, weak public health infrastructure and the onset of globalization have had a great impact on the well-being of poor people. In most LMICs, disease-specific programs receive substantial external funding; however, broader healthcare infrastructures remain relatively underfunded. The density of the population is higher in urban areas, and therefore public health initiatives will reach a larger population in these regions. In rural areas, access to healthcare facilities remains a problem because of travel distance.

Surgical Missions

Five years ago, a poignant article was published in the leading medical journal *The Lancet*, stating that the need for surgical care in the poorest regions of the world is currently not widely recognized [4]. In 2010, an estimated 16.9 million lives (32.9% of all deaths worldwide) were lost worldwide to conditions that required surgical care. This number far exceeded the deaths from HIV/AIDS (1.6 million), tuberculosis (1.2 million) and malaria (1.2 million) combined. Our surgical workforce will need to double within 15 years to prevent these deaths, meaning 2.2 million additional surgeons, anaesthesiologists, orthopaedic surgeons, midwives and gynaecologists will need to be trained and positioned in rural areas. This burden of surgical disease mainly concerns basic forms of surgery, such as open fracture treatment, caesarean section, hernias, perforated hollow organs and bowel obstruction, and also thyroid surgery [5].

The burden of surgical disease can be reduced in different ways. One option is by surgical missions. Traditionally, surgeons from high-income countries (HICs) plan short-term surgical volunteer missions. The outcomes of such missions for specific surgery are underreported. During these missions, well-trained doctors from affluent countries carry out interventions in a country where healthcare is less developed. They can provide essential medical interventions, which would not be available for many patients without the existence of these missions. However, the fact that the provided medical service is only carried out for short periods of time is also a great downside. Follow-up, evaluation and knowledge transfer are often absent.

In order to make a long-term contribution, such initiatives should meet certain conditions:

1. An organization should formulate a clear vision involving a local clinic. Are the procedures that are performed also taught to the local doctors? Is there a transfer of knowledge in such a way that the healthcare institution ultimately will be able to provide this care itself? What is the predicted time frame?
2. An organization conducting medical missions must report its own results. In the study by Hendriks et al., the results of short-term surgical missions have been reviewed [6]. Of the 41 articles they found, nine missions reported no information concerning complications and just ten organizations monitored their patients for up to 6 months. The study only investigated the missions that put efforts in recording and publishing their results; therefore, it likely overestimates the positive impact of surgical missions.
3. Mission work needs to be performed in close collaboration with local healthcare providers. Some missions operate with insufficient knowledge of the local culture and healthcare system, whereas local experience is crucial to provide appropriate treatment. Standard medical treatments carried out in high-income countries may sometimes have bad outcomes in other settings. An example is the treatment of burn wounds. It is customary for us to use techniques such as skin transplantation, but the higher risk of infection makes it not always a sensible treatment.
4. Direct post-operative care is crucial. Many missions take place in rural areas. Because of the temporary nature of the missions, some monitoring for post-operative complications should be at hand so that proper referral to more experienced urban hospitals is executed when the mission healthcare workers have departed.
5. Finally, there must be a financial plan for the long term to develop sustainable care for the local community. Providing patients with free healthcare creates structural dependence. The people in need of care must be willing to put an effort into receiving this care. This ultimately also offers the possibility to involve the local government in providing specific care.

We want to emphasize that surgical missions should only continue to exist when sustainable partnerships are developed. These partnerships should provide quality aftercare, perform outcome research and build the surgical capacity of local healthcare systems.

Differences in Thyroid Surgery in Low- and Middle-Income Countries Compared to High-Income Countries

The accessibility of and need for thyroid surgery depend on different pillars: local thyroid pathology, available diagnostics, treatment options and access to follow-up.

Pathology

Whereas in HICs thyroid surgery is mainly performed for goitres or (suspected) malignancy, a different range of indications exists in LMICs. Conversely, some diseases that indicate surgery in HIC may preferably be treated with conservative management in LMICs. One should remember that patients in LMICs always present in late phases of their disease, which is often related to their fear of medicine or the costs that are involved. For this reason, physicians will often encounter patients in LMICs with large goitres or advanced-stage disease, which is hardly seen in a HIC practice.

Goitre

There is a variance of thyroid pathology, particularly in regions with endemic goitre. A colloid goitre in iodine-deficient regions, for example, although seen less nowadays, will regress in most (98%) cases treated by iodine over a period of 3 months. Areas with iodine deficiency decreased to 19% globally in 2017 [7]. When patients present with obstructed breathing or swallowing, an extended hemithyroidectomy may be indicated (Fig. 16.2). Physiological goitres that present as uniform, smooth, painless swelling of the thyroid gland in women aged 12–20 years should be treated conservatively. They resolve spontaneously as the period of maximal hormonal activity passes.

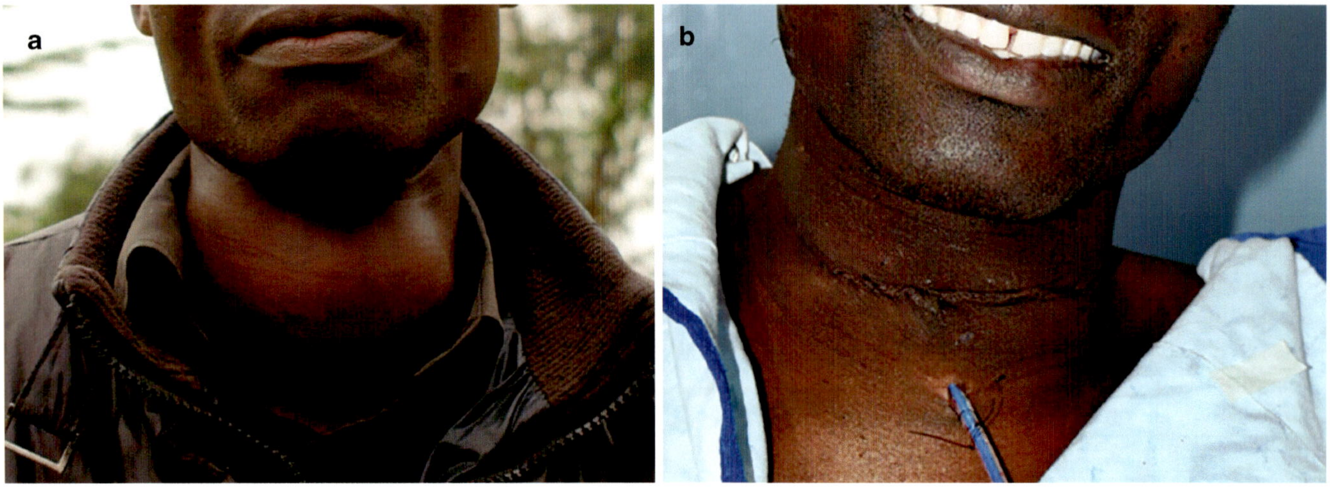

Fig. 16.2 Large goitre. Before (**a**) and after surgery (**b**)

Thyrotoxicosis and Auto-immune Disorders

Thyrotoxicosis, a clinical syndrome caused by the overproduction of triiodothyronine (T3) and thyroxine (T4), has two main potential causes in LMICs. The first is related to the introduction of iodine to the salt in an endemic goitrous area (idiopathic); the second cause is autoimmune with production of antibodies against thyroid stimulating hormone (TSH) receptors. Graves' disease is becoming more prevalent in African areas, which are transitioning from iodine deficient to iodine sufficient. The prevalence of autoimmune hypothyroid disorders is low, compared to European or North American countries [8]. With the absence of laboratory testing, thyrotoxicosis should be suspected when there is a combination of thyroid enlargement (diffuse or nodular) and clinical signs of hyperthyroidism, such as loss of weight, tremor, sweating, anxiety, hyperactivity, palpitations, tachycardia or exophthalmos. Sometimes the presenting symptoms are dramatic and characterized by complications of the condition, such as heart failure. Similar to HICs, the first choice of treatment in LMICs for almost all cases is the prescription of propranolol, to have a rapid control of the tachycardia, and carbimazole, to get the patient euthyroid over time. Radioactive iodine, which is the standard treatment in some HICs for older patients, is often unavailable in LMICs, and it may lead to hypothyroidism and the need for lifelong thyroid hormone replacement. This would be undesirable when chronic medication is scarcely available. Surgery will only be the choice of treatment in limited cases: in the case of a relapse of symptoms after long-term propranolol and carbimazole regimen, when alternative anti-thyroid drugs are unavailable or in case of severe thyrotoxicosis [9]. Patients should be euthyroid before the operation.

Thyroid Malignancy

Thyroid malignancy presence vary across the world, both between and within HICs and LMICs, though some patterns are seen. As papillary thyroid cancers (PTCs) tend to be the commonest in HICs, follicular thyroid cancers (FTCs) are the most common in areas where iodine deficiency is endemic [10]. In Sub-Saharan Africa and Nepal, the incidence of malignancy is higher among multinodular goitres (13–22.9%), which may favour surgery for goitres. Patient delay often leads to a presentation of large invasive tumors. Lymphomas originating from the thyroid gland are rare [11]. In the absence of fine-needle aspiration biopsy (FNAB) or experienced ultrasonography, most solitary nodules are an indication of hemithyroidectomy, reserving completion thyroidectomy for those that are aggressively malignant (when performed by an experienced surgeon).

Infection

Although highly rare, suspect a thyroid abscess when a thyroid gland becomes hot and tender accompanied with leukocytosis. It is often related to immunosuppression, or it is a rare presentation of extrapulmonary tuberculosis. Drainage by aspiration (to prevent open tuberculosis) and intravenous administration of antibiotic therapy may be adequate next to the treatment of the primary disease.

Diagnostics

The availability of diagnostics for thyroid pathology, such as ultrasonography, fine-needle aspiration biopsy (FNAB) and biochemical testing, varies widely between LMICs and between rural and urban clinics.

Clinical Signs

Symptoms suspicious for malignancy are hoarseness, a solid nodule, and lymphadenopathy. In rural settings, a pragmatic approach is often necessary: a solitary nodule without signs of hyperthyroidism is likely to be malignant [9]. Plain radiography of the neck gives important information about compression and deviation of the trachea. Chest X-ray may reveal retrosternal extension or signs of cardiomegaly or tuberculosis.

Ultrasound

Ultrasound machines are widely available in low-resource settings, and for many tropical diseases the best local diagnostic utility [12]. Although expertise is necessary, ultrasound courses for local otolaryngologists can be effective, even when of short duration [13]. In the absence of FNAB, some easy ultrasound clues can be useful: it shows at least whether a nodule is solid and/or cystic, single or multiple. If a cystic swelling turns out to have clear fluid on aspiration, it is unlikely to be malignant. It also helps identify lymphadenopathy. Handheld ultrasound probes are increasingly available and fairly affordable. These are specifically useful in low-resource settings as they can be connected with smartphones and are independent of a stable power source. Remember that ultrasound in inexperienced hands can lead to false diagnoses. We believe that ultrasonography is an indispensable diagnostic prior to thyroid surgery in low-resource conditions. When it is not available, referral to a larger medical centre is in place.

Cytology/Histology

Usually, a preoperative cytological diagnosis will only be available in large medical centres, where there is a pathologist and a physician who is comfortable performing FNAB with sufficient tissue for diagnosis. In general, surgeons working in conditions where FNAB or pathology are not available should be aware that malignancy appears more prevalent in nodules and goitres in LMICs than in HICs, possibly because when access to healthcare is scarce, patients will only visit a doctor when symptoms are severe (i.e., in case of malignancy).

Surgery

The indications for thyroid surgery are essentially no different than they are in HICs. The most frequently occurring diagnoses are obstructive multinodular or even partially malignant goitre, thyrotoxicosis and solitary thyroid nodules.

Considerations regarding perioperative capacity are important before one decides to perform thyroid surgery. Anaesthetic facilities differ per clinic. Thyroid surgery can be performed under locoregional anaesthesia (Fig. 16.3), although most surgeons and patients would prefer general anaesthesia.

Surgeons should bring their own tools—they are familiar with. It is advisable to bring their own set of headlights, surgical magnifier glasses and sometimes even specific operative instruments to get sterilized locally. As thyroid and perithyroidal tissues are well vascularized, the utilization of diathermia is important; however, advanced electrocautery instruments as used in HICs are often unavailable. Additives for haemostasis are swabs soaked in adrenaline solution, running absorbable suturing along the thyroid 'capsule' secured to the pre-tracheal fascia and placement of wound catheters next to the thyroid bed. Recurrent laryngeal nerve monitoring is unlikely to be present. Therefore, the general policy is that this nerve should be identified.

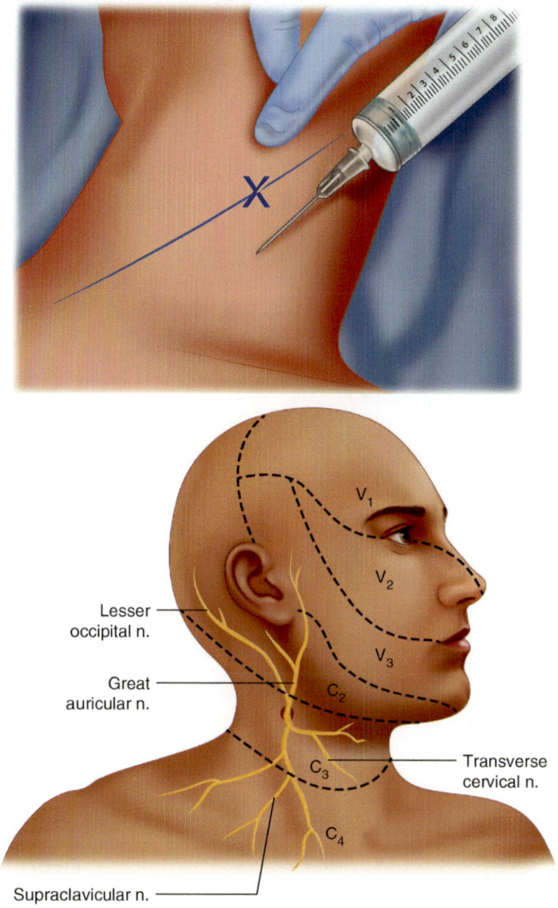

Fig. 16.3 Locoregional anaesthesia: sensory innervation of the cervical plexus is derived from C2-4. The superficial branches include the lesser occipital, greater auricular, transverse cervical and supraclavicular nerves. A superficial nerve block is performed by turning the head to the opposite side. The midpoint of the posterior border of the sternocleidomastoid muscle is identified. Infiltration in multiple vectors maximum 1–2 cm deep. Numbness of the ear suggests a successful nerve block. Infiltration directly in the incision line can be added to this

Generally, in LMICs the extent of surgery is limited to hemithyroidectomy or extended hemithyroidectomy, lowering post-operative risks of hypoparathyroidism and hypothyroidism. Analysis of these post-operative conditions and replacement therapy with calcium, vitamin D or thyroxine are often absent. Therefore, extended hemithyroidectomy is preferred over total thyroidectomy when surgery is indicated for multinodular goitre, even considering the higher 10-year recurrence risk of the prior (8.6% vs 0.6%) [14]. A classic subtotal thyroidectomy should not be performed for unilateral nodes or goitres as this leaves bilateral remnant thyroid tissue, which is inadequate treatment in case of (often unknown) malignancy (Fig. 16.4). Total thyroidectomy should be reserved for very large multinodular goitres with bilateral tracheal compression or advanced carcinomas. They should only be performed in well-equipped centres with experienced thyroid surgeons and access to chronic medication (i.e. for hypocalcaemia and hypothyroidism). Often, advanced thyroid cancer presents a therapeutic challenge that will be unresectable.

The aim of surgical treatment should have a similar outcome when performed in HICs. However, the treatment options are limited by the resources available (Fig. 16.5).

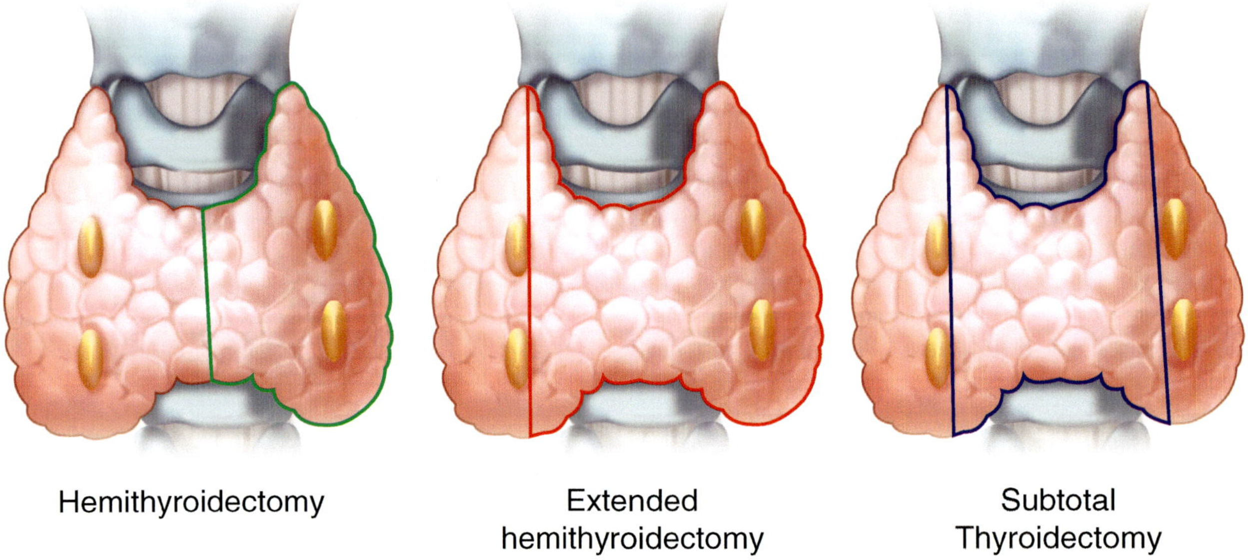

Fig. 16.4 Schematic illustration of the resected tissue for a hemithyroidectomy (highlighted in green), extended hemithyroidectomy (highlighted in red) and subtotal thyroidectomy (highlighted in blue)

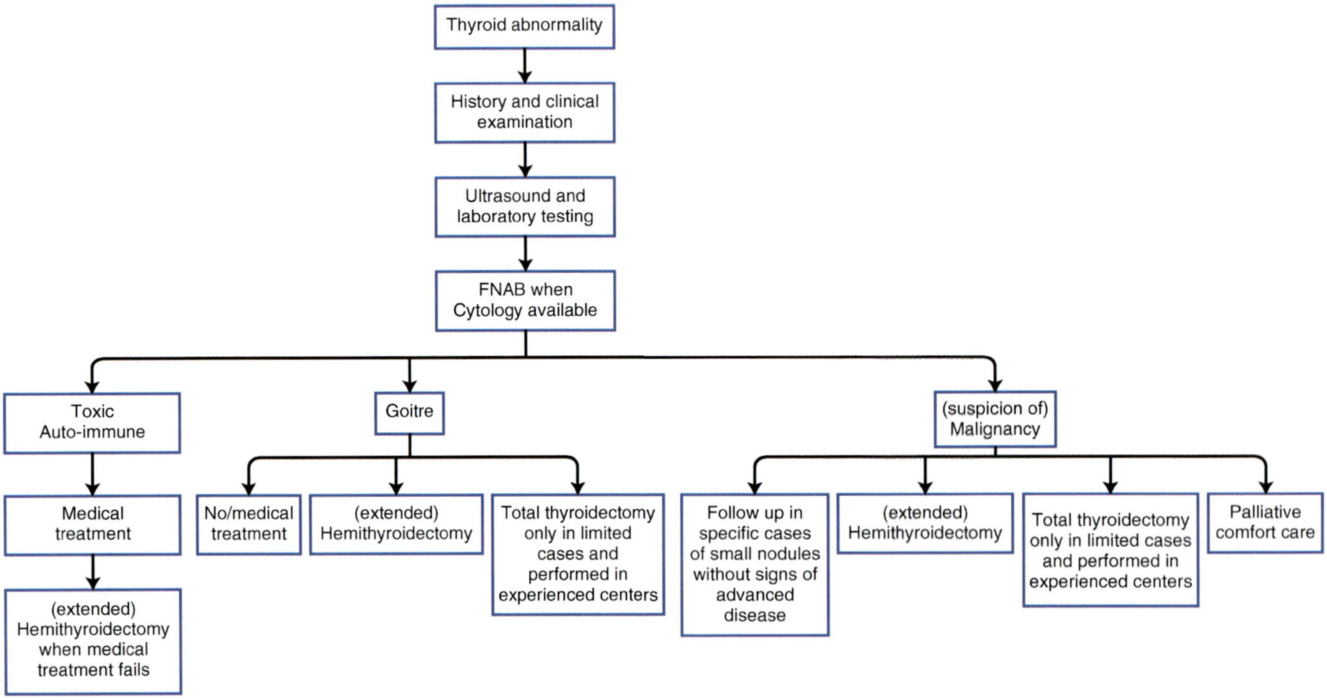

Fig. 16.5 Thyroid pathology management algorithm modified for low- and middle-income countries

Alongside experienced surgeons and trained personnel, the minimal available equipment should include absorbable gauzes, a suction device, electrocautery and an emergency tracheostomy set.

In the case of advanced fast-growing fixed carcinomas with acute respiratory obstruction, palliative comfort care should be the treatment of choice. Damage control surgery or tracheostomy will result in a deplorable situation for a patient with great morbidity. Often, there is insufficient experience how to nurse patients with a tracheostoma, especially when patients are being discharged to their home.

In general, there is evidence that thyroid surgery can be carried out safely with a minimum of complications even in remote mission hospitals with limited facilities for investigation. Standards can be set in terms of surgical outcomes, for example mortality (0%), permanent recurrent laryngeal nerve (RLN) injury (<2%), re-exploration for haematoma (<2%), permanent hypocalcaemia (<5%) and wound infection (2.5%) [15].

Follow-Up

Post-operative monitoring in hospitals in LMICs can be of poor quality. Wards are often overcrowded and equipped with poorly trained personnel. Laboratory tests for calcium or thyroid hormone levels are often not available. Therefore, clear instructions about the symptoms of hypocalcaemia or hypothyroidism should be given to nurses in the ward.

In the case of acute airway obstruction caused by cervical haematoma and bilateral recurrent laryngeal nerve palsy, sufficient recognition and timely action are necessary. There is suspicion of subfascial bleeding when a patient develops stridor and swelling in the neck. Nurses on the ward should know how to recognize this. Therefore, it is of utmost importance to train ward nurses before performing thyroid surgery. The surgeon should be in the near presence of the hospital during the first 24 hours after surgery. An option is to perform thyroid surgery in the morning to make sure that the first post-operative period is during the daytime.

In the case of post-operative haemorrhage, the wound – skin and fascia–should be reopened as soon as possible to evacuate blood clots and prevent airway obstruction. One should be cautious of essential anatomic structures during this emergency procedure. Poor operative light combined with changed anatomy after surgery can result in difficult recognition and subsequent damage to the recurrent laryngeal nerve or the parathyroid glands.

In-hospital recovery is more common in LMICs as patients often live far away from the clinic and because of inferior hygiene in their homes and limited possibility for travel back to the hospital in case of complications. Hypothyroidism is developed on a longer term and is characterized by fatigue, weight gain, cold intolerance, menstrual irregularity, or bradycardia. Hypothyroidism can only be acknowledged when patients take the initiative to come to the clinic for evaluation when they experience these symptoms. Hypothyroidism should be treated with levothyroxine, and the dosage should be adjusted on the basis of complaints.

The scarce availability of follow-up also plays a role in surgical decision-making. In HICs, there is a trend towards de-escalation of treatment for differentiated thyroid cancer with a low-risk profile. However, for this strategy long-term follow-up with high-quality ultrasound is required. When patients present with reasonably small goitre or nodule without signs of advanced-stage disease, non-surgical management can be the treatment of choice when the patient is willing and able to return to the hospital on a regular basis.

Take-Home Messages

1. When planning to work in an LMIC, it is important to evaluate the available facilities and diagnostic tools before commencing any treatment for thyroid pathology. If the necessary equipment for diagnosis, treatment, aftercare or follow-up is unavailable, referral to a better equipped medical centre should be considered.
2. Patients should only be referred to a different clinic when they (and their family) are able to travel the distance – physically as well as financially – and reasonably better disease outcomes can be expected.
3. Visiting surgeons should work in a team with local physicians, who are familiar with local medical dilemmas and culturally sensitive themes. There should be investment in teaching the local personnel about post-operative care.
4. When performing thyroid surgery in a low-resource setting, (extended) hemithyroidectomy will be the preferred and more safe strategy as it decreases the risk of complications, has a shorter recovery time and gives less post-operative drug dependency as compared to total thyroidectomy.
5. In the case of advanced thyroid carcinoma, palliative comfort care should be the treatment of choice as inadequate treatment is much worse than palliative treatment.

References

1. How does the World Bank classify countries? https://datahelpdesk.worldbank.org/knowledgebase/articles/378834-how-does-the-world-bank-classify-countries. Accessed 27 Oct 2020.
2. Human Development Index (HDI). http://hdr.undp.org/en/content/human-development-index-hdi. Accessed 27 Oct 2020.

3. Rosling H. Factfulness: ten reasons we're wrong about the world– and why things are better than up think. First. New York: Flatiron Books; 2016. 341 p.
4. Sullivan R, Alatise OI, Anderson BO, Audisio R, Autier P, Aggarwal A, et al. Global cancer surgery: delivering safe, affordable, and timely cancer surgery. Lancet Oncol. 2015;16(11):1193–224.
5. O'Neill KM, Greenberg SLM, Cherian M, Gillies RD, Daniels KM, Roy N, et al. Bellwether procedures for monitoring and planning essential surgical care in low- and middle-income countries: caesarean delivery, laparotomy, and treatment of open fractures. World J Surg. 2016;40(11):2611–9.
6. Hendriks TCC, Botman M, Rahmee CNS, Ket JCF, Mullender MG, Gerretsen B, et al. Impact of short-term reconstructive surgical missions: a systematic review. BMJ Glob Health. 2019;4(2):e001176.
7. UNICEF. UNICEF global databases, based on MICS, DHS and other nationally representative household surveys, with additional analysis by UNICEF, 2010–2018. https://data.unicef.org/topic/nutrition/iodine. Accessed 27 Oct 2020.
8. Ojo O, Ikem R, Kolawole B, Ojo O, Ajala M. Prevalence and clinical relevance of thyroid autoantibodies in patients with goitre in Nigeria. J Endocrinol Metab Diabetes S Afr. 2019;24(3):92–7.
9. King M, Bewes P, Cairns J, Thornton J. Primary surgery. Volume 1: non-trauma. UK: Oxford University Press; 2013. p. 348–50.
10. Kalk W, Sitas F, Patterson A. Thyroid cancer in South Africa – an indicator of regional iodine deficiency. S Afr Med J. 1997;87:735–8.
11. Ukekwe FI. Patterns of thyroid cancers in southeastern Nigeria: a 15 year histopathologic review (2000–2014). J Clin Diagn Res. 2017;11(8):EC16–9.
12. Stewart KA, Navarro SM, Kambala S, Tan G, Poondla R, Lederman S, et al. Trends in ultrasound use in low and middle income countries: a systematic review. Int J MCH AIDS. 2020;9(1):103–20.
13. Wood CB, Yancey KH, Okerosi SN, Wiggleton J, Seim NB, Mannion K, et al. Ultrasound training for head and neck surgeons in rural Kenya: a feasibility study. J Surg Educ. 2020;77(4):866–72.
14. Barczyński M, Konturek A, Hubalewska-Dydejczyk A, Gołkowski F, Nowak W. Ten-year follow-up of a randomized clinical trial of total thyroidectomy versus dunhill operation versus bilateral subtotal thyroidectomy for multinodular non-toxic goiter. World J Surg. 2018;42(2):384–92.
15. Watters DAK, Wall J. Thyroid surgery in the tropics. ANZ J Surg. 2007;77(11):933–40.

Total Thyroidectomy with Comprehensive Central and Lateral Neck Dissection for Differentiated Thyroid Carcinoma

17

Marco Raffaelli, Carmela De Crea, Luca Sessa, and Rocco Bellantone

Introduction

Total thyroidectomy with comprehensive central and lateral neck dissection represents the standard surgical treatment of differentiated thyroid carcinomas (DTCs) with lateral neck lymph node involvement (N1b) [1–7].

Lymph node metastases may negatively affect recurrence rate and survival [1–3] and occur in 30–80% of patients with papillary thyroid carcinoma (PTC) [8, 9] and, rarely (1–8%), in follicular thyroid carcinoma (FTC) patients [10].

Clinical evaluation and preoperative workup are of utmost importance to plan the correct initial surgical procedure, balancing a complete oncological removal of the tumor and nodal disease while minimizing the complication rate.

An accurate ultrasound evaluation, eventually performed by the surgeons, himself/herself [11], is essential in the evaluation of the thyroid tumor and nodal status. The loss of fatty hilum, calcifications, peripheral vascularity, hyperechogenicity, rounded rather than oval shape, cystic changes, and large size are all characteristics of lymph nodes suspicious for nodal metastases at ultrasound [4]. Preoperative fine-needle aspiration cytology confirms in many cases suspicion of nodal involvement. Thyroglobulin measurement in the washing fluid of the fine-needle aspirate can be helpful in the diagnosis of node-positive (N1) DTC, especially in the case of cystic lateral neck masses, where aspiration cytology is often paucicellular [4]. In the cases in which there is no cytologically/histologically proven nodal disease, a frozen section examination of suspiciously enlarged nodes can enable definitive intraoperative diagnosis, reducing the need for further operations for persistent/recurrent disease [11].

Cross-sectional imaging studies (computed tomography – (CT) or magnetic resonance imaging – (MRI)) with intravenous contrast could be sometimes helpful in the identification of nodal involvement, especially in the upper mediastinum and the retropharyngeal and parapharyngeal spaces [1, 4], and in confirming/excluding the invasion of adjacent organs/structures, including the esophagus, trachea, larynx, and vessels in selected cases (bulky tumors, tumors showing an unexpected rapid growth, signs and symptoms of local invasion – i.e., dysphonia, dysphagia, dyspnea, suspicious findings at preoperative ultrasonography). In suspicious cases, esophagogastroduodenoscopy and/or endotracheal endoscopy can be used to preoperatively confirm/exclude local invasion.

The preoperative workup should include the evaluation of inferior laryngeal nerves (ILNs), by means of direct laryngoscopy. Preoperative vocal fold paralysis may indicate gross invasion by tumor and/or lymph node metastasis or surgical injury during previous operations. The affected nerve can be confidently resected in similar situations in order to achieve adequate oncologic resection. On the contrary, if normal vocal fold motility is demonstrated at preoperative workup, any effort should be made to preserve the anatomic integrity and function of the ILN, even in the presence of macroscopic invasion by the tumor itself or by metastatic nodes with an extranodal growth pattern. However, in such challenging settings, every effort should be made to remove all gross diseases, while preserving ILN function. The benefits of preserving a functioning nerve should be always weighed against the risks of leaving structural disease, especially when facing aggressive histopathological variants of follicular-cell-derived tumors, less prone to respond to adjuvant treatment (i.e., radioiodine treatment).

Lymph node neck dissections are challenging operations associated with several possible complications, as many anatomic structures are at risk during the surgical dissection in a

M. Raffaelli (✉) · C. De Crea
Division of Endocrine and Metabolic Surgery, Fondazione Policlinico Universitario Agostino Gemelli IRCCS, Università Cattolica del Sacro Cuore, Rome, Italy
e-mail: Marco.Raffaelli@unicatt.it

L. Sessa
Division of Endocrine and Metabolic Surgery, Fondazione Policlinico Universitario Agostino Gemelli IRCCS, Rome, Italy

R. Bellantone
Center of Endocrine and Obesity Surgery, Fondazione Policlinico Universitario Agostino Gemelli IRCCS, Università Cattolica del Sacro Cuore, Rome, Italy

A. Shifrin (ed.), *Atlas of Thyroid Surgery*, https://doi.org/10.1007/978-3-030-93673-0_17

relatively small operative field. The trachea, esophagus, laryngeal nerves, and parathyroid glands are extensively exposed during central neck dissection (CND). Moreover, when a lateral neck dissection (LND) is performed, the internal jugular vein (IJV); common carotid artery (CCA); vagus, hypoglossal, phrenic, and spinal accessory nerves (SANs); sympathetic trunk; brachial plexus; and thoracic duct could be at risk of injury.

Knowledge of anatomic landmarks, nomenclatures, classifications, and surgical techniques is essential to offer the most appropriate surgery [7, 8].

Neck lymph nodes have been grouped in levels by the Committee for Head and Neck Surgery and Oncology of the American Academy of Otolaryngology-Head and Neck Surgery (AAO-HNS), with the specific aim of standardizing the nomenclature and reporting system of neck dissections. Level I includes submental (Ia) and submandibular nodes (Ib). Level II includes the upper jugular nodes (the SAN, which travels obliquely across this area, is used as a landmark to subdivide this group into IIb, the portion above and behind the nerve, and IIa, the portion that lays antero inferiorly to it). Level III includes the mid jugular nodes, and level IV includes the lower jugular nodes. Level V includes the lymph nodes of the posterior triangle of the neck (this level is further subdivided by a plane passing along the inferior border of the cricoid cartilage into level Va, superiorly, containing the spinal accessory nodes, and level Vb, inferiorly, containing the transverse cervical and supraclavicular nodes) [12, 13]. Level VI–VII nodes include the lymph nodes of the anterior cervical compartment (level VI) and the superior mediastinal nodes that can be reached via a cervical incision (previously reported as level VII), more commonly reported as central compartment. The boundaries of the anterior compartment (level VI) are defined superiorly by the hyoid bone, inferiorly by the sternal notch, and laterally by the medial aspect of the carotid sheath. Superior mediastinal nodes (level VII lymph nodes) that are removable by a trans cervical approach are those associated with the brachiocephalic vein and innominate artery. The boundaries of level VII are the suprasternal notch superiorly, the medial aspect of the carotid sheath laterally, and the innominate artery on the right (at its point of tracheal crossing) and the corresponding axial plane on the left [14].

Regarding the surgical technique, following the initial description by G. Crile in 1906 of a series of patients who successfully underwent radical neck dissection (RND) [15], which implied the removal of level I–V neck nodes *en bloc* with the IJV, sternocleidomastoid muscle (SCM), and SAN, several modifications have been proposed over the last century in order to minimize the unnecessary consequences and mutilation of Crile's procedure. Owing to high morbidity and anatomical deformity due to RND, in 1963, O. Suarez [16, 17] and, subsequently, Bocca and Pignataro [16] and Gavilan et al. [18–20] described a modified RND (MRND) as functional neck dissection [16, 21], in which satisfactory oncologic results could be obtained while preserving key anatomical structures, i.e., SAN, IJV, and SCM, using a technique of dissection, which follows the fascial planes of the neck.

Indeed, the cervical lymph nodes are without exception contained in the spaces delimited by the muscular fasciae and vascular aponeuroses. As a consequence, in the absence of direct muscular, vascular, and/or nervous invasion, neck dissection can be safely achieved by removing the fascial covering *en bloc* with the fibrofatty tissue containing the lymph nodes while preserving muscular, vascular, and nervous structures [16]. Classically four different fascial layers have been described in the neck: the superficial cervical fascia (SCF) and the deep cervical fascia (DCF). The latter further recognizes three more different layers: the superficial (SLDCF), middle (MLDCF), and deep layers of the DCF (DLDCF) [22, 23].

Then the crucial point in CND and LND is the fascial compartmentalization of the neck: the "wrapping cloth" (i.e., the whole aponeurotic system) can be removed in one piece, together with the packing material (i.e., the cellular and fat tissue contained therein), while preserving important and non affected structures [16].

CND and LND should comprehensively remove fibro fatty tissue in the target compartments, ensuring complete oncologic removal of all nodal diseases, while preserving the anatomical integrity and function of non lymphatic structures.

In the case of N1b DTC, to date, CND and selective LND, including levels IIa, III, IV, and Vb, are considered the standard of treatment in the absence of lymph node involvement at levels I, IIb, and Va [1].

In the present chapter, the authors described the technique for comprehensive CND (levels VI and VII) and LND (levels II–VB) using a fascial dissection approach.

Surgical Technique

Lymph node dissection for thyroid carcinoma should include a comprehensive, possibly *en bloc*, removal of all the target nodal basins: prelaryngeal, pretracheal, and paratracheal lymph nodes in CND and levels IIa–Vb in LND. The dissection of additional nodal groups (i.e., retropharyngeal, retroesophageal, level I, level IIb, and level Va) is selectively needed on the basis of the dissemination of nodal disease.

To achieve an adequate and comprehensive clearance of the target basins, it is particularly useful to follow the planes of coalescence of different fascial layers, which are avascular and allow to remove the target nodes *en bloc* with their investing fascial layers. That is the well-known principle of fascial dissection, theorized for LND by O. Suarez and popularized worldwide by Bocca and Pignataro [16] and Gavilan et al. [18, 20, 24]. Despite this concept having been primarily developed for LND dissection, it is applicable also for CND, owing to the fascial envelopments of the central (anterior) compartment.

When neck dissection is performed at the time of thyroidectomy, the central compartment would be preferably removed *en bloc* with the thyroid gland to respect the principles of oncologic resection. When LND is planned and performed at the same time as thyroidectomy and/or CND, it should be accomplished first to reduce the risk that traction on an empty thyroid bed (central compartment) would cause inadvertent injury to the ILN and/or parathyroid glands, which are no more protected by adjacent structures. For this reason, in the present chapter, the operative technique of LND will be discussed first.

The central and lateral compartments are separated by the carotid sheath. For this reason, *en bloc* resection of the lateral and central compartments is not suitable. Conversely, in the case of RND or extended radical neck dissection for locally advanced tumors, invading structures included in the carotid sheath, *en bloc* resection of the lateral and the central compartments could be feasible and advisable.

Patient's Preparation and Positioning

General anesthesia with orotracheal intubation is needed. Nerve-monitoring endotracheal tube is preferable. The patient is placed in supine position, and the neck is slightly hyperextended with the help of a shoulder roll (Fig. 17.1). After checking the nerve monitoring system, the patient is prepared and draped in the usual way. The trapezoidal operative field should include the chin, the inferior margin of the mandible, and the earlobe cranially, the anterior margin of the trapezius muscle laterally, and the sternal notch and the clavicle caudally (Fig. 17.2a).

In the case of LND, the head of the patient should be rotated on the opposite side to maximize exposure. During such maneuver, it is important to avoid any dislodgment of the orotracheal tube and its electrodes for intraoperative nerve monitoring.

Skin Incision and Flap Elevation

In a conventional procedure, a 4–5-cm collar incision about 2 fingers above the sternal notch, usually in a natural neck crease, is adequate to provide access and good exposure for total thyroidectomy and CND. In the case of LND, the incision should be prolonged on the side(s) of the dissection (Fig. 17.2b). The horizontal skin incision should be prolonged up to the posterior third/posterior margin of the ipsilateral SCM. The extended collar incision can offer adequate exposure for neck dissections required in thyroid carcinoma.

Monopolar cautery is used to elevate the subplatysmal flap (Fig. 17.3), preserving the SLDCF, the external and anterior jugular veins, and the greater auricular nerve. The flap should be extended cranially to expose the hyoid bone in the midline and the submandibular gland laterally if LND is planned. Inferiorly, the flap is elevated to the sternal notch in the midline and the clavicle laterally. The posterior border of

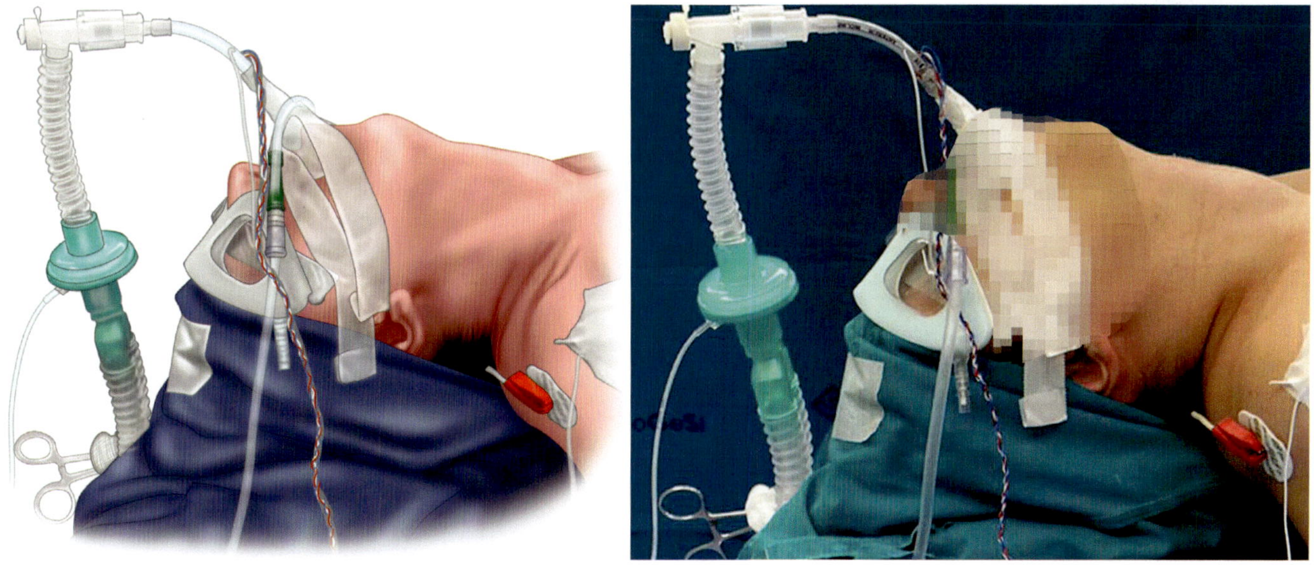

Fig. 17.1 Patient's position. The patient is placed in supine position, and the neck is slightly hyperextended with the help of a shoulder roll. General anesthesia with orotracheal intubation is needed. A nerve-monitoring endotracheal tube is advisable

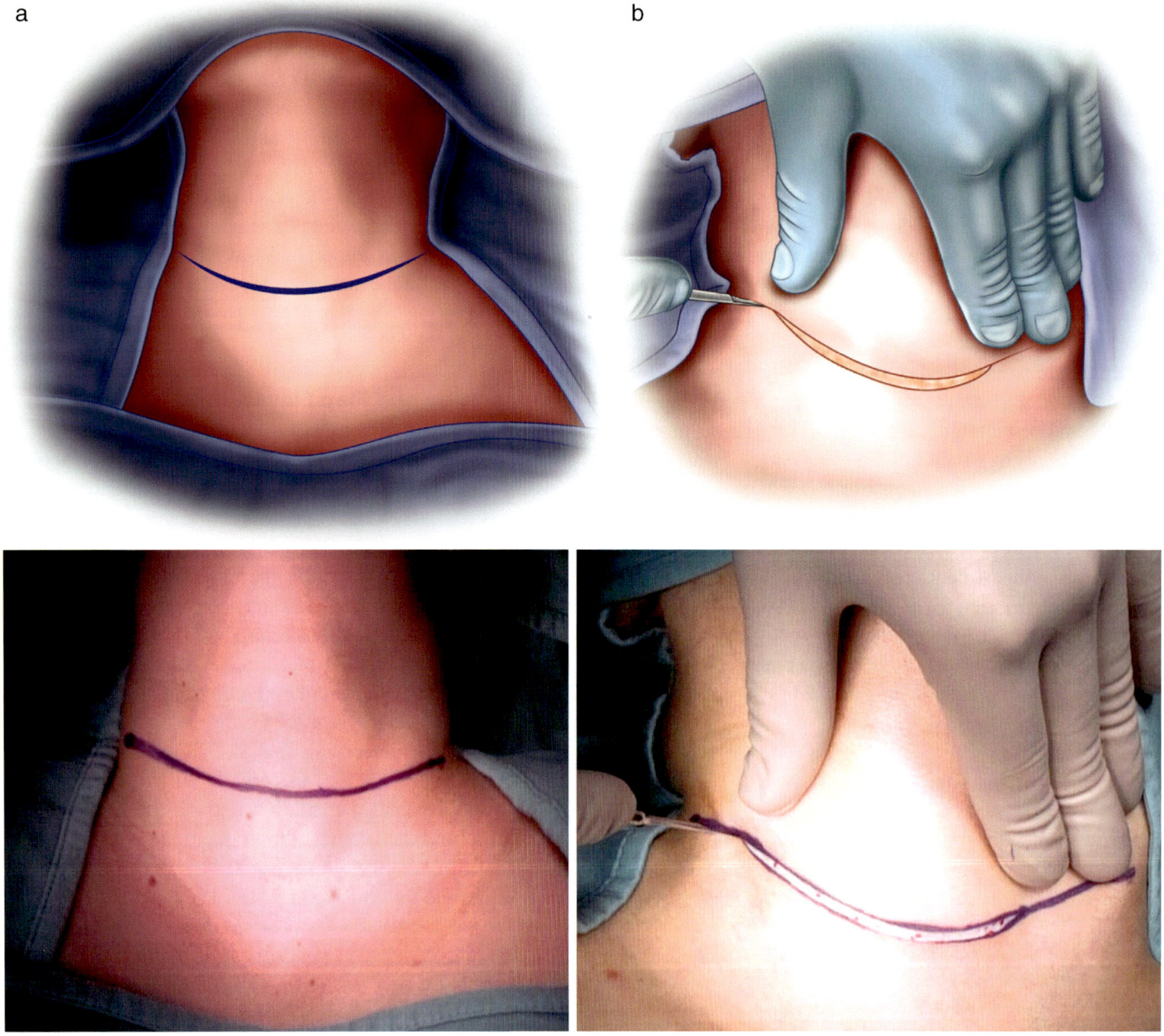

Fig. 17.2 (**a**), Operative field should include the chin, the inferior margin of the mandible and the earlobe cranially, the anterior margin of the trapezius muscle laterally, and the sternal notch and the clavicle caudally. (**b**) Horizontal skin incision is performed about 2 fingers above the sternal notch, ideally in a natural neck crease, and is prolonged laterally on the side of neck dissection until the posterior third/posterior margin of the ipsilateral sternocleidomastoid muscle

the SCM should be exposed as well if LND is planned (Fig. 17.4).

Selective Lateral Neck Dissection: Levels II–Vb

It should be underlined that the sequence of the steps usually reflects the operating surgeon's preference and experience. Usually, a medial to lateral approach is used by general and endocrine surgeons, while a lateral to medial approach is usually preferred by head and neck surgeons. Every approach has its own advantage(s). A combination of both a lateral to medial and a medial to lateral approaches can be useful, depending on the step of the procedure and the individual patients and tumor to be treated.

What is of utmost importance is the comprehensive removal of all the fibrofatty tissue *en bloc* and embedded within the investing fascial planes.

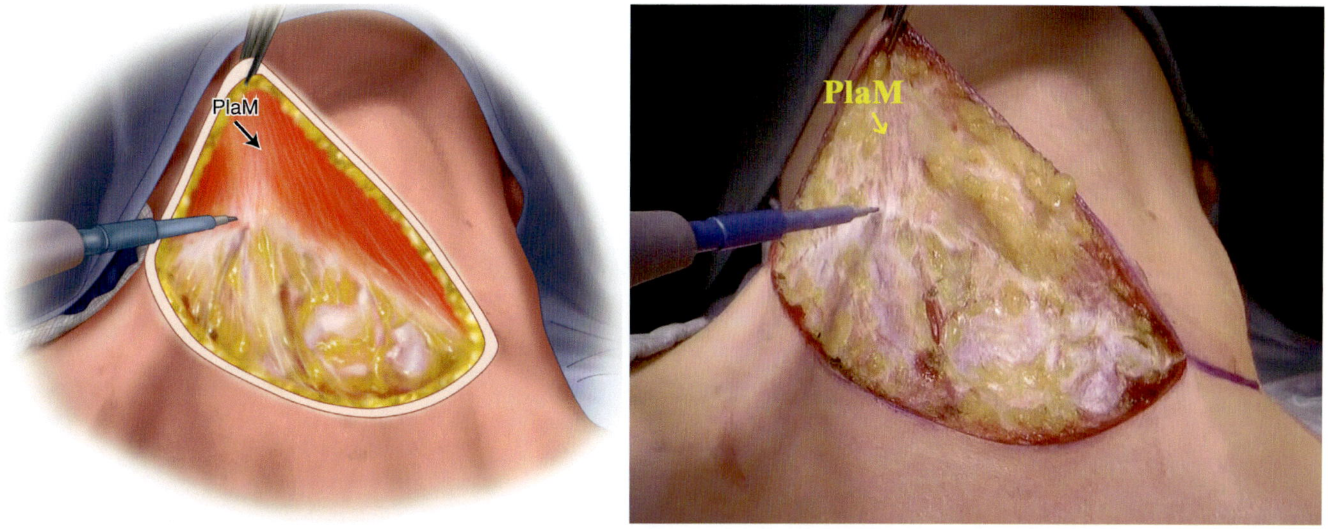

Fig. 17.3 A wide subplatysmal flap is elevated upward, paying attention to preserving the integrity of the superficial layer of the deep cervical fascia (see text). PlaM – platysma muscle

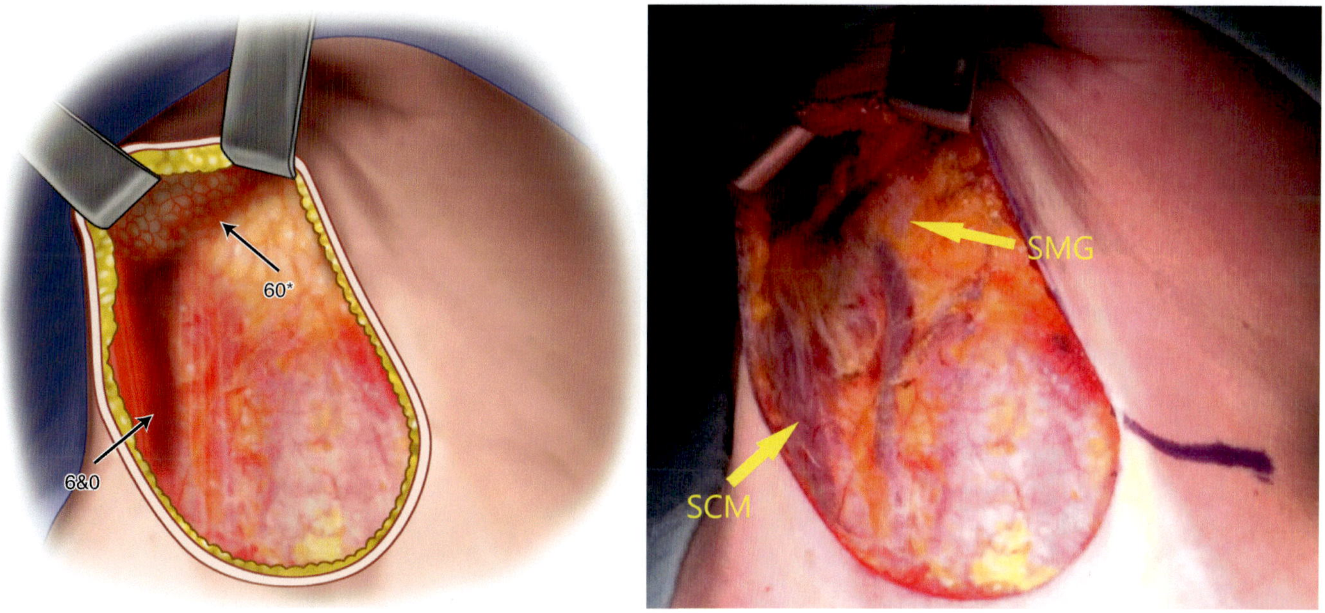

Fig. 17.4 The subplatysmal flap is accomplished, preserving the integrity of the superficial layer of the deep cervical fascia and the anterior jugular veins. It is extended cranially to expose the hyoid bone in the midline and the submandibular gland laterally and caudally to the sternal notch in the midline and the clavicle laterally. The posterior border of the SCM is exposed. SCM – sternocleidomastoid muscle, SMG – submandibular gland

Unwrapping the SMC

The dissection starts with vertical incision of the SLDCF investing the SCM along all the length of the SCM itself. The incision is preferably close to the posterior border of the SCM (Fig. 17.5). At this point, the SCM should be completely enwrapped. Although most surgeons usually prefer to proceed with subfascial dissection toward the anterior margin of the muscle, it could be preferable to prepare the dissection of the subclavicular triangle first, proceeding with a postero lateral direction. The incised fascia is then elevated by means of a pair of forceps and retracted postero laterally at the level of the distal third of the SCM. Dissection is achieved by means of monopolar electrocautery or bipolar scissors to avoid any minimal bleeding.

The SLDCF is detached from its infero anterior attachments at the level of the sternum and the medial third of the clavicle. Once the posterior border of the SCM is reached, dissection of the fascia proceeds anteriorly along the poste-

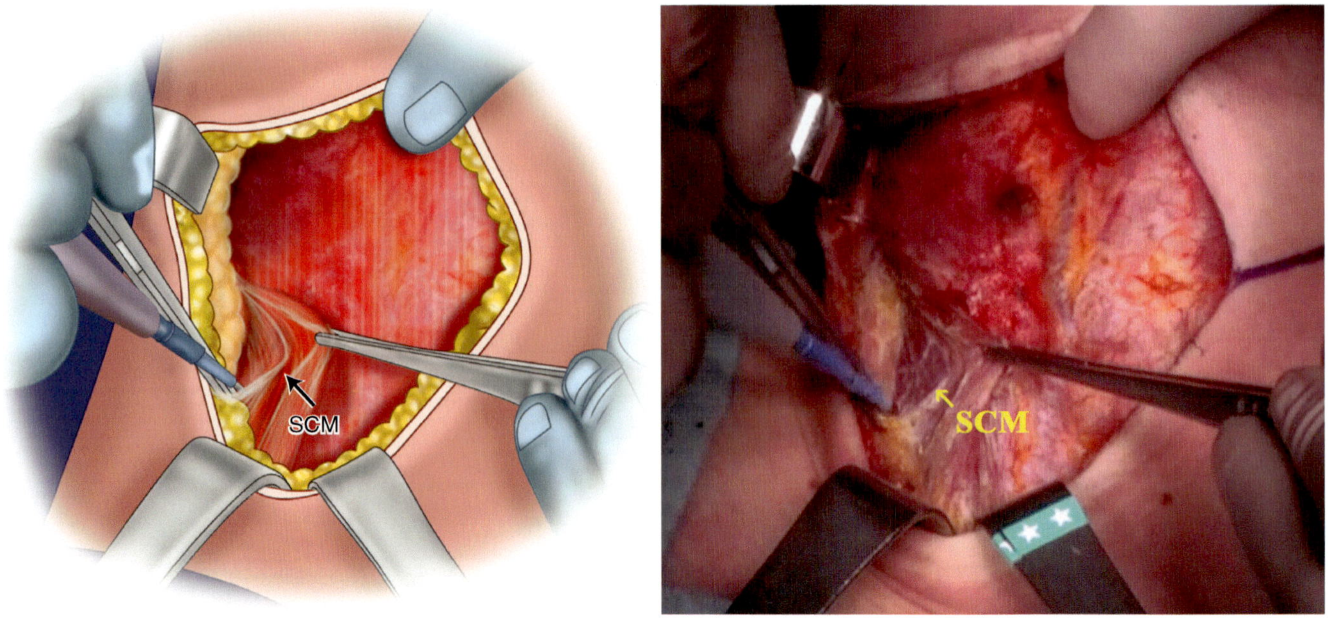

Fig. 17.5 Unwrapping the sternocleidomastoid muscle. The superficial layer of the deep cervical fascia is incised vertically along the sternocleidomastoid muscle, close to its posterior border, and subfascial dissection is accomplished using monopolar cautery. In the distal thirds of the sternocleidomastoid muscle, dissection proceeds first posteriorly along the posterior border and the inferior aspect of the sternocleidomastoid muscle (supraclavicular triangle). SCM – sternocleidomastoid muscle

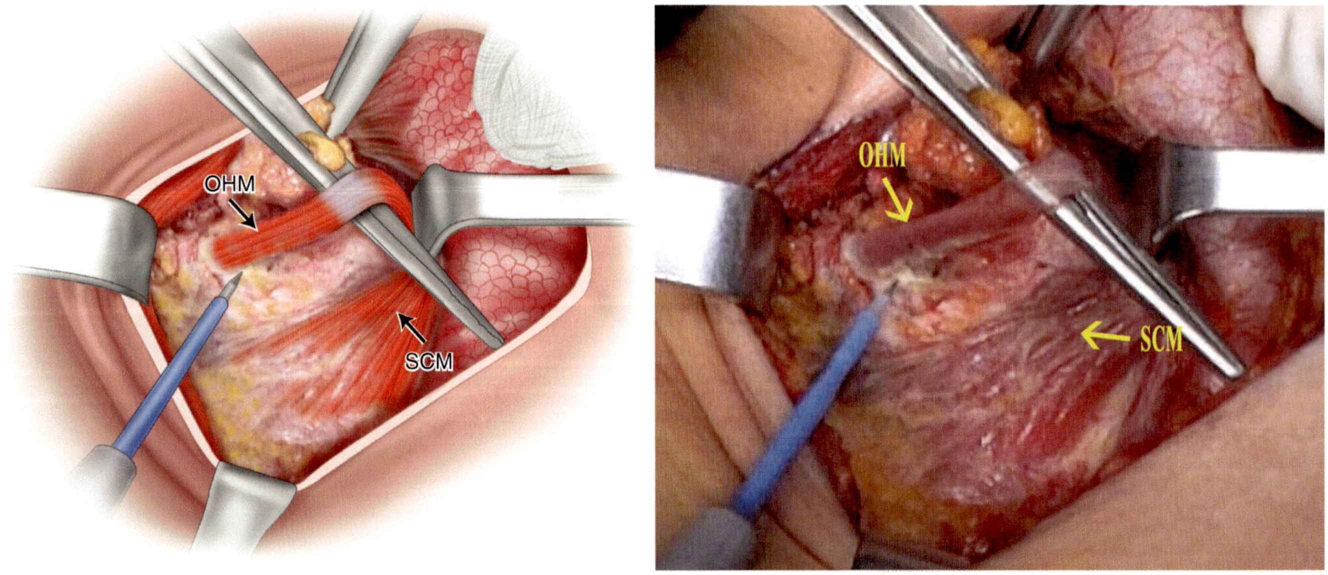

Fig. 17.6 Superficial dissection of the supraclavicular triangle. The inferior belly of the omohyoid muscle is identified and unwrapped of the investing middle layer of deep cervical fascia, from the intermediate tendon to the point where it crosses the trapezius muscle. OHM – omohyoid muscle, SCM – sternocleidomastoid muscle

rior aspect of the distal third of the muscle, which is retracted antero medially, allowing a progressive dissection of the fascial covering (Fig. 17.5). The posterior belly of the omohyoid muscle is then identified and unwrapped of its fascial coating from the intermediate tendon to its crossing with the trapezius muscle (Fig. 17.6). Unwrapping the omohyoid muscle will be continued anteriorly during the anterior dissection. It is essential to preserve the muscle and obtain adequate exposure, especially during supraclavicular triangle dissection. In addition, it should be underlined that omohy-

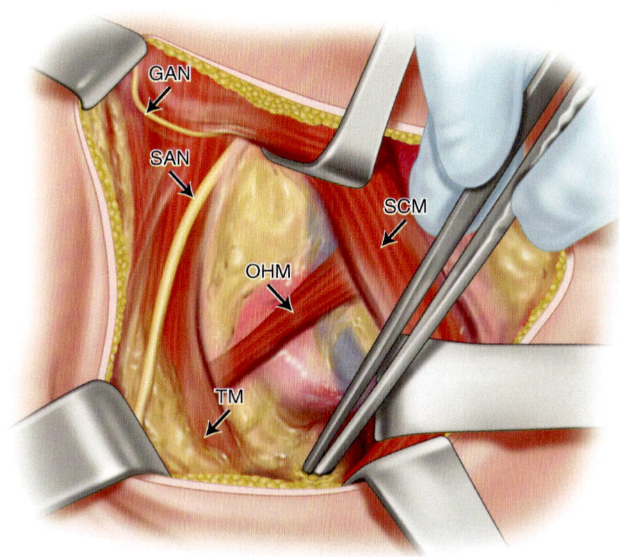

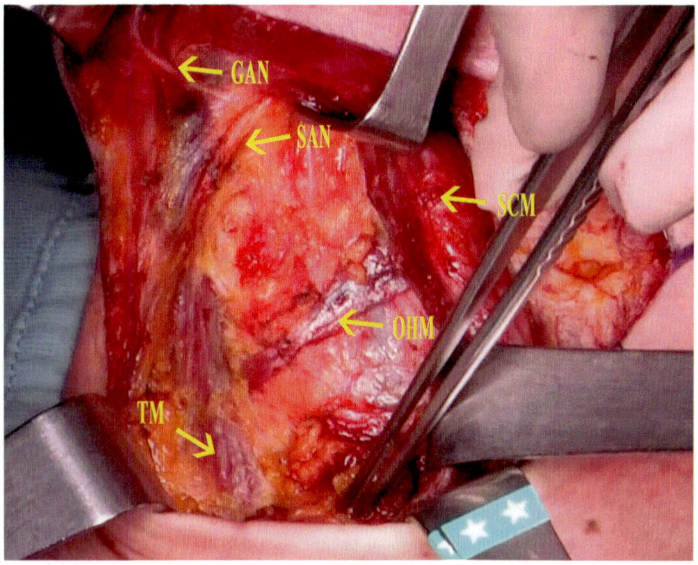

Fig. 17.7 Superficial dissection of the supraclavicular triangle completed. GAN – greater auricular nerve, OHM – omohyoid muscle, SAN – spinal accessory nerve, SCM – sternocleidomastoid muscle, TM – trapezius muscle

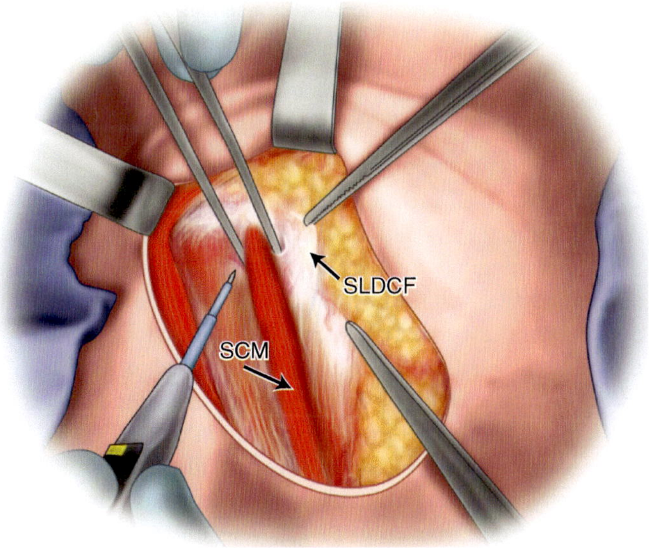

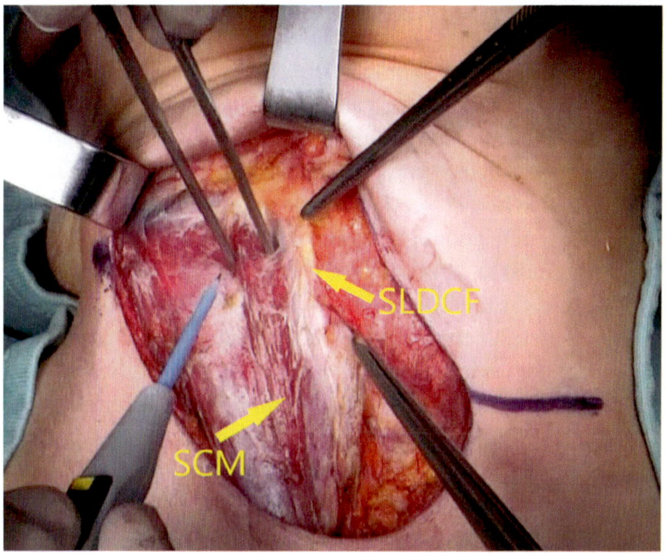

Fig. 17.8 Dissection of the superficial layer of the deep cervical fascia is continued along the anterior aspect of the sternocleidomastoid muscle and its anterior margin. The fascial layer is elevated with two forceps and dissection performed using monopolar cautery. SLDCF – superficial layer of the deep cervical fascia, SCM – sternocleidomastoid muscle

oid muscle is enveloped by the MLDCF that should be removed *en bloc* to ensure adequate clearance.

Once the achieved dissection of the posterior belly of the omohyoid muscle is achieved, the SLDCF is detached inferiorly from the clavicle and posteriorly from the trapezius muscle. The clavicle and the trapezius muscle are exposed. Dissection is then continued upward along the anterior margin of the trapezius muscle until exposure of the external jugular vein, which can be ligated or preserved (Fig. 17.7). If preservation of the external jugular vein is chosen, it should be freed from investing in fibrofatty tissue. At this point, the superficial dissection of the supraclavicular triangle is completed. A small gauze may be left at this level.

Dissection is then directed anteriorly. The SLDCF is detached along the anterior aspect of the SMC. When dissection reaches the anterior border of the SCM, the muscle is retracted posteriorly to continue dissection underneath, over its medial aspect, starting from the caudal portion upward, aiming to free the fascial covering from the posterior border of the SCM (Fig. 17.8). Inferiorly, the dissection reaches the

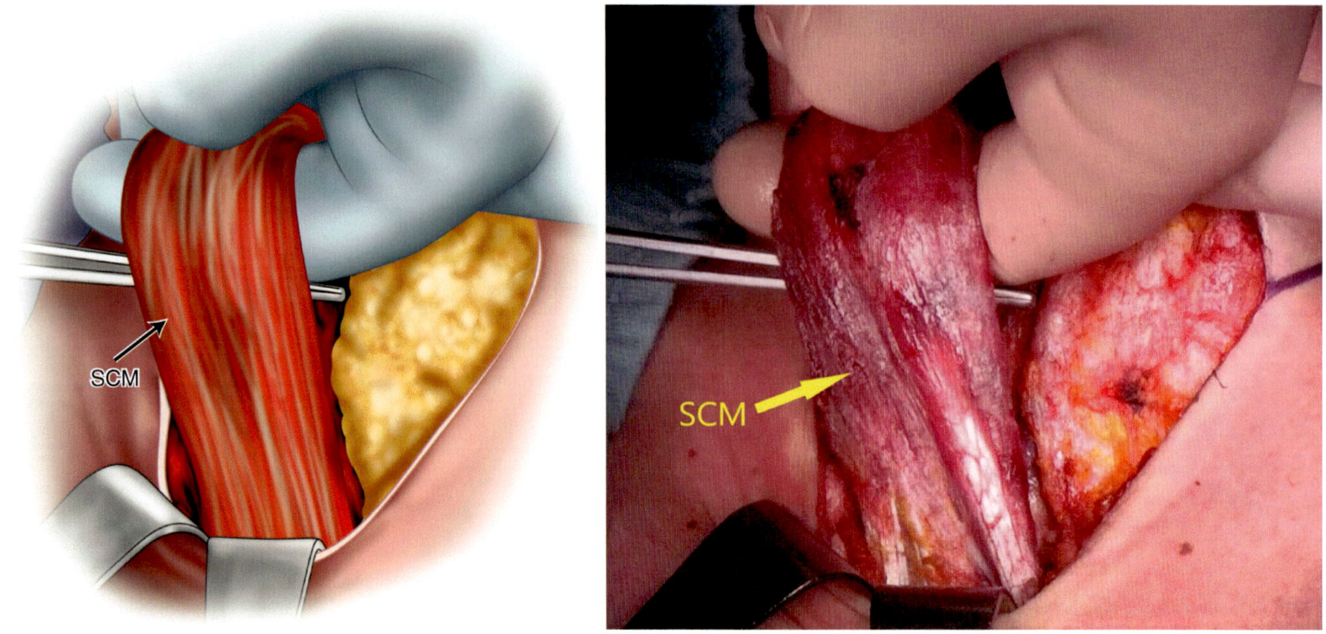

Fig. 17.9 The sternocleidomastoid muscle is completely unwrapped of its investing fascial layer, belonging to the superficial layer of the deep cervical fascia. That allows complete mobilization of the sternocleidomastoid muscle itself. SCM – sternocleidomastoid muscle

previously dissected supraclavicular triangle, as evidenced by the identification of the gauze left at that level.

Dissection over the medial surface of the SCM is then continued, allowing complete mobilization of the SCM (Fig. 17.9). When dissection reaches the cranial third of the muscle, special attention should be paid to the SAN that enters the muscle, approximately at the junction of its upper and middle thirds. To minimize the risk of SAN injury, it may be preferable to stop posterior dissection before reaching such a dangerous area. Dissection can be more safely accomplished after the dissection of the submandibular triangle and the identification of the SAN in its proximal tract below the posterior belly of the digastric muscle.

In summary, the first step of the procedure consists in the complete unwrapping of the SCM (Fig. 17.9) and of the inferior belly of the omohyoid muscle and the dissection of the SLDCF from its clavicular and sternal attachments and from the anterior border of the trapezius muscle. Below Erb's point, dissection is accomplished posterior to the SCM; in the upper two thirds, dissection is accomplished anterior to the SCM.

Preparing the Submandibular Triangle

At this point, the SLDCF is incised along the inferior margin of the submandibular gland (Fig. 17.10a). The gland is then retracted upward to expose the cranial boundary of the dissection represented by the posterior belly of the digastric muscle and the stylohyoid muscle. In the SND for thyroid carcinoma, the section of the facial vein is not required. However, it should be preferably unwrapped of the investing fascial layer, since small lymph nodes may be missed along its posterior aspect, below the inferior margin of the submandibular gland.

Dissecting the Medial Boundary

At this point, the dissection of the SLDCF is continued along the lateral margin of the sternohyoid muscle by preserving the anterior jugular veins. The SLDCF is dissected away from the antero lateral aspect of the sternohyoid muscle. This allows exposing the medial border of the LND, which is represented by the coalescence of the fascia covering the lateral border of the sternothyroid muscle with the carotid sheath (Fig. 17.11). Proceeding in a postero lateral direction, the superior belly of the omohyoid muscle is identified and completely unwrapped of its investing fascia (Fig. 17.12). This allows for complete mobilization of the muscle, very useful in the text steps of the dissection process and for complete exposure of the carotid sheath and the neurovascular bundle of the neck. By retracting postero laterally the medial border of the dissected SLDCF, the neurovascular bundle is unwrapped, caudal to cranial, until reaching the sagittal aponeurosis, posterior to the neurovascular bundle, and, consequently, the coalescence of the avascular plane with the DLDCF (Fig. 17.13). An effort should be made to preserve the descending branch of the *ansa cervicalis*, which should be followed upward till its travels along with the hypoglossal nerve. Moreover, during the most posterior part of the dissection, its ascending branch should be preserved as well since it represents an important landmark for the deepest plan of dissection (Fig. 17.13). During this step of the dissection, it is usually unnecessary to ligate

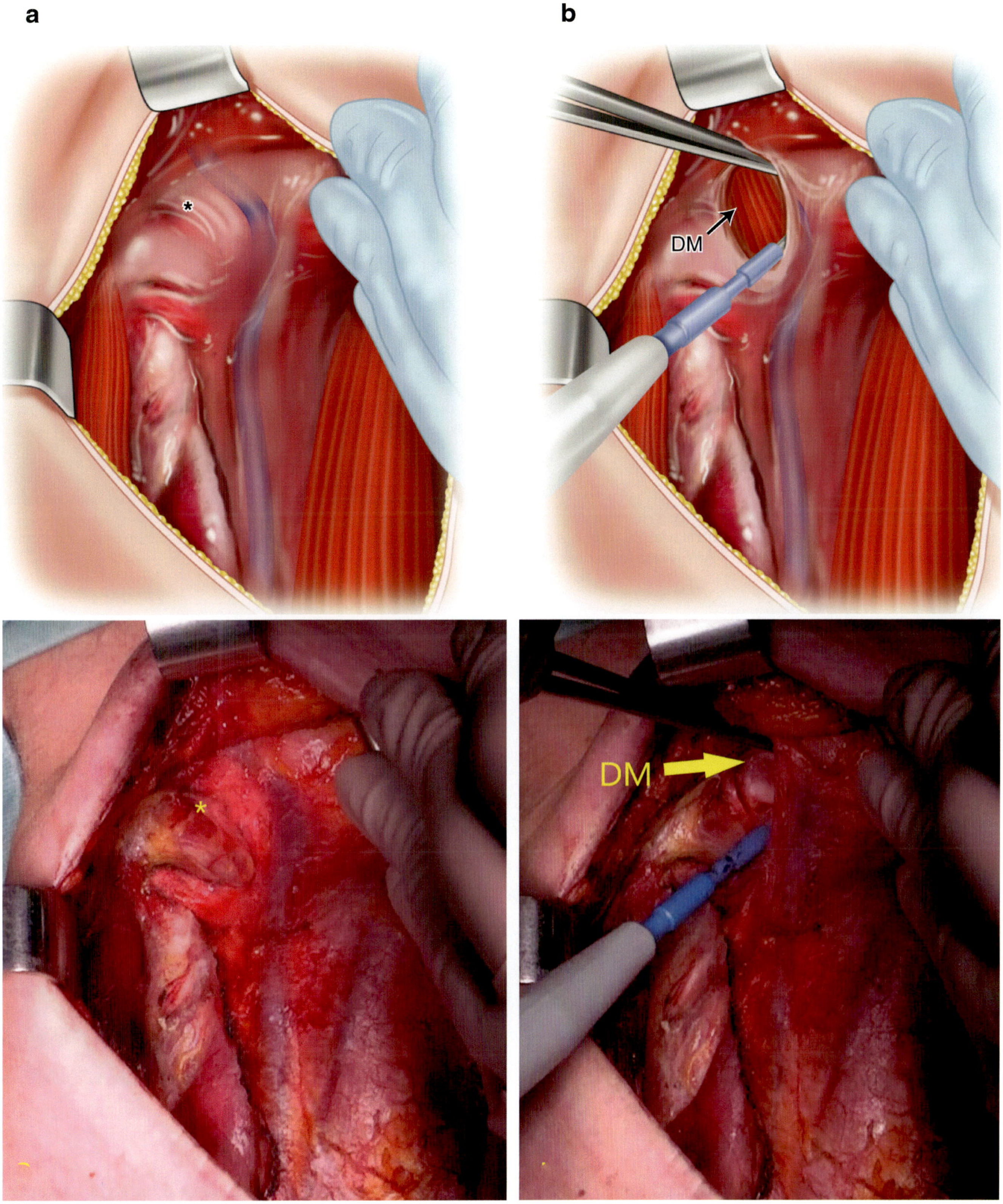

Fig. 17.10 Preparing the submandibular triangle. (**a**) The superficial layer of the deep cervical fascia (*) is incised along the inferior border of the submandibular gland. (**b**) The submandibular gland is retracted medially and upward to expose the cranial boundary of the dissection, represented by the posterior belly of the digastric muscle (DM) and the stylohyoid muscle

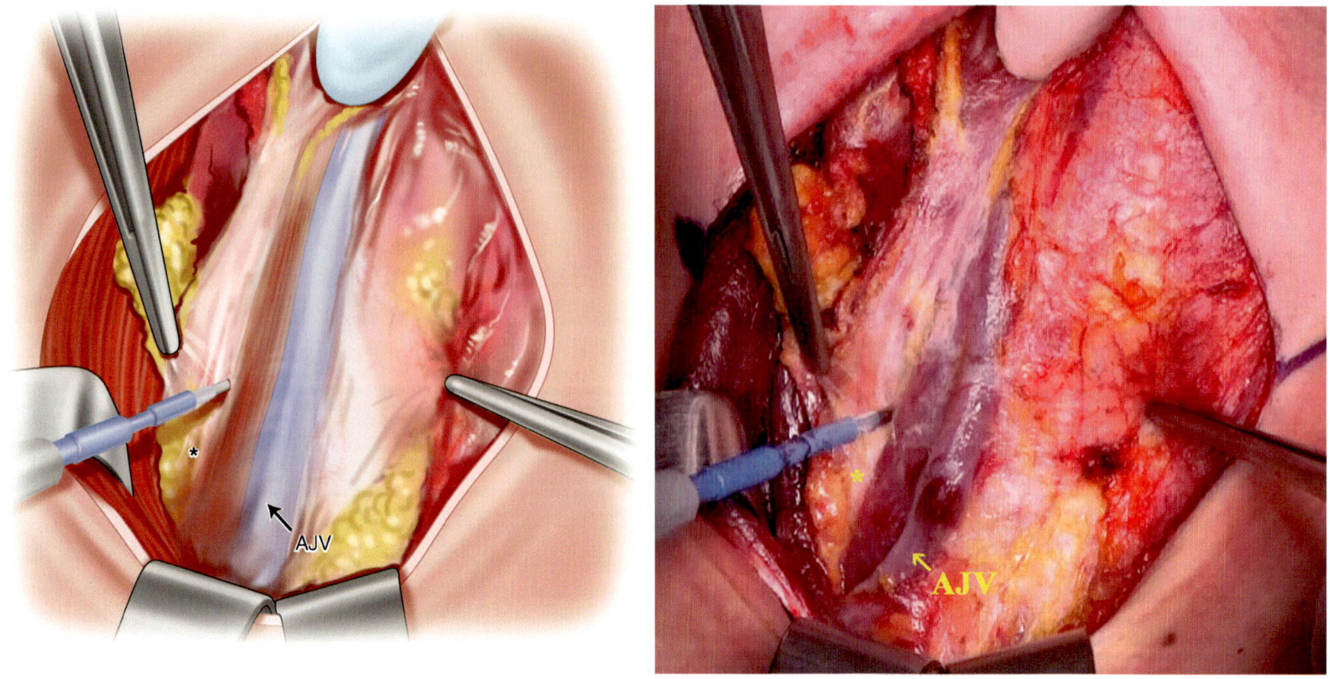

Fig. 17.11 The medial boundary of the lateral neck dissection is dissected: it is represented by the coalescence of the fascia investing the sternothyroid muscle and the carotid sheath (*). AJV – anterior jugular vein

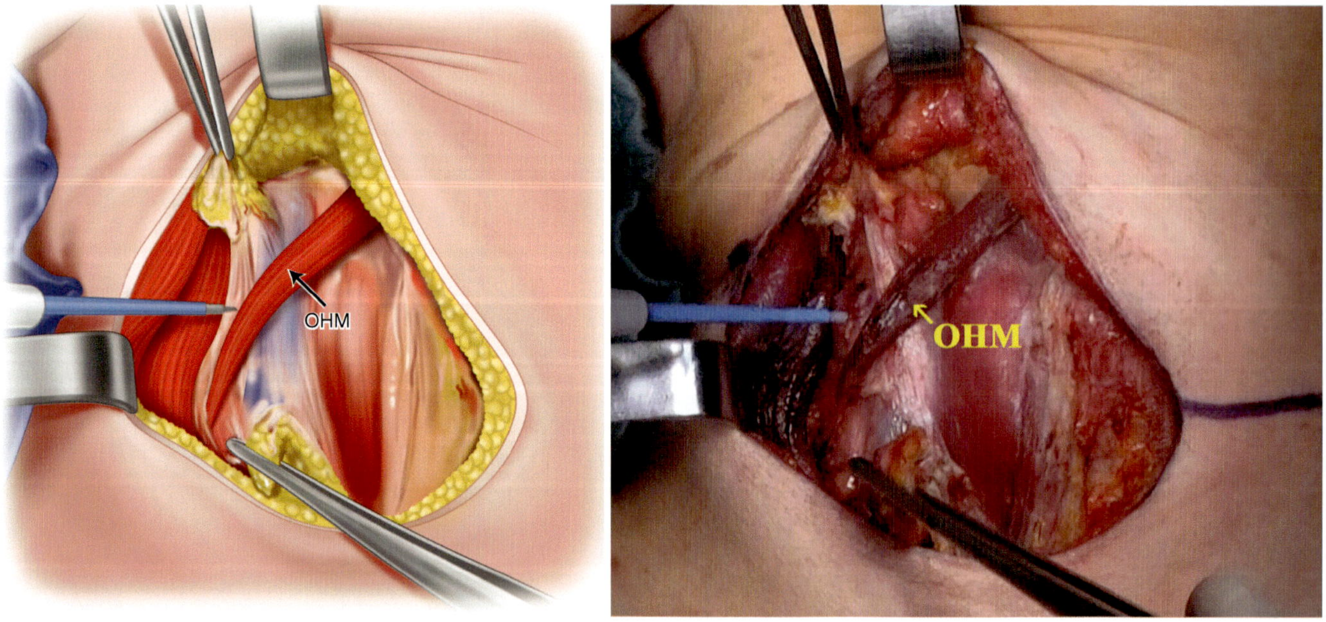

Fig. 17.12 The superior belly of the omohyoid muscle (OHM) is identified and completely unwrapped of the investing middle layer of the deep cervical fascia

the facial, lingual, and thyroid artery and veins, but they should be completely freed from the investing fascia.

In the caudal portion of the field, the IJV should be prepared till its confluence with the subclavian vein (Pirogoff's trunk), eventually preserving also the external and anterior jugular veins. At this level, attention should be paid to avoid injury to the thoracic duct on the left and the right lymphatic duct (if present) at their confluence on the Pirogoff's trunk.

During the dissection of the posterior aspect of the neuro vascular bundle, special attention should be paid to avoid inadvertent injury to the sympathetic chain, which can result in Horner's syndrome.

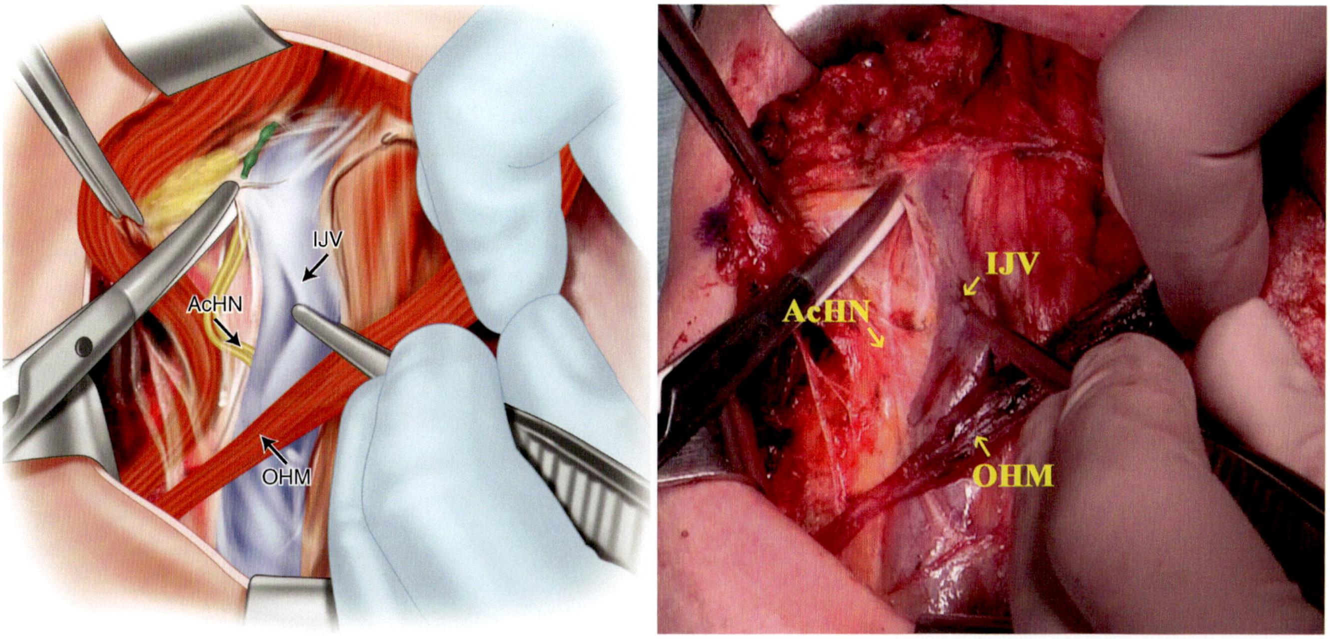

Fig. 17.13 The sagittal fascia posterior to the carotid sheet is incised, and the plane of coalescence of the superficial and deep cervical fascia layers is exposed. Dissection is continued along that avascular plane. The ascending branch of the *ansa cervicalis* is identified and preserved. AcHN – ascending branch of the *ansa cervicalis* of the hypoglossal nerve, IJV – internal jugular vein, OHM – omohyoid muscle

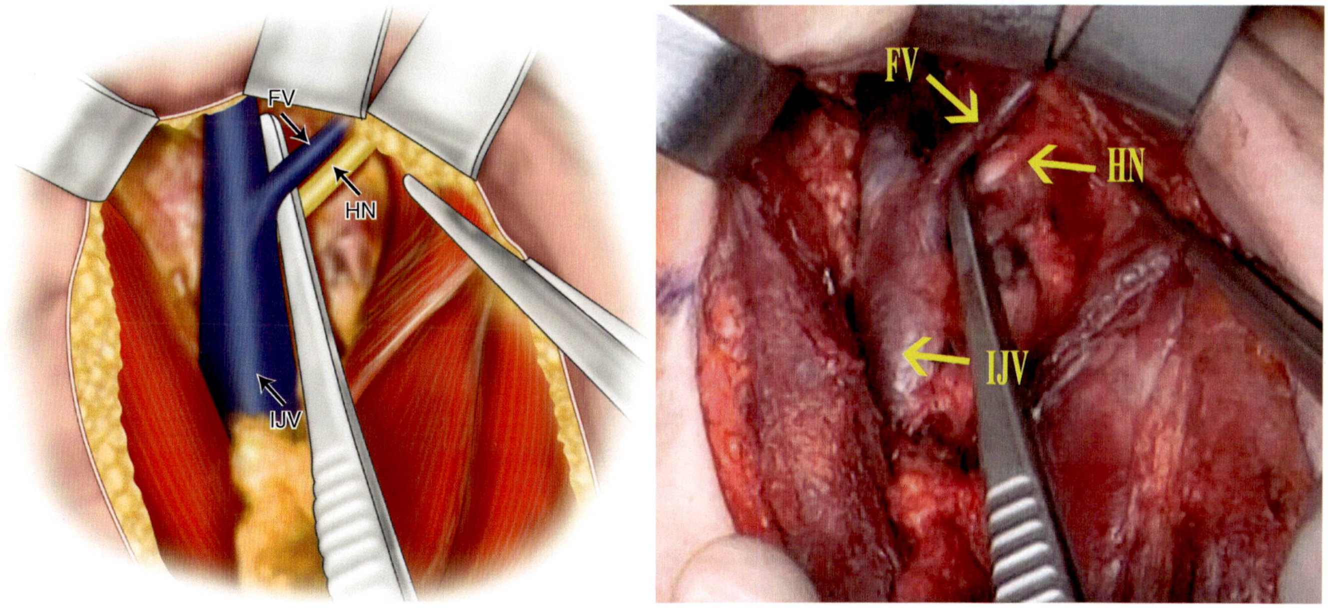

Fig. 17.14 Dissection of level II – submandibular triangle – the facial vein is unwrapped, and the hypoglossal nerve is identified. FV – facial vein, HN – hypoglossal nerve, IJV – internal jugular vein

Dissecting Level II

Proceeding upward, the fascia is incised along the posterior belly of the digastric muscle. Countertraction by the assistant over the uppermost portion of CCA facilitates the identification of the hypoglossal nerve (Fig. 17.14), following the descending branch of the *ansa cervicalis*. Dissection over the fascial plane is then continued laterally to complete the dissection of the anterior and lateral aspects of the IJV. At this point, the supero medial retraction of the posterior belly of the digastric muscle and the latero inferior retraction of the SCM muscle allow adequate exposition of the SAN between the SCM and IJV. The SAN has then to be completely dissected from its surrounding tissue since it crosses the intrafascial tissue, and it is completely embedded with lymph nodes containing fibrofatty tissue. In the absence of a gross involvement of such lymph nodes, it would be enough to dissect the tissue anterior to the nerve (IIa dissection). In the case that a level IIb dissection is needed, the SAN must be gently displaced to dissect the cranial and posterior fibrofatty tissue. Then the dissected IIb tissue has to be passed behind the nerve to be removed *en bloc* with the remaining specimen. Thus, in level IIb dissection, the splenius capitis and the levator scapulae muscles represent the most posterior aspect of the dissection in the cranial part of the operative field (Fig. 17.15).

Level III and IV Dissection

At this point, while the SCM is retracted laterally and the vascular bundle medially, the downward retraction of the specimen allows completing the dissection of the posterior boundary along the plane of coalescence of the SLDCF and DLDCF (Fig. 17.16) by preserving the roots of the

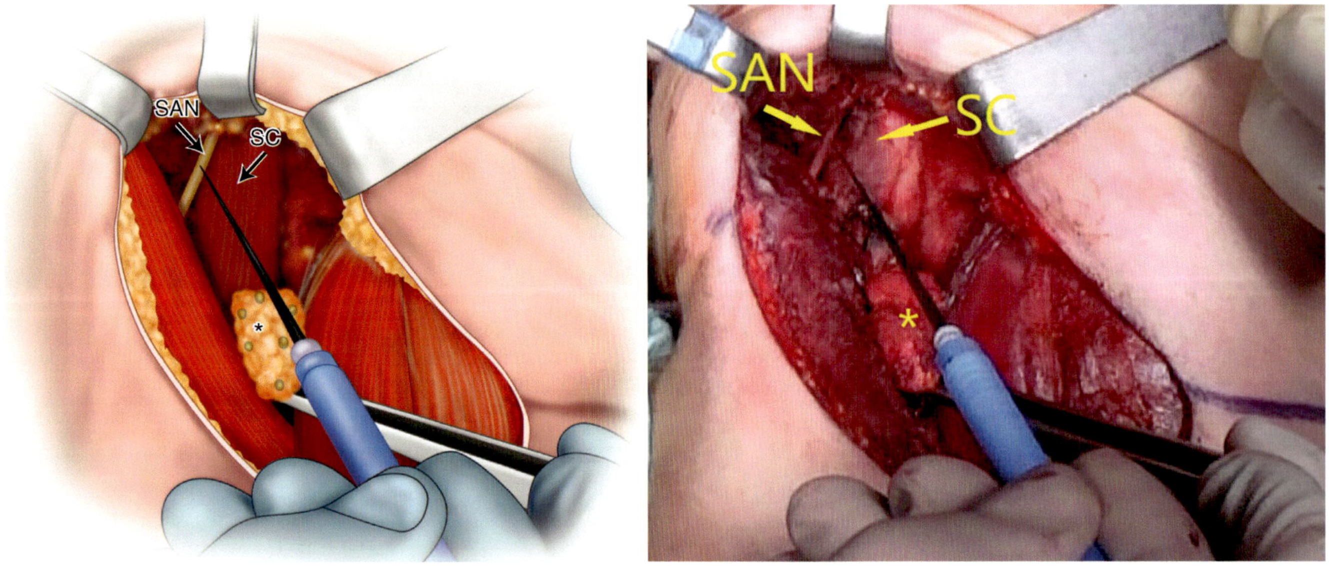

Fig. 17.15 Dissection of level II – the spinal accessory nerve has to be completely dissected from its surrounding tissue since it does not follow a fascial plane, but it crosses the intrafascial tissue and it is completely embedded with lymph nodes containing fibrofatty tissue. In case level IIb dissection is required, the splenius capitis and the levator scapulae muscles represent most of the posterior aspect of the dissection in the cranial part of the operative field. SAN – spinal accessory nerve, SC – splenius capitis, * – lymph nodes retracted downward

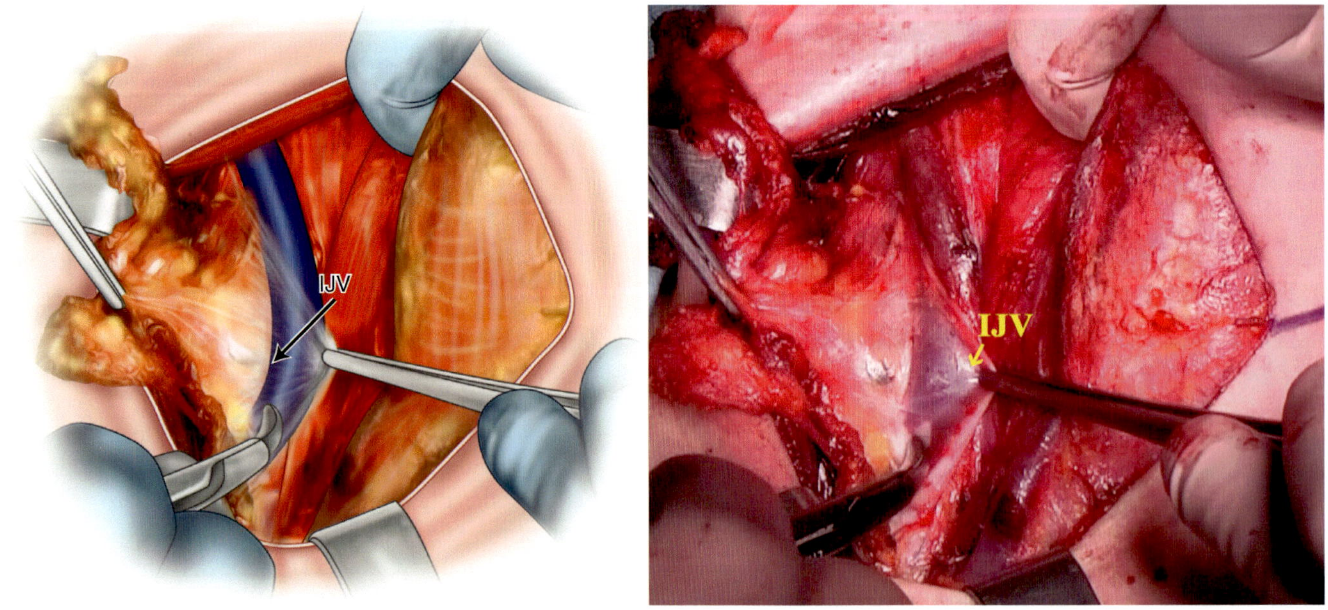

Fig. 17.16 Dissection of levels III and IV – the dissection of the posterior boundary is accomplished along the plane of coalescence of the superficial and deep layers of the deep cervical fascia, while the neurovascular bundle is retracted medially. IJV – internal jugular vein

cervical plexus (level III) (Fig. 17.17). The specimen is then passed behind the omohyoid muscle, and dissection is continued downward (level IV). Following the fascial plane allows preserving the integrity of the phrenic nerve and thyrocervical trunk. However, infrascalenic nodes can be safely removed *en bloc* after identifying the phrenic nerve. Small vascular branches arising from the thyrocervical trunk have to be ligated. Preserving the thyrocervical trunk is of utmost importance to reduce the risk of postoperative hypoparathyroidism.

In summary, during this step, since both the lateral and medial borders have been already prepared, it is possible to safely dissect the posterior aspect along the DLDCF, which should not be violated; Should be performed in an avascular plane, and the injury to the phrenic nerve should be avoided (Fig. 17.18).

Completing Level Vb Dissection (Supraclavicular Triangle)

At this point in time, the SCM is retracted medially, and the specimen is passed behind and transposed postero laterally

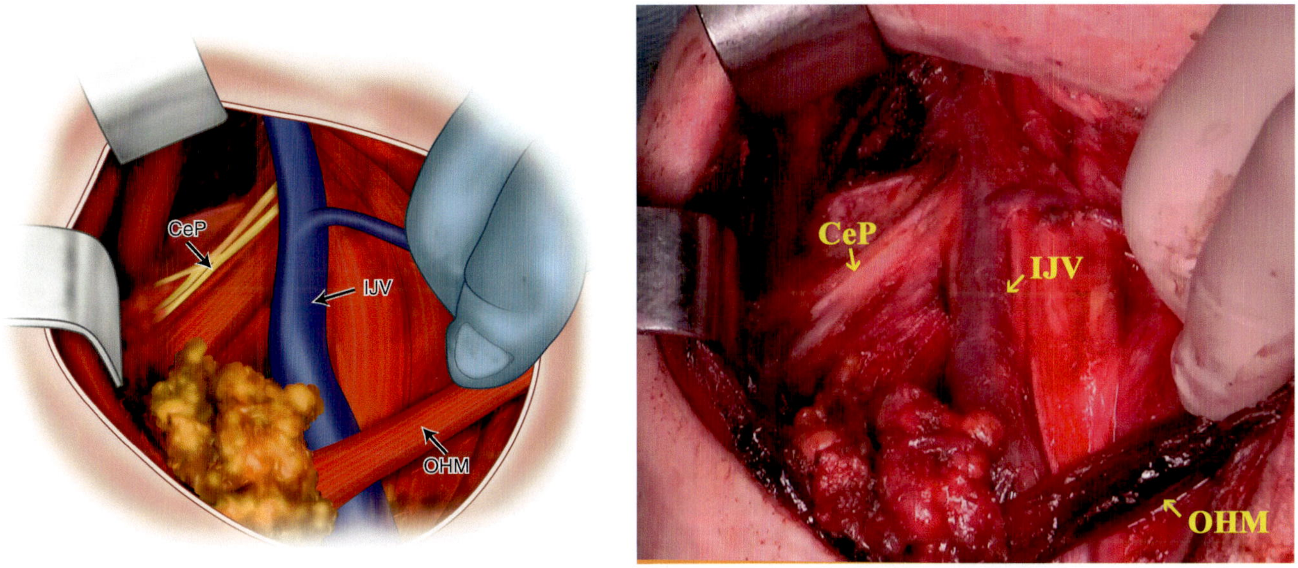

Fig. 17.17 Dissection of level III – dissecting along the fascial plane allows to preserving the roots of the cervical plexus. CeP – cervical plexus, IJV – internal jugular vein, OHM – omohyoid muscle

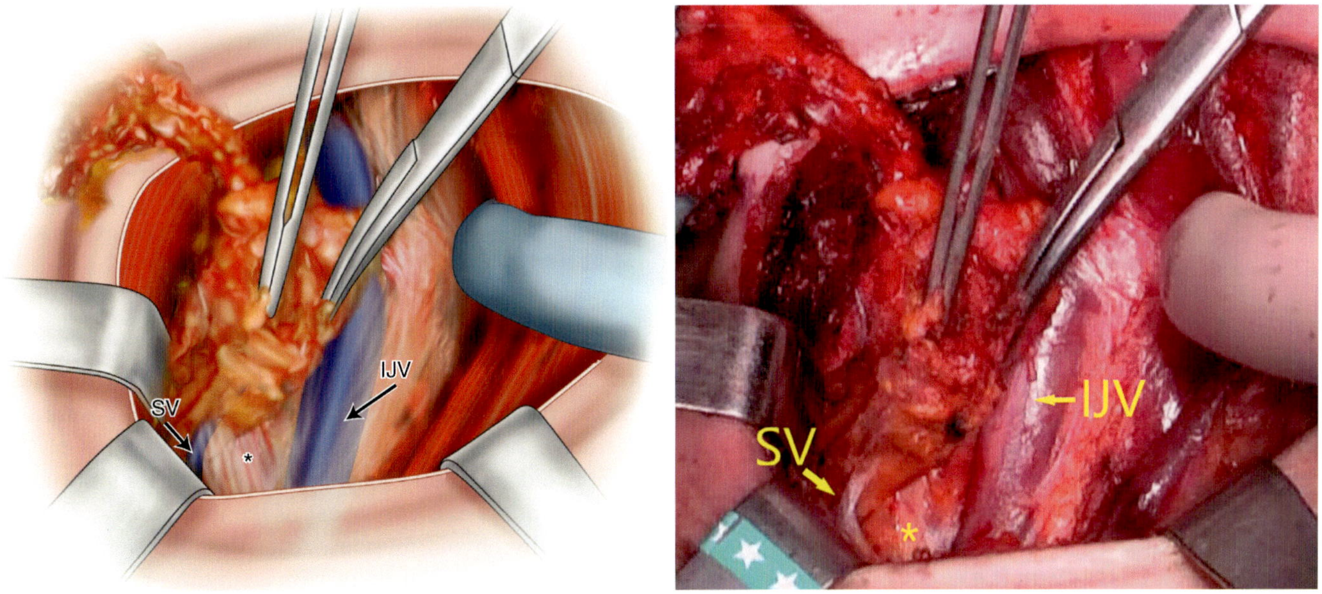

Fig. 17.18 Level IV dissection is completed along the superior aspect of the subclavian vein. IJV – internal jugular vein, SV – subclavian vein, * deep layer of the deep cervical fascia (prevertebral fascia)

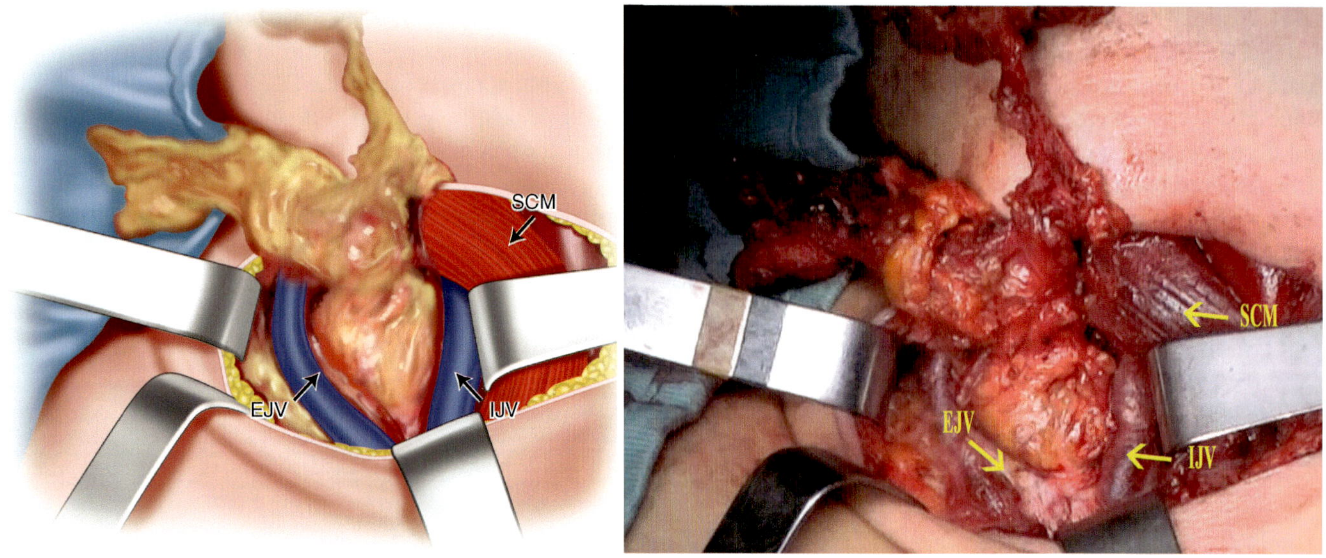

Fig. 17.19 Completing level IV–Vb dissection (supraclavicular triangle) – the sternocleidomastoid muscle is retracted medially and the specimen passed behind and transposed postero laterally. SCM – sternocleidomastoid muscle, EJV – external jugular vein, IJV – internal jugular vein

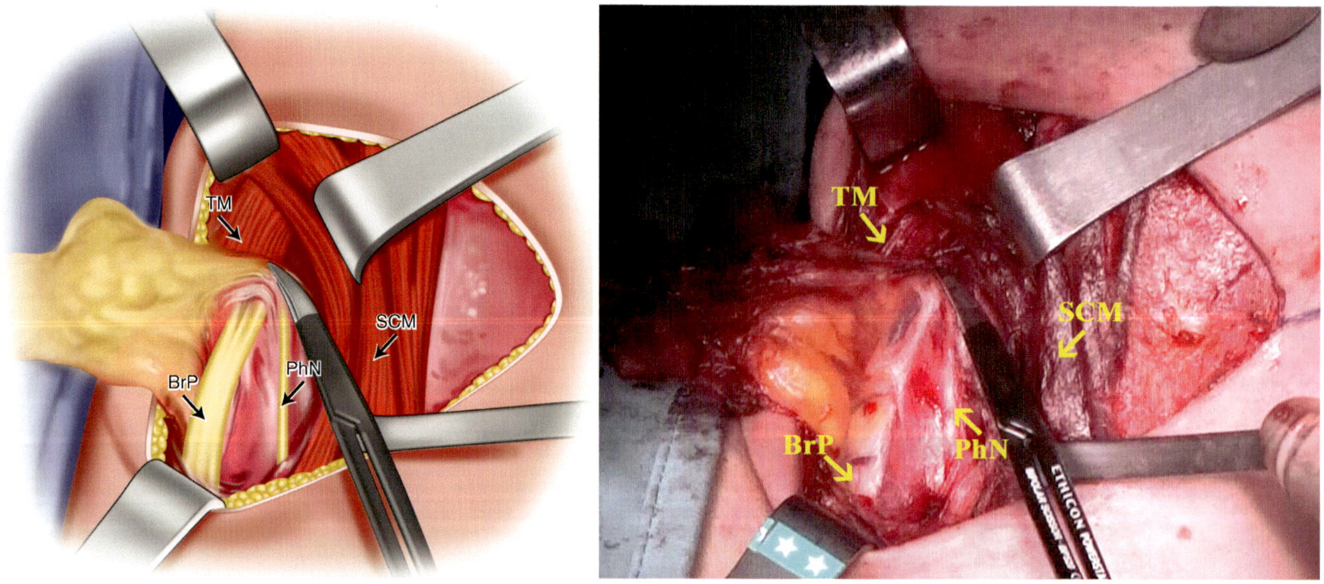

Fig. 17.20 Completing level IV–Vb dissection (supraclavicular triangle) – the brachial plexus is exposed posteriorly, the dissection is completed along the anterior margin of the trapezius muscle, and the specimen of the lateral neck dissection is removed. BrP – brachial plexus, PhN – phrenic nerve, SCM – sternocleidomastoid muscle, TM – trapezius muscle

(Fig. 17.19). The dissection continues along the superior aspect of the subclavian vein, exposing posteriorly the brachial plexus. Then the dissection is completed along the anterior margin of the trapezius muscle, and the specimen is removed (Fig. 17.20).

Central Neck Dissection (Levels VI–VII)

Strap Muscle Dissection

The strap muscles are separated along the midline as extensively as possible from the hyoid bone to the sternal notch. In the case of large infiltrating tumors and/or bulky lymph node metastases, *en bloc* resection of the sternothyroid muscles can be advisable since it ensures adequate exposure and clearance. In such cases, a complete mobilization of the sternohyoid muscle is reached by dissecting its posterior aspect from the anterior aspect of the ipsilateral sternothyroid and thyrohyoid muscles. After that, the sternothyroid muscle is sectioned at its proximal (thyroid cartilage) and distal (sternal) insertions (Fig. 17.21). If needed or preferred, the SLDCF, in its anterior portion, covering the strap muscles, can be removed *en bloc* with the central compartment. It is sectioned cranially at the level of the hyoid bone

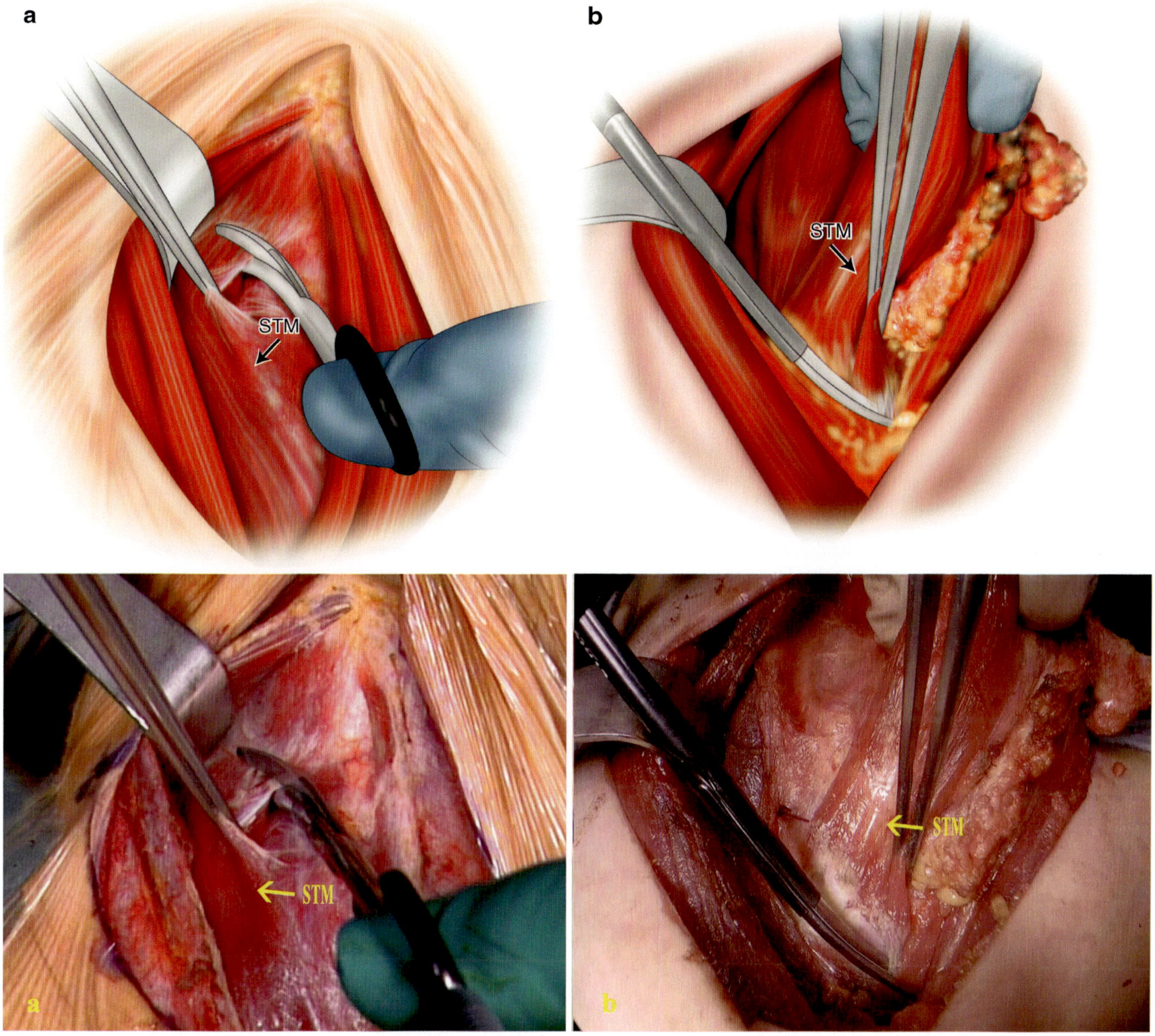

Fig. 17.21 Central compartment dissection. Once the sternohyoid muscle is freed from the ipsilateral sternothyroid and thyrohyoid muscles, the right sternothyroid muscle is sectioned at its proximal (**a**) and distal (**b**) insertions. STM – sternothyroid muscle

and caudally at the level of the sternal notch. Then the sternohyoid muscles are unwrapped from lateral to medial. When the dissection reaches the medial border of the sternohyoid muscles on each side, it changes direction, and the posterior aspect of the sternohyoid muscles is dissected as described above, leaving the fascial envelopment connected along the median raphe with the sternothyroid muscles and the "content" of the central compartment.

Dissection of the Lateral Boundary (Exposure of the CCA)

The dissection, using monopolar and/or bipolar cautery, follows the lateral margin of the sternothyroid muscle, along the carotid sheath (Fig. 17.22). Complete exposure should be obtained from the thyroid cartilage to the innominate trunk on the right side and as low as possible on the left side, depending on the patient's morphometric characteristics, but at least to the plane corresponding to the level where the innominate trunk crosses the trachea on the right side.

Identification of the ILN and Paratracheal Dissection

After the identification of the external branch of the superior laryngeal nerve and the selective dissection of the upper thyroid pedicle, the thyroid lobe is retracted medially to expose the tracheoesophageal groove. The ILN nerve is identified where it crosses the inferior thyroid artery or its branches, possibly using intraoperative nerve monitoring to confirm

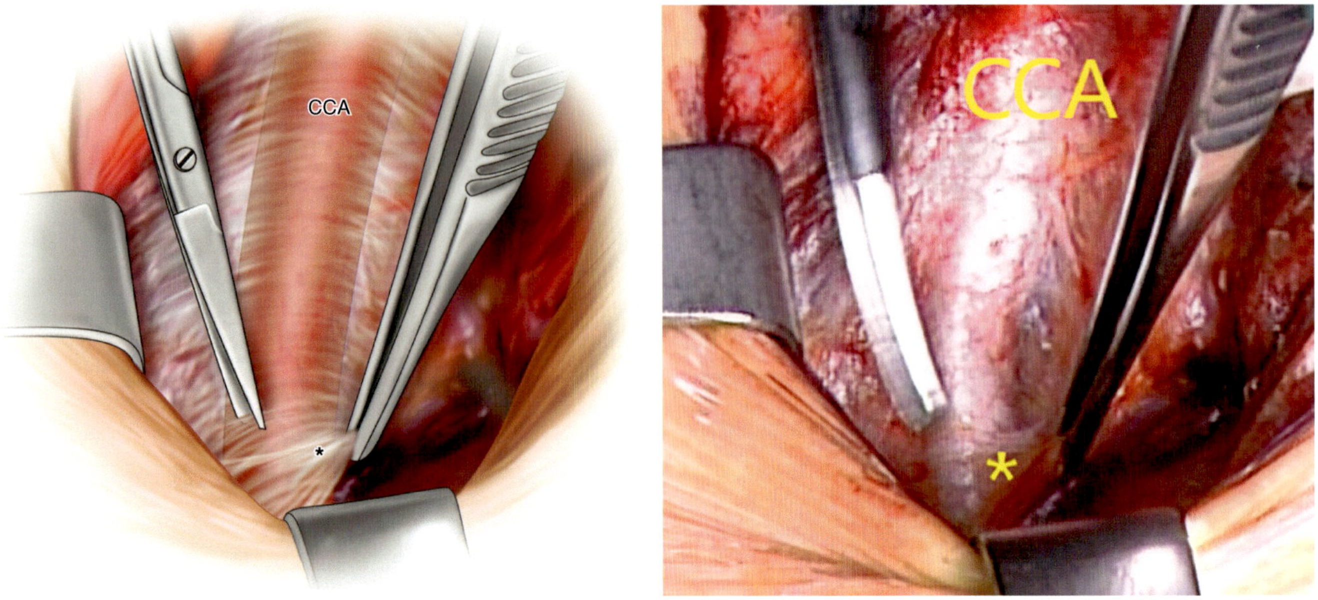

Fig. 17.22 Dissection of the lateral boundary of the central compartment (exposure of the common carotid artery). CCA – common carotid artery, *middle layer of the deep cervical fascia, investing the sternothyroid muscle at the conjunction with the carotid sheet

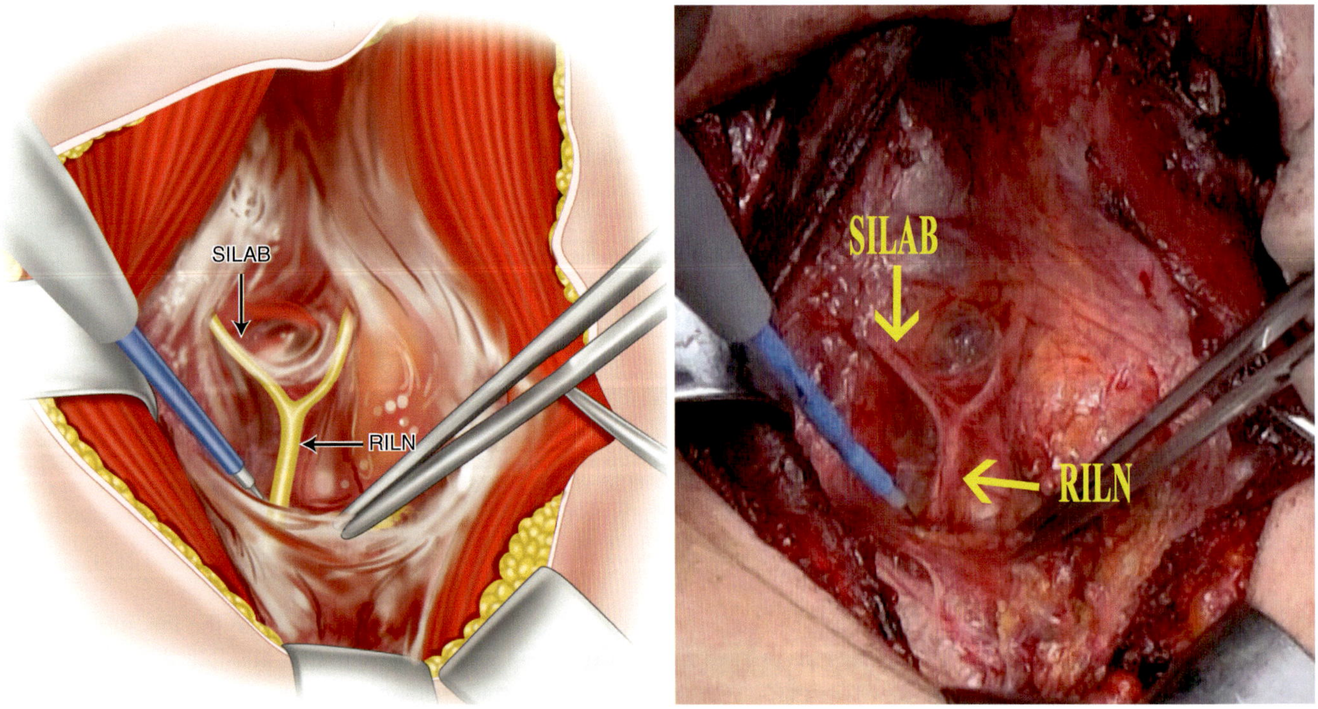

Fig. 17.23 After identifying the inferior laryngeal nerve, the sagittal aponeurosis is incised and the posterolateral fibrofatty tissue dissected from lateral to medial along the lateral aspect of the inferior laryngeal nerve, preserving its anastomotic branches with the sympathetic chain. RILN – right inferior laryngeal nerve, SILAB – sympathetic inferior laryngeal anastomotic branch

correct identification. Intraoperative nerve monitoring can also help in the identification of ILN. On the right side, the nerve should be dissected from the surrounding fibrofatty tissue along its entire cervical course from its origin behind the subclavian artery to its entrance into the larynx (Fig. 17.23). At this point, the sagittal aponeurosis posterior to the carotid sheath should be incised and the posterolateral fibrofatty tissue dissected with a lateral-to-medial direction along the lateral aspect of the ILN, preserving the small sympathetic-inferior laryngeal nerve connecting the branches (Fig. 17.23) [25]. Then the posterior aspect of the nerve is freed from the fibrofatty tissue. The ILN is cau-

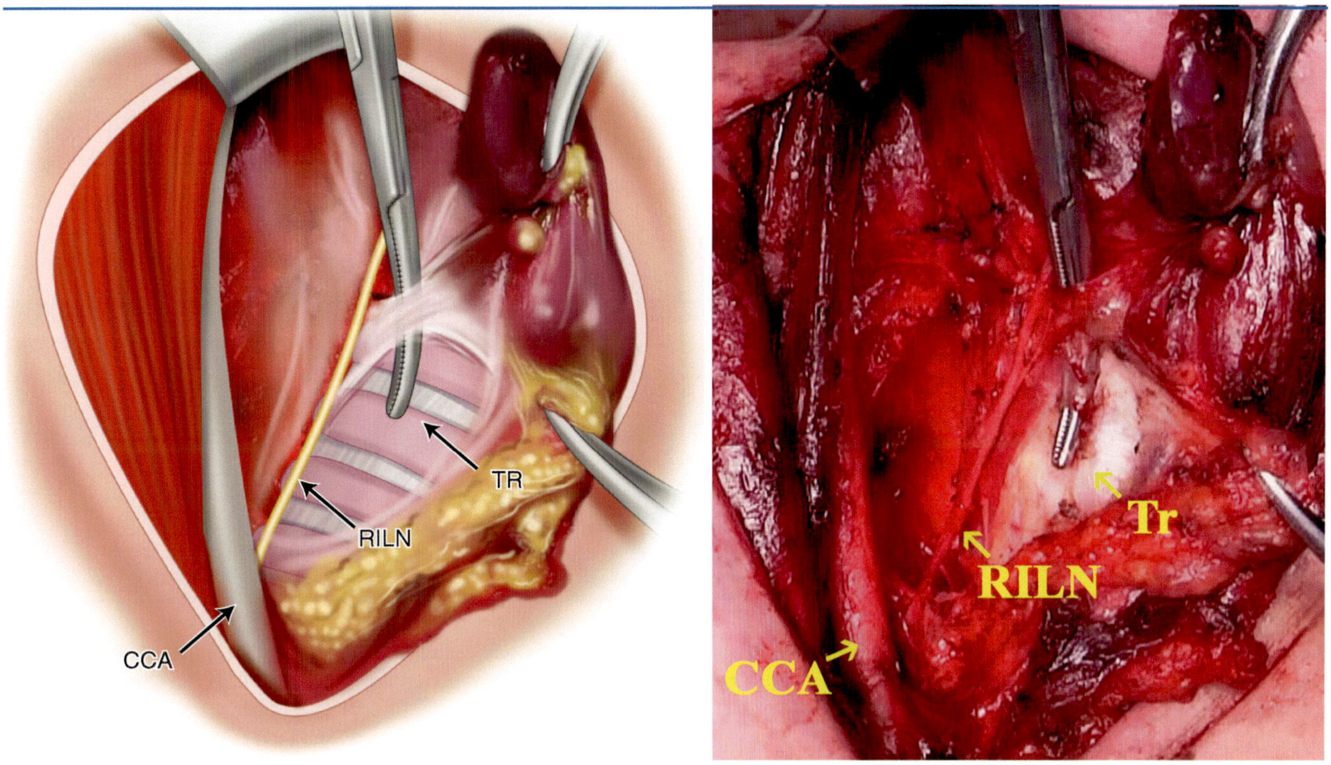

Fig. 17.24 Paratracheal dissection and thyroidectomy – the right inferior laryngeal nerve is dissected from the surrounding fibrofatty tissue all along its cervical course, and the right thyroid lobectomy is completed. CCA – common carotid artery, RILN – right inferior laryngeal nerve, Tr – trachea

tiously antero laterally displaced, and the posterolateral portion of the paratracheal nodes is transposed behind it medially (Fig. 17.24). The dissection is then continued in the antero medial portion of the paratracheal nodes, exposing the antero lateral aspect of the esophagus and the lateral aspect of the trachea. In most cases, the infero lateral part of the dissected field may expose the apex of the ipsilateral lung. On the left side, the nerve is identified where it crosses the inferior thyroid artery and followed in a caudal direction as deep as possible in the upper mediastinum. At this point, the sagittal aponeurosis is incised behind the carotid sheet. By lateral to antero medial retraction, the lymph node containing fibrofatty tissue is completely freed along the antero lateral aspect of the ILN, exposing the esophagus and the lateral margin of the trachea. Any effort should be done to preserve the superior parathyroid glands. First of all, a bloodless surgical field is essential since any bleeding could determine an alteration of the colors, which is essential for parathyroid identification. Once identified, the parathyroid glands should be preserved with their vascular pedicles as far as possible. This implies a very gentle, cautious, and sometimes time-consuming dissection.

Pretracheal Dissection

Just below the sternothyroid muscle, it is possible to identify the thymus. It should be explored for the identification of intrathymic parathyroid glands, which are often encountered or used as a landmark for the identification of inferior parathyroid glands embedded in the thyrothymic tract. The thymus, and the eventually identified inferior parathyroid gland, in the absence of overt involvement by the tumor or nodal disease, should be preserved since it lies in an anatomical plane anterior to the pretracheal nodes in order to preserve the viability of the inferior parathyroid glands. After that, the most inferior portion of the central compartment (upper mediastinal nodes) is dissected from the antero superior aspect of the innominate trunk, exposing the right brachiocephalic vein. Dissection is continued upward, dissecting the fibrofatty tissue embedded in the visceral portion of the MLDCF from the tracheal fascia (Fig. 17.24).

Prelaryngeal (Delphian) Nodes

Dissection then continues, en bloc with the thyroid gland and/or the resected sternothyroid muscles, in the prelaryngeal compartment, paying attention to avoid injury to the cricothyroid muscle, cricothyroid membrane, and thyroid cartilage, along with the pyramidal lobe in the case of synchronous thyroidectomy. Dissection should be continued extensively upward in order to expose the hyoid bone.

Wound Closure

After checking hemostasis and lymphatic leak (Fig. 17.25), the sternohyoid muscles are reapproximated along the mid-

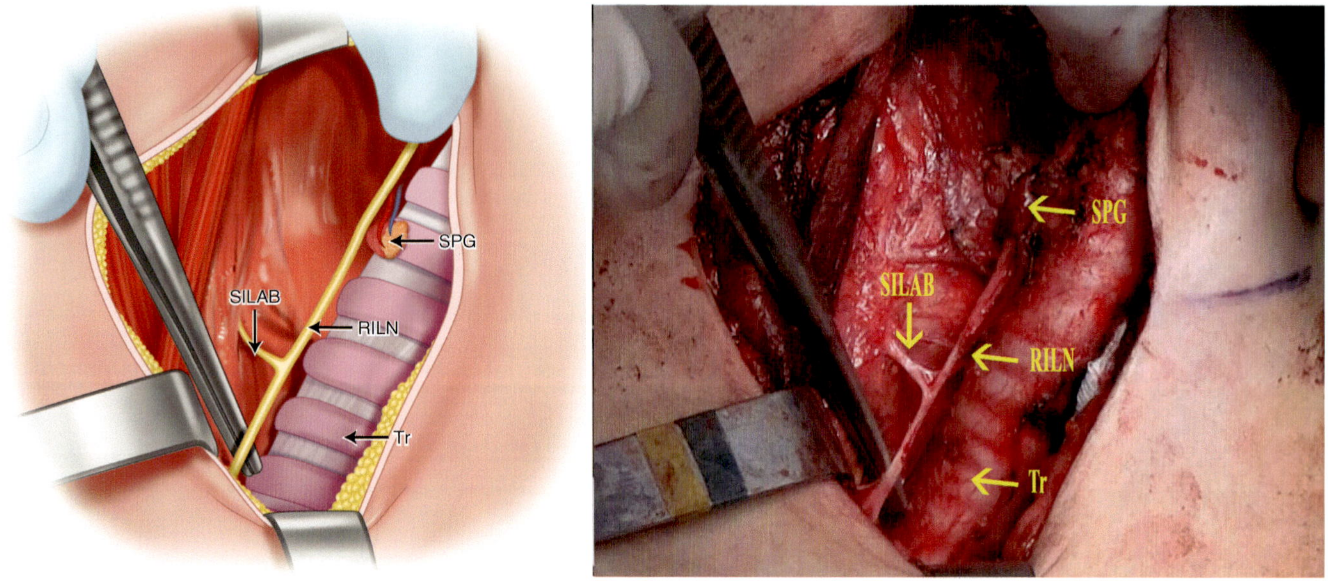

Fig. 17.25 Final view of the operative field. Checking hemostasis after thyroidectomy and central neck dissection is completed. RILN – right inferior laryngeal nerve, SILAB – sympathetic inferior laryngeal anastomotic branch, SPG – superior parathyroid gland, Tr – trachea

line. The wound is closed with subcuticular running sutures. Suction drains may be left inside.

Conclusion

Neck dissection is one of the most complicated surgeries of the human body since several nervous, muscular, and vascular structures are at risk during dissection. Thus, in patients with differentiated thyroid cancers, comprehensive central and lateral neck dissections should be performed only with a therapeutic intent (i.e., in the presence of proven lymph node metastases). Accurate knowledge of applied anatomy and embryology is essential to achieving a radical resection while minimizing the risk of complications. Since fibrofatty tissue containing lymph nodes is enveloped by the deep cervical fascia, to achieve an adequate and comprehensive clearance of the target basins it is particularly useful to follow the planes of coalescence of different fascial layers, which are avascular and allow to remove the target nodes en bloc with their investing fascial layers. Those layers are avascular and allow the surgeon to remove the target nodes *en bloc* along with their investing fascial layers. The technique of fascial dissection for both central and lateral compartments has been described in the present chapter.

References

1. Patel KN, Yip L, Lubitz CC, et al. The American Association of Endocrine Surgeons guidelines for the definitive surgical management of thyroid disease in adults. Ann Surg. 2020;271:E21–93.
2. Asimakopoulos P, Shaha AR, Nixon IJ, et al. Management of the neck in well-differentiated thyroid cancer. Curr Oncol Rep. 2021; https://doi.org/10.1007/s11912-020-00997-6.
3. Tuttle RM, Haugen B, Perrier ND. The updated AJCC/TNM Staging System for differentiated and anaplastic thyroid cancer, 8th edition: what changed and why? Thyroid. 2017;27:751–6.
4. Haugen BR, Alexander EK, Bible KC, et al. 2015 American Thyroid Association management. Thyroid. 2016;26:1–133.
5. Perros P, Boelaert K, Colley S, et al. Guidelines for the management of thyroid cancer. Clin Endocrinol. 2014;81:1–122.
6. Dralle H, Musholt TJ, Schabram J, et al. German Association of Endocrine Surgeons practice guidelines for the surgical management of malignant thyroid tumors. Langenbeck's Arch Surg. 2013;398:347–75.
7. Pacini F, Basolo F, Bellantone R, et al. Italian consensus on diagnosis and treatment of differentiated thyroid cancer: joint statements of six Italian societies. J Endocrinol Investig. 2018;41:849–76.
8. Shaha AR, Shah JP, Loree TR. Patterns of nodal and distant metastasis based on histologic varieties in differentiated carcinoma of the thyroid. Am J Surg. 1996;172:692–4.
9. Roh JL, Park JY, Park CI. Total thyroidectomy plus neck dissection in differentiated papillary thyroid carcinoma patients: pattern of nodal metastasis, morbidity, recurrence, and postoperative levels of serum parathyroid hormone. Ann Surg. 2007;245:604–10.
10. Alfalah H, Cranshaw I, Jany T, Arnalsteen L, Leteurtre E, Cardot C, Pattou F, Carnaille B. Risk factors for lateral cervical lymph node involvement in follicular thyroid carcinoma. World J Surg. 2008;32:2623–6.
11. Monteiro R, Han A, Etiwy M, Swearingen A, Krishnamurthy V, Jin J, Shin JJ, Berber E, Siperstein AE. Importance of surgeon-performed ultrasound in the preoperative nodal assessment of patients with potential thyroid malignancy. Surgery. 2018;163:112–7.
12. Stack BC, Ferris RL, Goldenberg D, Haymart M, Shaha A, Sheth S, Sosa JA, Tufano RP. American thyroid association consensus review and statement regarding the anatomy, terminology, and rationale for lateral neck dissection in differentiated thyroid cancer. Thyroid. 2012;22:501–8.
13. Robbins KT, Shaha AR, Medina JE, Califano JA, Wolf GT, Ferlito A, Som PM, Day TA. Consensus statement on the classification

and terminology of neck dissection. Arch Otolaryngol – Head Neck Surg. 2008;134:536–8.
14. Carty SE, Cooper DS, Doherty GM, et al. Consensus statement on the terminology and classification of central neck dissection for thyroid cancer. Thyroid. 2009;19:1153–8.
15. Crile G. Excision of cancer of the head and neck: with special reference to the plan of dissection based on one hundred and thirty-two operations. J Am Med Assoc. 1906;XLVII:1780–6.
16. Bocca EPO. A conservation technique in radical neck dissection. Ann Otol Rhinol Laryngol. 1967;76:975–87.
17. Ferlito A, Rinaldo A. Osvaldo suárez; often-forgotten father of functional neck dissection (in the non-spanish-speaking literature). Laryngoscope. 2004;114:1177–8.
18. Gavilán J, Herranz J, Gavilán C. Functional neck dissection. Otolaryngol Head Neck Surg. 1995;112:P73.
19. Gavilán J, Herranz J, Martín L. Functional neck dissection: the Latin approach. Oper Tech Otolaryngol – Head Neck Surg. 2004;15:168–75.
20. Gavilán J, Moñux A, Herranz J, Gavilán J. Functional neck dissection: surgical technique. Oper Tech Otolaryngol – Head Neck Surg. 1993;4:258–65.
21. Ferlito A, Robbins KT, Silver CE, Hasegawa Y, Rinaldo A. Classification of neck dissections: an evolving system. Auris Nasus Larynx. 2009;36:127–34.
22. Guidera AK, Dawes PJD, Fong A, Stringer MD. Head and neck fascia and compartments: no space for spaces. Head Neck. 2014;36:1058–68.
23. Skandalakis LJ, Skandalakis JE, Skandalakis PN. Surgical anatomy and technique. Surg Anat Tech. 2009; https://doi.org/10.1007/978-0-387-09515-8.
24. Ferlito A, Rinaldo A, Silver CE, et al. Neck dissection: then and now. Auris Nasus Larynx. 2006;33:365–74.
25. Raffaelli M, Iacobone M, Henry JF. The "false" nonrecurrent inferior laryngeal nerve. Surgery. 2000;128:1082–7.

Thyroidectomy for Substernal Goiter

18

Marco S. Demarchi and Frédéric Triponez

Introduction

Substernal goiter (SG) affects up to 1 in 5000 patients [1] and was first described by Haller [2] in 1749, and since then it has been given various names: intrathoracic, retrosternal, substernal, subclavicular, mediastinal, among others. Substernal goiters are usually classified as primary if they result from an abnormal embryologic migration of the thyroid and receive intrathoracic blood supply (less than 1% of cases) or secondary if the thyroid tissue descends into the mediastinum, maintaining proper thyroid vessel blood supply [3].

Many definitions of substernal goiter have been proposed (Table 18.1) [4], but it can generally be defined as a goiter that partially or totally extends in the anterior or posterior mediastinum and that requires a mediastinal dissection for its extraction.

From an anatomical point of view, substernal goiters can be described according to their relationship with intrathoracic vessels, trachea, and esophagus: in 85%, they are localized in the anterior mediastinum (type I) with the mass extending anteriorly to the subclavian and innominate vessels, and in 15% of cases, they are localized posteriorly to these vessels (type II). Regarding posterior mediastinal goiters, some authors further differentiate them according to their relationship with the trachea and esophagus (Table 18.2) [5].

The differentiation between anterior and posterior substernal goiters is of paramount importance to predict the localization of the recurrent laryngeal nerve (RLN), which can be located anterior to the goiter or even entrapped inside the thyroid tissue in type II substernal goiters [6].

Table 18.1 Substernal goiter according to different definitions

Author	Year	Definition
Hsu	1995	A thyroid gland (clinically or radiologically) below the sternal manubrium
Kocher	19xx	A thyroid gland in which some portion remains permanently retrosternal
Torre	1995	Goiter with its lower position permanently remaining below the sternal notch with the neck in hyperextension
Eschapase	1989	Goiter totally or partially located in the mediastinum that, in operating position, has its edge at least 3 cm below the sternal manubrium
Lahey	1920	Goiter that needs exeresis to be performed in the upper mediastinum
Lindskog	1957	Thyroid growth up to the level of the fourth thoracic vertebrae on X-ray examination
Crile	1939	Thyroid growth up to the aortic arch
Katlic	1985	Goiter in which at least 50% is retrosternal

Table 18.2 Substernal goiter classification

Type		Location	Anatomy
I		Anterior mediastinum	Anterior to RLN, trachea, and great vessels
II		Posterior mediastinum	Posterior to RLN, trachea, and great vessels
IIA		Ipsilateral extension	
IIB		Contralateral extension	
	B1	Extension posterior to both trachea and esophagus	
	B2	Extension between trachea and esophagus	
III		Isolated mediastinal goiter (or primary)	Possible mediastinal blood supply

From Randolph [5], with permission

The lack of a unique definition for substernal goiter leads to highly variable prevalence reports, ranging from 0.2% to 45%, of thyroidectomies [7]. In a large series of 355 patients in 2011, Raffaelli et al. [8] reported a rate of 15.7% of substernal goiters, defined as an enlarged thyroid gland with more than 50% of the gland or of any thyroid nodule located in the mediastinum, as evaluated during the surgical procedure with the neck extended.

Supplementary Information The online version contains supplementary material available at [https://doi.org/10.1007/978-3-030-93673-0_18].

M. S. Demarchi · F. Triponez (✉)
Department of Thoracic and Endocrine Surgery, Geneva University Hospitals and University of Geneva, Geneva, Switzerland
e-mail: Frederic.Triponez@hcuge.ch

A. Shifrin (ed.), *Atlas of Thyroid Surgery*, https://doi.org/10.1007/978-3-030-93673-0_18

The majority of patients present a visible neck mass (77–90%), although a significant number of substernal goiters are found incidentally on imaging studies performed for other reasons.

Symptoms of substernal goiter may range from complete absence to compressive effects on neurovascular or aerodigestive structures.

The most common symptoms associated with substernal goiter are dysphagia, dyspnea, orthopnea, cough, and globus sensation.

The large majority of substernal goiters can be successfully managed by thyroidectomy through a cervical approach. A concomitant partial or complete sternotomy or other thoracic approaches are needed in a minority of patients, ranging between 1% and 11% of cases [7]. Sternotomy, while conditioning the postoperative hospital stay, does not seem to aggravate a patient's mortality and morbidity [9].

Regarding postoperative complications, hypoparathyroidism and RLN palsy remain the most common complications after thyroidectomy for substernal goiter. Several studies reported higher morbidity after thyroidectomy for substernal goiter, particularly when a thoracic approach is necessary [10, 11]; however, other authors do not report a higher risk of postoperative complications if thyroidectomy is performed in high-volume centers [8].

Procedure

A 53-year-old woman presented to the endocrine surgery service for a large substernal goiter with subclinical hyperthyroidism. The patient reported progressive symptoms of

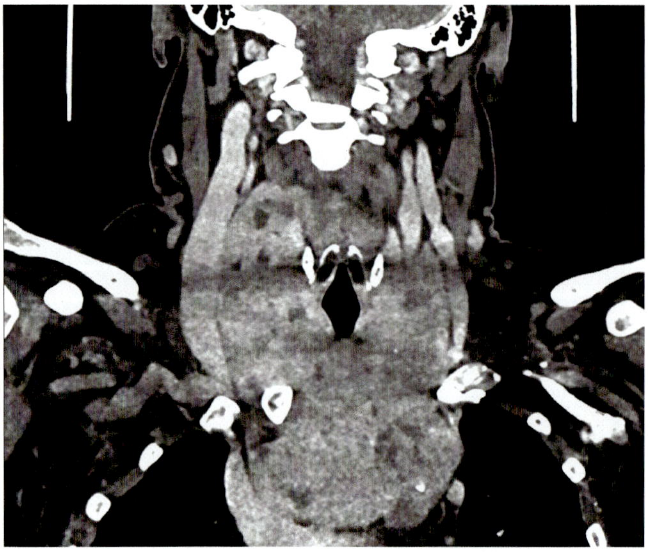

Fig. 18.1 Coronal CT scan image showing the presence of a large type IIA goiter

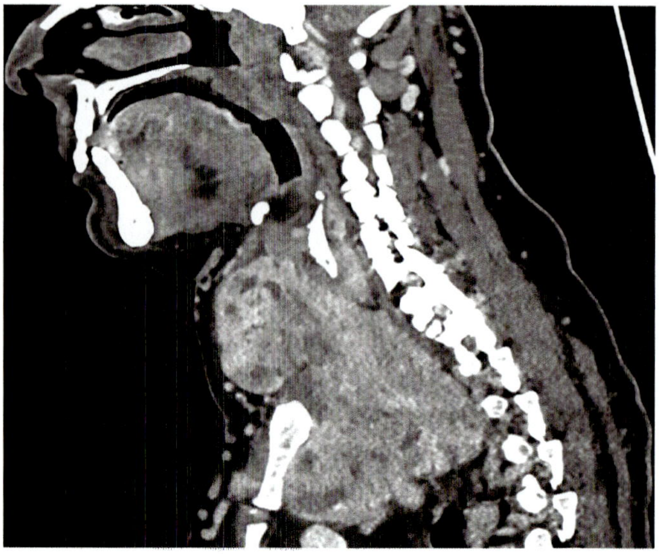

Fig. 18.2 Sagittal CT scan image showing the anatomical relations with the big type IIA goiter

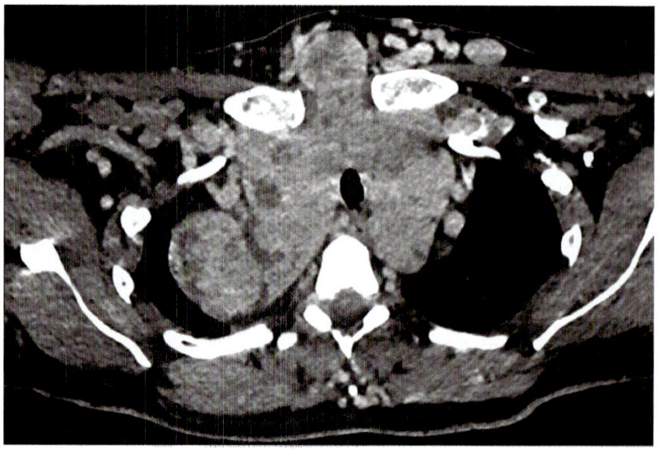

Fig. 18.3 Axial CT scan image showing the large goiter and the slight reduction of the trachea lumen size

dysphagia to solids and dyspnea mostly in supine position. A computed tomography (CT) scan (Figs. 18.1, 18.2, and 18.3) showed the presence of a large type IIA goiter with only a slight reduction of the tracheal size.

Positioning

The patient under general anesthesia is positioned supine with gentle neck extension. Orotracheal intubation with electromyographic (EMG) endotracheal tube is usually performed with the use of a fiber-optic laryngoscope in our institution.

The patient is positioned with both arms tucked by his/her sides in 25–30° of flexion of the trunk with an inflat-

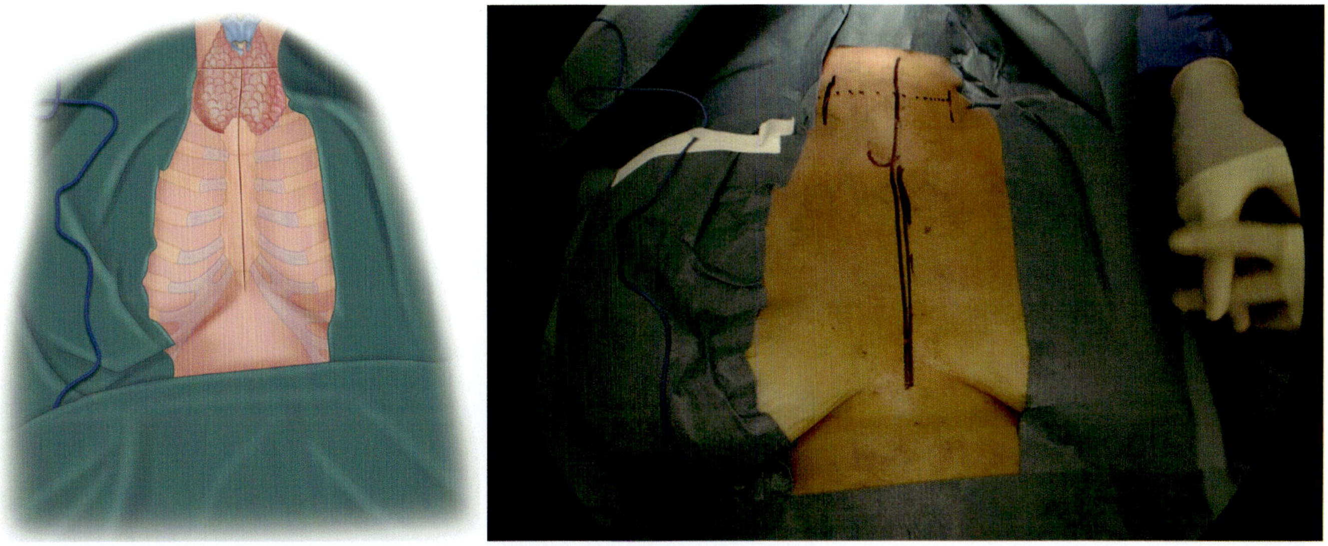

Fig. 18.4 Patient preparation. Supine position with partial cervical extension. Cervical incision site is drawn. Midline sternal landmark is drawn in case of sternotomy conversion

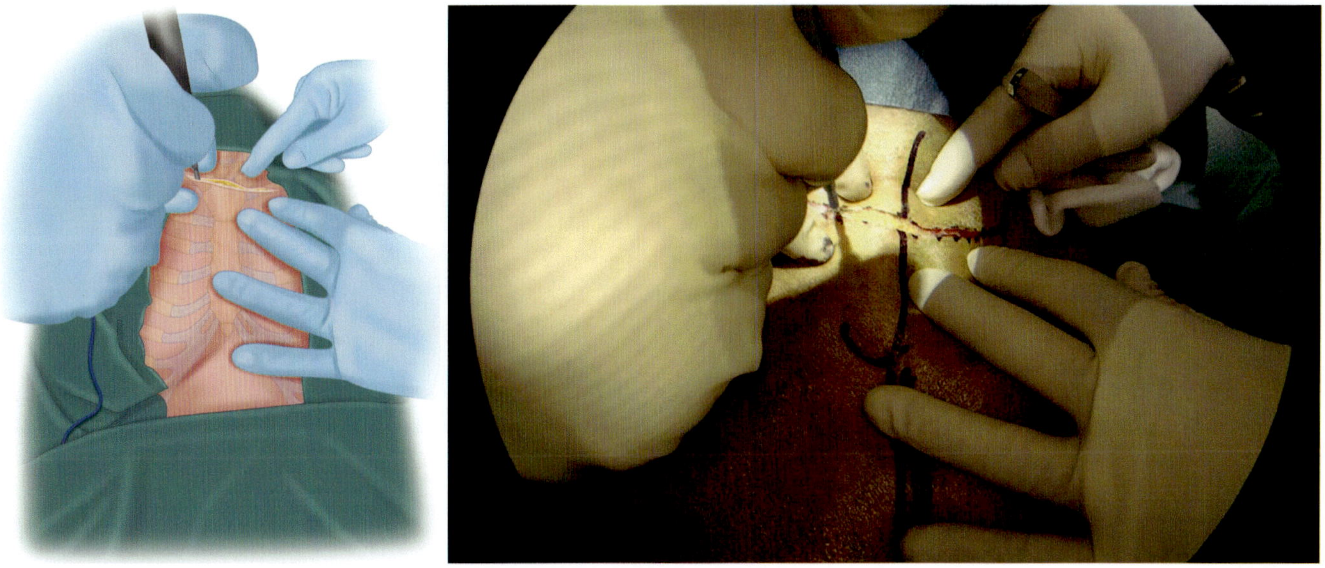

Fig. 18.5 Skin incision: a transverse Kocher incision is centered 2 fingerbreadths above the sternal notch

able straight tube or a folded blanket behind the scapula to allow for a moderate passive cervical extension. The chest should be prepared in all patients with SG, even when a sternotomy is unlikely, to allow for mediastinal access in case of unexpected difficulties (unexpected adherences due to cancer or inability to mobilize the inferior part of the SG or vascular lesion in particular) (Fig. 18.4).

Incision and Exposure

A 6- to 10-cm transverse Kocher incision is centered 2 fingerbreadths above the sternal notch (Fig. 18.5). The platysma is divided and a superior subplatysmal flap is raised to the thyroid cartilage and an inferior flap is dissected to the sternal notch (Figs. 18.6, and 18.7). The "midline" of the strap muscles is then identified, which is often deviated by an asymmetric goiter. Strap muscles are separated in the midline from the sternal notch to the thyroid cartilage (Fig. 18.8), exposing the anterior surface of thyroid lobes. Sternohyoid and sternothyroid muscles are usually sectioned transversely in large goiters (Fig. 18.9); this will not create postoperative functional consequences.

The smaller thyroid lobe can sometimes be left in situ, and a unilateral thyroid lobectomy can be sufficient in many cases of large SG in elderly patients with clearly asymmetric goiters. In case of bilateral SG or when total or near-total

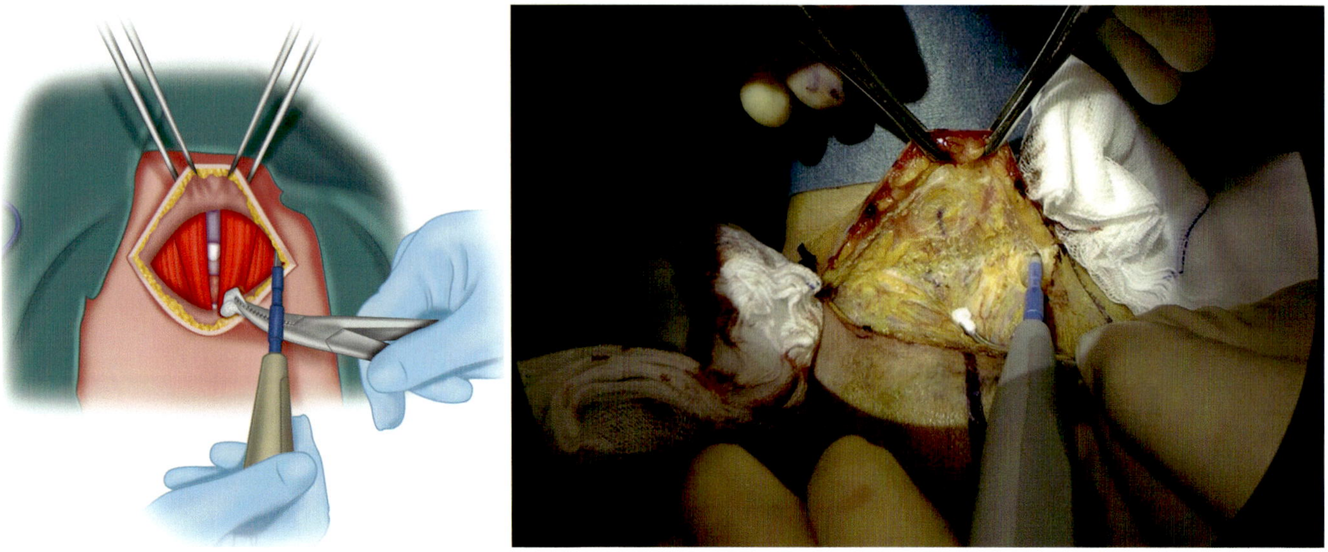

Fig. 18.6 Superior subplatysmal flap raised to the thyroid cartilage

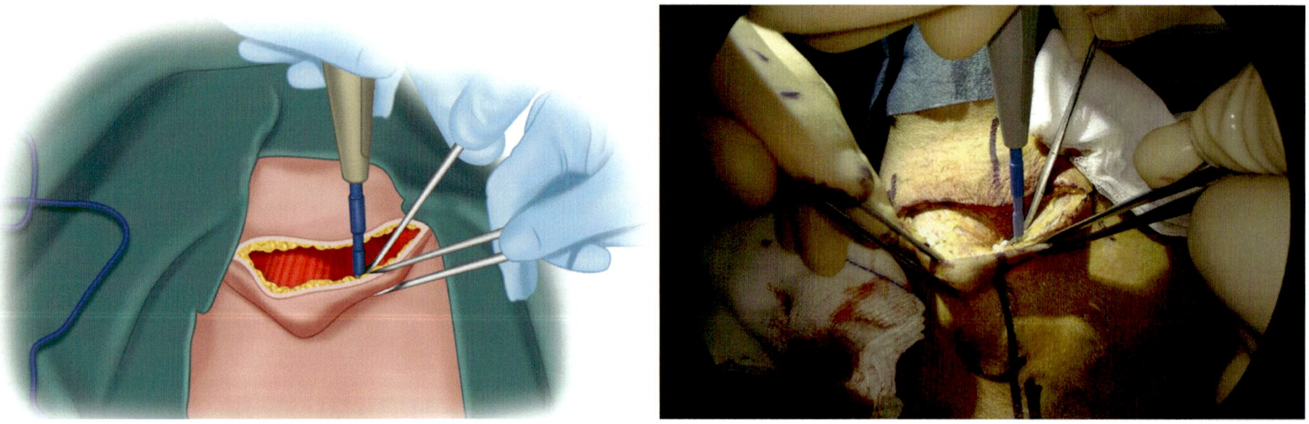

Fig. 18.7 Inferior subplatysmal flap dissected till the sternal notch

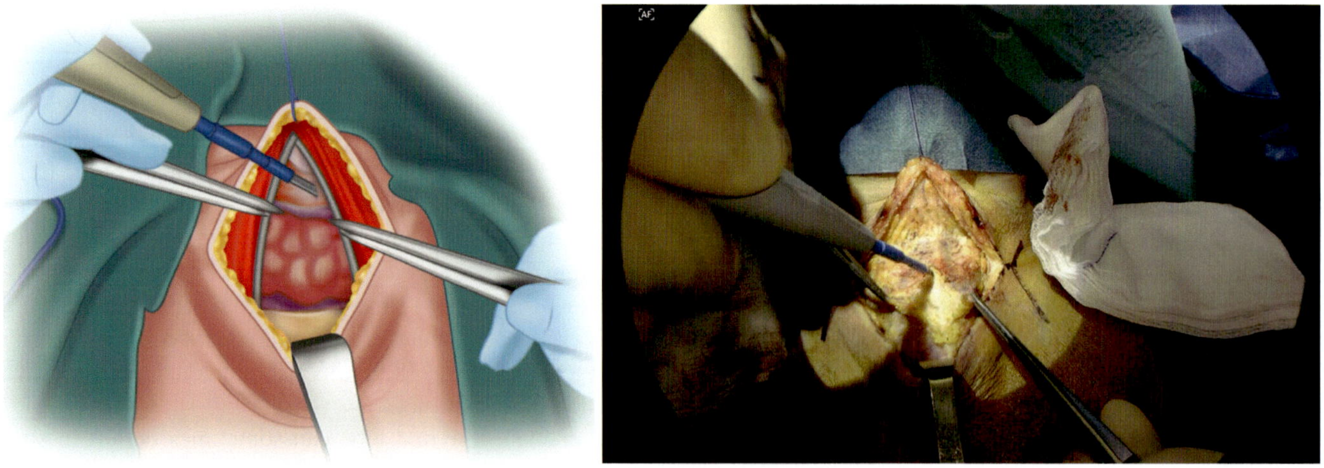

Fig. 18.8 Longitudinal separation of strap muscles in the midline from the sternal notch to the thyroid cartilage

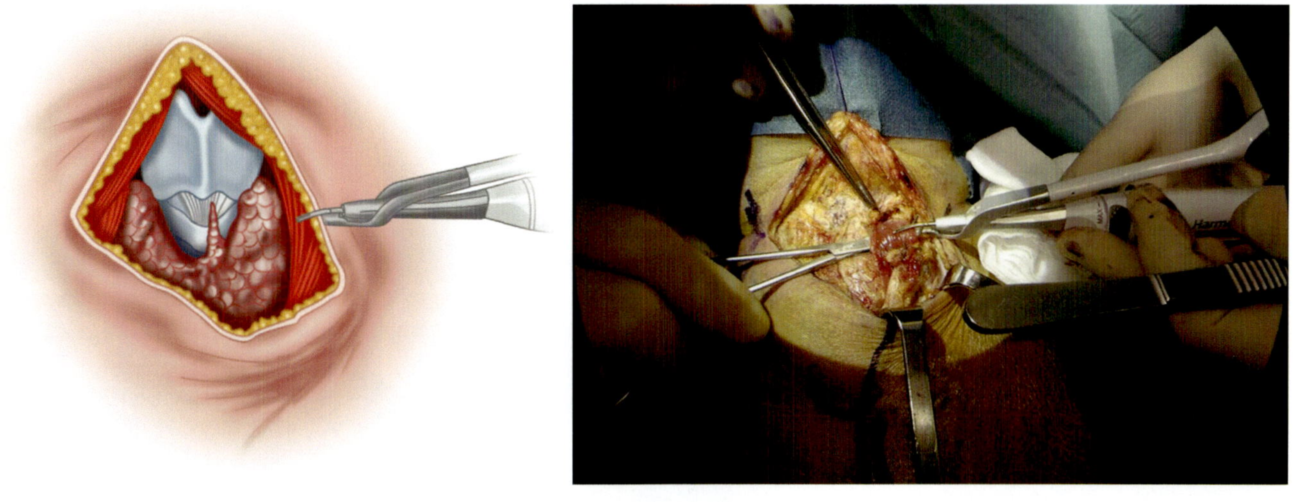

Fig. 18.9 Transverse section of the sternohyoid and sternothyroid muscles

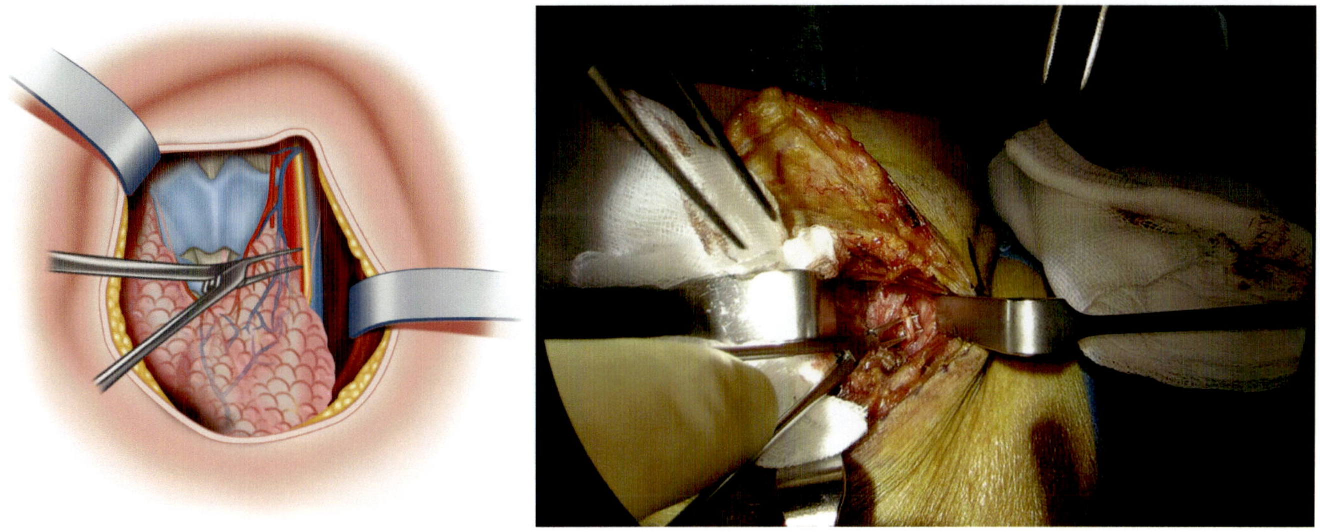

Fig. 18.10 Dissection and isolation of the vagal nerve

thyroidectomy is necessary, we suggest to begin with the larger side first to be able to interrupt the surgery after the first side in case of RLN neuromonitoring signal loss [12]. However, in some situations, it can be helpful to begin with the smaller side to have easier access to the larger side; this will depend upon surgeons' preferences.

The middle thyroid veins are ligated, the lobe is lateralized and the carotid sheath is then dissected, the vagal nerve is identified, and the neuromonitoring signal is tested on it. The vagal nerve is then gently dissected and isolated (Fig. 18.10), and a continuous EMG neuromonitoring electrode is positioned on it (Fig. 18.11). This will allow a continuous monitoring of the EMG signal to recognize reductions in the amplitude (and increased latencies) of the neuromonitoring signal caused by the stretching or traction of the RLN, which could lead to temporary or definitive RLN lesions.

The position of the orotracheal tube can be optimized with the collaboration of the anesthesia team to have an amplitude of the neuromonitoring signal of at least 500 mV (Fig. 18.12).

Thyroid Isthmus Division

The thyroid isthmus is then exposed, and the arborizing venous network on the superior and inferior parts of the isthmus is ligated to expose the avascular plane at the midline of the deviated trachea posteriorly to the isthmus. If possible, the isthmus is then dissected with a clamp beneath the gland

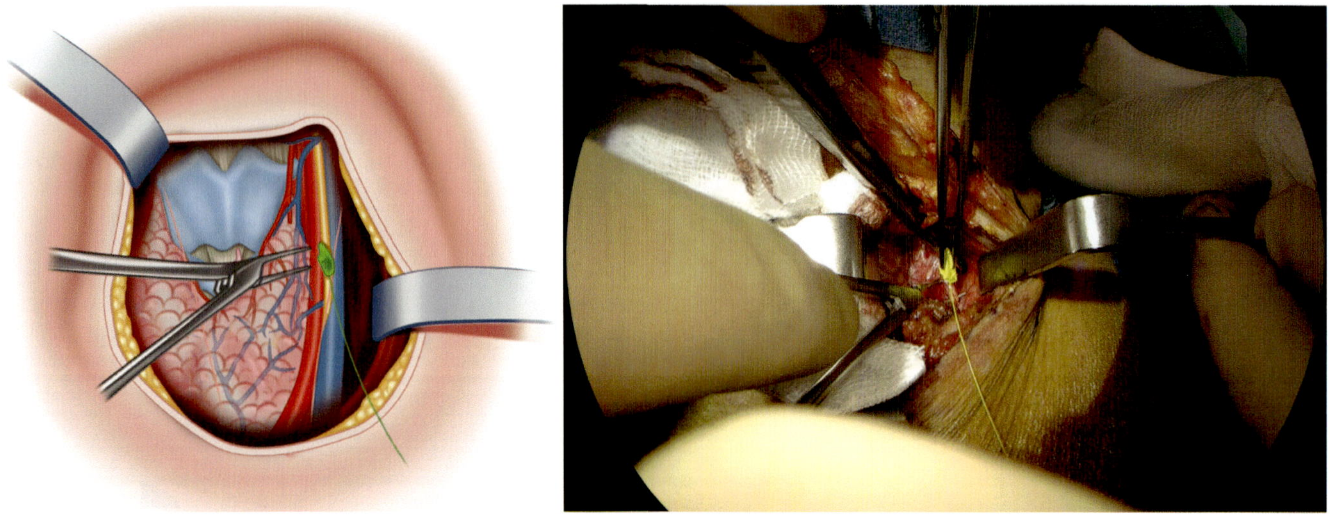

Fig. 18.11 Continuous EMG neuromonitoring electrode positioning on the vagal nerve

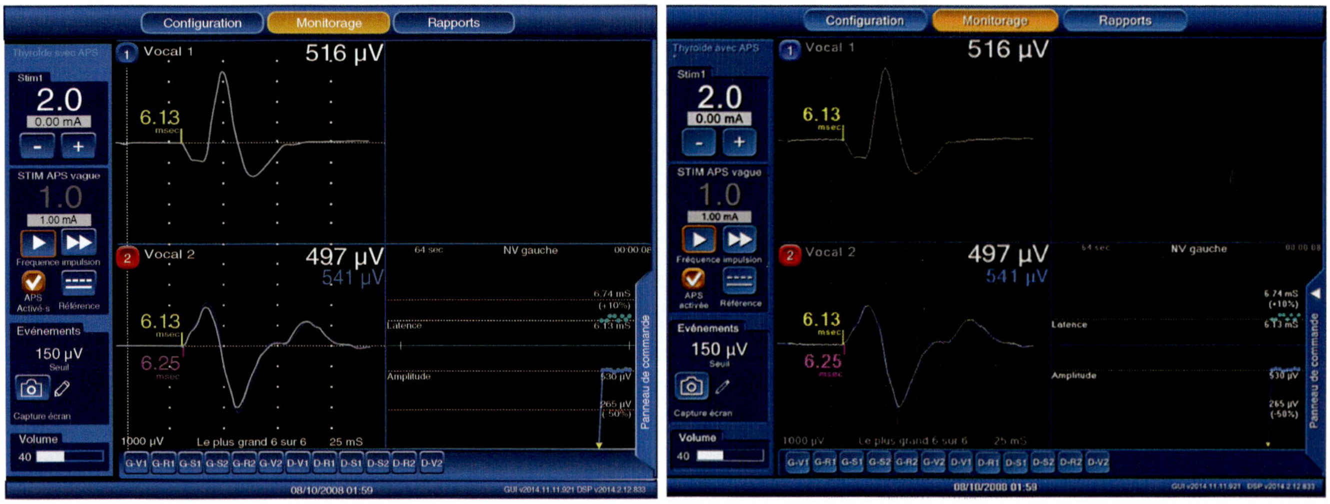

Fig. 18.12 Screenshot of continuous neuromonitoring showing the amplitude and latency values of the RLN

and divided with electrocautery or a vessel sealer (e.g., LigaSure, Harmonic scalpel). The division of the isthmus greatly facilitates the mobilization of the goiter and gives clear anatomical landmarks (at this stage, the carotid artery and trachea are clearly dissected free) (Fig. 18.13).

Superior Pole Ligation

The superior pole of the thyroid is then exposed with the identification and preservation of the external branch of the superior laryngeal nerve. With a gentle lateral retraction of the upper portion of the thyroid gland with Babcock forceps, superior thyroid vessels are isolated, divided, and ligated (Fig. 18.14) immediately adjacent to the thyroid (to avoid injury to the external branch of the superior laryngeal nerve). The superior parathyroid gland is frequently identified on the posterior surface of the upper pole and should be preserved blood supply.

Medial Dissection with "Toboggan" Technique

After dissection of the anterior and lateral surfaces of the goiter and after the section of the superior vessels, instead of medializing the thyroid lobe, the superior pole is moved aside laterally and dissection is started at the level of Berry's ligament.

At this point, the gland becomes more mobile, improving the exposure of the medial laryngo-thyroid space allowing for the search of the recurrent laryngeal nerve at its entry point into the larynx (Fig. 18.15) close to the inferior horn of the thyroid cartilage. Intermittent neuromonitoring can be

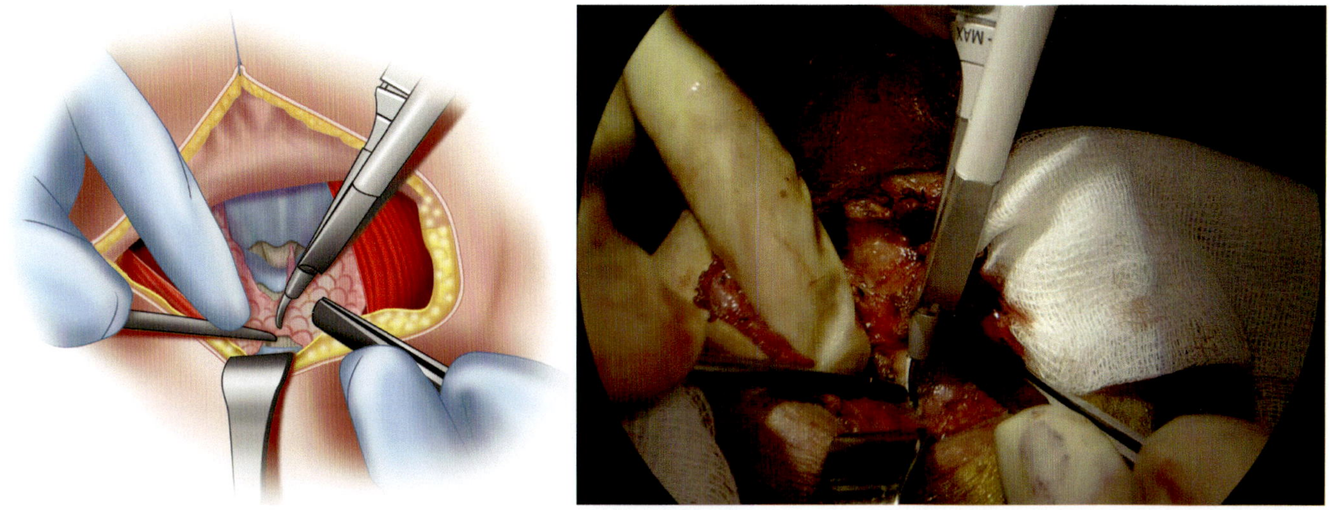

Fig. 18.13 Section of the isthmus with a Harmonic vessel sealer

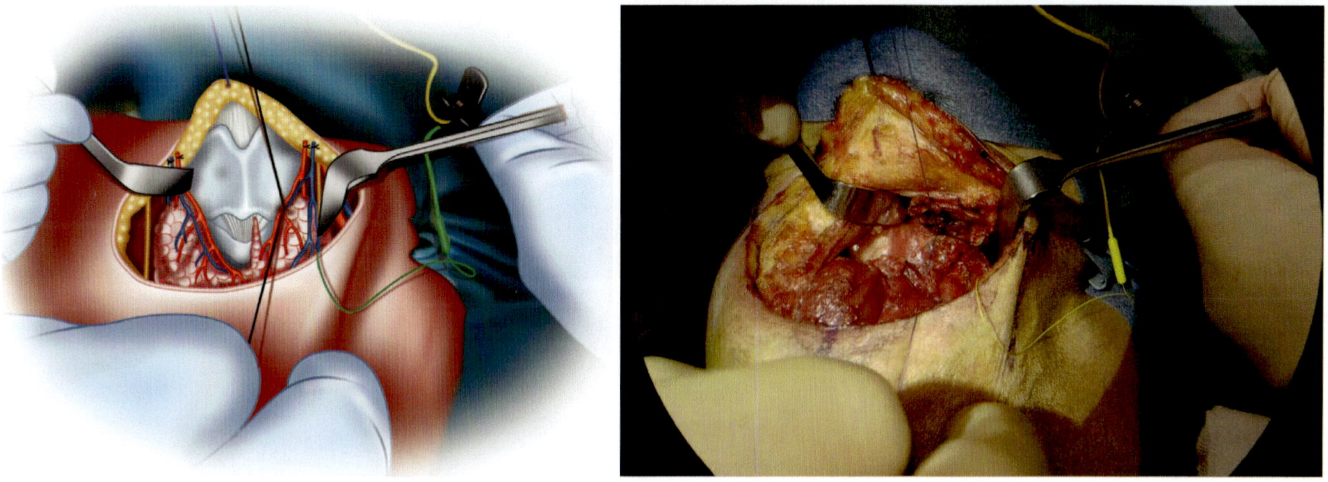

Fig. 18.14 Isolation, ligation, and section of upper pole vessels

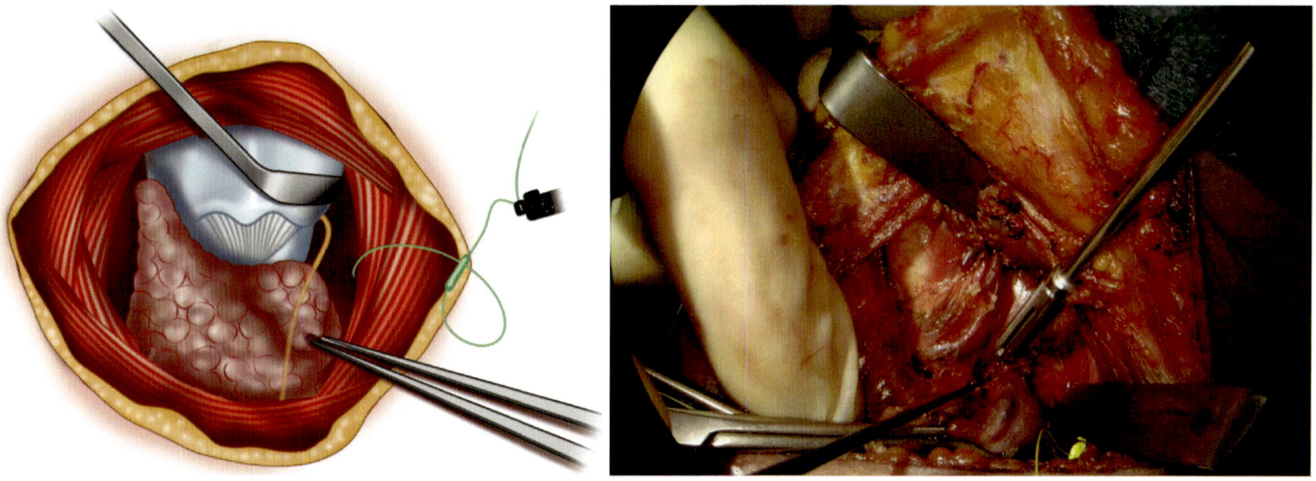

Fig. 18.15 Search of the recurrent laryngeal nerve at its entry point into the larynx with neuromonitoring probe

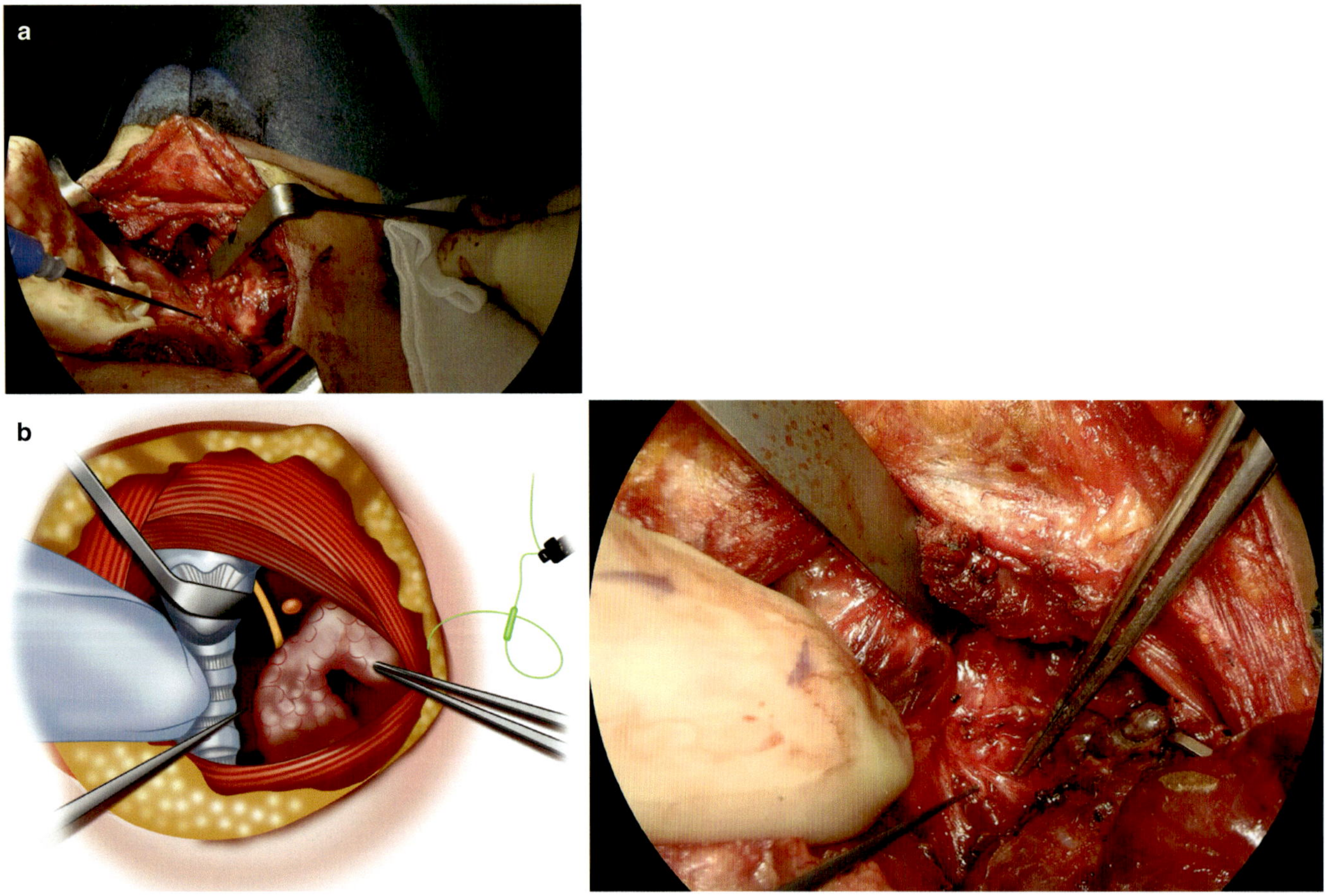

Fig. 18.16 (**a**) lateralization of the upper part of the thyroid lobe and search of the nerve, (**b**) dissection continues progressively in the prenervous plane in caudal direction between the nerve and the posterior part of the thyroid gland, descending as on a toboggan

used to help search for the RLN in this vessel-rich area. Once the nerve is identified, the dissection continues progressively in the prenervous plane in a caudal direction between the nerve and the posterior part of the thyroid gland, descending as on a "Toboggan" (slide) (Fig. 18.16).

The dissection of the first centimeter is sometimes laborious due to the presence of a lot of small vessels in this sometimes dense area ("ligament" of Berry), but once the dissection is well engaged, it is quite easy to pursue it as low as possible. Besides controlling the nerve, this maneuver will also allow the identification of the superior parathyroid gland (Fig. 18.17). The localization of the parathyroid gland can be facilitated with the use of novel fluorescence probes able to detect parathyroid autofluorescence (Fig. 18.18) [13, 14].

A finger or retractor is placed in the cervicothoracic space following the dissection of the posterior part of the lobe to control the location of the nerve and to progressively free the surrounding adhesions. When the Berry ligament and most of the middle thyroid lobe adhesions are liberated, the thyroid lobe can be progressively mobilized and exteriorized without traction on the RLN (Figs. 18.19 and 18.20).

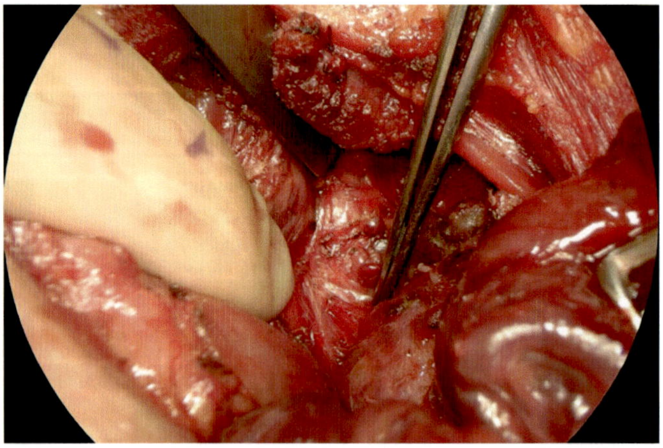

Fig. 18.17 Identification of the superior parathyroid gland with the RLN progressively dissected

If exteriorization seems still difficult, a longitudinal caudal extension of the skin incision on the midline until the sternal notch can be performed (a T-shape incision) to allow the exteriorization of the goiter. The subcutaneous plane is dissected, the platysma muscle is opened, and multiple prominent anterior jugular branches are controlled and ligated (Fig. 18.21).

With gentle traction on the thyroid lobe, the substernal part of the goiter can be progressively exteriorized, and the surrounding adhesions become progressively less tight and can be gradually controlled. During the entire intervention, but mostly in this phase, it is of paramount importance to reduce traction in case of reduction of the amplitude of continuous neuromonitoring signal to avoid traction lesions on the RLN.

When the entire lobe is extracted, an accurate search of the inferior parathyroid gland on the posterolateral surface of the thyroid lobe should be performed to avoid incidental parathyroid resection (Fig. 18.22). In case of an inadvertent resection or devascularization of a parathyroid gland, this one should be fragmented and autotransplanted in the sternocleidomastoid muscle at the end of the procedure.

After the complete resection of the first lobe and in absence of signal loss, the contralateral side can be removed in an identical way, with the benefit of creating more room for mobilization and exposition.

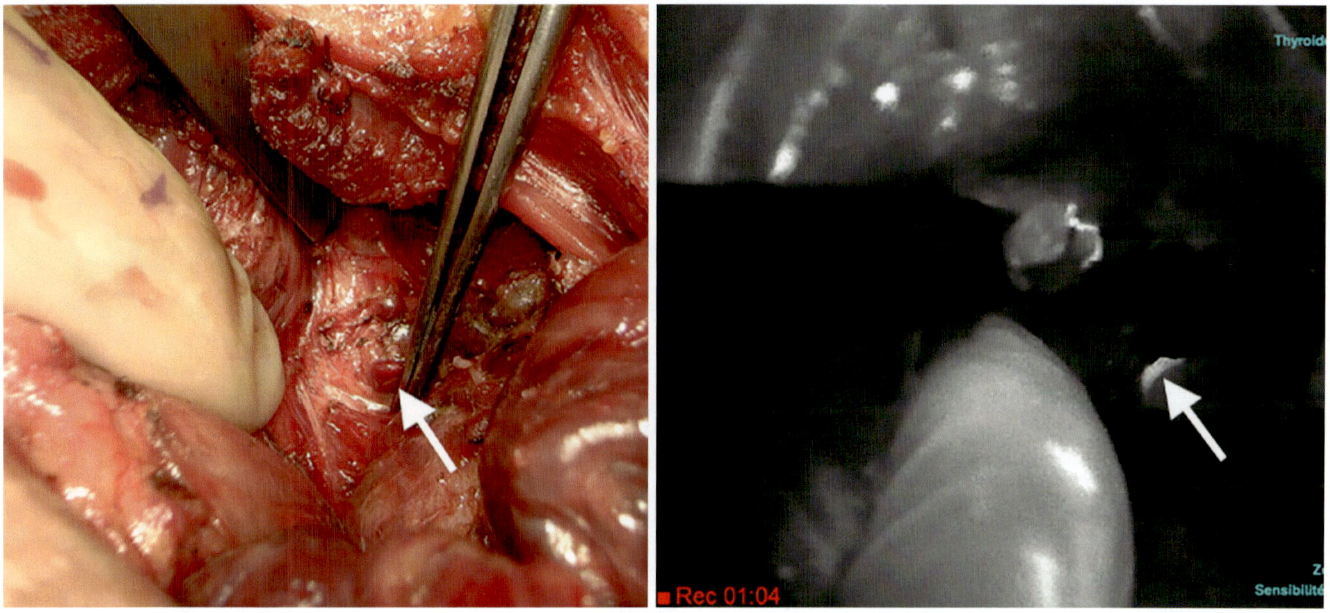

Fig. 18.18 Localization of the parathyroid gland can be facilitated by using novel fluorescence probes that are able to detect parathyroid autofluorescence and confirm the localization of parathyroid gland (arrow in black and white images)

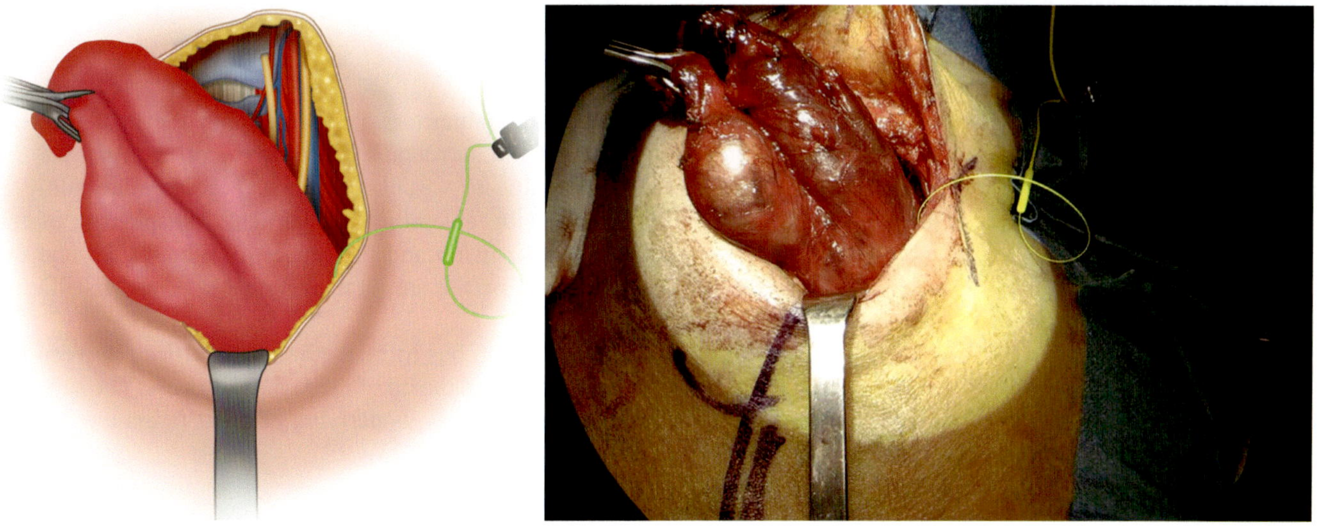

Fig. 18.19 Most of the middle thyroid lobe adhesions forming Berry's ligament are freed; the thyroid lobe can be progressively mobilized and exteriorized without traction on the RLN

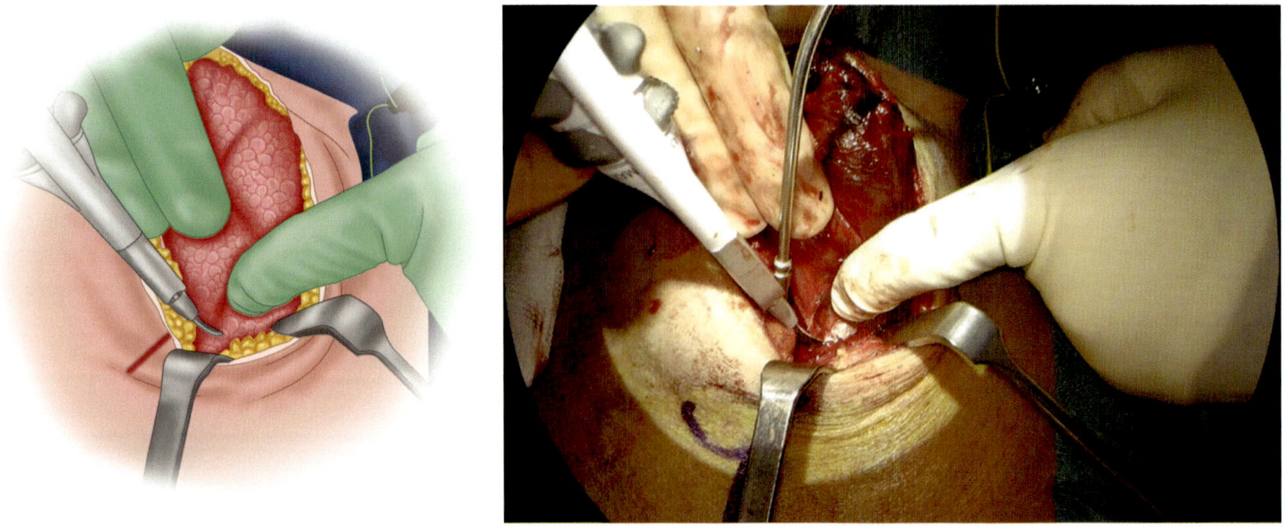

Fig. 18.20 Section of the inferior adhesions after exteriorization of the thyroid lobe

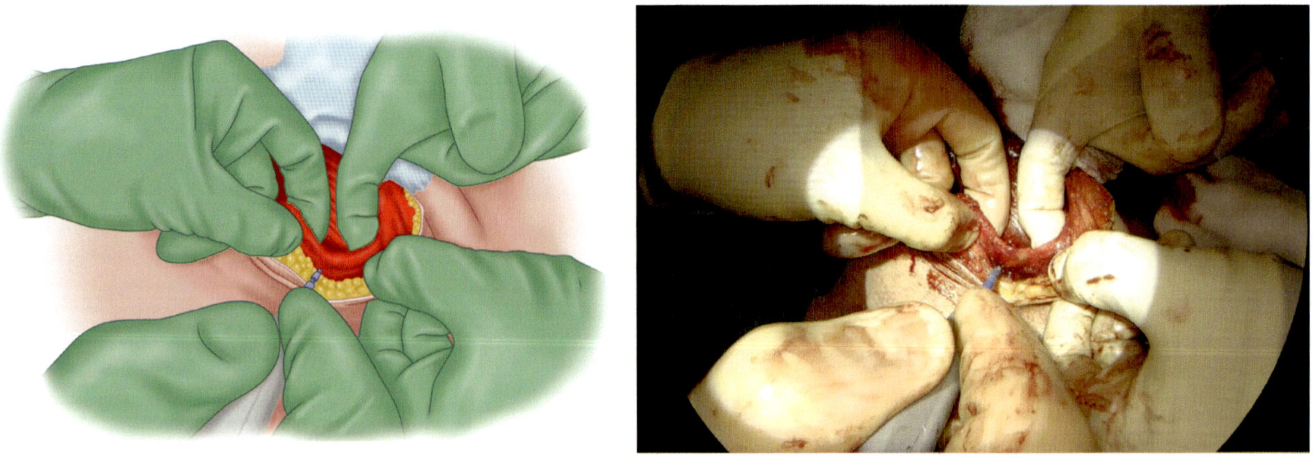

Fig. 18.21 T-shape midline longitudinal skin incision to allow better exteriorization of the goiter

In case of loss of RLN neuromonitoring signal at the stimulation of the vagal nerve at the end of the first side, a two-stage surgical resection should be taken into consideration to avoid the risk of a bilateral lesion of RLN.

In Case of Sternotomy

The operation begins routinely via a neck approach, and the need for a thoracic extention through partial upper sternotomy or total sternotomy is taken intraoperatively in case of failure in retrieving the gland (caused by adherences between the abnormal neo-vascularized capsule of the mass and the surrounding structures) or to minimize the bleeding due to vascular damage. Median sternotomy is performed by extending the vertical T-shape part of the cutaneous incision and the section of manubrium and the upper third of the sternum using a motorized oscillating surgical saw.

The incision has to be median and vertical between the sternal notch and the tip of the xiphoid process. The subcutaneous tissue and the underlying pectoral fascia are divided with cautery. (Fig. 18.23).

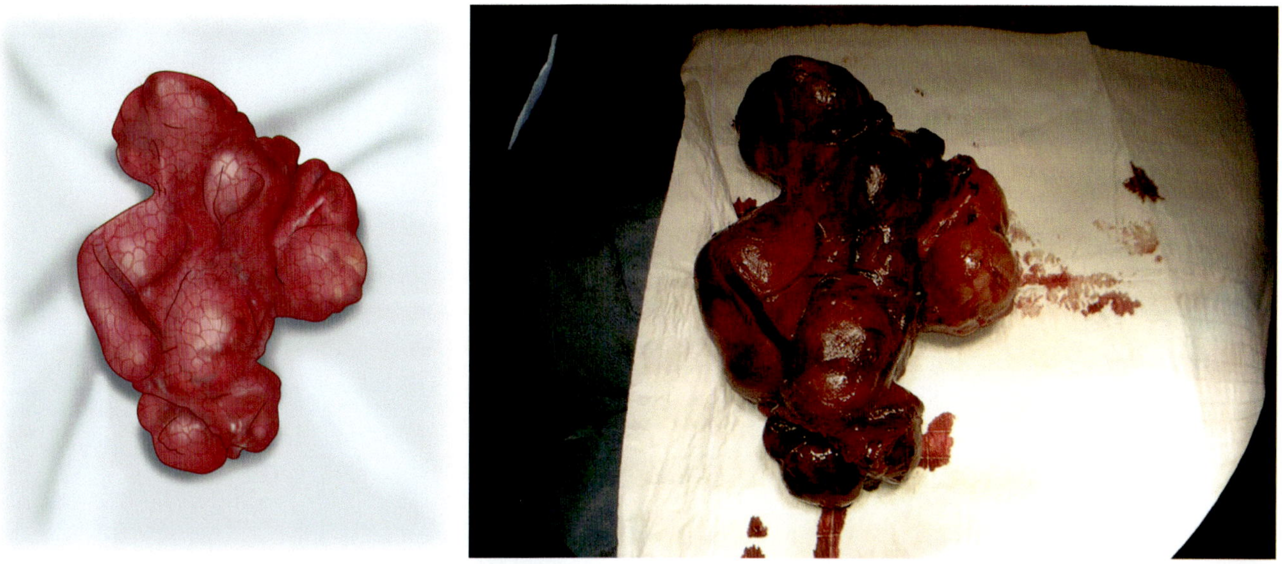

Fig. 18.22 Accurate search of the inferior parathyroid gland on the posterolateral surface of the thyroid lobe to avoid incidental parathyroid resection. This procedure could be facilitated by using novel fluorescence probes that are able to detect parathyroid autofluorescence

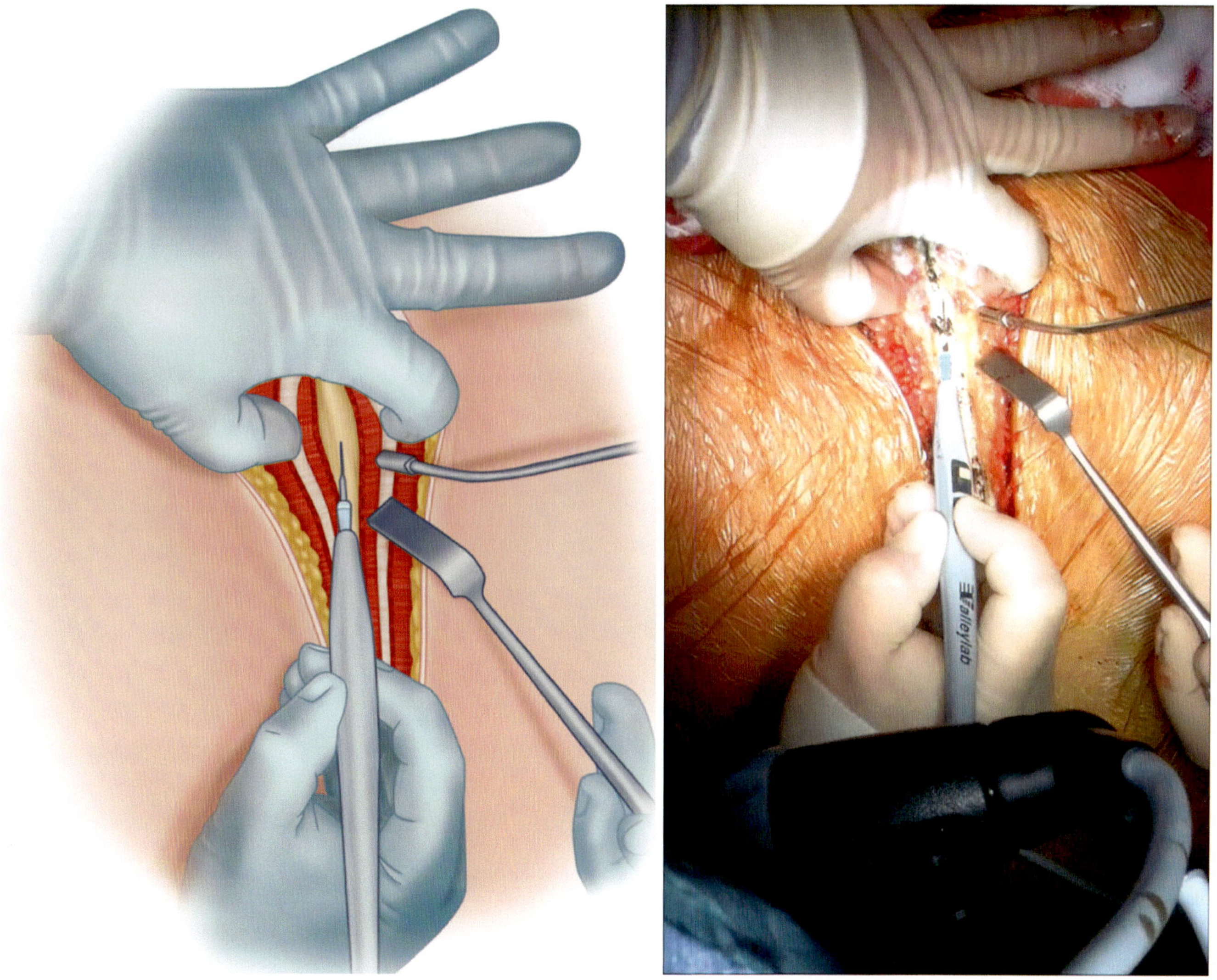

Fig. 18.23 To prepare for sternotomy, an incision is made between the sternal notch. The subcutaneous tissue and the underlying pectoral fascia are divided. The tip of the xiphoid process in cauterized

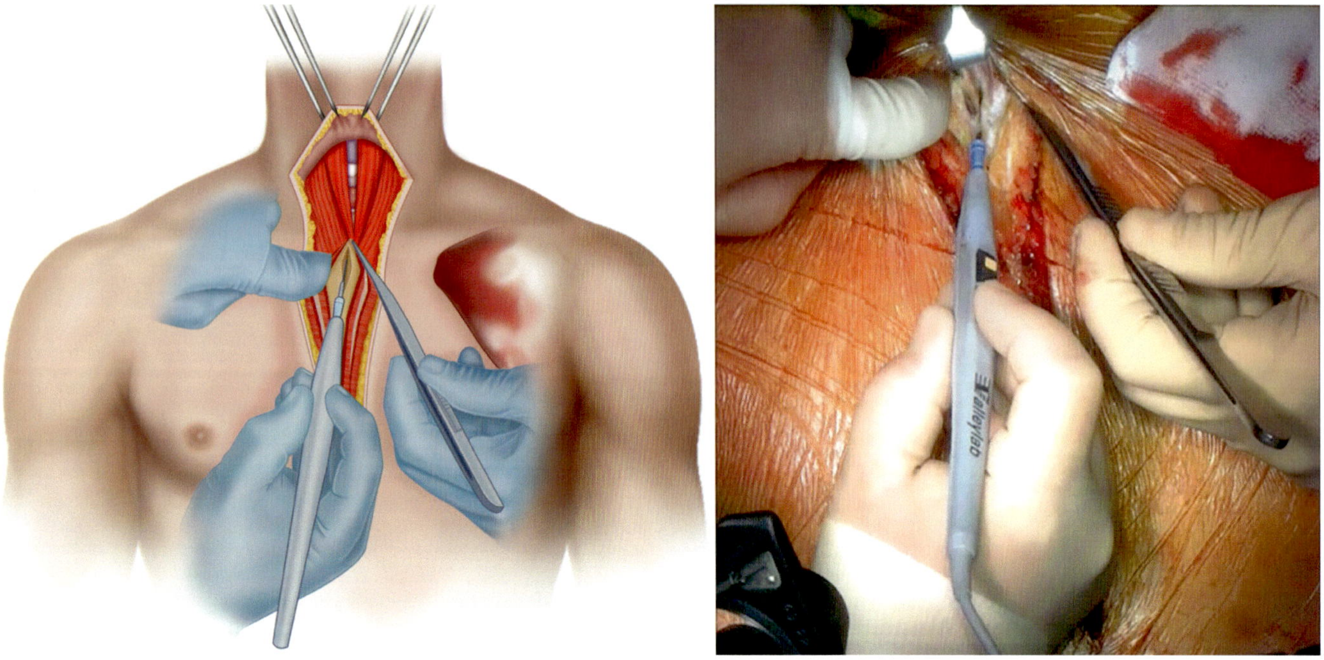

Fig. 18.24 Division of the interclavicular ligament

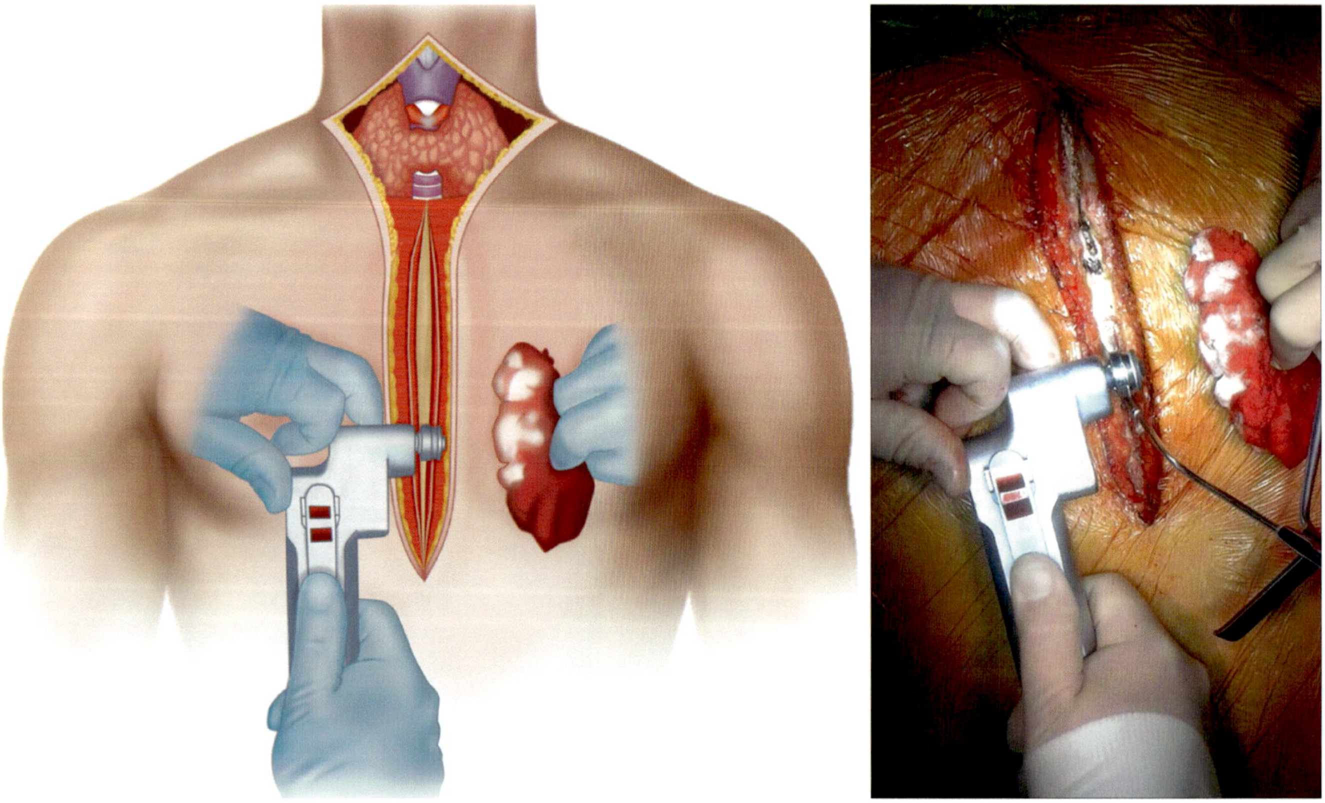

Fig. 18.25 Sternotomy is performed with an oscillating saw, paying attention to avoid injury to underlying structures (pleura, pericardium, innominate vein)

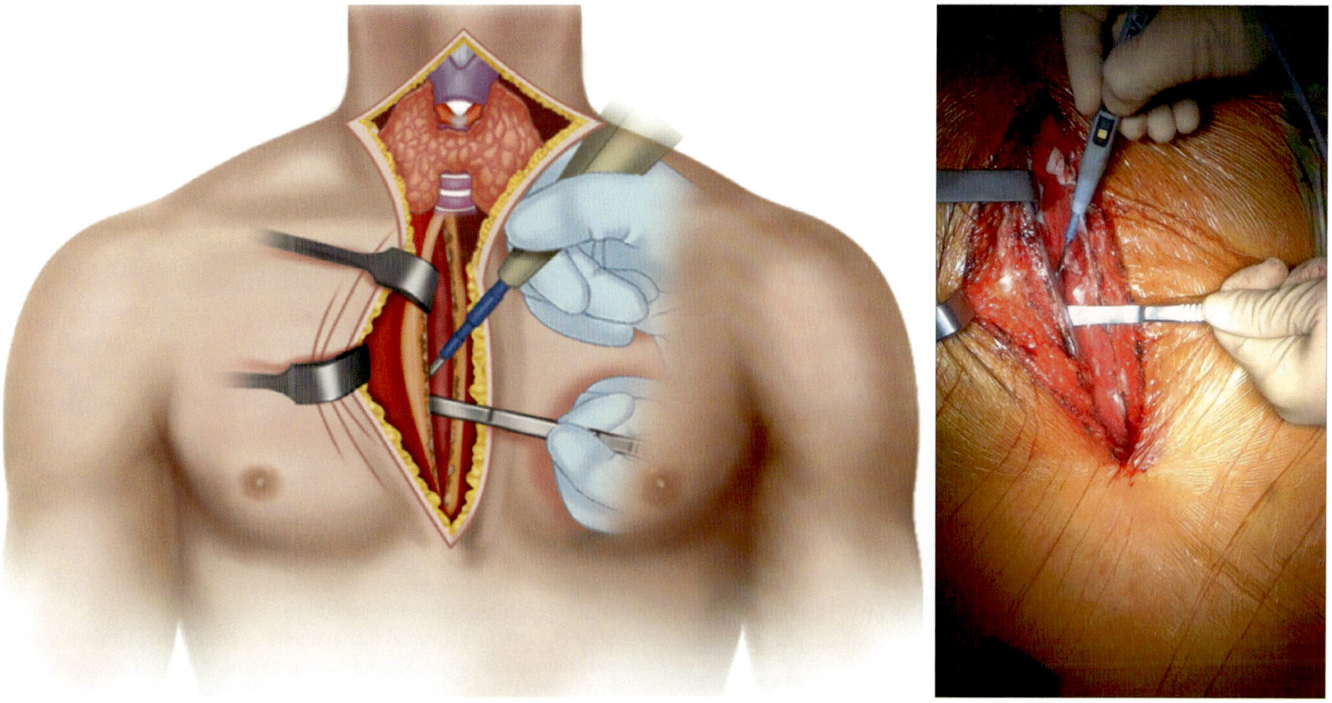

Fig. 18.26 Bleeding control with cautery of the periosteum

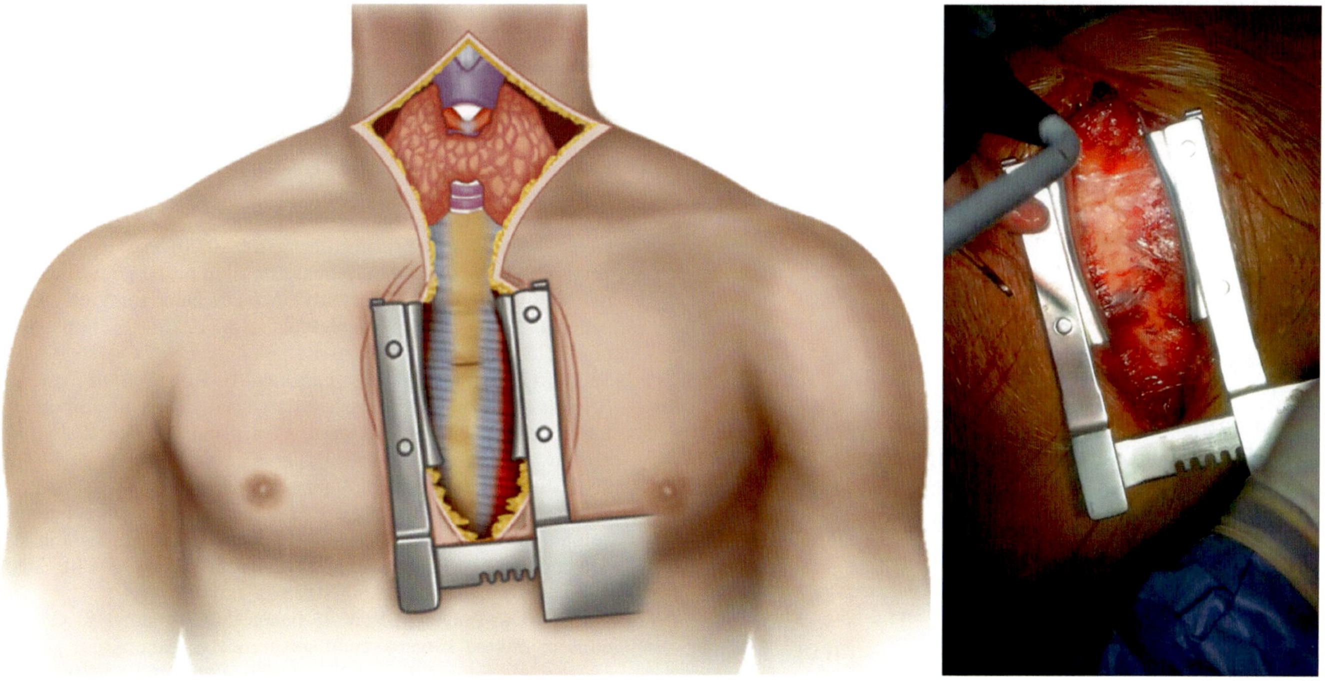

Fig. 18.27 Placing Finochietto retractor and progressive sternum retraction

The interclavicular ligament has to be divided (Fig. 18.24). Once the periosteum is reached, the midline should be identified by palpating the sternochondral junctions and the intercostal spaces at both sides of the sternum.

An oscillating saw is used for sternotomy, stopping the ventilation to avoid injury to the underlying structures (pleura, pericardium) (Fig. 18.25). The osteotomy can be complete or limited to the manubrium and upper third of the sternum.

Bleeding is controlled with cautery of the periosteum and/or the use of bone wax to seal the bone marrow (Fig. 18.26). Towels are placed around the sternal edges to control bleeding, a Finochietto retractor is placed, and the sternum is retracted progressively to avoid fractures to the ribs (Fig. 18.27).

This procedure will give access to the mediastinal part of the goiter and provide enough room to control eventual bleeding and allow for the dissection of mediastinal adhesions.

At the end of the procedure, sternotomy is closed first with 4–8 discontinuous sutures using a number 1 polyglactinic acid thread with triangular needle or stainless-steel wires passing perpendicularly through the entire thickness of the bone. Sutures or wires are firmly tightened after proper approximation, avoiding a too tight approximation that could cause malperfusion of the bone that in turn could lead to wound infection or nonunion.

Wound closure is completed by suturing the muscular and subcutaneous planes and skin.

We strongly suggest that endocrine surgeons ask for specialized assistance to perform sternotomy, as this is key to avoid catastrophic complications at opening (essentially bleeding) and long-term complications at closing (essentially nonunion and infections).

Closure

The insertion of a single 7-French suction drain running through both thyroid beds and exiting laterally to the edge of the skin incision is recommended at the end of the procedure to avoid the accumulation of liquid and blood in the remaining large mediastinal cavity.

Sternohyoid and sternothyroid muscles are reapproximated longitudinally with 3-0 Vicryl sutures. The strap muscles are then sutured in the midline with interrupted 3-0 Vicryl suture. The platysma is reapproximated with interrupted 3-0 Vicryl suture, and the skin is closed with a running 4-0 subcuticular Prolene suture without knots and Steri-Strips are applied with a loose bandage (Video 18.1).

References

1. Reeve TS, Rubinstein C, Rundle FF. Intrathoracic goitre: its prevalence in Sydney metropolitan mass radiography surveys. Med J Aust. 1957;44(5):149–56.
2. Haller A. Disputatones anatomic selectae. Gottingen: Vendenhoceck; 1749. p. 96.
3. Mack E. Management of patients with substernal goiters. Surg Clin N Am. 1995;75(3):377–94. https://doi.org/10.1016/S0039-6109(16)46628-4.
4. Ríos A, Rodríguez JM, Balsalobre MD, Tebar FJ, Parrilla P. The value of various definitions of intrathoracic goiter for predicting intra-operative and postoperative complications. Surgery. 2010;147(2):233–8. https://doi.org/10.1016/j.surg.2009.06.018.
5. Randolph GW. Surgery of the thyroid and parathyroid glands. 3rd ed. Philadelphia: Elsevier, Inc; 2020.
6. Shin JJ, et al. The surgical management of goiter: part I. Preoperative evaluation: the surgical management of goiter: part I. Laryngoscope. 2011;121(1):60–7. https://doi.org/10.1002/lary.21084.
7. Doulaptsi M, et al. Substernal goiter: treatment and challenges. Twenty-two years of experience in diagnosis and management of substernal goiters. Auris Nasus Larynx. 2019;46(2):246–51. https://doi.org/10.1016/j.anl.2018.07.006.
8. Raffaelli M, De Crea C, Ronti S, Bellantone R, Lombardi CP. Substernal goiters: incidence, surgical approach, and complications in a tertiary care referral center. Head Neck. 2011;33(10):1420–5. https://doi.org/10.1002/hed.21617.
9. Di Crescenzo V, et al. Surgical management of cervico-mediastinal goiters: our experience and review of the literature. Int J Surg. 2016;28:S47–53. https://doi.org/10.1016/j.ijsu.2015.12.048.
10. Pieracci FM, Fahey TJ. Substernal thyroidectomy is associated with increased morbidity and mortality as compared with conventional cervical thyroidectomy. J Am Coll Surg. 2007;205(1):1–7. https://doi.org/10.1016/j.jamcollsurg.2007.03.010.
11. Testini M, et al. Does mediastinal extension of the goiter increase morbidity of total thyroidectomy? A multicenter study of 19,662 patients. Ann Surg Oncol. 2011;18(8):2251–9. https://doi.org/10.1245/s10434-011-1596-4.
12. Sadowski SM, Soardo P, Leuchter I, Robert JH, Triponez F. Systematic use of recurrent laryngeal nerve neuromonitoring changes the operative strategy in planned bilateral thyroidectomy. Thyroid. 2013;23(3):329–33. https://doi.org/10.1089/thy.2012.0368.
13. Demarchi MS, Karenovics W, Bédat B, Triponez F. Intraoperative autofluorescence and indocyanine green angiography for the detection and preservation of parathyroid glands. J Clin Med. 2020;9(3):830. https://doi.org/10.3390/jcm9030830.
14. Falco J, Dip F, Quadri P, de la Fuente M, Rosenthal R. Cutting edge in thyroid surgery: autofluorescence of parathyroid glands. J Am Coll Surg. 2016;223(2):374–80. https://doi.org/10.1016/j.jamcollsurg.2016.04.049.

Index

A
Allis clamp, 11, 33, 55
Autoimmune disorders, 194
Automated periodic stimulation (APS) electrode, 150

B
Benign thyroid nodule, 29
Berry's ligament, 12, 13, 17, 24, 26, 28, 84, 226, 227
Bilateral axillo-breast approach (BABA) robotic thyroidectomy, 163–165
Bipolar energy devices, 23

C
Central neck dissection
  ILN and paratracheal dissection, 213, 215
  lateral boundary dissection, 213
  prelaryngeal (Delphian) nodes, 215
  pretracheal dissection, 215
  strap muscles dissection, 212
  wound closure, 216
Central neck lymph nodes dissection (CNLND), 75–77, 88
  EBSLN, 80
  irrigation, followed by muscles and skin closure, 88, 89
  left inferior parathyroid gland identification, 84
  left recurrent laryngeal nerve identification, 80, 84
  left superior parathyroid gland identification, 84
  left thyroid lobe, lateral mobilization of, 80
  muscle incision, 77, 78
  old scar excision, 77, 78
  patient positioning, 77, 78
  thoracic duct injury, 90
  thyroid lobe off the trachea, 84
  transection of Berry's ligament, 84
Contra-lateral hemithyroidectomy, 122
Contralateral lobectomy, 107, 177
CS-14 Ultracision Harmonic Scalpel® model, 148
Cytology/histology, 195

D
Dermabond, 21
Differentiated thyroid carcinomas (DTC), 199, 200
  central neck dissection, 212–216
  patient's preparation and positioning, 201
  selective lateral neck dissection, 202–204, 206, 208–211
  skin incision and flap elevation, 201, 202
  surgical approach, 200, 201

E
Endotracheal tube, 31
Erb's point dissection, 206
External branch of the superior laryngeal nerve (EBSLN), 1, 8–10, 80, 102

F
Farabeuf retractor, 151
Finochietto retractor, 231

G
Gelpi retractor, 44
Goitre, 193
Graves' disease, 194

H
Hand-held stimulating probe, 131
Harmonic Focus device, 6, 16–18, 84, 88
Health care system, 192
Hematoma, 21
Hemi-thyroidectomy, 129, 135, 136, 138, 139
  See also Right thyroid lobectomy
High-income countries (HIC), 193, 194
  clinical signs, 194
  cytology/histology, 195
  follow-up, 197
  pathology, 193, 194
  surgery, 195, 197
  ultrasound, 195
Hook electrocautery, 189
Human Development Index (HDI), 192
Hurthle cell neoplasm, 31
Hyperextension, 24

I
Infection, 194
Inferior parathyroid gland, identification and preservation of, 11
Inferior subplatysmal flap, 33, 100, 110, 222
Inferior thyroid artery (ITA), 3
Intraoperative RLN monitoring (IONM), 1, 76
Ipsilateral central lymph node dissection, 117–119, 121, 122, 126, 127
Isthmectomy, 175
Isthmusectomy, 109, 110

A. Shifrin (ed.), *Atlas of Thyroid Surgery*, https://doi.org/10.1007/978-3-030-93673-0

J
Joll's space, 176

K
Kelly clamp, 27
Kocher and Langenbeck retractors, 118
Kocher incision, 221
Kocher's vein, 131

L
Large type IIA goiter, 220
Lateral mobilization of the left thyroid lobe with division of the middle thyroid vein, 5, 6, 80
Lateral neck dissection
  dissecting level ll, 209, 210
  level III and IV dissection, 210, 211
  level Vb dissection, 212
  medial boundary dissection, 206, 208
  SCM, unwrapping, 203–206
  submandibular triangle preparation, 206
Left inferior parathyroid gland identification, 84
Left recurrent laryngeal nerve identification, 80, 84
Left superior parathyroid gland identification, 84
Left thyroid lobectomy, 43
  cervical incision and landmarks, 44
  closure, 51
  CNLND, 75–77, 88
    EBSLN, 80
    irrigation, followed by muscles and skin closure, 88, 89
    left inferior parathyroid gland identification, 84
    left recurrent laryngeal nerve identification, 80, 84
    left superior parathyroid gland identification, 84
    left thyroid lobe, lateral mobilization of, 80
    muscle incision, 77, 78
    old scar excision, 77, 78
    patient positioning, 77, 78
    thoracic duct injury, 90
    thyroid lobe off the trachea, 84
    transection of Berry's ligament, 84
  isthmusectomy and, 109, 110
  mobilization of
    inferior pole, 46
    superior pole, 46
    thyroid, 47
  obtaining exposure, 44, 45
  parathyroid assessment and transplantation, 48
  patient positioning, 44
  pyramidal lobe, identification and inclusion of, 46
  RLN identification, 45
  tips and pitfalls, 51
LigaSure™, 19, 32, 33, 35, 37, 38, 117, 125
Lobectomy, 105
Low and middle income countries (LMIC), 191, 192
  advanced thyroid carcinoma, young patient with, 191
  vs. high-income countries, thyroid surgery in, 193, 194
    clinical signs, 194
    cytology/histology, 195
    follow-up, 197
    pathology, 193, 194
    surgery, 195, 197
    ultrasound, 195
  surgical missions, 192, 193
Low-risk medullary thyroid cancer, 129, 135, 136, 138, 139
Low-risk papillary thyroid cancer, 129, 135, 136, 138, 139
Lymph node neck dissections, 199

M
Middle thyroid vein, 25
Minimally invasive thyroidectomy, 143
Modified RND (MRND), 200
Myocutaneous (subplatysmal) flaps, 97

N
Nanoscope™ System, 145
Neural integrity monitoring (NIM), 23, 117
Non-recurrent laryngeal nerve (NRLN), 2

O
Open right thyroid lobectomy, 23
  hemostatic agents, 29
  Kelly clamp, 27
  orogastric tube placement, 23
  patient positioning, 24
  subplatysmal flaps, 24
  transverse curvilinear incision, 24
Orotracheal tube, 223
Overholt clamps, 132

P
Papillary thyroid carcinoma (PTC)
  ipsilateral central lymph node dissection for, 117–119, 121, 122, 126, 127
  total thyroidectomy for, 117–119, 121, 122, 126, 127
Papillary thyroid microcarcinoma (mPTC), 97
Parathyroid gland, 3
Platysma, 5, 20, 41, 114, 127
Postoperative hypocalcemia, 21
Prelaryngeal (Delphian) nodes, 215
Pretracheal dissection, 215
Pyramidal lobe, 27, 46

R
Radioactive iodine (RAI) therapy, 117, 194
Recurrent laryngeal nerve (RLN), 1–3, 21, 45, 46, 103, 113
Richardson retractor, 55
Right recurrent laryngeal nerve, identification and preservation of, 11, 12
Right superior parathyroid gland, identification and preservation of, 12, 13
Right thyroid lobectomy
  anatomical considerations
    inferior thyroid artery, 3
    parathyroid gland, 3
    recurrent (inferior) laryngeal nerve, 1, 3
    tubercle of Zuckerkandl, 3
  EBSLN, 8, 9
  inferior parathyroid gland, identification and preservation of, 11
  instruments set, 3, 4
  lateral mobilization of thyroid lobe with division of middle thyroid vein, 5, 6
  management of complications
    hematoma, 21
    postoperative hypocalcemia, 21
    RLN injury, 21
  muscle and skin closure, 16, 17
  patient's preparation, intubation and positioning, 4
  right recurrent laryngeal nerve, identification and preservation of, 11, 12

right superior parathyroid gland, identification and preservation of, 12, 13
skin mark and skin incision, 4
surgical pearls, 17–20
thyroid lobe off the trachea with isthmus and pyramidal lobe, 15
transection of Berry's ligament, 13

S
Senn retractor, 53
Steri-Strip™, 41, 126
Sternocleidomastoid muscle (SCM), 44, 203–206
Sternohyoid and sternothyroid muscles, 120
Sternotomy, 228, 229, 232
Subplatysmal flaps, 5, 6, 24, 79, 119
Substernal goiter (SG), 219
anatomical point of view, 219
anterior and posterior, 219
classification, 219
definition of, 219
incision and exposure, 221, 223
medial dissection with "toboggan" technique, 224, 226–228
patient positioning, 220
patient preparation, 221
sternotomy, 228, 232
superior pole ligation, 224
symptoms, 220
thyroid isthmus division, 223
total thyroidectomy for, 69–72, 74
wound closure, 232
Superior platysma flap, 130
Superior subplatysmal flap, 33, 44, 54, 100, 221, 222
Sutureless thyroidectomy, 117

T
Thoracic duct injury, 90
Thyroidectomies, 1
Thyroid isthmus, 60
Thyroid lobectomy, 23
Allis clamp placement, 33
anatomic landmarks, 32
inferior subplatysmal flap, 33
intraoperative nerve monitoring, 34
LigaSure™, 32, 35, 37, 38
patient positioning, 31
prelaryngeal space, 34
superior subplatysmal flap, 33
surgical instruments, 32
Thyroid lobectomy counter traction placement, 32
Thyroid lobe off the trachea with isthmus and pyramidal lobe, 15
Thyroid malignancy, 194
Thyrotoxicosis, 194
Toboggan technique, 224, 226–228
Total thyroidectomy, 1, 53, 55–57, 60–63, 97, 196
carotid sheath exposure, 101
control of the superior vascular pedicle, 102
in-depth dissection, 99
inferior parathyroid gland, 104
initial vagus nerve functional evaluation, 101
inter-cricothyroid space dissection, 102
landmarks, 98
mobilization of strap muscles, 101
for papillary thyroid carcinoma, 117–119, 121, 122, 126, 127
patient positioning, 53
patient preparation, 98
platysma muscle closure, 108
post-lobectomy surgical field assessment, 106
skin closure, 108
skin incision, 99
specimen assessment, 105
strap muscles approximation, 107
strap muscles midline incision, 100
for substernal goiter, 69–72, 74
superior parathyroid gland, 103
surgical procedure, 97, 99, 103
thyroid isthmus transection, 105
with comprehensive central and lateral neck dissection, for DTC, 199, 200
central neck dissection, 212–216
patient's preparation and positioning, 201
selective lateral neck dissection, 202–204, 206, 208–211
skin incision and flap elevation, 201, 202
surgical approach, 200, 201
Transection of Berry's ligament, 13, 84
Transoral endoscopic thyroidectomy vestibular approach (TOETVA), 173, 181
contraindications of, 173
contralateral resection, 177
flap formation, 174
incision, 174
indications of, 173
lateral dissection, 176
lower pole ligation and resection of the gland, 177
midline dissection and isthmectomy, 175
patient positioning and preparation, 174
procedure, 181, 185, 187
recurrent laryngeal nerve identification and preservation, 177
specimen retrieval, 177
suture and stitch-out, 177
tips and pitfalls, 188
upper pole ligation, 176
Tubercle of Zuckerkandl, 3, 12, 15, 58, 119

U
Ultrasound, 195
Unilateral thyroid lobectomy, 221

V
Vagus nerve, 33
Valsalva maneuver, 19
Vein of doom, 64
Video-assisted thyroidectomy (VAT), 143
advantage, 144
indications for, 144
operative techniques
anesthesia, 145
APS electrode, 150
inferior parathyroid gland preservation, 152
patient and surgical team positions, 145
skin incision, 148
surgical instruments for, 145, 148
thyroid lobe extraction, 152
Vocal cord paralysis (VCP), 117

W
Weitlaner retractor, 7, 53

GPSR Compliance

The European Union's (EU) General Product Safety Regulation (GPSR) is a set of rules that requires consumer products to be safe and our obligations to ensure this.

If you have any concerns about our products, you can contact us on ProductSafety@springernature.com

In case Publisher is established outside the EU, the EU authorized representative is:

Springer Nature Customer Service Center GmbH
Europaplatz 3
69115 Heidelberg, Germany

Batch number: 10756390

Printed by Printforce, the Netherlands